National
Dental Hygienist
Licensure Exam
Third Edition

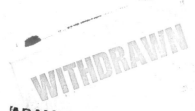

National Dental Hygienist Licensure Exam

Third Edition

by Paula Tomko, RDH

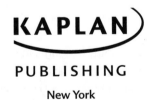

PUBLISHING

New York

© 2009 by Paula A. Tomko

Published by Kaplan Publishing, a division of Kaplan, Inc.
1 Liberty Plaza, 24th Floor
New York, NY 10006

Printed in the United States of America

10 9 8 7 6 5 4 3 2 1

ISBN-13: 978-1-4195-5269-4

Kaplan Publishing books are available at special quantity discounts to use for sales promotions, employee premiums, or educational purposes. Please email our Special Sales Department to order or for more information at kaplanpublishing@kaplan.com, or write to Kaplan Publishing, 1 Liberty Plaza, 24th Floor, New York, NY 10006.

Table of Contents

Available Online

FOR ANY TEST CHANGES OR LATE-BREAKING DEVELOPMENTS

kaptest.com/publishing

The material in this book is up-to-date at the time of publication. However, the American Dental Association may have instituted changes in the test after this book was published. Be sure to check the website when you register for the test.

If there are any important late-breaking developments—or any changes or corrections to the Kaplan test preparation materials in this book—we will post that information online at kaptest.com/publishing. Check to see if there is any information posted there regarding this book.

FEEDBACK AND COMMENTS

kaplansurveys.com/books

We'd like to hear your comments and suggestions about this book. We invite you to fill out our online survey form at **kaplansurveys.com/books**. Your feedback is extremely helpful as we continue to develop high-quality resources to meet your needs.

About the Author

Paula Tomko, RDH, is the owner of PTRDH Dental Hygiene National Board Review, which runs review courses for the exam across the country. She is a former instructor at Wake AHC for the University of North Carolina at Chapel Hill, where she taught a variety of dental hygiene topics, including Infection Control and Sterilization, OSHA updates, and Radiology. She currently holds review courses around the United States. Visit her at www.denhyg.com/.

Acknowledgments

The author wishes to thank Patricia A. Hogan, RDH, BSHS for her expertise and authorship of Chapters 16 and 18 on Instrumentation for Client Assessment and Community Health. Her contributions are invaluable.

Thanks are also extended to the following for their permission to reprint radiographs and photographs throughout the book: Dr. Michael W. Finkelstein, College of Dentistry at the University of Iowa; Dr. Akitoshi Katsumata, Department of Oral Radiology, Asahi University in Japan; Dr. Richard Monahan, University of Illinois; Dr. Brad Potter, Medical College of Georgia; Dr. Richard Cray, Periodontist; Dr. P. Alexander Bollendorf, DDS, and the Eastman Kodak Company.

Kenneth Tomko, Esquire also deserves special mention for his ongoing support and advice, as do Kyle, Noah, Jack, and Morgan, for their continual enthusiasm and inspiration.

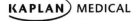

Preface

Preparing for and doing well on the National Board Dental Hygiene Exam is an essential requirement on the road to becoming a practicing dental hygienist. Dental hygiene licensure requirements vary in each jurisdiction, though all jurisdictions have 3 requirements: an educational requirement, a written exam requirement, and a clinical exam requirement.

The National Board Exam addresses the requirement for the written exam, though acceptance of National Board scores is completely at the discretion of the individual state. Though scores are provided in a 49 to 99 range, a score if 75 is required to pass. Additionally, a state or regional written exam may be required.

The skills needed for preparation and execution on multiple-choice tests have little to do with the day-to-day practice of dental hygiene, but are required hurdles that you must overcome to advance your dental hygiene career. This guidebook is intended to help you with this process.

- Section I provides an overview of the National Board Exam. It will help you gain a better understanding of the scope, format, and design of the exam. In addition, it offers crucial insights to help you do your best on test day.

- Section II provides a detailed content review of the topics covered on the exam. Keep in mind that the review is not intended to be comprehensive in scope, but rather, focused in the areas of practical dental hygiene that appear with regularity on the exam.

- Section III is a full-length practice test of a National Board Exam. It includes the full range of questions, in addition to questions based on case studies. We recommend that you wait until you complete your review of the subject content before taking an exam. Once you have taken this practice test, all parts of the exam will feel more natural to you.

As you work through this book, note the areas that you are most weak in and practice until you feel more at ease. For more information on the exam, go to the test site, at ada. org/prof/ed/testing/natboardhyg/index.asp.

Good luck on your exam.

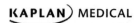

The Basics

Chapter One: **Overview**

According to the dental laws of each state, a dental hygienist must be licensed. To become licensed, the dental hygienist must pass the National Board Exam as well as a state or regional exam.

The National Board Exam is offered several times a year by the American Dental Association (ADA). It is offered to students of accredited programs (and non-accredited programs if they are equivalent), and to dental hygienists who may have let their licenses expire or are moving to a state that requires recent exam scores.

HISTORY OF THE NATIONAL BOARD EXAM

Today, the ADA thrives with more than 147,000 members, but it was originally founded in 1859 by 26 dentists. At the turn of the 20th century, each state had its own written and clinical exams, and because of the great variation in each exam, the dentists of that time pushed to have them standardized.

In response to that push, in 1928 the ADA created a National Board of Dental Examiners. It comprised three ADA members, three members of the American Association of Dental Examiners (AADE), and three members of the American Association of Dental Schools. By 1933, the first National Board Exam for dentists was administered.

In the 1950s, dental hygiene education programs realized the advantage of standardization, and the American Dental Hygienists' Association (ADHA) went about establishing a national board exam for dental hygienists. Eventually, with the help of the AADE, a national exam was developed.

In 1962, the first National Dental Hygiene Board Exam was administered. It included 12 subjects: anatomy, physiology, histology, pathology, radiology, chemistry, microbiology, nutrition, pharmacology, preventive measures, and dental materials. In 1973, the subjects of clinical dental hygiene and community dental health were added.

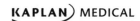

In 1996, the exam was revised to include case-based questions and dental-hygiene functions. Two years later, a case booklet was added; in order to test candidates' ability to assess and manage patients, they were given extensive patient information: medical history, dental history, radiographs, periodontal pocket depth charting, and clinical photographs.

STATE AND REGIONAL EXAMS

Passing the National Dental Hygiene Board Exam fulfills only *one part* of the requirements for licensure. Each state has the discretion to accept completely or partially the National Dental Hygiene Board Exam score. Some state boards accept the National Board scores as long as the exam was taken within the previous 10–15 years.

Similarly, each state has its own legislative requirements for licensure of dentists and dental hygienists. There are many variations from state to state. Each state's practice act clarifies the scope of practice for dentists, dental hygienists, and dental assistants. The state board of dental examiners administers the regulations within each state.

Currently, 42 states conduct regional testing within their jurisdictions. Eleven states offer their own independent testing. Pooling the resources of several jurisdictions allows for more expertise in the written and clinical portions of the test, and it broadens the geographic base for the exam.

Regional Testing Agency	NERB	CRDTS	SRTA	WREB	Own Test	Reciprocity
Alabama					X	
Alaska		Accepts		Member		
Arizona				Member		
Arkansas			Member			
California					X	
Colorado		Member		Accepts		
Connecticut	Member	Accepts	Accepts	Accepts		
Delaware						
District of Columbia	Member					
Florida					X	
Georgia			Member			
Hawaii					X	
Idaho		Accepts		Member		
Illinois	Member	Member	Accepts	Accepts		
Indiana					X	

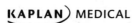

Regional Testing Agency	NERB	CRDTS	SRTA	WREB	Own Test	Reciprocity
Iowa		Member		Accepts		
Kansas	Accepts	Member	Accepts	Accepts		X
Kentucky	Accepts	Accepts	Member	Accepts		
Louisiana					X	
Maine	Member	Accepts	Accepts	Accepts		X
Maryland	Member					
Massachusetts	Member	Accepts	Accepts	Accepts		
Michigan	Member					
Minnesota	Accepts	Member	Accepts	Accepts		
Mississippi					X	
Missouri	Accepts	Member	Accepts	Accepts		X
Montana		Accepts		Member		
Nebraska		Member		Accepts		
Nevada					X	
New Hampshire	Member	Accepts	Accepts	Accepts		
New Jersey		Accepts		Member		
New Mexico		Accepts		Member		
New York	Member					
North Carolina					X	
North Dakota	Accepts	Member	Accepts	Accepts		
Ohio	Member	Accepts	Accepts	Accepts		
Oklahoma		Accepts		Member		
Oregon		Accepts		Member		
Pennsylvania	Member					
Rhode Island	Member					
South Carolina			Member			
South Dakota		Member				
Tennessee			Member			
Texas		Accepts		Member		
Utah	Accepts	Accepts	Accepts	Member		
Vermont	Member	Accepts	Accepts	Accepts		
Virginia	Member					
Washington		Member		Member		
West Virginia	Member	Accepts	Accepts	Accepts		X
Wisconsin		Member		Accepts		
Wyoming		Member	Accepts	Member		

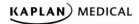

Regional Boards

NERB

North East Regional Board of Dental Examiners
Phone: (301) 563-3300
Web: nerb.org/

The NERB is comprised of 15 state member dental boards that accept the results of this test. Non-member states that accept NERB test results include Colorado, Kansas, Kentucky, Minnesota, Missouri, Nebraska, Tennessee, Utah, and Virginia.

CRDTS

Central Regional Dental Testing Service
Phone: (785) 273-0380
Web: crdts.org

The CRDTS is composed of 12 state boards of dentistry, and tests both dentists and dental hygienists. Other states that accept CRDTS results include Alaska, Connecticut, Idaho, Kentucky, Maine, Massachusetts, Montana, New Hampshire, New Mexico, Ohio, Oklahoma, Oregon, Texas, Utah, Vermont, and West Virginia.

SRTA

Southern Regional Testing Agency
Phone: (757) 318-9082
Web: srta.org

The SRTA has 6 member states: Arkansas, Georgia, Kentucky, South Carolina, Tennessee, Virginia, and West Virginia. Non-member states accepting SRTA test results are Connecticut, Illinois, Kansas, Maine, Massachusetts, Minnesota, Missouri, New Hampshire, North Dakota, Ohio, Utah, Vermont, West Virginia, and Wyoming. Hygienists are required to perform a partial dental prophylaxis in addition to providing a periodontal assessment.

WREB

Western Regional Examining Board
Phone: (602) 944-3315
Web: wreb.org

The WREB has 11 member states. Non-member states accepting WREB test results are Colorado, Connecticut, Illinois, Iowa, Kansas, Kentucky, Maine, Massachusetts, Minnesota, Missouri, Nebraska, New Hampshire, North Dakota, Ohio, South Dakota, Vermont, West Virginia, and Wisconsin.

State Boards

Alabama Board of Dental Examiners
Web: dentalboard.org
Phone: 205/985-7267
E-mail: BDEAAL@bellsouth.net

Alaska Board of Dental Examiners
Web: dced.state.ak.us/occ/pden.htm
Phone: 907/465-2542
E-mail: wandafleming@dced.state.ak.us

Arkansas State Board of Dental Examiners
Web: www.asbde.org
Phone: 501/682-2085
E-mail: asbde@mail.state.ar.us

Arizona State Board of Dental Examiners
Web: www.azdentalboard.org/
Phone: 602/242-1492

Dental Board of California
Web: dbc.ca.gov
Phone: 916/263-2300

Colorado Board of Dental Examiners
Web: www.dora.state.co.us/dental
Phone: 303/894-7758

Connecticut Department of Public Health,
   Dental Licensure
Web: www.ct-clic.com
Phone: 860/509-7561

Delaware State Board of Dental Examiners
Web: professionallicensing.state.de.us/boards/dental
Phone: 302/739-4522, ext. 220

Florida Board of Dentistry
Web: doh.state.fl.us/mqa/dentistry/dn_home.html
Phone: 850/245-4474
E-mail: MQA_Dentistry@doh.state.fl.us

Georgia Board of Dentistry
Web: www.sos.state.ga.us/plb/dentistry
Phone: 478/207-1680
E-mail: ajpitts@sos.state.ga.us

Hawaii State Board of Dental Examiners
Web: hawaii.gov/dcca/areas/pvl/boards/dentist
Phone: 808/586-2689

Idaho State Board of Dentistry
Web: www2.state.id.us/isbd/index.htm
Phone: 208/334-2369
E-mail: smiller@isbd.state.id.us

Illinois Department of Professional Regulation
Web: dpr.state.il.us/WHO/dent.asp
Phone: 217/785-0800

Indiana State Board of Dentistry Health
   Professions Bureau
Web: www.state.in.us/hpb/boards/isbd
Phone: 317/234-2057
Email: hpb7@hpb.state.in.us

Iowa Board of Dental Examiners
Web: www.state.ia.us/dentalboard/
Phone: 515/281-5157
E-mail: ibde@bon.state.ia.us

Kansas Dental Board
Web: accesskansas.org/kdb/
Phone: 785/273-0780
E-mail: dental@ink.org

Kentucky Board of Dentistry
Web: dentistry.ky.gov/
502/423-0573

Louisiana State Board of Dentistry
Web: lsbd.org/
Phone: 504/568-8574

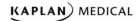

Maine Board of Dental Examiners
Web: mainedental.org/
Phone: 207/287-3333

Maryland State Board of Dental Examiners
Web: dhmh.state.md.us/dental/
Phone: 410/402-8511

Massachusetts Board of Registration in Dentistry
Web: mass.gov/dpl/boards/dn/
Phone: 617/727-9928

Michigan Board of Dentistry
Web: michigan.gov/mdch
Phone: 517/335-0918

Minnesota Board Dentistry
Web: www.dentalboard.state.mn.us/
Phone: 612/617-2250

Mississippi State Board of Dental Examiners
Web: www.msbde.state.ms.us/mainpg.htm
Phone: 601/944-9622

Missouri State Dental Board
Web: http://pr.mo.gov/dental.asp
Phone: 573-751-0040
E-mail: dental@pr.mo.gov

Montana Board of Dentistry
Web: http://mt.gov/dli/bsd/license/hc_index,asp
Phone: 406/841-2390

Nebraska Board of Dentistry
Web: www.hhs.state.ne.us/crl/crlindex.htm
Phone: 402/471-2115
E-mail: marie.mcclatchey@hhss.state.ne.us

Nevada State Board of Dental Examiners
Web: nvdentalboard.org/
Phone: 702/486-7044
E-mail: nsbde@govmail.state.nv.us

New Hampshire Board of Dental Examiners
Web: state.nh.us/dental/
Phone: 603/271-4561

New Jersey Board of Dentistry
Web: www.state.nj.us/lps/ca/medical/dentistry.htm
Phone: 973/504-6405

New Mexico Board of Dental Health Care
Web: www.rld.state.nm.us/b&c/dental/index.htm
Phone: 505/476-7125

New York Office of the Professions
Web: www.op.nysed.gov/dent.htm
Phone: 518/474-3817
E-mail: op4info@mail.nysed.gov

North Carolina State Board of Dental Examiners
Web: ncdentalboard.org/default.asp
Phone: 919/678-8223
E-mail: info@ncdentalboard.org

North Dakota State Board of Dental Examiners
Web: nddentalboard.org/
Phone: 701/258-8600

Ohio State Dental Board
Web: dental.ohio.gov/
Phone: 614/466-2580

Oklahoma Board of Dentistry
Web: www.dentist.state.ok.us/
Phone: 405/524-9037
Email: dentist@oklaosf.state.ok.us

Oregon Board of Dentistry
Web: egov.oregon.gov/Dentistry
Phone: 503/229-5520
E-mail: information@oregondentistry.org

Pennsylvania State Board of Dentistry
Web: www.dos.state.pa.us
Phone: 717/787-8503
E-mail: st-dentistry@state.pa.us

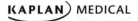

Rhode Island Board of Examiners in Dentistry
Web: www.healthri.org/hsr/professions/dental.php
Phone: 401/222-2827
E-mail: GailG@doh.state.ri.us

South Carolina Board of Dentistry
Web: llr.state.sc.us/POL/dentistry/INDEX.ASP
Phone: 803/896-4599
E-mail: joness@mail.llr.state.sc.us

South Dakota State Board of Dentistry
Web: state.sd.us/doh/dentistry/
Phone: 605/224-1282
E-mail: sdsbd@dtgnet.com

Tennessee Board of Dentistry
Web: www2.state.tn.us/health/Boards/Dentistry/
index.htm
Phone: 615/532-3202

Texas State Board of Dental Examiners
Web: tsbde.state.tx.us/
Phone: 512/463-6400

Utah Board of Dentists and Dental Hygienists
Web: dopl.utah.gov/licensing/dental.html
Phone: 801/530-6628

Vermont Board of Dentistry
Web: vtprofessionals.org/opr1/dentists/
Phone: 802/828-2390
E-mail: dlafaill@sec.state.vt.us

Virginia Department of Health Professions
Web: www.dhp.state.va.us/default.htm
Phone: 804/662-763-6804

Washington State Dental Health Care Quality
Assurance Commission
Web: https://fortress.wa.gov/doh/hpqa1/
Phone: 360/236-4859

Washington, D.C.
District of Columbia Board of Dentistry
Web: http://dchealth.dc.gov/prof_license/services/
main.asp
Phone: 202/442-4764

West Virgina Board of Dental Examiners
Web: wvdentalboard.org
Phone: 877/914-8266

Wisconsin Board of Dental Examiners
Web: http://drl.wi.gov/index.htm
Phone: 608/266-2811

Wyoming Board of Dental Examiners
Web: http://plboards.state.wy.us/dental
Phone: 307/777-6529
E-mail: dbridg@state.wy.us

CONTINUING EDUCATION

Medicine and dentistry are constantly changing, with new research and technological changes taking place every day. Continuing education is a necessary part of keeping up with those changes. Updating professional skills and knowledge through continuing education is a requirement in most states.

Continuing Ed Requirements

State	Required Hours	Cycle Length
Alabama	12	1 year
Alaska	14	2 years
Arizona	54	3 years
Arkansas	40	2 years
California	25	2 years
Colorado	NA	–
Connecticut	16	2 years
Delaware	24	2 years
D.C.	15	2 years
Florida	24	2 years
Georgia	22	2 years
Hawaii	20	2 years
Idaho	12	1 year
Illinois	24	2 years
Indiana	14	2 years
Iowa	30	3 years
Kansas	30	2 years
Kentucky	15	1 year
Louisiana	24	2 years
Maine	20	2 years
Maryland	25	2 years
Massachusetts	20	2 years
Michigan	36	3 years
Minnesota	40	5 years
Mississippi	20	2 years
Missouri	30	2 years

State	Required Hours	Cycle Length
Montana	36	3 years
Nebraska	30	2 years
Nevada	12	1 year
New Hampshire	20	2 years
New Jersey	20	2 years
New Mexico	45	3 years
New York	24	3 years
North Carolina	6	1 year
North Dakota	16	2 years
Ohio	12	2 years
Oklahoma	30	3 years
Oregon	24	2 years
Pennsylvania	20	2 years
Rhode Island	30	3 years
South Carolina	14	2 years
South Dakota	75	5 years
Tennessee	30	2 years
Texas	12	1 year
Utah	30	2 years
Vermont	12	2 years
Virginia	15	1 year
Washington	15	1 year
West Virginia	12	2 years
Wisconsin	NA	–
Wyoming	BLS CPR only	–

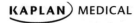

FORMAT OF THE NATIONAL BOARD EXAM

Today's National Board Exam contains 350 multiple-choice questions. It is an all-day exam. Though the number of questions remains constant each year, the number of questions within each topic changes. The morning session, Component A, consists of 200 questions. The afternoon session, Component B, includes 150 questions, based on the cases of 12 to 15 patients.

COMPONENT A (200 questions)

Component A addresses three major topic areas: scientific basis for dental hygiene practice; provision of clinical dental hygiene services; and community health/research principles.

The distribution of items is defined by the following outline. A small percentage of these items simultaneously address behavioral science and professional responsibility (ethics and risk management).

I. Scientific Basis for Dental Hygiene Practice (approximately 60 questions)

Anatomic Sciences
- Anatomy
- Histology and embryology

Physiology

Biochemistry and Nutrition (including nutritional deficiencies)

Microbiology and Immunology

Pathology
- General
- Oral

Pharmacology

II. Provision of Clinical Dental Hygiene Services (approximately 120 questions)

Assessing Patient Characteristics
- Medical and dental history (including vital signs and behavioral factors)
- Head and neck examination (including technique and normal and abnormal findings)
- Periodontal evaluation (including deposits and stains)
- Oral evaluation
- Occlusal evaluation
- Clinical testing (e.g., thermal vitalometer, percussion)

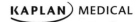

Obtaining and Interpreting Radiographs

- Principles of radiophysics and radiobiology
- Principles of radiologic health (including radiation protection and measurement)
- Technique (including evaluation of quality of radiographs)
- Recognition of normalities and abnormalities

Planning and Managing Dental Hygiene Care

- Infection control (application)
- Recognition of emergency situations and provision of appropriate care
- Individualized patient education
- Anxiety and pain control
- Recognition and management of compromised patients

Performing Periodontal Procedures

- Etiology and pathogenesis of periodontal diseases
- Prescribed therapy (including adjunctive therapies, instruments, and instrumentation)
- Reassessment and maintenance (e.g., implant care)

Using Preventive Agents

- Fluorides—systemic and topical
- Pit and fissure sealants
- Other preventive agents

Providing Supportive Treatment Services

- Properties and manipulation of materials
- Polishing natural and restored teeth
- Making of impressions and preparation of study casts
- Other supportive services (including placement and removal of temporary restorations, rubber dams, and matrices; margination and debonding)

III. Community Health/Research Principles (approximately 20 questions)

Promoting Health and Preventing Disease within Groups

Participating in Community Programs

Analyzing Scientific Literature, Understanding Statistical Concepts, and Applying Research Results

COMPONENT B (150 questions based on 12 to 15 patient cases)

Component B includes actual dental hygiene cases, either child or adult. These cases present information by means of patient histories, dental charts, radiographs, and sometimes intra- and extra-oral photographs. Each exam includes at least one special case, such as geriatric, adult periodontal, pediatric, special needs, or medically compromised.

The case-based items address knowledge and skills required in:

- Assessing patient characteristics
- Obtaining and interpreting radiographs
- Planning and managing dental hygiene care
- Performing periodontal procedures
- Using preventive agents
- Providing supportive treatment service.

Eligibility

If you are a student, you may take the exam if you are enrolled in an **accredited program** and are designated as "prepared" by the program director. You must also be eligible to graduate from your accredited school within 4 months of taking the exam.

If you are a dental hygienist who has graduated from an accredited program, you may take the exam once you provide a letter stating such from the director of that program.

Candidates with a documented disability may make special arrangements to take the test, but must do so 60 days in advance.

A candidate who is a graduate of an unaccredited program may take the exam if the program is equivalent to an accredited program. In that case, a letter from the dean/director of an accredited program *and* a letter by the board of dentistry of a U.S. licensing jurisdiction must accompany the application.

Note: When taking the clinical portion of the state or regional exam, train your dental patient to keep track of the time and say, "It's been 30 minutes; dry my teeth." One of the first things the examiners will do after you are finished with the clinical exam is to dry the patient's teeth to observe remaining calculus. Make sure to look for those little remaining areas before the examiners do by drying the patient's teeth often.

If the state in which you are taking your clinical exam allows you to choose your teeth for scaling, do not pick a hard place. You don't need to impress anyone; you just need to pass the test. If, radiographically, it is observed that you have subgingival spicules of calculus on #1 distal, #2 undetectable calculus radiographically, #3 distal and mesial spicules, #4 distal and mesial spicules, and #5 distal and mesial spicules, do not pick #1 distal to be included.

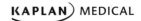

Scoring

A score of 75 is required for passing.

The range of scores for the National Board Exam is 49–99. However, a score of 75 is required as a minimum passing score by the Joint Commission on National Dental Exams. A score below 75 is considered a failure and does not earn National Board credit.

On each National Board Exam, 10–15% of the test questions are "experimental." That is, they are included to see whether they are appropriate for future National Board Exams. These experimental questions are not scored and do not affect your real score.

Two factors affect your score: the number of correct answers you selected and the conversion scale for the exam. There is no penalty for a wrong answer. If two or more answer choices are marked for the same test item, no credit is given. Your score is then converted to a scaled score, based upon the performance of the others taking the exam.

Your score report will arrive in approximately 6–8 weeks. Scores are sent directly to you, your school, and up to three licensing boards or states provided you included that information on your application form.

Registration

To register for the National Board Exam, you will have to complete an application from the Joint Commission on National Dental Exams.

American Dental Association
(312) 440-2500
www.ada.org

HOW TO PREPARE FOR THE EXAM

Preparing for the exam requires ample study and review. Establish a study schedule long before your scheduled test date and stick to that schedule. Start 3–6 months beforehand—review class notes, flashcards (whether purchased or homemade), hand outs, or class books.

Develop Realistic Goals

Form study groups and always attend, making sure that your environment is free of distractions. Cramming at the last minute is useless and nonproductive.

As you review, think about what you are reading rather than just skim over it. Can you come up with examples other than those in the material? Can you express the author's point in your own words? Quiz yourself with some of the practice questions without looking at the answers.

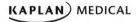

Master Multiple-Choice Questions

Focus on the question and do not read into it. Each question contains an item stem and possible answer choices. Mark off the answer choices you know are wrong and then select the one that is right.

Read the question and formulate an answer in your mind. Then, look for the answer. If it is not there, look for the answer that most closely resembles the one you formulated. If you cannot decide between two answers, then consider which one fits the stem words best.

Never Leave a Question Blank

Eliminate all the wrong answer choices that you can; then pick the best of the answers that remain. If there are two answer choices that are the complete opposite of each other, one of them is most likely to be correct. For example:

1. Symptoms of fluoride toxicity include all the following EXCEPT:
   A. Cramping and diarrhea
   B. Tachycardia
   C. Increased salivation
   D. Decreased salivation

Perhaps you remember that some type of salivation is a symptom of fluoride toxicity but aren't sure whether it is increased or decreased. Since these two answer choices, (C) and (D) are opposites, there's a 50 percent chance that one of the two is right. In this case, decreased salivation is the exception, so (D) is correct.

If you cannot come up with an answer, leave the question blank for the moment and circle that question number in the test booklet. Make sure to skip the appropriate space on the answer sheet; otherwise, your entire scoring grid will be off.

Every so often, check to make sure that the number of a question matches with the correct number on the answer sheet (check every 10–20 questions). If you accidentally placed an answer in a wrong number on the answer sheet, the following answers will subsequently be placed in the wrong numbers as well on the answer sheet. Occasionally, an answer that you were not sure of may pop up in another question.

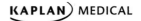

Do Not Change Your First Answer

According to statistics, your first choice is usually the right answer. Do not go back and change the answer unless you are absolutely sure that changing the answer is the right thing to do. Research shows that students most often change a right answer to a wrong answer.

Be Careful of Qualifiers

Watch out for words such as *always*, *never*, *all*, *only*, and *none*. These words require 100 percent of the question to be true. If everything in that question is not always true, then the answer has to be false. Similarly, be careful of the word EXCEPT, since it requires you to find the exception to the rule.

Qualifiers such as *sometimes*, *frequently*, *often*, or *generally* usually indicate a correct answer.

Multiple-Choice Questions

There are 200 multiple-choice questions in the morning and 150 in the afternoon. There are different kinds of multiple-choice questions:

All of the Above Questions

In an *All of the Above* question, if you are sure that at least two answer choices are correct but aren't sure about the others, then pick the *All of the Above* answer choice. This is frequently the correct answer.

Umbrella Questions

Umbrella questions can have answers that are all correct (and *All of the Above* is not an answer choice). One answer choice encompasses all of the others, and it is your job to figure out which one that is.

2. Which of the following can cause tooth erosion?

   A. Sucking on lemons
   B. Sipping cola all day long
   C. Acidic chemical forces
   D. Reflux disease

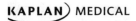

The answer is (C), *acidic chemical forces*. We know that erosion is not from bacteria breaking down tooth structure. Lemons have citric acid, cola is acidic, and stomach acid from reflux disease is hydrochloric acid. Therefore, sucking on lemons, sipping cola all day, and reflux disease can all erode teeth. So *acidic chemical force*s encompasses lemons, cola and acid reflux disease.

Distractor Questions

In certain questions, you may not recognize certain words in the answer choices. These unfamiliar words are planted there by the test maker to distract you from the correct answer. The test makers are hoping you'll focus on that unknown word rather than on finding the correct answer. To make sure this doesn't happen, cover up the answer choices and reread the question, then formulate an answer in your mind.

3. Of the following types of medical emergencies that can occur in the dental office, which would involve immediate difficulty in breathing?

    A. Chronic bronchitis
    B. Apoplexy
    C. Anaphylaxis
    D. Thyroid storm

The answer is (C); *anaphylaxis* comes on suddenly. But did you wonder what (B), *apoplexy* was? The test makers were hoping you would focus on that word. *Apoplexy* has to do with crippling by a stroke. *Thyroid storm* symptoms (D), don't include difficulty in breathing. *Chronic bronchitis* (A), is just that—chronic—and though there is difficulty in breathing, it is not sudden.

Case Study Questions

All students get excited or nervous about the case studies. The case studies tie in all the information you have learned. These questions need not be intimidating.

You will have a list of items that you can take into the exam. Two of them are paper clips and a magnifying glass. *Paper clips* should be used during the case study portion: If you use the paper clips properly, you will avoid accidentally opening to the wrong pictures.

Paperclip page 1 of the first case study booklet pictures to the front cover of the book. Paper clip the last page of that same case study to the back cover of the book. This permits access to only the case study pictures that you are working on. When you get to the next case study, move the paper clips. Then, moving ahead, paperclip page 1 of the second case study pictures to the front cover and the last page of that same case study to the back cover.

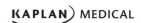

A *magnifying glass* is essential for looking at the pictures or radiographs. Not every picture will be obvious, and it may be very hard to pick out the part you are being asked about. Most office supply stores carry magnifying glasses.

Erasing Your Original Answer

You will be using a #2 pencil to fill out your answers on a Scantron answer grid. This grid will be fed into a computer for scoring. So if you have to erase an answer, make sure you erase the original *thoroughly*. If you don't, the Scantron may misread your incomplete erasure. In that case, your first answer will be marked, indicating you gave multiple answers for the question.

Test Failure and Scantron

If you fail your test by only a few points, ask to have it hand graded. If any incomplete erasures were picked up as multiple answers and marked as wrong, then hand grading may give you the extra points you need to pass.

WHAT TO TAKE ON TEST DAY

To be permitted into the test, you are required to present the admittance ticket issued by the ADA that also has a recent photograph attached. In addition, two recent photo ID's are required, such as a driver's license, school ID, or passport.

There are a few things you must take with you to the exam:

- No. 2 pencils (so that the Scantron answer sheets can be read by the computer)
- A magnifying glass (not required but strongly suggested). Many office supply stores sell a credit card size magnifying glass that works well.
- Two or three paper clips for use during the case-based study questions

You may *not* bring a calculator, cell phone, pager, pen, highlighter, dictionary, or extra scrap paper into the exam room. Additionally, no food or drink is allowed.

Test materials are not allowed out of the room under any circumstances nor are they allowed to be copied.

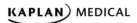

HOW TO GET IN PEAK SHAPE FOR TEST DAY

Proper nutrition is necessary for good brain function. Even if you are anxious about the test and don't feel like eating, do not go into the test without something in your stomach. Avoid caffeine and eat slow-release carbohydrates such as whole grain pastas, starchy vegetables like sweet potatoes or corn, and fresh fruits. Candy will give a quick rise in sugar, but it will also give you a low when it is used up.

Lack of exercise results in loss of body tone, which in turn makes you less alert. Go for a walk every day or work out at the gym.

Cramming the Night Before

Do not study on the day before the exam. If you do not know the material by this point, then cramming won't help. Go to a movie or out for dinner. Relax and do something nice for yourself.

Visiting the Test Site Ahead of Time

Check out the testing site ahead of time, even if an appointment is required. By familiarizing yourself with the setup, you will have an edge before you walk in the door.

Sleep

Lack of sleep impairs thinking and memory. It can also cause visual fatigue. Get a good night's rest the night before the exam.

Anxiety and Panic

Panic only blocks concentration and the recollection of facts. Take a deep breath and concentrate on rational thoughts. Don't schedule stressful events just before the exam. Avoid people who can be irritating. Arrive early since you will not be allowed into the exam if late. The big key is try to relax and not let anxiety prevent you from reasoning things out. Remember, an answer you may not be able to reason out may be in another place in the test.

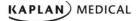

YOUR LICENSE: NEVER GIVE IT UP

Never, ever give up your license. Some people do so, thinking that they will never be a hygienist again to find years later that they want to regain their license. Even if you suffer a major crisis in your personal life or have career burnout, do not give up your license. It is an enormous task to regain it. It is worth every effort to take the continuing education requirements and pay the yearly renewal fee. It is a small price to pay because you never know when you may decide to return to this career later in life.

Dental Hygiene Review

Chapter Two: **Histology and Embryology**

Histology is the study of cells and their function. Cells hold distinctive physiological properties such as the ability to become excitable, as in cardiac tissue, or the ability to transport nutrients (endocytosis) and wastes (exocytosis) across their cell membranes. Cells reproduce by mitosis and possess the ability to communicate with one another.

Embryology is the study of human development from the time an egg is fertilized and until the time a fetus is born. Fetal development may be perfectly normal or can occur with abnormalities. Development of the oral cavities and their related structures can help the dental hygienist to better understand the environment that she will be working in. Knowledge of developmental abnormalities can also help the dental hygienist formulate a treatment plan for a patient with abnormalities.

HISTOLOGY

The human body is made up of various **organ** systems. Each organ in an organ system is composed of specialized **tissue**, which in turn is made up of **cells**. Each cell is surrounded and protected by a **cell membrane** or **plasmalemma** made up of proteins and lipids that microscopically appear to be a trilaminar structure. The proteins reinforce the structural trilaminar layer in the **cytoskeleton**.

Cell Parts and Functions

The lipid layer consists of phospholipids that have hydrophilic ends located toward the outside of the membrane and hydrophobic ends forming the middle of the trilaminar layer. The cell membrane is selectively semi-permeable to allow different things to enter into each cell—such as nutrients, hormones, immunoglobulins, neurotransmitters, and oxygen for cell respiration.

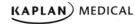

Cells in the body lacking a nucleus are erythrocytes and thrombocytes.

Within the cell membrane is cytoplasm, an aqueous gel that holds many organelles that perform different functions. It also contains spaces called vacuoles. In human cells, the **nucleus** contains the **46 chromosomes** of DNA which store the cell's genetic code. As the master copy, it acts like an instruction manual to tell the RNA how to copy the DNA. **Chromatin** within the nucleus is the main nucleoprotein. The midpoint of a chromosome is the **centromere**.

The **nucleus** holds one or more spherical structures called nucleoli. Made up of RNA, DNA, and protein, it contains a nuclear matrix of ions, metabolites, and proteins. Chromosomes are contained with the nuclear matrix. The nucleolus consists primarily of RNA and is the site where RNA and ribosomes are compiled.

There are three types of RNA necessary for protein synthesis:

- **Messenger RNA** is a template of DNA for protein synthesis. It transcribes (copies) small portions of DNA as it travels through ribosomes connected to the endoplasmic reticulum. **Transcription** is the way in which messenger RNA uses DNA as a template; that is, to copy the genetic code for transfer into the messenger RNA.

- **Transfer RNA** carries out the genetic code from messenger RNA to channel amino acids for synthesizing new proteins.

- **Ribosomal RNA** aids in protein synthesis and may be free-floating in cytoplasm or attached to the endoplasmic reticulum. **Ribosomes**, which produce protein, are small organelles derived from the RNA of the nucleolus. Some roam free in the cytoplasm while others attach to the endoplasmic reticulum. The fate of these proteins is to become secretions or to be included in the membranes. Yet others are simply put into storage.

The **endoplasmic reticulum** is a three-dimensional maze within the cytoplasm that contains a network of parallel membrane channels and spaces. It is made up of two types: **rough endoplasmic reticulum (RER)** and **smooth endoplasmic reticulum (SER)**. RER has ribosomes attached. Its function is to modify proteins for export to the Golgi complex. SER does not have ribosomes attached and synthesizes steroids but also aids in metabolism and detoxification of substances. The **Golgi complex** is a curved, membranous stack of sacs that packages and distributes newly modified protein to be exported out of the cell, but also synthesizes lysosomes. **Lysosomes**, also found within the cytoplasm, are the digestive system of the cell that breaks down foreign substances and old cell components. This process is termed phagocytosis and utilizes over 40 hydrolytic enzymes. The Golgi complex produces lysosomes. Each cell contains one or more **mitochondria** that are the "powerhouse" of the cell.

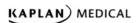

Mitochondria generate adenosine triphosphate (ATP) during Krebs cycle, as the cell's chief energy source. **Cristae** are folds within the mitochondria that allow for additional work surface areas during aerobic cellular respiration. The amount of mitochondria within a cell is dependent upon the amount of energy that a particular cell must produce. Heart muscle cells produce vast amounts of metabolic activity and each cell contains numerous mitochondria.

Other cell parts include thread-like structures called **microfilaments** and **microtubules** that help to maintain the shape of the cell, cylindrical **centrioles** that aid in chromosome separation in the mitosis of cell division, and inactive structures accumulated in cytoplasm and utilized when called for.

Cell Replication

Mitosis is the process of cell division. **Prophase**, the first phase, occurs when chromatin coils (spiralizes) and compresses into chromosomes, the nuclear membrane is lost, and the centrioles help to arrange the mitotic spindles as they migrate toward opposite poles.

Metaphase is the second stage. Chromosomes align their centromeres at the midpoint as mitotic spindles form. **Anaphase**, the third stage, occurs when the chromatids of each chromosome join at the centromere. The spindles then migrate toward opposite poles of the cell.

Telophase is the last stage of mitosis when nuclear division is complete. Chromatids uncoil into two new nuclei surrounded by new nuclear membranes. **Cytokinesis** is the division of the cytoplasm into two new daughter cells, each containing about the same organelles of the original or parent cell.

Interphase is the cell stage between cell division when the DNA replicates and centrioles get ready to start the process over again.

Cell Membrane Physiology

Diffusion is the movement of molecules across a cell membrane from high to low concentration without energy use. When the movement of a substance is directed from an area of higher concentration toward an area of lower concentration, it is termed **diffusion gradient**. **Facilitated diffusion** or **passive transport** is the movement of water-soluble molecules across the lipid layer of a semi-permeable cell membrane. A **carrier protein** binds with the water-soluble molecule to assist it across the lipid layer (water and fat do not mix) to the other side and then drops it off. Energy is *not* required to do this.

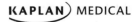

Active transport also uses proteins to force molecules in or out of cells. As these molecules are pumped in and out of cells, they require ATP energy to do so. **Osmosis** is the movement of fluid across the cell membrane from an area of higher concentration to lower concentration.

Cell Junctions

Junctional epithelium attaches to the tooth surface by hemidesmosomes.

Desmosomes joins cells together. Tight junctions adhere cells together to prevent any undesired substances from passing into the cells. Gap junctions consist of passageways that allow for the transfer of ions and molecules between cells. **Hemidesmosomes** attach a **cell to a non-cellular** surface.

Tissues

There are four types of body tissues: **epithelial tissue**, which covers and protects the external and internal body surfaces; **connective tissue** that includes several body systems; **muscle**, which includes voluntary and involuntary systems; and **nerves**, which carry messages to and from the brain.

Basic Tissues	Types	
Connective Tissue	Blood	Plasma, platelets, RBCs, WBCs
	Bone	Flat, irregular, long, short
	Cartilage	Elastic, fibrous, hyaline
	Fat or adipose	Insulates under skin, around organs
	Lymph	Lymph nodes, tonsils
Epithelial	Simple	Columnar, cuboidal, squamous, pseudostratified
	Stratified	Columnar, cuboidal, squamous, transitional
Muscle	Cardiac	Involuntary, striated
	Skeletal	Voluntary, striated
	Smooth	Involuntary, smooth
Nerve	Central	Brain, brain stem, spinal cord
	Peripheral	Cranial nerves (12), spinal nerves (31)
	Autonomic	Sympathetic, parasympathetic
	Somatic	Voluntary

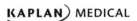

Epithelial Tissue

In embryo, **epithelial** tissue is derived from the ectoderm, mesoderm, and endoderm. The ectoderm gives rise to **epithelial** tissue, hair, and nails. The **endothelium** from endoderm lines the GI tract and lungs, while the **mesothelium** from the mesoderm lines the peritoneal cavity, renal tubules, blood vessels, and lymph vessels. The purpose of epithelial tissue is to maintain **homeostasis** in the body by protecting the body from the outside environment, provide endocrine and exocrine secretions from glands, sensory reception, and absorption as in the digestive tract. Epithelial tissue is unique in that it has very tightly attached cells that rest on the basement membrane of connective tissue. There are also different types of simple and stratified epithelial cells. Squamous cells are flat cells while cuboidal cells are shaped like cubes and columnar cells are column shaped.

Since epithelial tissue is located in so many varied places in the body, there are specialized types of epithelial tissue—simple and stratified. Simple epithelial tissue is involved in the internal organs. Stratified epithelial tissue is involved with the skin, glands, and some internal linings near the body's entrances and exits. Simple epithelial is one cell layer due to the tissue being located in areas that receive little friction. Stratified epithelial tissue has more layers due to being in areas receiving higher friction.

Type of Epithelial Tissue	Locations
Simple Columnar	Lines stomach, small intestine, colon, gallbladder
Simple Cuboidal	Kidney tubules, ovary surface, small ducts of endocrine glands
Simple Squamous	Lines respiratory tract, vascular system, Bowman's capsules
Pseudostratified	Lines bronchia, trachea
Stratified Columnar	Large ducts of exocrine glands
Stratified Cuboidal	Sweat glands, ducts, large ducts of exocrine glands
Stratified Squamous	Epidermis, esophagus, oral cavity, vagina
Transitional	Bladder, ureter, urethra

Connective Tissue

Many forms of connective tissue are derived from the **mesenchyme** in embryo. Connective tissue includes blood, bone, cartilage, lymph, adipose, elastic, fibrous, and reticular connective tissues. **Cartilage** is a connective tissue that is noncalcified and firm. It is present in most joints at the articular surfaces. It is avascular and receives nutrients from the surrounding tissues. Cartilage is produced by chondroblasts and then matures into chondrocytes. Like in bone, the chondrocytes are encased in cartilage and surrounded by lacuna.

The three types of cartilage are hyaline, elastic, and fibrocartilage. The most abundant is **hyaline cartilage**, which is comprised of only collagen fibers. It is found in the "C" rings of the trachea, nasal septum, and the articular ends of bone. **Elastic cartilage** is similar

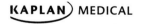

to hyaline cartilage but contains more elastic fibers. As flexible support, it is found in the ear, auditory canal, and epiglottis. **Fibrocartilage** supports and withstands compression as it merges with hyaline cartilage. It is found in the intervertebral discs and the pubic symphysis.

Bone is produced by **osteoblasts** and broken down by **osteoclasts**. Bone cells are **osteocytes**. Bone ossification occurs by both **intramembranous osteogenesis** and **endochondral osteogenesis.**

Intramembranous osteogenesis occurs when osteoblasts enter into dense connective tissue and form osteoids. Bone apposition occurs when osteoids form concentric layers of bone matrix upon one another. **Endochondral osteogenesis** occurs in existing hyaline cartilage. First, chondrocytes detach themselves from their nourishment and die. As the cartilage calcifies, it is degenerated by osteoclasts and replaced by osteoblasts that proliferate bone matrix.

Compact bone is comprised of bone **matrix** where **osteoblasts deposit matrix** in thin sheets termed **lamella**. Lamellae, in turn, form cylindrical circles around a blood vessel to become an **osteon**. These concentric circles of osteons make up the **haversian canal system**. As osteoblasts produce bone matrix, they become entrapped in the matrix to become **osteocytes**. Osteocytes have cytoplasmic processes termed **canaliculi** that **radiate** outward into the bone matrix. The canaliculi communicate with other osteocytes to pass on information, nutrients, and/or wastes. A space in the bone matrix surrounding the osteocyte is called a **lacuna**.

The haversian system, lacunae, and canaliculi connect with each other in the osteon which then connects them to **Volkmann's canals** located at the exterior segment of the haversian system. These canals provide nerve, blood, and nutrients to the bone as well as allowing for communication between osteons.

Cancellous or **spongy** bone consists of **trabecular** bony plates that are irregular and contain the red bone marrow. **Compact bone** is very dense bone that appears to be an accumulation of a solid mass of bone.

Bone marrow produces platelets, red blood cells, granulocytes (neutrophils, basophils, eosinophils), monocytes, and lymphocytes. At birth until about age 3, bone marrow is present throughout most of the bones, but by age 21, it is replaced by inactive yellow lymphoid marrow. In adults, blood cells are produced in the cranial bones, pelvis, ribs, sternum, and vertebrae.

Lymph tissue is a series of glands that are an essential component of the immune system. They originate from mesenchyme and are located throughout the body, but can be found in clusters under the arm, in the inguinal area, and in the cervical regions of the body. **Reticular fibers** are not often seen, but can be found between connective tissue and other tissues. These fibers can provide a support framework for organs. **Adipose** connective tissue insulates the body and protects organs.

Muscle

In embryo, muscle is derived from the mesoderm which then differentiates into three types of body muscles—skeletal, cardiac, and smooth. The contractile units of **myofibrils** or muscle cells are sarcomeres. **Sarcomeres** are found in skeletal and cardiac muscle tissue.

Each muscle cell contains **myofibril** bands of light and dark areas. The light areas are called I bands and the dark areas, A bands. Near each I band, there is a Z line where adjacent sarcomeres adjoin. Within each **sarcomere** are the protein filaments of **actin** and **myosin**. Sarcomeres contract when actin and myosin filaments slide over each other.

> The contractile unit of muscle is the sarcomere.

Skeletal muscle is **striated** muscle that works by conscious thought for body movement. Skeletal muscle also provides body stability. Neuron stimulation is what allows for movement. Calcium ions stored in the sarcoplasmic reticulum of the myofibril aid in the muscle contraction. **Cardiac** muscle is very specialized in that it has the ability to conduct electricity. It is **striated involuntary** muscle that is controlled by the autonomic nervous system. Cardiac cells are joined together by **intercalated disks** that allow for electrical impulses to methodically spread to other cells. **Smooth** muscle is found in glands, organs, and the lining of blood vessels.

Nerves

Nerves are a pathway for cells to communicate. In embryo, neural tissue is derived from neuroectoderm. Neural stem cells produce neuroblasts that form both neurons and **glia** that act as guide wires for neurons.

The **neuron** is the communicator of the nervous system; it can both receive and deliver messages. It is made up of a neural cell body, dendrite, and axon. The **neural cell body** contains the nucleus and maintains the homeostasis within the cell. The **dendrite** has numerous branches that increase surface reception capacity to receive signals and carry them back to the cell. The **axon** carries away a signal as it transmits an electrochemical signal over a **synapse** to another neuron. The **myelin sheath** that protects the axon has an outer covering of **Schwann cells** that prevent exposure to neighboring non-neural cells.

Blood

Blood is a connective tissue fluid but does not contain fibers. Hemoglobin in erythrocytes delivers oxygen to cells and transports CO_2 back to the lungs. Blood also provides nutrients to cells, takes away waste, carries antibodies, transports electrolytes, and conveys hormones necessary for body function. The fluid portion of plasma contains proteins, clotting factors, and the formed elements or blood cells.

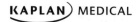

Red blood cells and thrombocytes are cells in the body that **lack a nucleus**.

Thrombocytes or **platelets** are fragments of cytoplasm whose function is to aid in blood clotting. Each cubic centimeter of blood has 250,000–500,000 of thrombocytes. **Erythrocytes** or red blood cells contain hemoglobin, which transports oxygen to cells and carries CO_2 back to the lungs. Iron combines with protein to form hemoglobin. If there is a deficiency of iron, anemia can result. The bone marrow produces red blood cells which have a life of about 120 days. They are removed by phagocytosis in the liver or spleen. Women have 4–5 million erythrocytes per cubic millimeter of blood while men have 5–6 million.

Neutrophils are also involved with **acute** inflammation.

Leukocytes include all the white blood cells of both granulocytes and agranulocytes. **Granulocyte leukocytes** contain cytoplasmic granules. These cells, produced in the bone marrow, include basophils, eosinophils, and neutrophils. **Neutrophils** or **polymorphonuclear (PMN)** leukocytes have a lifespan of about one week and are the most common white blood cell. Their nucleus is **multilobulated** into segments with **no nucleolus** present. Their job is the phagocytosis of invading pathogens when injuries occur. Neutrophils are attracted by chemotactic factors and are the first cells to invade the early stages of inflammation.

Granular leukocytes = BEN (basophils, eosinophils, and neutrophils)

Eosinophils are involved in allergic responses and parasitic infections. They have two lobes in the nucleus. In allergic responses, they secrete chemical mediators that cause bronchoconstriction. **Basophils** contain basophilic granules and are the least numerous white blood cells. They play an important role along with mast cells in inflammatory and allergic responses. When IgE from an allergic response is released, basophils release histamine along with mast cells.

Mast cells are not seen in normal circulation. They are activated when an allergen causes the release of IgE. The amount of histamine released depends on the amount and type of stimuli.

Agranulocytes include lymphocytes and monocytes and lack cytoplasmic granules.

Monocytes are the largest leukocytes and become large **macrophages** when they leave the capillaries. Monocytes hide in tissues as macrophages after circulating for 5-8 days where they lie in wait for invading pathogens. They are involved in **chronic** inflammation and take longer to get to the site of an infection than do neutrophils.

Lymphocytes are the smallest white blood cells and contain a very large nucleus. As the second most common white blood cell, lymphocytes are involved in an immune response. They are found both in blood and lymph circulation but are formed in the bone marrow by stem cells. As lymphocytes enter into circulation, about half of them journey to the **thymus** to mature into **T cells** or **T lymphocytes**. Others mature in the bone marrow as **B cells** or **B leukocytes**. T cells are incapable of producing antibodies while B cells can produce antibodies.

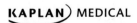

ABO Classification of Blood

The **ABO classification** system is based on the antigen that produces agglutinogens from protein and is present on the surfaces of red blood cells. In this system, there are four major blood types: **Type A** blood has the A antigen or agglutinogen while **Type B** blood has the B antigen or agglutinogen. **Type AB** blood possesses both the A and B antigens or agglutinogens. **Type O** blood has neither.

Type	Agglutinogen	Anti-Agglutinogen
O	None	Anti-A / Anti-B
A	A	Anti-B
B	B	Anti-A
AB	A & B	None

There is a protein in blood that indicates a person's Rh factor. If you have this protein, you are Rh+. If you don't, you are Rh−. For an Rh− mother during her first pregnancy, the Rh− factor usually does not interact with the blood of the baby. The mother can receive a shot of **Rh immune-globulin (RhoGAM)** in the 28th week of pregnancy and another within 72 hours of the delivery. The Rh immune-globulin serves as a vaccine to suppress antibodies from forming against a future Rh+ baby. If the mother does not receive the RhoGAM shot, should she carry another baby that is Rh+ in the future, her Rh− antibodies can migrate across the placenta to destroy the baby's Rh+ blood cells. The antibodies destroy the baby's red blood cells.

Type O blood is the universal donor.

Type AB blood is the universal recipient.

Lymph Glands

Lymph nodes, which are derived from the mesoderm, are an essential part of our immune system. They hold lymphocytes, which filter invading antigens in the body. Connective tissue capsules that contain the cortex and medullary areas of lymph glands surround each node. The cortex consists of tightly packed lymphocytes that form spherical lymphoid follicles. The medullary area is divided into the **medullary trabeculae** as well as the **medullary cords** and **sinuses**. The **trabeculae** extend toward the medullary region, subdividing it into lobules that aid in giving shape to the lymph node. The medullary sinuses and cords are composed of reticular cells. **Reticular cells** create a filtering mesh for lymph. The **sinuses** drain lymph fluid into the efferent lymphatic vessels. The medullary **cords** channel plasma and B lymphocytes to the hilum, which is where the blood vessels enter and exit the lymph node.

Tonsils start developing around the eighth week of gestation when the mesenchyme differentiates into tonsillar lymphoid tissue. Epithelial tissue forms nodular structures that invaginate into tonsillar crypts. The **palatine tonsils** located in the lateral wall of the oropharynx are comprised of lymphocytes contained in epithelial crypts that are encompassed by lymph nodes. They are surrounded by squamous epithelial tissue. The **lingual tonsils** are located in the base of the tongue and

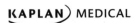

contain lymphoid tissue. The palatine and lingual tonsils contain deep crypts of lymphoid tissue containing mostly B lymphocytes to fight off any invading antigens. The **pharyngeal tonsils** or adenoids are located in the nasopharynx and are covered by pseudostratified columnar epithelium. They do not contain crypts, as do the lingual tonsils, but they do filter out invading antigens.

As exocrine glands, the **salivary glands** are derived from connective and epithelial tissue. As the glands are forming, epithelial tissue invaginates into connective tissue and forms into lobules. Each lobule forms a duct to channel its secretions from either mucous acini, serous acini, or mucoserous acini into a lumen where saliva collects.

Endocrine Glands

Some endocrine glands (pineal and pituitary) are derived from ectoderm along with sweat glands and salivary glands. Little is known about the **pineal** gland except that it releases melatonin. The **pituitary gland**, derived from ectoderm, is the master gland that regulates most of the other endocrine glands. The anterior portion that contains nests of cuboidal cells of the pituitary gland or **adenohypophysis** secretes the hormones ACTH (adrenocorticotropic hormone), GH (growth hormone), TSH (thyroid stimulating hormone), FSH (follicle stimulating hormone), and LH (luteinizing hormone). The posterior portion contains nerve tissue called **neurohypophysis** where terminal axons extend down from hypothalamus. The posterior portion stores ADH (antidiuretic hormone) and oxytocin produced by the hypothalamus. The pituitary gland also later secretes the ADH and oxytocin when needed. It contains cells called pituicytes.

A stalk at the posterior part of the pituitary gland connects it to the **hypothalamus**, which has a strong influence on the pituitary gland. The **hypothalamus** is a collection of gray matter that regulates blood pressure, body temperature, and body fluids. It is derived from neuroectoderm. The **thalamus** is also a collection of gray matter that receives signals from various parts of the brain and after processing them it sends the signals to the cerebral cortex. The **thyroid** is cuboidal epithelial tissue surrounded by colloid filled lumen and is derived from the endoderm. In the thyroid, parafollicular cells contain C cells that secrete **calcitonin**, which regulates calcium necessary for bone structure and muscle function. The thyroid also produces thyroxine, which stimulates metabolic rate.

On both sides of the thyroid gland lie the **parathyroid glands**, also derived from endoderm. The parathyroid gland is surrounded by a thin fibrous capsule and is divided into parenchymal lobules containing **chief cells** and oxyphil cells. The chief cells secrete parathyroid hormone which regulates calcium homeostasis.

Also derived from the endoderm is the **thymus**, which is comprised of lymphatic tissue. It has an outer cortex and inner medulla that contains densely populated lymphocytes to be matured into T cells or T lymphocytes.

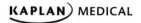

EMBRYOLOGY

Embryology is the study of the development of embryos in their prenatal period. **Preimplantation** occurs when the sperm penetrates the ovum and becomes a **zygote**, traveling down the fallopian tube. As it divides into about 32 cells, the zygote becomes a **morula** or globular mass of blastomeres. As these cells undergo mitosis, the morula becomes an outer shell that nourishes the baby. The inner cells become the **blastocyst**.

About five days later, the blastocyst implants into the mother's uterine wall. The **embryonic period** begins at that point, when the transfer of nutrients from the endometrium of the mother begins. The blastocyst then becomes an **embryo** until the **eighth week**, as cells start to **differentiate** (identical cells become different tissues), **proliferate** (controlled multiplication of cells), and undergo **morphogenesis** (embryonic cells interact with one another as they migrate to become new types of cells).

There are two layers of cells: the inner cells of the embryo, and the outer cells of the placental formation which then form a third middle layer by cell migration called **gastrulation**. Gastrulation produces the ectoderm, mesoderm, and endoderm from which morphogenesis occurs. At the third week, the neural system starts to develop as the ectoderm thickens and invaginates as a midsagittal groove forming the neural folds. These folds fuse together to become the neural tube and future site of the brain and spinal cord. In the ninth week, the embryo becomes a fetus until birth at about 40 weeks.

Head and Neck Formation

In the embryonic period of the fourth week, the face starts to develop. It develops from all three layers of ectoderm, mesoderm, and endoderm as well as the neural crest cells. By the twelfth week, the face is completed; during this time, neural crest cells begin to differentiate into connective tissue that will become cartilage, bone, and ligaments.

Five branchial arches give rise to facial formation in the fourth week, when five bulges or primordia start to surround the **stomodeum** or primitive mouth. The **first branchial arch** gives rise to the **frontonasal** process (1), 2 **mandibular** processes, and 2 **maxillary** processes but is also known as the mandibular arch. The **mandibular processes** fuse at the mandibular symphysis first to form the mandible and lower face. Neural crest cells derived from mesenchyme will differentiate into various tissues. Meckel's cartilage develops first in the mandible before intramembranous ossification occurs to form the bone of the mandible. Meckel's cartilage also contributes to the formation of the middle ear.

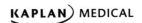

Period	Organs	Developing
Week 1	Zygote	
Week 2	Blastocyst	
Week 3	Embryo	Brain
		Heart (begins beating 22 days)
		Spinal cord
		Gastrointestinal tract
Weeks 4–5	Embryo	Cranial nerves
		Eyes and ears
		Vertebra, some bones
		Blood vessels
		Arm and leg buds
Week 6	Embryo	Lungs
		More brain development
		Digits on hands and feet
		Heart and circulation more developed
Weeks 7–8	Embryo	Facial features
		Hair follicles
		All major organs developing
Weeks 9–12	Fetus	Tooth buds
		Urogenital tract complete
		Genitals appear
Weeks 12–40	Fetus	All organs mature

At the end of the fourth week, the tongue starts to develop from the 1st through the 4th branchial arches. Branchial arch 1 forms the body of the tongue, while arches 2 and 3 form the base of the tongue. This is also when the **thyroid gland** starts to develop in the **foramen cecum** of the tongue; at week five, it starts to regress downward and the trigeminal nerve begins to innervate the tongue.

Around the fifth week, the mandibular arch gives rise to the muscles of mastication. The cells start to differentiate into the lateral and medial pterygoid along with the masseter and temporalis. At the tenth week, the developing trigeminal nerve innervates into the maturing muscles of mastication.

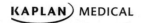

The maxillary arches become more prominent in the fifth week as they develop from the mandibular arch anteriorly and superiorly to the stomodeum. Neural crest cells also derived from mesenchyme differentiate into the tissues that make up the midface, cheeks, sides of the upper lip, lateral palatine processes, posterior maxilla, maxillary canines, and maxillary posterior teeth. The maxillary arches also give rise to the zygoma and part of the temporal bones.

In the fourth week, the **upper jaw** develops from five main buds. The median **frontonasal process** gives rise to the upper face of the forehead, primary palate, nasal septum, and dorsum of the nose. The **frontonasal process** fuses with the **two medial processes** and **both lateral nasal processes** to form the middle and sides of the nose respectively.

The **medial nasal process** also fuses with the stomodeum to form the premaxilla or **intermaxillary segment** which then gives rise to the primary palate, all four maxillary incisors, and the nasal septum. When the medial nasal process fuses with the maxillary process, the upper lip is completed in the sixth week. If the two maxillary processes and medial nasal process fail to fuse by then, **cleft lip** can occur. It can be unilateral or bilateral.

Cleft lip can occur in the 4–7 week range of the embryonic period.

Palatal formation occurs by the twelfth week, while lip formation occurs by the sixth week. The primary palate forms in the 5–6 week period with the fusion of the premaxillary segment and the medial nasal process. In the 6–12 weeks of prenatal development, the secondary palate is the fusion of the two palatal shelves of the maxillary processes. During the twelfth week of development, the secondary palate fuses with the primary palate. If the palatel shelves fail to fuse, then **cleft palate** can occur.

Cleft palate can occur in the 8–12 week range of fetal development.

Types of Clefts
Tip of uvula
Bifid uvula
Soft palate
Soft and hard palate
Unilateral lip
Bilateral lip
Unilateral lip and palate
Bilateral lip and palate

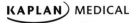

The neck starts to develop in the fourth week from branchial arches 1–6, with the 5th branchial arch not forming in humans. The **second branchial arch**—the **hyoid arch**—forms cartilage called Reichert's cartilage that gives rise to the root of the tongue, the hyoid bone, styloid process of the temporal bone, stapes of the middle ear, stapedius muscle of the middle ear, muscles of facial expression, and suprahyoid muscle. Other tissues that develop here are the hyoid arteries and palatine tonsils. The facial nerve innervates here.

The **third branchial arch** gives rise to portions of the hyoid bone, the root portion of the tongue, the thymus hypopharynx, and the inferior portion of the parathyroid glands. The glossopharyngeal nerve innervates here. The thymus is the most active in childhood and atrophies in adulthood but is the producer of T-lymphocytes.

The **fourth** and **sixth branchial arches** are innervated by the vagus nerve and give rise to thyroid cartilage, other laryngeal cartilages, the pharyngeal muscles, and the superior portion of the parathyroid glands. The fourth branchial arch gives rise to the epiglottis.

During the embryonic period of 4–8 weeks, the **tongue** begins to develop from the first four branchial arches. The first branchial arch gives rise to the body of the tongue. The second, third, and fourth branchial arches give rise to the root of the tongue. The hypoglossal nerve that innervates the tongue provides for movement of the tongue, while the innervation of the glossopharyngeal nerve provides for taste sensation to the posterior $\frac{1}{3}$ of the tongue.

The thyroid gland initially develops as a depression in the foramen cecum of the tongue.

The **thyroid**, the first endocrine gland to form, develops from endoderm in the **foramen cecum** of the tongue at about the fourth week in embryo. It then descends from the foramen cecum of the tongue as it regresses downward around the fifth week. In the seventh week, it completes its travel to the area of the second and third tracheal cartilage.

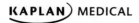

TOOTH DEVELOPMENT

In the seventh week in embryo, **odontogenesis** starts to form the 20 teeth of the primary dentition. Each tooth is derived from mesenchyme that comes from neural crest cells, and ectoderm that gives rise to epithelial tissue. Epithelial tissue gives rise to the enamel organ, ameloblasts, and enamel matrix. The **ectomesenchyme** gives rise to the dental papilla, dentin matrix, pulp cavity, dental sac, cementum, periodontal ligament, and alveolar bone.

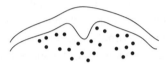

During the **initiation stage**, epithelial tissue begins to thicken and migrates into the mesenchyme (ectomesenchyme), producing the dental lamina. It is this stage of tooth development that can produce anomalies such as supernumerary teeth, partial or complete anodontia, or mesiodens. The **bud stage** occurs around week 8, when rapid proliferation of the dental lamina begins to form the primary dentition tooth buds. Here, the underlying mesenchyme becomes denser. Dental anomalies in this stage would be microdontia or macrodontia.

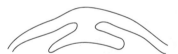

During the **cap stage**, proliferation occurs rapidly, as tissues start to morphodifferentiate into ectoderm and mesenchyme tissue. The ectoderm becomes the **enamel organ** that produces enamel. Mesenchyme proliferates into the **dental papilla** and **dental sac**. The dental papilla becomes the dentin and pulp tissue. The dental sac becomes the tooth's supporting structure of the periodontal ligament, alveolar bone, and cementum. During the cap stage, the successional dental lamina proliferate or bud off from the deciduous dentition to start forming the permanent dentition.

Dental anomalies of the cap stage would include dens in dente, fusion, gemination, or tubercles.

To remember which tooth structures are derived from which embryonic tissue, just remember that the endoderm is not involved in tooth structure at all. Tissues of the tooth are derived from the mesoderm and ectoderm. The mesoderm develops into the dental papilla (pulp and dentin) and dental sac (periodontal ligament, alveolar bone, and cementum). Then, remember that everything else of the tooth structure comes from the ectoderm.

The permanent molars are **NOT** succedaneous teeth.

Dental SAC = PAC =
Periodontal ligament,
Alveolar bone, Cementum

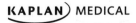

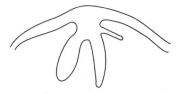

The stratum intermedium and stellate reticulum lie between the inner enamel epithelium and the outer enamel epithelium.

It is at the **bell stage** when the enamel organ, dental papilla, and dental sac differentiate more extensively into specific tissues of the tooth. The enamel organ determines the shape of the crown, and develops into the **outer enamel epithelium** that protects the enamel organ and inner enamel epithelium. The **inner enamel epithelium** is where the **ameloblasts** perform a secretory process (**Tomes' process**) that deposits enamel. The star-shaped **stellate reticulum's** function is to supply blood vessels to the enamel organ. The **stratum intermedium** also supplies vessels to the developing inner enamel epithelium.

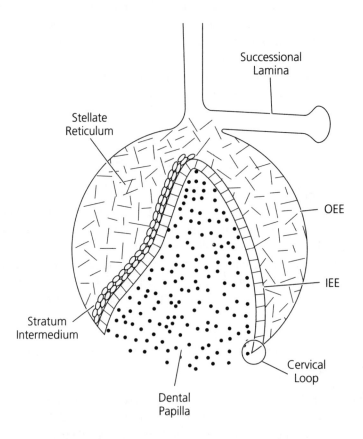

The outer enamel epithelium joins with the inner enamel epithelium to form the **cervical loop**, which then goes on to form Hertwig's sheath. **Hertwig's sheath** gives **shape** to the root of the tooth; then, it disintegrates into the **rests of Malassez** as the root formation reaches its full length.

Bell stage disturbances would include accessory roots, concresence, dilaceration, enamel pearls, and enamel dysplasia.

	Inorganic	Organic	Water
Enamel	95%	1%	4%
Dentin	70%	18%	12%
Cementum	65%	23%	12%
Bone	60%	25%	15%

Maturation

Maturation occurs as dental tooth structures reach their final stages of apposition. This occurs when ameloblasts, odontoblasts, and cementoblasts begin to lay down layers upon layers of each tooth structure: enamel, dentin, and cementum. The enamel organ determines the shape of the crown. The **inner enamel epithelium** elongates into **preameloblasts** and then **ameloblasts**, which then forms enamel by **amelogenesis**. Enamel and dentin originate in the same area but proliferate in opposing directions.

It takes 4 ameloblasts to form 1 enamel rod.

Microscopic Appearance of Teeth

Enamel rods microscopically have a **prism** appearance. **Perikymata** are grooves often located in the maxillary incisors that are associated with the lines of Retzius. The **lines of Retzius** are concentric imbrication lines on **enamel** surfaces—evidence of the deposition of successive layers of enamel matrix during apposition. Imbrication **lines of Von Ebner** are incremental lines found in **dentin** that correspond to the variations of apposition of dentin.

Enamel lamella is an organic defect that extends from the DEJ to the surface of the enamel. **Enamel tufts** also extend from the DEJ to approximately one-third of the thickness of the enamel lamella. This is thought to be a defect of mineralization. **Enamel spindles** are remnants of odontoblasts that cross prism boundaries a short distance into the enamel and are located in cusp tips.

Root Formation

After the crown is complete, the tooth starts to erupt into the oral cavity as the root forms. The cervical loop is the convergence of inner enamel epithelium (**IEE**) and outer enamel epithelium (**OEE**). The cervical loop then migrates deeper into the mesenchyme of the dental sac as it forms Hertwig's sheath. It is **Hertwig's sheath** that determines the **shape of the root** of a particular tooth. When root formation is complete, Hertwig's sheath disintegrates into the **rests of Malassez**. Occasionally, the rests of Malassez develop into a dentinal cyst.

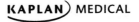

As a tooth erupts and enamel formation ceases, the outer enamel epithelium, the stratum intermedium, and the stellate reticulum combine to form the **reduced enamel epithelium** that covers the newly erupted tooth. This tissue becomes part of a membrane called **Nasmyth's membrane** that can sometimes stain green on newly erupted teeth.

The outer **dental papilla** forms odontoblasts that go on to produce **dentin**. The central cells of the dental papilla form the soft connective tissue of the **pulp** that supplies the blood vessels and nerve endings to the tooth.

The **dental sac** gives rise to the periodontal ligament that also gives rise to alveolar bone and the cementum. The **periodontal ligament** originates from the mesenchyme of the **dental sac** that differentiate into **fibroblasts** that proliferate collagen fibers. The fibers that are imbedded into the bone and cementum are called **Sharpey's fibers**.

The **cementum** is produced by **cementoblasts** derived from the dental sac or follicle after the crown of the tooth is formed. **Acellular cementum** is the first layer of cementum produced over the dentin. **Cellular cementum** is thickest at the apical third of the tooth and forms throughout life.

The **cementoenamel junction** can occur where the cementum slightly overlaps the enamel, or the two can meet edge to edge or cementum and enamel may just miss converging with each other allowing some dentin to be exposed.

Cementum is the tooth structure that most resembles bone.

Teeth are anchored into **alveolar bone proper** that is produced from **osteoblasts** derived form the mesenchyme of the dental sac. **Lamina dura** is a radiographic term for a **radiopaque line** that follows the shape of the root in the alveolar bone proper. Bone located between teeth is called **interdental bone**. Bone located between the roots of multi-rooted teeth is called **inter-radicular bone**.

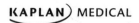

REVIEW QUESTIONS

1. Muscles of mastication are derived from which branchial arch?

   A. First branchial arch
   B. Second
   C. Third
   D. Fourth

2. When the endoplasmic reticulum modifies new protein, it send the new proteins to the

   A. Nucleolus
   B. Cytoplasm
   C. Centrioles
   D. Golgi complex
   E. Mitochondria

3. The urinary bladder is lined with which type of cells?

   A. Simple squamous
   B. Simple columnar
   C. Stratified cuboidal
   D. Transitional pseudostratified columnar
   E. Simple cuboidal

4. Some substances require energy to cross a cell membrane. Other substances give off energy when they cross the membrane. Which of the following terms indicates a movement that requires energy to move molecules across the membrane?

   A. Active transport
   B. Osmosis
   C. Facilitated diffusion
   D. Action potential
   E. Pinocytosis

5. Blood cells that aid in blood coagulation are

   A. Neutrophils
   B. Erythrocytes
   C. Leukocytes
   D. Eosinophils
   E. Thrombocytes

6. In compact bone, which of the following canals is the central vascular canal supplying osteons with nutrients?

   A. Lamellae
   B. Haversian canals
   C. Volkmann's canals
   D. Supraciliary canal
   E. Howship's lacuna

7. Which type of cartilage covers articulating surfaces of bone?

   A. Cricoid cartilage
   B. Elastic cartilage
   C. Fibrocartilage
   D. Hyaline cartilage

8. Hertwig's sheath determines the

   A. Shape of the crown
   B. Shape of the root
   C. Length of the root
   D. Size of the crown

9. Which of the flowing blood types is the Universal Donor?

   A. O
   B. A
   C. B
   D. AB

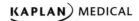

10. Which of the following structures connects epithelium to the basement membrane?

    A. Rete ridges
    B. Hemidesmosomes
    C. Lamina propria
    D. Stratum intermedium
    E. Prickle cells

11. At which week in utero do the tonsils develop from mesenchyme?

    A. 6
    B. 8
    C. 10
    D. 12
    E. 16

12. The human nucleus contains how many chromosomes?

    A. 23
    B. 36
    C. 46
    D. 48
    E. 52

13. Which of the following holds the master plan of the genetic code?

    A. Messenger RNA
    B. Transfer RNA
    C. Ribosomal RNA
    D. DNA

14. During which phase of cell replication do the mitotic spindles begin to align, so as to form a centromere before mitosis occurs?

    A. Prophase
    B. Metaphase
    C. Telophase
    D. Interphase
    E. Anaphase

15. Which of the following blood cells becomes a macrophage when it exits the capillaries?

    A. Neutrophil
    B. Leukocyte
    C. Mast cell
    D. Monocyte
    E. Plasma cell

16. When the root is completely formed, Hertwig's sheath disintegrates into what types of cells?

    A. Nasmyth's membrane
    B. Tomes' layer
    C. Rests of Mallassez
    D. Lines of Retzius
    E. Imbrication lines of von Ebner

17. Ameloblasts are derived from which of the following layers?

    A. Outer enamel epithelium
    B. Inner enamel epithelium
    C. Stratum intermedium
    D. Stellate reticullum

18. Which of the following cells is associated with humoral immunity?

    A. Lymphocytes
    B. B-cells
    C. T-cells
    D. Monocytes

19. Oral ectoderm gives rise to which of the following tissues?

    A. Enamel
    B. Bone
    C. Salivary glands
    D. Bronchioles
    E. Smooth muscle

20. Which of the following terms is associated with the concentric imbrication lines on the enamel surface—evidence of enamel deposition?

    A. Lines of vonEbner
    B. Lines of Retzius
    C. Perikamata
    D. Enamel lamellae

21. Which of the following is the main type of tissue in the body?

    A. Epithelial
    B. Muscle
    C. Bone
    D. Connective

22. Of the following blood cells, which has a nucleus that is segmented into multilobules and does not have a nucleolus?

    A. Erythrocytes
    B. Mast cells
    C. Eosinophils
    D. Basophils
    E. Neutrophils

23. Which of the following endocrine glands is the first to start developing in utero?

    A. Thalamus
    B. Adrenal
    C. Thyroid
    D. Pituitary
    E. Pancreas

24. If the medial nasal process and maxillary process fail to fuse, the result is

    A. Cleft lip
    B. Cleft palate
    C. Bifid tongue
    D. Cleft uvula

25. The greater cornu of the hyoid bone develops from which branchial arch?

    A. 1st
    B. 2nd
    C. 3rd
    D. 4th
    E. 5th

ANSWER EXPLANATIONS

1. A

The first branchial arch gives rise to the muscles of mastication.

B. The second branchial arch gives rise to the muscles of facial expression.

C. The third branchial arch gives rise to stylopharyngeal muscle.

D. The fourth branchial arch gives rise to the laryngeal cartilages and muscles of the pharynx & larynx.

2. D

The endoplasmic reticulum sends newly modified proteins to the Golgi complex.

A. The nucleus holds the master plan of the genetic code and controls the cell's function.

B. The cytoplasm also synthesizes proteins and transports nutrients

C. The centrioles take part in cell replcation

E. The mitochondria is the power house of the cell that oxidizes nutrients for use within the cell.

3. D

The urinary bladder is lined with transitional pseudostratified columnar epithelium.

A. Simple squamous epithelial cells lines respiratory tract, vascular system, Bowman's capsules.

B. Simple columnar epithelial cells lines stomach, small intestine, colon, gall bladder.

C. Stratified cuboidal epithelial cells are found in sweat glands, ducts, large ducts of exocrine glands.

E. Simple cuboidal lines the ovaries

4. A

Active transport utilizes energy to transport a substance into a cell against a concentration gradient.

B. Osmosis occurs with water moving across a semi-permeable membrane from an area of higher concentration to an area of lower concentration.

C. Facilitated diffusion or passive transport does not require energy to transport a substance across a cell membrane and releases it on the other side.

D. Action potential has to do with nerve cells conducting electrical current.

E. Pinocytosis is fluid movement into a cell

5. E

Blood clotting or coagulation is the result of thrombocytes (platelets) adhering to each other at an injury site.

A. Neutrophils or polymorphonuclear (PMN) are white blood cells that become phagocytes against invading antigens. They are the first line of defense in acute infections

B. Erythrocytes are red blood cells that lack a nucleus and transport oxygen to cells and carbon dioxide out of cells

C. Lymphocytes differentiate into T-cells and B-cells to fight off infections

D. Eosinophils release histamine during an allergic response

6. B

The central vascular canal that supplies osteons with nutrients are the haversian canals.

A. Lamellae are the sheets of bone matrix of the osteon.

C. Volkmann's canals are located at the exterior portion of bone that communicates with the haversian system.

D. Supraciliary canal is a small opening present near the supraorbital notch, which transmits a nutrient artery and a branch of the supraorbital nerve to the frontal sinus.

E. Howship's lacuna house osteoclasts that break down bone in resorption.

7. D

The type of cartilage that covers the articulating surfaces of bone is the hyaline cartilage or articular cartilage. It is the most abundant cartilage that covers the articulating surfaces of synovial joints of long bones. It is also found in the external ear, trachea, larynx, and costal areas of the ribs.

A. Cricoid cartilage is a specific cartilage found in the trachea

B. Elastic cartilage is a more opaque and flexible cartilage that is found in the external ear, parts of the larynx and the epiglottis.

C. Fibrocartilage has little intracellular substance that merges with hyaline cartilage to connect tendons and ligaments.

8. B

Hertwig's sheath determines the shape of the root.

A. Shape of the crown is determined in the bell stage.

C. Length of the root is a part of the shape of the root determined by Hertwig's sheath.

D. Size of the crown is determined in the bell stage.

9. A

Type O blood is the universal donor.

D. Type AB blood is the universal recipient.

10. B

Hemidesmosomes are a cellelular junction of cell to a non-cellular surface and attach the epithelium with the basal lamina.

A. Rete pegs is the layer of tissue that extends from the epithelium into connective tissue.

C. Lamina propria is highly vascular tissue under the basement membrane.

D. Stratum intermedium is one of two layers located between the inner enamel epithelium and the outer enamel epithelium.

E. Prickle cells are the superficial layer of the basal layer.

11. B

The tonsils start to develop at 8 weeks in utero.

12. C

Each human nucleus has 46 chromosomes.

13. D

The master plan containing the genetic code is found in DNA, which is located in the nucleus.

A. Messenger RNA transcribes (copies) small portions of DNA and is a template for protein synthesis.

B. Transfer RNA carries specific amino acids.

C. Ribosomal RNA can be free floating or attached to the endoplasmic reticulum.

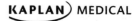

14. B

It is during the metaphase that chromosomes align at a mid point as the mitotic spindles form at the centromere or midpoint of the chromosomes.

A. Prophase chromatin coils or spiralizes and compresses into chromosomes, the nuclear membrane is lost, and the centrioles aid in the arrangement of the mitotic spindles as they migrate towards opposite poles.

C. Telophase is the last stage of mitosis when nuclear division is complete. Chromatids uncoil into two new nuclei surrounded by new nuclear membranes.

D. Interphase cell stage occurs between the cell division when the DNA replicates and centrioles get ready to start the process over again.

E. Anaphase occurs when the chromatids separate where they are joined at the centromeres.

15. D

Monocytes become large macrophages when they leave the capillaries. They are involved in chronic inflammation and take longer to get to a site of infection than neutrophils.

A. Neutrophils or polymorphonuclearcytes (PMN) perform phagocytosis of invading pathogens when injuries occur. Neutrophils are also involved with acute inflammation.

B. Lymphocytes enter into circulation, where about half journey to the thymus to mature into T cells or T lymphocytes. Other leukocytes mature in the bone marrow as B cells or B leukocytes.

C. Mast cells are not seen in normal circulation but appear when an antigen enters the body. They release histamine depending on the severity of the reaction.

E. Plasma cells are involved with humoral immune responses

16. C

Hertwig's sheath disintegrates into the Rests of Malassez.

A. Nasmyth's membrane is formed by the remnants of the enamel cuticle and reduced enamel epithelium that covers a newly erupted tooth. It can stain green.

B. Tomes' layer is inner enamel epithelium when ameloblasts perform a secretory process of depositing enamel.

D. Lines of Retzius are imbrication lines that are in the enamel of anterior teeth.

E. Imbrication lines of von Ebner are imbrication lines in the dentin

17. B

Ameloblasts are derived from the inner enamel epithelium.

A. Outer enamel epithelium is a protective barrier for tooth formation.

C. Stratum intermedium lies between the stellate reticulum and inner enamel epithelium.

D. Stellate reticullum consists of star shaped cells that lies between the outer enamel epithelium and stratum intermedium.

18. B

Humoral immunity is associated with the B-cells that release antibodies against pathogens

A. Lymphocytes become B-cells (matured in bone marrow) and also T-cells (matured in the thymus) for immunity.

C. T-cells are involved in cell-mediated immunity responding to specific antigens.

D. Monocytes become macrophages that perform phagocytosis.

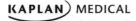

19. A

Oral ectoderm produces enamel from the neural crest cells.

B. Bone is a connective tissue that arises from cartilage. It is also derived from mesenchyme but not from oral mesenchyme.

C. Salivary glands are derived from epithelial proliferations.

D. Brochioles are derived from endodermal tissue that becomes endothelium.

20. B

The concentric imbrication lines on the enamel surface are the lines of Retzius.

A. Lines of vonEbner are imbrication lines in the dentin.

C. Perikamata are grooves associated with the lines of Retzius.

D. Enamel lamellae are organic defects that extend from the DEJ to the surface of the enamel.

21. D

Connective tissue is the most abundant tissue by weight in the body. Collagen is the most abundant fiber.

22. E

Neutrophils are blood cells with a segmented multilobulated nucleus.

A. Erythrocytes have no nucleus.

B. Mast cells have irregularly shaped double lobulated nucleii.

C. Eosinophils have two lobes in their nucleus.

D. Basophils have a double-lobulated irregular nucleus.

23. C

The thyroid gland starts at 4 weeks in embryo in the foramen cecum of the tongue. It descends into the area of 2nd and 3rd tracheal cartilage at the 7th week, leaving a depression in the tongue.

A. Thalamus gland starts at about week 5.

B. Adrenal gland starts at about week 6.

D. Pituitary gland starts at week 6.

E. Pancreas starts at week 10.

24. A

If the medial nasal process and maxialIary process fail to fuse, cleft lip results at 4–7 weeks in embryo.

B. Cleft palate occurs at 8–12 weeks, when the palatal shelves fail together or fuse with the posterior portion of the primary palate.

C. Bifid tongue occurs as an improper fusion of the lateral lingual swellings.

D. Cleft uvula is the result of the soft palate, not fusing.

25. C

The greater cornu develops from the 3rd branchial arch.

A. 1st branchial arch gives rise to the sphenoid bone and ear structures.

B. 2nd branchial arch gives rise to middle ear structures stylohyoid process of temporal bone, lesser cornu of the hyoid bone as well as the upper potion of the hyoid bone.

D. 4th branchial arch give rise to the laryngeal cartilages.

E. 5th and 6th branchial arch give rise to the laryngeal cartilage as well

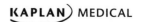

Chapter Three: **General Anatomy**

The oral cavity is part of the digestive system, one of many organ systems in our bodies. Because these organ systems are interconnected and reliant on each other, the dental hygienist must have a solid understanding of these areas.

DIGESTIVE SYSTEM

The digestive system provides the body with nutrients, water, and electrolytes needed for cell life. **Starch digestion begins in the mouth**, by the enzyme salivary **amylase**. When food is swallowed, the **hyoid bone** moves **upward**, and the **larynx elevates**. The hyoid bone is a U-shaped bone that supports the tongue.

Food passes through the digestive tract by way of the pharynx, then by **peristalsis** down the esophagus and into the stomach through the cardiac sphincter. The stomach contains parietal cells that produce hydrochloric acid; this acid kills microorganisms and creates ideal conditions for protein digestion. It also contains goblet cells—surface mucous cells—which produce mucous to protect the stomach lining from the hydrochloric acid. Chief cells in the stomach produce pepsinogen for protein digestion.

Intrinsic factor, which is a **protein** in the stomach, aids in the absorption of **Vitamin B12.**

Alcoholics lack intrinsic factor to absorb vitamin B12, and are susceptible to pernicious anemia.

The only thing absorbed by the stomach is water, a few ions, and some drugs. The main function of the stomach is to liquefy food into chyme, which is a semi-solid. Enzymes in the stomach that help food to digest are **pepsinogen**, which is converted into pepsin by hydrochloric acid. Pepsin, in turn, splits proteins into more absorptive peptides.

Gastric lipase hydrolyzes fatty acids from triglycerides. There are **no starch digestive** enzymes in the stomach. Chyme first leaves the stomach by way of the **pyloric sphincter** (preventing back-flow from the intestine), and then enters the small intestine, which consists of the duodenum, jejunum, ileum, and cecum. Peristalsis moves the food along in the **small intestine**, where **pancreatic amylase, sucrase, lactase,** and **maltase** help in starch digestion. **Trypsin** hydrolyzes proteins into polypeptides. **Pancreatic lipase** hydrolyzes fatty acids from triglycerides. Lecithinase hydrolyzes lecithin into fatty acids and monoglycerides.

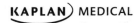

Chyme is absorbed into the capillary network by the villi and microvilli of the small intestine. Here, villi act as valves to allow solids, liquids, and/or acids to pass into the bloodstream and onto the liver by way of the hepatic portal vein. In the large intestine, water, electrolytes, and vitamins are absorbed. Any **Vitamin K** that is **absorbed** by the bacterial flora goes to the liver to produce prothrombin, necessary for blood clotting.

With the **exception of the veins from the small intestines,** all veins go directly back to the heart by way of the superior or inferior vena cava. The intestinal veins drain directly into the hepatic portal vein, then to a second set of capillary beds into the **liver**. This is where monosaccharides are converted into glycogen in the liver. Amino acids may be sent into general circulation or enter into cellular respiration, to be oxidized as energy with urea waste product. Many other things, as well, are detoxified in the liver, such as ingested drugs or toxins.

An accessory organ of the digestive system is the **liver**. It is the body's **largest visceral organ**. Blood goes into the liver through the hepatic artery, and is carried away by the hepatic portal vein (where veins from the small intestine join in the liver).

The liver has many other functions, including the production of **prothrombin from vitamin K**, storage of iron, and phagocytosis of old blood cells. The **bile** it produces contains amphiphilic acids, which emulsify fats. The negatively-charged portion of the hydrophobic steroid interacts with water molecules to help them repulse each other. **Bilirubin** is the breakdown of hemoglobin in red blood cells by the liver. If the bilirubin cannot be broken down in the liver and builds up in the bloodstream instead, the patient becomes jaundiced.

Bile from the liver travels to the gallbladder for storage and concentration. Then, with the **sphincter of Oddi** controlling the flow of bile out of the gallbladder, its duct joins with the pancreatic duct (**duct of Wirsung**) into the small intestine.

The digestive system is governed by both the sympathetic and the parasympathetic nervous systems. The **parasympathetic** nervous system is the vegetative stage that we live in most of the time and that governs the digestive system during that time. The **sympathetic** nervous system inhibits digestive activity during stressful situations, to shunt blood back to the heart, muscles, and brain.

SKELETAL SYSTEM

The skeletal system contains bone and cartilage that both support and protect the body. Bone and cartilage are connective tissues and are derived from the mesenchyme. The types of bone in the human body are:

- long bones (such as the femur and humerus)
- short bones (such as the carpals and tarsals)
- flat bones (such as the scapula and cranial bones)
- irregular bones (such as the vertebrae)

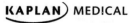

Long bones have an **epiphysis** at either end, and a **diaphysis** which surrounds each medullary cavity. They also have a **metaphysis** area lying between them. The epiphysis is covered by articular cartilage. The **periosteum** surrounds and protects bone.

Tendons attach bones to muscle. **Ligaments** attach bone to bone. Synovial fluid allows joints to work by hinge movement, ball and socket motion, gliding, pivoting, and saddle motion.

The skeleton contains both the axial and appendicular skeletal systems, which comprise **206 bones**. The **axial** skeletal system is comprised of the skull, spinal column, sternum, and ribs. The spinal column contains the cervical (7), thoracic (12), lumbar (5), sacral (5), and coccygeal (4-5) vertebrae. The first vertebrae of the cervical spine is the **atlas**, which allows for **up-and-down** motion of the head. The second cervical vertebra is the **axis**, which houses the **dens** for **side-to-side** or pivotal movement.

The **appendicular** skeletal system consists of the upper and lower extremities. The upper extremities include the shoulders, scapulae, clavicles, humeri, radii, ulnae, carpals (8), metacarpals (5), and phalanges (14). The lower extremities include the hips (pelvic girdle), femurs, patellas, tibias, fibulas, tarsals (7), metatarsals (5), and phalanges (14).

ENDOCRINE SYSTEM

The **endocrine system** contains glands that are **ductless** and that produce hormones that help to maintain the body's homeostasis. It is also involved in the body's immune system.

Another accessory organ of the digestive system is the pancreas. It has the unique distinction of containing both **endocrine** and **exocrine** function. The **endocrine** portion of the pancreas contains the Isles of Langerhans, which consist of 500,000–1,000,000 islets. The islets have **alpha** cells that produce **glucagon**, as well as **beta** cells that produce **insulin**.

Glucagon plays an important role at times when glucose in blood—needed for cells to survive—becomes too low. The **glucagon changes the glycogen**, stored in the **liver** to glucose to be utilized by cells to maintain life. **Insulin** plays a crucial role in allowing glucose to enter the cells.

Alpha cells in the pancreas produce glucagon. Glucagon goes after the glycogen, stored in the liver, if glucose in the blood gets too low. Cells need glucose to live.

As part of the digestive system, the **exocrine** portion of the pancreas produces a pancreatic fluid, made up of:

- Sodium bicarbonate (to neutralize pH)
- Pancreatic lipase (to hydrolyze fats into fatty acids and monoglycerides)
- Pancreatic amylase (to hydrolyze starches into maltose)
- Proteases (to digest proteins)

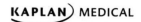

Proteases include **trypsin** that renders peptide bonds into arginine and lysine; chymotrypsin that renders peptide bonds into phenylalanine, tryptophan, & tyrosine; and carboxypeptidase, which removes amino acids from the C-terminal of peptides. Proteases are potent enzymes and are stored in their inactive forms. Enterokinase activates the potent trypsinogen, while trypsin activates chymotrypsinogen and some trypsinogen.

The **largest lymphoid organ** is the **spleen**, whose job is to filter out old red blood cells. Humans can survive without their spleen if needed, since the liver can perform this same job.

The **thymus**—responsible for part of immune response—is located beneath the sternum and cannot be palpated. It is divided into two parts: the outer cortex and the inner medulla. The **medulla** is involved in cell-mediated responses by **developing immature lymphocytes** into **immunocompetent T cells**. It is most active in childhood and atrophies with age.

Antipyretic pharmaceuticals take effect on body temperature in the hypothalamus.

The **hypothalamus** regulates our body's homeostasis. Specifically, it produces the hormones **oxytocin** (for uterus contraction) and **antidiuretic hormone** (ADH) that allows for reabsorption of water back into the bloodstream. These hormones are sent to the posterior pituitary. It also regulates body temperature, the circulatory system, electrolytes, and urine formation. This is where antipyretics in pharmacological medications take effect.

The **pituitary gland,** the **master gland,** lies beneath the hypothalamus and works in conjunction with the hypothalamus. It secretes growth hormone (somatotropin); adrenocorticotropic hormone (ACTH) which activates the adrenal cortex; thyroid stimulating hormone (TSH) all from the anterior pituitary; oxytocin; and antidiuretic hormone (ADH) from the posterior.

The **thyroid gland** regulates the physiological functions of the body; it is a bi-lobed organ located on both sides of the trachea, connected by an isthmus. It secretes **thyroxine** and triiodothyronine, which control the body's metabolism by increasing the activity of mitochondria in cells. It also produces **calcitonin**, which participates in calcium and phosphorus metabolism. The **parathyroid** gland contains four ductless glands; it produces parathyroid hormone (PTH) which increases the calcium ion concentration in blood. Calcium is necessary for nerve conduction and muscle contraction. Both calcium and phosphorus are necessary for bone and tooth formation.

Testosterone, the sex hormone in males from the testes, helps to produce mature male characteristics. Estrogen, in females from the ovaries, produces mature female characteristics, and the hormone progesterone thickens the uterine lining to prepare for pregnancy.

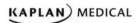

RENAL SYSTEM

The **renal system** plays an important role in the filtration of blood and also in the maintenance of the body's pH-balance. The renal fascia and adipose capsule surround and protect the kidney. The outer portion is the cortex, which covers the medulla. The cortex contains renal columns that separate the medulla, which contains the renal or medullary pyramids. Within the medullary pyramids are the cortical (85%) and juxtamedullary (15%) nephrons or functional portion of the kidney.

The **nephrons** are composed of the glomerulus, which is surrounded by **Bowman's capsule**. It is the **glomerulus** that does the actual filtration. The tubules exiting the glomerulus where plasma is filtered are called the proximal and distal tubules, and **loop of Henle**. It is there that minerals are secreted and then reabsorbed.

Loop diuretics of pharmacology take effect in the glomerulus in the Loop of Henle.

The glomerulus and loop of Henle are where nutrients and electrolytes pass in and out. The **loop of Henle** has both a descending and ascending convoluted tubule where the actual filtration takes place. Here, molecules can pass back and forth between the blood vessels and the convoluted tubules.

Loop diuretics that a patient may be taking have a pharmacologic effect in the loop of Henle. Water has a strong affinity toward sodium. In the loop of Henle, the loop diuretic drug "kicks out" the sodium and does not allow it to pass back into circulation. Water follows the sodium out of circulation and into the urine, for a concentrated salty urine.

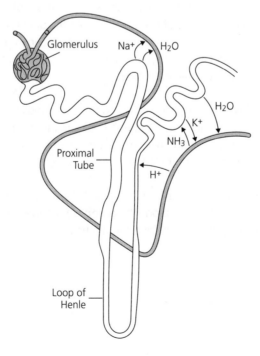

The Glomerulus

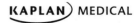

CIRCULATORY SYSTEM

The circulatory system maintains homeostasis by supplying nutrients to cells and by transporting waste away. The hemoglobin in red blood cells also provides oxygen to cells and transports CO_2 back to the lungs.

The heart starts beating in utero at **22 days**. In utero, there is an opening between the two atria called the **fossa ovalis**, since at that point, the lungs do not oxygenate the blood. Heart muscle is very specialized and has the ability to conduct electricity in an organized way. It is **involuntary, striated muscle** and myocardial cells that join together by **intercalated discs**.

A **pericardial sac** surrounds the heart to protect and lubricate it. The outer heart layer of muscle is the **epicardium**, which is continuous with the **myocardium**. The myocardium makes up the majority of the heart muscle. The innermost lining of the heart muscle is the **endocardium**.

Dental hygienists need to be aware of inflammations of the heart muscle. Pericarditis is an inflammation of the pericardial sac, while myocarditis is an inflammation of the myocardial muscle. In dentistry, patients at risk for the bacterial infection **endocarditis** must be premedicated with an antibiotic.

Arteries always carry oxygenated blood, with one exception: pulmonary arteries. Pulmonary arteries carry *de*oxygenated blood to the lungs.

Blood returns from systemic circulation to the heart by way of the **inferior vena cava** (from the lower portion of the body) and the **superior vena cava** (from the upper portion of the body). It then travels to the **right atrium** and passes through the **tricuspid valve** into the right ventricle. Finally, the blood passes through the **pulmonic valve** into the **pulmonary arteries**, which carry it to the lungs to drop off carbon dioxide and absorb oxygen. This is the only time in the circulatory system when arteries carry deoxygenated blood.

Veins always carry *de*oxygenated blood, with one exception: pulmonary veins. Pulmonary veins carry oxygenated blood from the lungs.

Pulmonary veins return oxygenated blood from the lungs to the **left atrium**. The blood passes from the left atrium through the **bicuspid** or **mitral valve** into the **left ventricle**. This part of the heart has a greater amount of heart muscle so that blood can be pumped out to the body.

Blood passes out of the left ventricle, through the **aortic valve** and into the aorta, and then to arteries into circulation. The **coronary arteries** branch off from the aorta and carry oxygen-enriched blood to the heart muscle.

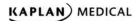

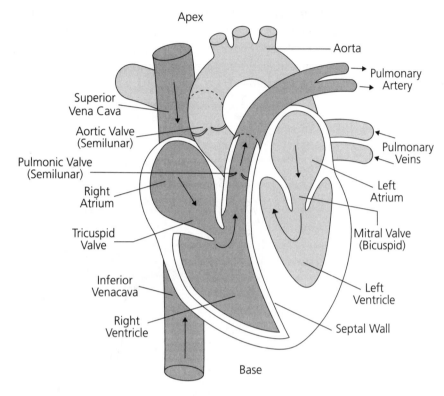

Apex

Aorta

Pulmonary Artery

Superior Vena Cava

Aortic Valve (Semilunar)

Pulmonic Valve (Semilunar)

Right Atrium

Tricuspid Valve

Inferior Venacava

Right Ventricle

Pulmonary Veins

Left Atrium

Mitral Valve (Bicuspid)

Left Ventricle

Septal Wall

Base

The Heart

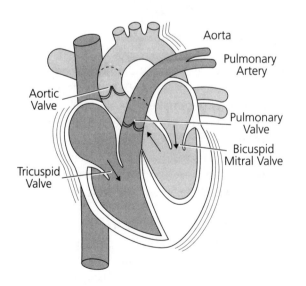

Aorta

Pulmonary Artery

Aortic Valve

Pulmonary Valve

Tricuspid Valve

Bicuspid Mitral Valve

The Heart Valves at Rest

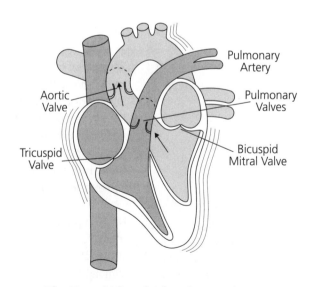

Pulmonary Artery

Aortic Valve

Pulmonary Valves

Tricuspid Valve

Bicuspid Mitral Valve

The Heart Valves During Contraction

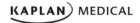

There are **four valves** in the heart. If the tricuspid and bicuspid valves are open at the same time, then the two valves exiting the heart—the aortic and pulmonic valves—will be closed at the same time. And vice versa: If the tricuspid and bicuspid valves are both closed, the aortic and pulmonic valves that exit the heart will both be open at the same time.

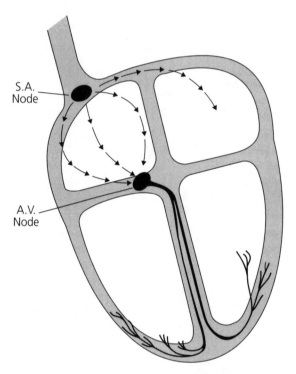

S.A.
Node

A.V.
Node

The Heart's Natural Pacemaker

The heart muscle is involuntary striated muscle that has the ability to conduct electricity. The actual beating of the heart begins at a rate of 60–100 beats per minute at the **sinoatrial node**, the body's **natural pacemaker**. The electrical current then travels down to the **atrioventricular** node, which, in the event that the SA node gets knocked out, can also conduct electricity to the heart muscle (though at a slower rate of 40–60 beats per minute). The electrical current is then transmitted to the **bundle of His,** which divides off into the left and right bundle branches. The current then travels to the **Purkinje fibers** at the apex of the heart.

Bradycardia is when the heart is beating at less than 60 beats per minute. Tachycardia is when it is beating faster than 100 beats per minute.

Nerve impulses for the electrical stimulation of the heart are transmitted by the **medulla oblongata** down the vagus nerve to the heart. Sympathetic nervous-system stimulation increases the heart rate, while parasympathetic nervous-system stimulation will decrease the heart rate. The heart is governed most of the time by the parasympathetic nervous system.

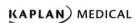

RESPIRATORY SYSTEM

The respiratory system consists of the upper and lower respiratory tracts along with the lungs. The **upper respiratory tract** contains the **nose, pharynx,** and **larynx,** which contains the vocal cords. The **lower respiratory tract** consists of the **trachea, bronchi, bronchioles,** and **alveoli.** The trachea is housed by hyaline cartilage, which contains goblet cells that produce mucous, which traps inhaled substances. The left and right bronchi split at the carina. Air then enters into each bronchial tree and branches out into smaller alveoli. There, carbon dioxide is eliminated and oxygen is taken in for cells to survive.

NERVOUS SYSTEM

The main function of the nervous system is to control and coordinate function by maintaining **homeostasis,** along with the endocrine system. The nervous system is the messenger system that sends communications out from the central nervous system to the peripheral nervous system for all body functions. Sensory nerves transmit information back to the brain via the spinal cord, and the brain can also transmit messages back out to the muscles for movement.

The **central nervous system** consists of the brain and spinal cord. The largest portion of the brain contains the cerebrum, which contains gray matter and is responsible for conscious thought. The **cerebellum,** the second largest portion, is responsible for coordination of muscle movement. The **diencephalon** is located between the cerebral hemispheres and midbrain. It surrounds the thalamus and the hypothalamus, which also play an important role in the body's homeostasis.

The brain stem, containing the **medulla oblongata, midbrain,** and **pons,** is located between the diencephalons and the spinal cord. The **medulla** regulates the **respiratory system** and **circulatory system.** The **pons** relays messages from the cerebrum to the cerebellum, and contains the body's sleep center. In addition, the pons regulates breathing along with the medulla. The midbrain is involved in audio and visual pathways.

The **peripheral nervous system** consists of **12** pairs of **cranial nerves** and **31** pairs of **spinal nerves** which, together, control the autonomic and the somatic nervous systems. Our somatic nervous system controls our muscles and dermatomes, but it also reacts to the changes of our external environment. The 31 pairs of spinal nerves have a dorsal root and ventral root: the **dorsal root** carries **sensory** sensations and is **afferent,** while the **ventral** root conveys **motor** function and is **efferent.**

Sensory = Dorsal
Afferent = Dorsal
Motor = Ventral
Efferent = Ventral

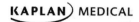

The autonomic nervous system contains the sympathetic and the parasympathetic nervous systems that oversee the body's involuntary systems. In an emergency or stressful situation, the **sympathetic** nervous system produces our **fight-or-flight** reaction: It releases **norepinephrine** over the synapses and will increase heart rate, raise blood pressure, and shunt blood away from the digestive tract. The **parasympathetic** nervous system, in contrast, maintains our **vegetative** state; it counteracts the sympathetic nervous system to restore and conserve energy. Using **acetylcholine** as a neurotransmitter over the synapses, it decreases the heart rate, returns blood pressure to normal, returns the digestive system back to normal function, and responds to our functional needs.

> Our bodies circulate acetycholine most of the time, since we live mostly in a vegetative state.

Nerve fibers exiting the spinal cord recombine to form nerve plexuses that then travel to a specific body part. These nerves convey motor, proprioceptive, and sensory impulses. Nerve cells—**neurons**—contain a nucleus, dendrites, and axons that convey nerve impulses between other neuron cells. **Dendrites** within the neuron have branching fibers that extend out from the cell body to receive incoming impulses. **Axons** are single and long, with fibers thicker than dendrites; they carry the impulse away from the cell body to other neurons.

> Dendrites receive information. Axons carry information away.

The axon is protected by an insulating myelin sheath composed of a fatty layer. **Synapses** are the tiny spaces between dendrites of one neuron and the axon of another neuron. This is where chemical neurotransmitters communicate to excite the next neuron. The most common neurotransmitters are acetylcholine, norepinephrine, and dopamine.

Cranial Nerves

#	Cranial Nerve		Function	Foramen
I	Olfactory	Afferent	Sensation smell impulses from nasal mucosa	Cribiform plate of ethmoid
II	Optic	Afferent	Sensation visual impulse from retina	Optic canal of sphenoid
III	Oculomotor	Efferent	Motor eye muscle contraction	Superior orbital fissure of sphenoid
IV	Trochlear	Efferent	Motor eye superior oblique muscle	Superior orbital fissure of sphenoid
V1	Trigeminal Ophthalmic			Superior orbital fissure of sphenoid
	Frontal nerve	Afferent	Sensation scalp & forehead	Supraorbital foramen of sphenoid
	Lacrimal nerve	Afferent	Sensation lacrimal glands & eyelid	
	Nasociliary nerve	Afferent	Sensation nose & nasal mucosa	
V2	Trigeminal Maxillary			Foramen rotundum of sphenoid
	Infraorbital	Afferent	Sensation upper lip, cheek, & eyelid	Infraorbital foramen
	Anterior superior alveolar	Afferent	Sensation pulp & tissue maxillary anteriors	Infraorbital canal joins infraorbital nerve
	Middle superior alveolar	Afferent	Sensation pulp & tissue maxillary premolars & MB root of 1st molar	Infraorbital canal joins infraorbital nerve
	Posterior superior alveolar	Afferent	Sensation pulp & tissue of maxillary molars except MB root of 1st molar	Posterosuperior alveolar foramina
	Greater palatine	Afferent	Sensation hard palate	Greater palatine foramina
	Lesser palatine	Afferent	Sensation soft palate and palatine tonsils	Lesser palatine foramina
	Nasopalatine	Afferent	Sensation anterior hard palate & linguals of maxillary anteriors	Incisive foramen
	Zygomatic	Afferent	Sensation cheek and temple	
V3	Trigeminal Mandibular			Foramen ovale of sphenoid
	Auriculotemporal	Afferent	Sensation ear and scalp	
	Buccal	Afferent	Sensation bucccal mucosa & gingiva, cheek	
	Inferior alveolar	Afferent	Sensation pulp & tissue all mandibular teeth	
	Lingual	Afferent	Sensation anterior $\frac{2}{3}$ of tongue, mouth floor, lingual mand. gingiva	
	Motor muscular branches	Efferent	Motor muscles of mastication	
	Mylohyoid	Efferent	Motor muscles of mastication	Foramen ovale of sphenoid
VI	Abducens	Efferent	Motor lateral eyeball muscle	Superior orbital fissure of sphenoid
VII	Facial			Internal acoustic meatus of temporal
	Chorda tympani	Afferent	Sensation taste anterior $\frac{2}{3}$ of tongue	
	Facial	Efferent	Motor muscles of facial expression	
	Greater petrosal	Efferent	Motor muscles lacrimal gland, nasal cavity, hard & soft palates	
	Greater petrosal	Afferent	Sensation taste palate	
VIII	Vestibulocochlear	Afferent	Sensation hearing and balance	Internal acoustic meatus of temporal
IX	Glossopharyngeal	Afferent	Sensation taste posterior $\frac{1}{3}$ tongue, pharynx, tonsils	Jugular foramen between occipital & temporal
	Glossopharyngeal	Efferent	Motor muscles stylopharyngeus (swallowing)	Jugular foramen between occipital & temporal
X	Vagus	Afferent	Sensation ear, epiglottis	
	Vagus	Efferent	Motor muscles soft palate, larynx, pharynx	
XI	Accessory Nerve	Efferent	Motor muscles trapezius, sternocleidomastoid, soft palate, pharynx	Jugular foramen between occipital & temporal
XII	Hypoglossal	Efferent	Motor muscles intrinsic and extrinsic tongue	Hypoglossal canal of occipital

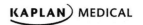

REVIEW QUESTIONS

1. There are 12 pairs of spinal nerves in all. Each has a dorsal efferent root and a ventral afferent root.

   A. Statement one is true. Statement two is false.
   B. Statement one is false. Statement two is true.
   C. Both statements are true.
   D. Both statements are false.

2. A trapezoid-shaped bone forming the lower part of the nasal septum is called

   A. Occipital
   B. Xiphoid process
   C. Zygomatic process
   D. Vomer
   E. Sphenoid

3. Humans possess the ability to move in different ways and directions. Which of the following vertebra articulates with condyles of the occipital bone for movement?

   A. C1
   B. C2
   C. C3
   D. Sacral vertebra
   E. Coccygeal vertebra

4. The heart contains valves to prevent backflow so that blood can keep moving forward. Which of the following valves prevent backflow of deoxygenated blood?

   A. Pulmonary and aortic valves
   B. Pulmonary and right atrioventricular valves
   C. Right and left atrioventricular valves
   D. Aortic and left atrioventricular valves

5. Which of the following cells secretes hydrochloric acid?

   A. Goblet
   B. Stem
   C. Chief
   D. Acinus
   E. Parietal

6. Which cells line the blood vessels of the body?

   A. Stratified squamous epithelium
   B. Pseudostratified epithelium
   C. Simple squamous
   D. Transitional epithelium
   E. Stratified cuboidal

7. Cartilage cells are replaced by osteoblasts in long bones as the organic matrix is calcified. As calcium and phosphate are deposited, this process is known as

   A. Intramembranous ossification
   B. Endochondral ossification
   C. Appositional growth
   D. Osteon
   E. Interstitial growth

8. Actin and myosin are proteins contained within

   A. Fascicles
   B. Copula
   C. Myofibril
   D. Sarcoplasmic reticulum
   E. Endomysium

9. Stomach contents usually have a pH of

   A.   0

   B.   1

   C.   7

   D.   14

10. Which area of the brain controls respiration and cardiovascular function?

   A.   Brain stem

   B.   Medulla

   C.   Cerebellum

   D.   Cerebrum

   E.   Hindbrain

11. The autonomic nervous system controls

   A.   Smooth muscle

   B.   Respiration

   C.   Cardiac muscle

   D.   All of the above

12. All of the following terms are associated with haversian systems in bone EXCEPT

   A.   Osteons

   B.   Canaliculi

   C.   Volkman's canals

   D.   Lamellae

   E.   Perichondrium

13. Antidiuretics such as furosemide eliminate water from the body. This takes place in

   A.   Bowman's capsule

   B.   Calyces

   C.   Loop of Henle

   D.   Nephron

14. Which of the following enzymes hydrolyzes polysaccharides?

   A.   Amylase

   B.   Lipase

   C.   Protease

   D.   Pepsin

15. Blood pressure is lowest in which of the following blood vessels of the cardiovascular system?

   A.   Arteries

   B.   Arterioles

   C.   Capillaries

   D.   Venules

   E.   Veins

16. Prothrombin is necessary for blood clotting. Which of the following organs is responsible for the production of prothrombin?

   A.   Pancreas

   B.   Liver

   C.   Spleen

   D.   Glomerulus

   E.   Hypothalamus

17. If the natural pacemaker of the heart should not function properly, which of the following nodes would take over?

   A.   Sinoatrial node

   B.   Atrioventricular node

   C.   Bundle of His

   D.   Purkinje fibers

18. Insulin, a critically important hormone, is produced in the pancreas by

   A.   Kupffer cells

   B.   Alpha cells

   C.   Beta cells

   D.   Islets of Langerhans

   E.   Bowman's capsules

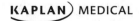

19. Intrinsic factor is important for B$_{12}$ Vitamin absorption. Which of the following organs contains intrinsic factor for this absorption?

    A. Spleen
    B. Liver
    C. Pancreas
    D. Stomach
    E. Thalamus

20. Most of the time, humans live in a vegetative state (as opposed to a flight-or-fight state). Which of the following neurotransmitters acts mostly to maintain our vegetative state?

    A. Acetylcholine
    B. Norepinepherine
    C. Catecholamine
    D. Dopamine
    E. Serotonin

21. Valves in our digestive system prevent backflow during food digestion. Pyloric stenosis restricts the flow of food from entering the

    A. Esophagus
    B. Stomach
    C. Small intestine
    D. Large intestine

22. When a woman has hot flashes during pregnancy and menopause, which of the following endocrine glands is involved?

    A. Thalamus
    B. Hypothalamus
    C. Thyroid
    D. Parathyroid
    E. Adrenal

23. Should a person's blood-sugar level drop, the body can seek out the liver's storage of

    A. Glucose
    B. Glucagon
    C. Glycogen
    D. Glucan

24. If an alcoholic has cirrhosis, which of the following body organs is affected?

    A. Spleen
    B. Kidneys
    C. Adrenal glands
    D. Liver
    E. Lungs

25. Which of the following defines the body's ability to maintain a stable state?

    A. Homeopathy
    B. Homeothermic
    C. Homeostasis
    D. Homogenous

ANSWER EXPLANATIONS

1. D

Statement 1 is false since there are 12 cranial nerves but 31 spinal nerves. Statement 2 is also false since sensory and afferent are the dorsal root. The motor and efferent are the ventral root. SAME: SA = Dorsal, ME = Ventral.

2. D

A single trapezoid midline bone that forms the posterior part of the nasal septum is the vomer bone.

A. Occipital is a single bone at the back of the skull.

B. Xiphoid is the protuberance at the end of the sternum.

C. Zygomatic process occurs when paired bones join with each other and to the hard palate. They form the cheekbones.

E. Sphenoid bone is a single bone that articulates with the ethmoid, frontal temporal, parietal, vomer, palatal, maxillary, and occipital bones.

3. A

C1 (cervical-1) is the vertebra that articulates with the condyles of the occipital bone for up-and-down movement at the atlas.

B. C2 articulates with C1 ring at the dens for side-to-side movement at the axis.

C. C2–3 have intervertebral discs that can deform during flexion and extension.

D. There are five sacral bones in the lower back.

E. There are four fused coccygeal bones at the end of the spine.

4. B

The heart valves that prevent backflow of deoxygenated blood are the pulmonary valve, which goes from the right ventricle to the lungs, and the right AV valve, which lies between the right atrium and the right ventricle.

A. The pulmonary valve transports deoxygenated blood from the right ventricle to the lungs; the aortic valve transports oxygenated blood from the left ventricle out to the body.

C. The right atrium transports deoxygenated blood through the right AV valve (tricuspid) to the right ventricle; the left atrium transports oxygenated blood through the left AV valve (bicuspid) to the left ventricle.

D. The aortic valve transports oxygenated blood to the body from the left ventricle; the left AV valve (bicuspid) transports oxygenated blood from left atrium to the left ventricle.

5. E

Hydrochloric acid is produced by the parietal cells in the stomach.

A. Goblet cells secrete mucous.

B. Stem cells are used in research.

C. Chief cells secrete pepsinogen enzyme which digests protein.

D. Acinus cells located in the saliva glands secrete saliva.

6. C

The endothelium of blood vessels is composed of simple squamous cells.

A. Stratified squamous epithelium consists of two or more layers and is found in superficial skin and the oral mucosa.

B. Pseudostratified epithelium lines the upper respiratory tract including the trachea and nasal cavity.

D. Transitional epithelium is found in the bladder.

E. Stratified cuboidal epithelium is found in sweat glands, ducts, and large ducts of exocrine glands.

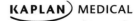

7. **B**

The process by which long bones form is called endochondral ossification. Osteoid-replacing cartilage allows the bones to lengthen.

A. Intramembranous ossification is the formation of small fragments of bone by osteoblasts that eventually coalesce into larger pieces of bone. This occurs in the maxilla and mandible.

C. Appositional growth is a part of intramembranous ossification growth that occurs in layers to the outer tissue mass.

D. Osteons are concentric circles of tightly apposed sheets of bone tissue.

E. Interstitial growth occurs as the initial stage of endochondral ossification when cartilage forms the shape of the bone.

8. **C**

Actin and myosin are protein filaments found in myofibrils.

A. Fascicles are numerous bundles of striated muscle.

B. Copula are the two swellings of the third and fourth branchial arches that form a portion of the base of the tongue.

D. Sarcoplasmic reticulum stores calcium necessary for muscle contraction.

E. Endomysium is the sheath that covers the myofibrils.

9. **B**

The stomach's pH is 1 since it is in the range of strong acid.

C. 7 is a neutral pH.

D. 14 is an alkaline pH, and the stomach contains hydrochloric acid.

10. **A**

The area of the brain that controls respiration and cardiovascular function is the pons. The brain stem contains the medulla oblongata, pons, and midbrain.

B. The medulla also regulates the cardiac/respiratory center but it relays the message from the brain stem to the spinal cord.

C. The cerebellum is the center for motor coordination.

D. The cerebrum is the center for conscious thought.

E. The hindbrain consists of the cerebellum, pons, and medulla oblongata.

11. **D**

The autonomic nervous system controls all involuntary systems (cardiac, respiratory, smooth muscle) in the body through the sympathetic and parasympathetic nervous systems.

12. **E**

The haversian system in bone does not contain the perichondrium that is the dense connective tissue surrounding cartilage.

A. Osteocytes are the bone cells or osteons within the haversian system.

B. Canaliculi are the tunnels that allow for communication between the osteocytes.

C. Volkmann's canals carry the blood vessel and nerve supply to osteons.

D. Lamellae create concentric circles around the osteons.

13. **C**

An antidiuretic eliminates water from the body at the loop of Henle. The pharmaceutical physically forces out sodium. Water follows the sodium out, because it is attracted by sodium.

A. Bowman's capsule surrounds the glomerulus which contains the loop of Henle.

B. Calyces encase the pyramids of the kidney.

D. Nephron is the functional unit of the kidney that contains many glomeruli.

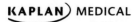

14. A

Polysaccharides are carbohydrates that are broken down or hydrolyzed by an amylase. Salivary starch digestion begins in the mouth and then goes on into the small intestine, where pancreatic amylase continues to metabolize it.

B. Lipase is found in the stomach and small intestine to hydrolyze fat.

C. Protease is an enzyme that hydrolyzes protein.

D. Pepsin hydrolyzes the peptide bonds of proteins.

15. E

The lowest amount of pressure in the cardiovascular system is in the veins. The veins are last in the line of blood vessels; they are the farthest away from the original pumping station of the heart, where the pressure is the greatest.

A. The pressure is the highest the arteries. If someone injures an artery, it spurts out blood since the pressure is greatest.

B. Arterioles have high pressure, though not as high as arteries.

C. Capillaries seep blood since there is less pressure.

D. Venules will ooze blood since the pressure drops here.

16. B

Prothrombin is produced in the liver. Vitamin K is absorbed in the large intestine and then goes to the liver.

A. The pancreas produces glucagon by the alpha cells and insulin by the beta cells in the islets of Langerhans.

C. The spleen filters out old red blood cells and is a reservoir for lymphocytes.

D. The glomerulus—in the kidney—is where filtering occurs.

E. The hypothalamus is responsible for producing oxytocin and antidiuretic hormone, and for regulating body temperature, the circulatory system, electrolytes, and urine formation.

17. B

If the natural pacemaker of the sinoatrial (SA) node malfunctions, the atrioventricular (AV) node will take over, though at a slower rate of 40–60 beats per minute.

A. The sinoatrial node is the natural pacemaker of the heart that beats at 60 to 100 beats per minute.

C. The bundle of His is just below the AV node and branches off into the right and left bundle branches. These branches go down to the Purkinje fibers.

D. The Purkinje fibers will try to take over if the SA node and the AV node are not functioning, but their rate is very slow at 20 to 40 beats per minute.

18. C

Insulin is produced by the beta cells of the pancreas. Insulin acts as a key that unlocks cells to allow glucose to enter.

A. Kupffer cells are phagocytic cells lining the sinusoids in the liver.

B. Alpha cells produce glucagons.

D. The islets of Langerhans are in the pancreas and contain the alpha and beta cells.

E. Bowman's capsules are contained in the kidney.

19. D

Intrinsic factor is a substance produced in the stomach that aids in the absorption of vitamin B12. Alcoholics lack intrinsic factor and are prone to pernicious anemia because they cannot absorb vitamin B12.

20. A

The neurotransmitter that maintains our vegetative state is acetylcholine. Norepinepherine, catecholamine, and dopamine are all amines based in the sympathetic nervous system, and arise in a fight-or-flight situation. Serotonin is involved in emotion and mood.

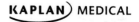

21. C

The pyloric valve lies between the stomach and small intestine. Stenosis would impede the flow of food from exiting the stomach and entering the small intestine.

A. The esophagus and stomach are separated by the cardiac sphincter. Stenosis here would affect food exiting the esophagus and entering the stomach.

B. The stomach has both of the above-named sphincters or valves.

D. The large intestine is separated from the small intestine by the ileocecal sphincter.

22. B

The endocrine gland that regulates body temperature and hot flashes is the hypothalamus gland which acts as the body's thermostat.

23. C

If a person's blood-sugar level drops, the body has the ability to go after the liver's storage of glycogen.

A. Glucose is what cells need to survive and circulates in our blood.

B. Glucagon is produced by the alpha cells in the pancreas. Glucagon goes after the stores of glycogen stored in the liver if blood glucose become too low.

D. Glucan is a polysaccharide that is a polymer of glucose.

24. D

Cirrhosis in an alcoholic affects the liver. It is a chronic, progressive, degenerative liver disease.

25. C

The body's ability to maintain a stable state is termed homeostasis.

A. Homeopathy is a method for treating disease in small doses with a remedy that produces symptoms similar to that of a healthy person.

B. Homeothermic means warm-blooded.

D. Homogenous refers to something that is the same or similar in nature.

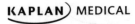

Chapter Four: **Head and Neck Anatomy**

A thorough patient exam of the head and neck requires an understanding of all the landmarks of bones of the cranium and muscle, or lymph node and nerve locations. With this total assessment, the dental hygienist will be better able to recognize any abnormalities.

BONES OF THE HEAD AND FACE

The bones of the head and face consist of 8 cranial bones with 14 facial bones. The **cranium** itself consists of two temporal bones, two parietal bones, and one each of sphenoid, ethmoid, frontal, and occipital bones.

The **facial bones** include two zygomatic, two maxillae, one mandible, two small lacrimal bones, two small nasal bones, one vomer, and one hyoid bone along with 3 small bones in the ear.

Except for the mandible, which is movable, all of the bones of the skull **articulate** with one another as the bones join together at immovable joints called **sutures**. The bones contain features such as **foramina** or openings for blood vessels and nerves to pass through, apertures which are other openings or orifices, **fissures** that are narrow openings or clefts, **canals** that are passageways, **meati** which are a type of canal, and **sinuses** which are air-filled cavities. **Processes** are where attachments occur and a **fossa** is a depression in a bone.

Bones of the Cranium

The **occipital** bone is a large single bone that forms the base or back of the cranium. It houses the cerebellum and the occipital lobes of the cerebrum of the brain. It also contains the **foramen magnum** that is the passageway for the spinal cord, accessory nerve, and vertebral arteries. On either side of the foramen magnum are two hypoglossal foramina where the hypoglossal nerve exits to the tongue. The **occipital bone articulates with the first cervical vertebra**, the **atlas** (where the skull is able to move up and down), paired parietal, paired temporal, and sphenoid bones.

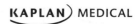

Bones of the Cranium

Bone	#	Location	Articulation	Suture or Joint	Opening	Nerve	Vessel
Ethmoid	1	Cranial	Frontal		Cribriform plate	Olfactory (I)	
			Lacrimal		foramen		
			Maxilla				
			Sphenoid				
			Vomer				
Frontal	1	Cranial	Ethmoid				
			Lacrimal				
			Maxilla				
			Nasal				
			Zygoma				
			Sphenoid				
			Parietal	Coronal			
Occipital	1	Cranial	1st cervical vertebrae	Foramen Magnum	Spinal cord,	Vertebral arteries	
			Sphenoid		spinal accessory (XI)		
			Temporal		Hypoglossal canal	Hypoglossa (XII)	
			Parietal	Lambdoidal	Jugular foramen	Glossopharyngeal (X)	Internal jugular vein
					(with temporal bone)	Vagus (X)	
						Spinal Accessory (XI)	
Parietal	2	Cranial	Sphenoid				
			Frontal	Coronal			
			Occipital	Lambdoidal			
			Parietal	Sagittal			
			Temporal	Squamosal			
Sphenoid	1	Cranial	Ethmoid		Foramen ovale	Mandibular of Trigeminal (V)	
			Frontal		Foramen rotundum	Maxillary of Trigeminal (V)	
			Maxilla		Inferior orbital fissure	Infraorbital nerve,	Infraorbital artery,
			Occipital		(with maxilla)	zygomatic nerves	Ophthalmic vein
			Palatine		Foramen spinosum		Middle meningeal artery
			Parietal		Optic canal & foramen	Optic nerve	Ophthalmic artery
			Temporal		Pterygoid canal	Pterygoid (vidian) nerve	Pterygoid (vidian) vessels
			Vomer		Superior orbital fissure	Occulomotor (III)	Ophthalmic artery
			Zygomatic			Trochlear (IV)	
						Abducent (VI)	
						Optic nerve	

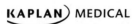

Bone	#	Location	Articulation	Suture or Joint	Opening	Nerve	Vessel
Temporal	2	Cranial	Sphenoid		Carotid canal	Internal carotid artery	
			Mandible		Ext. acoustic meatus	Tympanic cavity opening	
			Occipital		Jugular foramen	Glossopharyngeal (IX)	
			Parietal	Squamosal	(with occipital)	Vagus (X)	
			Zygomatic	Temporozygomatic		Spinal Accessory	
					Int. acoustic meatus	Facial (VII)	
						Auditory (VIII)	
					Petrotympanic fissure	Chorda tympani	
					Styloid mastoid foramen	Facial (VII)	
Lacrimal	2	Facial	Ethmoid				
			Frontal				
			Maxilla				
Maxilla	2	Facial	Ethmoid				
			Frontal				
			Lacrimal				
			Nasal bone				
			Nasal concha				
			Palatine				
			Sphenoid				
			Vomer				
			Zygomatic				
Mandible	1	Facial	Temporal	Tempromandibular			
Nasal Bones	2	Facial	Frontal				
			Maxilla				
Nasal Conchae	2	Facial	Ethmoid				
			Lacrimal				
			Maxilla				
			Palatine				
Vomer	1	Facial	Ethmoid				
			Maxilla				
			Palatine				
			Sphenoid				
Zygomatic	2	Facial	Frontal				
			Maxilla				
			Sphenoid				
			Temporal	Temporozygomatic			

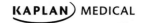

The **frontal** bone of the cranium forms the forehead and houses the anterior cerebrum and frontal sinuses. It also forms the supraorbital ridge or upper boundary of the orbit of the eye. The frontal bone articulates with the paired parietal bones at the coronal suture, paired lacrimal bones, paired maxilla bones, paired nasal bones, paired zygomatic bones, single sphenoid bone, and single ethmoid bone.

The **sphenoid** bone connects the cranial and facial skeletons. It contributes to the support of the medial orbits of the eyes and separates the right and left nasal septum. There are four apertures within the sphenoid bone:

- The **foramen ovale** conveys the **mandibular division** of the trigeminal nerve;

- The **foramen rotundum** conveys the **maxillary branch** of the trigeminal nerve;

- The **foramen spinosum** conveys the arteries that supply blood to the meninges;

- The **superior orbital fissure** conveys cranial nerves III, IV, VI and a portion of cranial nerve V (opthalmic branch).

The sphenoid articulates with the paired parietal, temporal, zygomatic, and maxillary bones as well as the single frontal, occipital, ethmoid, palatine, and vomer bones.

The **ethmoid** bone is a single, midline, rhomboid-shaped bone that forms the floor of the orbits and cranium. It contains the cribriform plate that allows for the passage of the olfactory nerve. The ethmoid bone articulates with the frontal, lacrimal, maxillary, sphenoid, and vomer bones.

The paired **temporal** bones are the lateral wall supports of the cranium and have three sections.

- The first section is the squamous portion that forms the zygomatic process where it adjoins the zygomatic bone. The squamous portion contains the **articular** or **mandibular fossa** and the **articular eminence** to accommodate the mandibular condyle of the **temporomandibular joint**.

- The second section is the tympanic portion of the temporal bones; this houses the external acoustic meatus and petrotympanic fissure through which the chorda tympani emerges.

- The third section of the temporal bones, the petrous portion, includes the **mastoid process** and the **styloid process** where muscles and ligaments attach. Also found here is the stylomastoid foramen as the passageway of the facial nerve. The temporal bones articulate with the parietal bones, the zygomatic bones, occipital bone, sphenoid bone, and mandible.

The **parietal** bones of the cranium articulate with each other to form the sagittal suture. They also articulate with the frontal, occipital, sphenoid, and temporal bones.

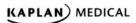

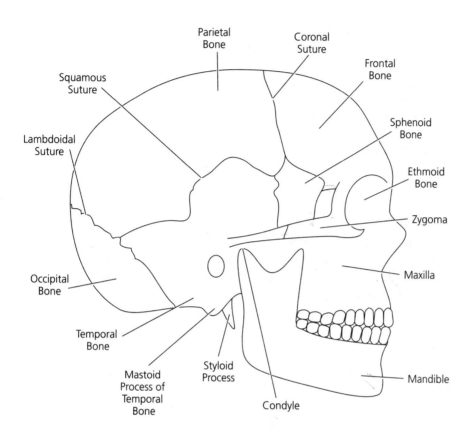

Bones of the Skull

FACIAL BONES

The facial bones shape our facial features and oral cavity, and also house the teeth.

Maxilla

The paired **maxillary** bones are fused together and contain four processes. The **alveolar processes** house the roots of the maxillary teeth. Cortical bone is on the facial and lingual surfaces of teeth. **Alveolar bone proper**, also referred to as the **cribriform plate** or **lamina dura**, is the bone that outlines the root of the tooth and is seen radiographically as a radiopaque line.

The **frontal process** articulates with the frontal bone and lacrimal bones. When it articulates with the frontal bone, it forms the medial orbital rim. The **palatine processes** are the two palatal bones fused together at the median palatine suture to form the **anterior** hard palate. The incisive foramen located here is the passageway for the right and left nasopalatine nerves and corresponding blood vessels.

Lamina propria is a very vascular epithelial connective tissue beneath the basement membrane and is not seen radiographically. Lamina dura is a radiopaque bone that follows the outline of the root of a tooth and is seen radiographically.

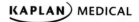

The **zygomatic processes**, which are the fusion of the temporal and zygomatic bones, form a part of the infraorbital rim.

Foramina of the maxilla include the incisive foramen for the nasopalatine nerve and the posterior superior alveolar foramen that exits from the maxillary tuberosity with the posterior superior alveolar nerve.

The **maxillary tuberosity** located at the posterior of the most distal maxillary molar appears radiographically as a radiopaque rounded prominence.

Palatine Bones

The two **palatal** bones fuse at the continuance of the median palatine suture to form the **posterior** hard palate and serve to unite the maxilla and sphenoid bones. The greater palatine foramen is the passageway for the greater palatine nerve. The lesser palatine foramen is the passageway for the lesser palatine nerve.

Mandible

The mandible is the only bone in the skull that contains a movable joint. The mandible articulates at the temporal bone with the condyle as the temporomandibular joint. The body of the **mandible** contains the alveolar processes that anchor the roots of the mandibular teeth. When it forms in utero, the mandible is fused at the mandibular **symphisis**.

Also located in this area is the **mental protuberance** that gives shape to the chin. In this same area, though on the internal surface of the mandible, are the **genial tubercles** that serve as muscle attachment for the **genioglossus muscle**. More landmarks on the internal surface are the sublingual and submandibular fossae that house their corresponding glands along with the **mandibular foramen** where the **inferior alveolar nerve** passes through the **mandibular canal**.

The mental foramen is located near the root tip of the first and second premolars and is sometimes mistaken for an abscess.

Close by is the mylohyoid ridge which is the mode of attachment for the mylohyoid muscle. The mylohyoid groove is the passageway for the mylohyoid nerve and corresponding blood vessels. Moving posteriorly from the center of the exterior surface of the mandible is the **mental foramen** through which the **mental nerve** passes. The soft tissue of the retromolar pad covers the **retromolar triangle** that is distal to the third molars.

Moving posteriorly, the ramus ascends rearward along the **external oblique line** that unites the ramus with the body of the mandible. The most posterior and inferior portion of the mandible is the **angle** that projects upward to the condyle. The **condyle** is the articulator of the temporomandibular joint with the temporal bones. The **coronoid process** that is the anterior portion of the ramus is the site of muscle attachment for the temporalis and masseter muscles. The **coronoid** or **mandibular notch** is a concavity between the condyle and coronoid process.

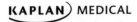

Temporomandibular Joint

A joint is a merger of two bones that allows for movement between the bones. The **temporomandibular joint** (TMJ) is the bilateral juncture of the **condyles** of the mandible with the **articular fossa** and **articular eminence** of the **temporal bones**. When closed, the condyle lies within the articular fossa of the temporal bone, but when opened, it moves anteriorly into the articular eminence of the temporal bone.

The **meniscus,** a fibrous structure that separates the condyle from the temporal bone, provides a gliding surface for the condyle to produce smooth joint movements. The TMJ is a **synovial joint** (filled with synovial fluid) that allows for **rotation** and **translation** motions for movement of the lower jaw.

Upon **opening**, the **rotation** occurs first, and then allows for **translation** or gliding of the condylar head anteriorly along with the meniscus. When closed, the meniscus lies slightly anterior above the head of the condyle.

Many **TMJ disorders** can occur. One vital role of dental professionals is to perform an extraoral examination by palpating the TMJ. Signs and symptoms may include popping noises, deviations upon opening, bruxism, clenching, facial pain, and joint tenderness. The **popping** noise of the TMJ occurs when the meniscus is displaced out of its normal position. **Subluxation** is the dislocation of the TMJ should a patient open wider than normal.

Zygoma

The paired **zygomatic** bones articulate with the temporal bones to form the zygomatic process of the cheekbones. They also articulate with the frontal, maxillary, sphenoid, and temporal bones.

Vomer

The **vomer** bone is a single midline bone that forms the posterior segment of the nasal cavity. It articulates with ethmoid bone, maxilla, and sphenoid bone.

The vomer bone has **no** muscle attachments. Most of the anterior nasal septum is cartilage.

Nasal and Lacrimal Bones

The paired **nasal bones** articulate with each other to form the bridge of the nose. They also articulate with the frontal bone and maxilla. The paired **lacrimal bones** aid in forming a portion of the orbit for the eye, and articulate with the ethmoid bone, the frontal bone, and the maxilla.

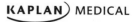

BONES OF THE NECK

The **first cervical** vertebra is the **atlas** that allows for **up and down** movement. The atlas articulates with the occipital condyles of the occipital bone and supports the head. The **second cervical** vertebra is the **axis** that allows for **pivoting** movement of the head. The **dens** found anteriorly on the second vertebra articulates with the anterior arch of the atlas of the first vertebra.

The **hyoid bone** is a U-shaped bone of the neck that is suspended and does not articulate with any other bones. It is the mode of attachment for the geniohyoid muscle, mylohyoid muscle, omohyoid muscle, sternohyoid muscle, stylohyoid muscle, thyrohyoid muscle, and the suprahyoid muscle group.

NERVES OF THE HEAD AND NECK

The nervous system—the gatekeeper of the body—consists of the **central nervous system** (CNS) of the brain and spinal cord as well as the **peripheral nervous system** (PNS) which includes the **cranial nerves** and the **spinal nerves**. The PNS carries messages to and from the central nervous system.

Afferent receptors are involved in getting **sensory** information back to the CNS. **Efferent** receptors get the message from the CNS out to the body. Involved in efferent output are the somatic nervous system and the autonomic nervous system (ANS).

The **somatic nervous system** carries messages from the spinal cord to all voluntary skeletal muscles for muscle contraction. It also controls nerve fibers that keep the body in touch with changes in the external environment.

The ANS is made up of two systems: the **sympathetic nervous system** and the **parasympathetic nervous system**. The **parasympathetic nervous system** governs the body the majority of the time, and **acetylcholine** is the usual neurotransmitter for neuron communication.

When we are under great stress, our bodies change, and that is when the **sympathetic nervous system** takes over: our heart rate and blood pressure increase, and our GI tract decreases its ability to function.

The body has **12 cranial nerves** and **31 spinal nerves**. The **spinal nerves** consist of 8 cervical, 12 thoracic, 5 lumbar, 5 sacral, and 1 coccygeal nerve. The spinal nerves carry motor function messages to various parts of the body, and also receive proprioceptive sensations from the neck, trunk, and extremities.

CRANIAL NERVES

The cranial nerves are part of the peripheral nervous system. They are designated by Roman numerals (CN III, CN V, CN VII, CNIX, and CN X). The cranial nerves have the ability to function as sensory or motor, or both sensory and motor. They may also carry parasympathetic fibers.

Cranial Nerve I: Olfactory

The olfactory nerve is a sensory afferent nerve that receives smell impulses from the nasal mucosa. The olfactory bulb relays the neural signal to the neurons as they pass through the foramen of the cribriform plate.

Cranial Nerve II: Optic

The optic nerve is a sensory afferent nerve that transmits visual impulses from the retina. It exits the brain through the optic canal of the sphenoid bone.

Cranial Nerve III: Oculomotor

The oculomotor nerve is a motor efferent nerve that controls the muscle movement of the eye. This nerve also supplies parasympathetic function to control the iris opening. It passes through the superior orbital fissure of the sphenoid bone.

Cranial Nerve IV: Trochlear

The trochlear nerve, the **smallest cranial nerve**, is a motor efferent nerve that controls eye muscle contraction at the superior oblique muscle. It passes through the superior orbital fissure of the sphenoid bone.

Cranial Nerve V: Trigeminal

The **trigeminal nerve** is the *largest* nerve in the body and has three main nerve branches: the V1 ophthalmic division (sensory afferent); the V2 maxillary division (sensory afferent); and the V3 mandibular division (sensory afferent and motor efferent nerves). Each of these divisions has additional subdivisions:

Trigeminal V1: Ophthalmic Division

The V1 **ophthalmic** division of the maxillary nerve is an **all-sensory afferent** division that contains the **frontal division** which transmits sensations from the **scalp** and **forehead**. The **lacrimal division** of the V1 regulates the **lacrimal gland** (parasympathetic stimulation) and **eyelid** while the **nasociliary division** conveys sensation from the **nose** and **nasal mucosa**. The **lacrimal** nerve also supplies **parasympathetic** stimulation to the lacrimal gland. The **ophthalmic** division passes through the **superior orbital fissure** of the **sphenoid** bone.

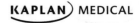

The maxillary (upper) division of the trigeminal nerve travels through the foramen rotundum. Think of a rotunda, as in a capital building, that is a dome overhead. The mandibular (lower) division exits by the foramen ovale. Ovale = Down in the valley for the lower mandibular division.

Trigeminal V2: Maxillary Division

The V2 **maxillary division** is an all **sensory afferent** division whose passageway is through the **foramen rotundum**. The V2 maxillary division consists of the eight (8) following divisions of the V2 nerve.

- The **infraorbital nerve** (IO) conveys afferent sensation from the lower eyelid, cheek, side of nose, and upper lip. It eventually **joins** with the **anterior superior alveolar** nerve by way of the **infraorbital canal**.

- The **anterior superior alveolar** (ASA) division conveys pulpal afferent sensation from all of the **maxillary incisors** and **canines** including their **surrounding tissues**. The **ASA ascends** into the **infraorbital canal** where it **joins** the **infraorbital nerve**. When considering the use of local anesthesia, the ASA will often cross the midline.

- The **middle superior alveolar** (MSA) conveys pulpal afferent sensation from the maxillary premolars and the **mesial buccal root of the maxillary first molars** including their surrounding tissues. It also ascends to the infraorbital canal to join the infraorbital nerve.

- The **posterior superior alveolar** (PSA) division that conveys pulpal afferent sensation from the **maxillary molars** *except* the **mesial buccal root of the first molar** and corresponding **periodontium** and **buccal gingiva**. It ascends along the maxillary tuberosity as it exits through various **posterior superior foramina** then travels to the pterygopalatine fossa where it rejoins the maxillary nerve.

- The **greater palatine nerve** conveys afferent sensation from the posterior hard palate and posterior lingual tissues. Its entrance into the oral cavity is through the greater palatine foramen of the palatal bone in the vicinity of the maxillary molars.

- The **lesser palatine nerve** conveys afferent sensation from the **soft palate** and **palatine tonsil area**. These two nerves both enter the **pterygopalatine canal** to join the **maxillary nerve**.

- The **nasopalatine nerve** conveys afferent sensation from the **anterior hard palate** and the **lingual** tissues of all of the **maxillary incisors** and **canines**. The nasopalatine nerve passes through the **incisive foramen** and also corresponds with the greater palatine nerve.

- The **zygomatic nerve** conveys **afferent sensation** from the **cheek** and **temple area**, but also brings **parasympathetic** fibers to the **lacrimal gland**. The zygomatic nerve exits by way of the inferior orbital fissure to unite with the maxillary nerve.

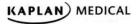

Trigeminal V3 Mandibular Division

The mandibular V3 division has six branches as follows:

- The **auriculotemporal nerve** conveys afferent sensation from the **scalp** and **ear**, but also supplies **parasympathetic** fibers to the **parotid gland** (parasympathetic fibers from CN IX travel with the auriculotemporal nerve).

- The **buccal** or **long buccal nerve** conveys **afferent sensation** from the **buccal mucosa**, buccal gingiva of the posterior mandibular teeth, and the cheek. It descends from the trigeminal nerve as it branches out over the surface of the buccinator muscle to supply the skin and mucous membranes.

- The **inferior alveolar nerve** (IA) is formed by the convergence of the **mental nerve** and **incisive nerve**. It also joins with nerve branches from the mandibular posterior teeth to form the **dental plexus** and conveys afferent pulpal and surrounding tissue sensations to all the mandibular teeth. The **IA** nerve passes through the **mandibular canal** along with the inferior alveolar artery and vein and exits the mandible via the **mandibular foramen**. It later unites with the **mylohyoid nerve**.

- The **incisive nerve** conveys **afferent pulpal sensation** and surrounding **periodontium** sensation from the **mandibular anterior teeth**. The incisive nerve joins the mental nerve at the **mental foramen** near the roots of the mandibular premolars to become the IA nerve.

- The **mental nerve** conveys afferent sensation to the **lower lip**, **chin**, and mandibular **anterior buccal mucosa**. It joins with the incisive nerve at the **mental foramen** to form the IA nerve.

- The **lingual nerve** conveys afferent sensation for the **floor of the mouth**, **lingual mandibular gingival surfaces**, and **two thirds** ($\frac{2}{3}$) of the anterior surface of the **tongue**. The lingual nerve also provides **taste sensation** for the same **two thirds** of the tongue by carrying fibers of chorda tympani. It provides **parasympathetic** fibers to the **submandibular** and **sublingual glands** (parasympathetic fibers from CN VII travel with the lingual nerve).

- **The motor muscular nerve** branches of the mandibular division of the trigeminal nerve provide **efferent motor** nerve transmission to the muscles of mastication that include the **masseter**, **lateral pterygoid**, **medial pterygoid**, and **temporalis muscles**. The usually paired nerves consist of the temporal nerve, masseteric nerve, and the medial and lateral pterygoid nerves.

- The **mylohyoid nerve** provides **efferent motor** nerve transmission to the **mylohyoid muscle** and anterior **digastric muscle**. It unites with the inferior alveolar nerve at the **foramen ovale**.

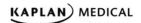

Cranial Nerve VI: Abducens

The **abducens** nerve is a **motor efferent** nerve that controls **movement** to the lateral eyeball. It passes through the **superior orbital fissure** of the **sphenoid bone**.

Cranial Nerve VII: Facial

The **facial nerve** has **both afferent sensation** and **efferent motor** branches and exits the brain by way of the **internal acoustic meatus** in the temporal bone. The **greater petrosal nerve** branch conveys both afferent and efferent functions. The **afferent** sensation is the conveyed taste **sensation** from the **palate**. The **greater petrosal nerve** functions with **efferent parasympathetic** transmission to the **minor salivary glands** of both the hard and soft palates, the **lacrimal glands** and the **nasal cavity**. The **chorda tympani nerve** branch provides **afferent taste sensation** for the anterior $\frac{2}{3}$ body of the **tongue**, but also supplies **parasympathetic** fibers for the **submandibular** and **sublingual glands**.

Other branches of the **efferent motor** portion of the **facial nerve** include buccal, cervical, mandibular, temporal, and zygomatic nerves that innervate their respective muscles for facial expression.

Cranial Nerve VIII: Vestibulocochlear

The vestibulocochlear nerve conveys afferent sensation to the semicircular canals of the inner ear for balance and to the sensory fibers of the inner ear for hearing. It exits the cranium by way of the internal acoustic meatus of the temporal bone.

Cranial Nerve IX: Glossopharyngeal

The **glossopharyngeal nerve** has both afferent sensation and efferent motor functions. Its afferent branch provides both general sensory and **taste sensation** for the **posterior one third** of the **tongue**, and also provides afferent sensation for the **pharynx** and **tonsils**. The **efferent motor** portion of this nerve controls the **stylopharyngeal muscle** that **elevates** the **larynx** anteriorly during swallowing.

Cranial Nerve X: Vagus

The **vagus nerve** is the *longest* of all the cranial nerves and extends out to the trunk of the body. It has both afferent and efferent components. The **vagus nerve** provides **afferent sensation** to the **ear** and **epiglottis**. It also provides **sensation** to the larynx, pharynx, digestive system, respiratory system, and heart. The vagus nerve provides **efferent motor** innervation to the **muscles** of the **larynx**, **pharynx**, and **soft palate**. It exits the cranium through the **jugular foramen** that is located between the occipital and temporal bones and provides **parasympathetic** fibers to the **respiratory system**, **digestive system**, and the **heart**.

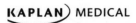

Cranial Nerve XI: Accessory

The accessory nerve is an efferent motor nerve that controls the muscles of the soft palate, trapezius, sternocleidomastoid, and pharynx. It leaves the skull by way of the jugular foramen.

Cranial Nerve XII: Hypoglossal

The **hypoglossal nerve** is an **efferent motor** nerve that controls the **muscles** of the **tongue**, both **intrinsic** and **extrinsic**, except for the palatoglossus muscle (controlled by the vagus nerve). The extrinsic muscles are the genioglossus, genio-hyoideus, hyoglossus, and styloglossus muscles.

NERVE AILMENTS AFFECTING THE HEAD AND FACE

Facial paralysis may occur after a cerebral vascular accident, where one half of the body is paralyzed, or as a result of nerve disorder that disrupts the 5th or 7th cranial nerve, respectively, with trigeminal neuralgia or Bell's palsy.

> Bell's Palsy affects the facial nerve (VII). Trigeminal Neuralgia affects the trigeminal nerve (V).

Trigeminal Neuralgia (Tic douloureux)

Trigeminal neuralgia is a **trigeminal nerve disorder** that could be an irritation of the trigeminal nerve and is usually **unilateral**. It is a debilitating, **shock-like**, **stabbing pain** that comes on **suddenly**—often described as a sudden **lightning** or **burning sensation** that lasts seconds or minutes. It is **triggered** by some mild stimulation to the face, such as brushing teeth, shaving, talking, or eating. The patient may experience pain for days, weeks, or months until it disappears. There can be remissions and recurrences. Since it is caused by a trigger point, the patient may not be able to perform proper hygiene.

> <u>T</u>rigeminal neuralgia = <u>T</u>ic Delaroux = <u>T</u>ic = facial spasm
> <u>T</u>rigeminal nerve (V) involved
> <u>T</u>rigger point sets it off

Bell's Palsy

Bell's palsy is facial paralysis caused by damage to the **facial nerve (VII)**. It may be caused by a virus—possibly Herpes Simplex I virus. Its symptoms include **unilateral motor deficits, facial asymmetry, drooling, sagging eyebrow,** and **taste impairment**. Some patients experience diminished saliva production. Patients may get better in as little as 3 weeks, or up to 6 months. On occasion, Bell's palsy causes permanent damage. The facial paralysis makes it harder for the patient to maintain good oral hygiene, and as such, the dental hygienist should help advise on appropriate adjuncts. Any elective dental treatment should be postponed until the paralysis has subsided.

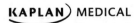

CIRCULATION OF THE HEAD AND NECK

The circulatory system consists of the heart (the pump), blood vessels (a system of pipes), and blood (the fluid in the pipes). Blood is a connective tissue that supplies nutrients and oxygen necessary for cell life. Blood also carries away waste and carbon dioxide from cells. The head and neck have many circulatory plexuses (networks of blood vessels) to supply nutrients and oxygen to cells.

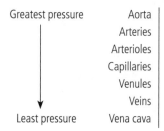

| Greatest pressure | Aorta |
| Arteries |
| Arterioles |
| Capillaries |
| Venules |
| Veins |
| Least pressure | Vena cava |

Arteries carry oxygenated blood and nutrients away from the heart to cells. Veins, on the other hand, transport carbon dioxide and waste back to the heart and then lungs. **Arteries** contain the **greatest pressure** within vessels. As they become smaller arterioles, the pressure lessens. Capillaries are the smallest vessels where the actual exchange of gases, nutrients, and waste takes place. Venules connect the capillaries to the veins as they start the blood's trip back to the heart. It is in the veins where the pressure of circulation is the least.

Arteries of the Head and Neck

Circulation away from the heart starts at the aorta, from which the common carotid artery branches off. The **brachiocephalic artery**—the first branch of the aorta—goes on to divide into the **right common carotid** artery and **right subclavian** artery. The **left common carotid** artery arises from the aorta. Both common carotid arteries go on to divide into the external and internal carotid arteries.

Internal Carotid Artery

The **internal carotid artery** enters the skull by way of the carotid canal near the sphenoid bone to **supply the brain**, eye, and orbital cavities.

External Carotid

The **external carotid artery** supplies blood to the neck, exterior head, and face. It divides into several arteries:

- The **facial artery** that branches off from the external carotid supplies blood to the **muscles** of the **face** and nasal area. It branches off into the **ascending palatine artery** that supplies the **palatine muscles, palatine tonsils,** and **soft palate**. The facial artery also has a **submental artery** branch, which supplies the **digastric muscles,** mylohyoid, submandibular lymph nodes, and submandibular salivary gland.

- Another facial artery branch includes the **inferior** and **superior labial arteries,** which supply the lower and upper **lips**, respectively, with the inferior artery supplying **muscles** of **facial expression.**

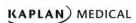

- The **lingual artery** is an anterior branch of the external carotid that arises above the hyoid bone. It supplies blood to the **floor of the mouth**, to the **suprahyoid muscles**, and, anteriorly, to the **apex** of the **tongue**. It then branches off into the **sublingual artery** to supply blood to the **mucous membranes in the floor of the mouth**, the **mylohyoid muscle**, and the **sublingual salivary gland**.

- The **maxillary artery** is a large vessel that branches off from the external carotid artery near the **condyle** of the mandible. It traverses the infratemporal fossa then crosses the lateral pterygoid muscle before it disappears into the **pterygopalatine fossa**. After entering this fossa, it branches off into more arteries.

- The **middle meningeal artery** of the maxillary artery supplies blood to the **bones** of the skull and **meninges** of the brain.

- The **inferior alveolar artery** branch of the maxillary artery enters the mandibular canal by way of the mandibular foramen to supply blood to **floor** of the mouth, **mandibular teeth**, and **mental region** of the mandible. The **incisive artery** is a branch of the inferior alveolar artery traveling in the mandibular canal and supplies blood to the **pulp tissue** and **periodontium** of the anterior mandibular teeth.

- The **mental artery**, also a branch of the inferior alveolar artery, exits the mandibular canal by way of the mental foramen and supplies blood to the **chin** and the **anastomoses** (network between vessels) of the inferior labial artery. The **mylohyoid artery**, another branch of the inferior alveolar artery, passes through the mandibular foramen to enter the mandibular canal. It supplies blood to the floor of the mouth and the mylohyoid muscle.

- Another branch of the maxillary artery is the **infraorbital artery**, which enters into the orbit by way of the infraorbital fissure. It supplies blood to the **orbit** and then branches off into the anterior superior alveolar artery.

- The **anterior superior alveolar artery** branch of the infraorbital artery supplies blood to the **pulp tissue** and **periodontium** of the maxillary anterior teeth as well as the **anastomoses** of the **posterior superior alveolar artery**.

- The **greater** and **lesser palatine artery** branches of the maxillary artery pass through greater and lesser palatine foramina to supply blood to the **hard** and **soft palates**. Arteries that correspond to their muscles of mastication include the **buccal artery** (buccinator muscle), **masseteric artery** (masseter muscle), **pterygoid artery** (medial and lateral pterygoid muscles), and **temporal artery** (temporalis muscle).

- The **posterior superior alveolar artery** branch of the maxillary artery supplies blood to the **pulp tissue** and **periodontium** of the maxillary posterior teeth as well as joining with the anastomoses of the anterior superior alveolar artery.

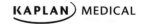

- The **occipital artery** branch of the external carotid artery traverses the ramus of the mandible then proceeds toward the posterior segment of the scalp, and supplies blood to the **meningeal tissues, sternocleidomastoid muscle,** and **suprahyoid muscle.**

- The **posterior auricular artery** is also a branch of the external carotid artery. It originates just above the stylohyoid muscle and ascends along the temporal bone to supply blood to the **ear, tympanic membrane,** and **scalp** in that region.

- The **superficial temporal artery** is one of the terminal branches of the external carotid artery. It supplies blood to the **parotid gland** and the **temporalis muscle.**

- The **superior thyroid artery** branch of the external carotid artery branches off into many other branches that supply blood to the **hyoid bone,** infrahyoid muscles, and thyroid gland.

Veins of the Head and Neck

- The **facial vein** drains blood from the superficial structures of the face such as the **lips** and **chin** as well as draining the **corner** and **orbit of the eye**. The facial vein drains into the **internal jugular vein**. This vein communicates with the **cavernous venous sinus** which has important structures running through it.

- The **external jugular vein** drains the **exterior cranium, neck,** and deep parts of the **face**. It lies outside of the sternocleidomastoid muscle and also merges with the subclavian artery.

- The **internal jugular vein** exits the skull through the **jugular foramen** and drains blood from the **brain** (interior cranium) and **facial area** by way of the facial vein. It also drains the **lingual vein, sublingual vein,** and **pharyngeal vein**. When it **merges** with the **subclavian vein,** it becomes the brachiocephalic vein.

- The **maxillary vein** receives blood from the **pterygoid plexus** of veins of the pterygoid muscle that arises from the maxillary artery supplying blood to that area. It also receives drainage from the inferior alveolar vein that drains the periodontium and pulp tissue of the mandibular teeth. The maxillary vein also drains the posterior superior alveolar vein which receives blood from the periodontium and pulp tissue of the maxillary teeth.

- The **pterygoid plexus** is a collection of **anastomoses** (network between vessels) situated in the pterygoid muscle. It receives drainage from the **alveolar, buccinator, masseteric, palatal, pterygoid, deep temporal,** and **middle meningeal** (from the brain) veins. It then drains into the internal maxillary vein.

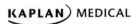

- The **retromandibular vein** arises from the union of the **maxillary vein** and **super-ficial temporal vein** at the parotid gland. It communicates with the internal and external jugular veins but also divides into a posterior and anterior branch. The **posterior branch** drains the **maxillary vein, posterior auricular vein,** and the **temporal vein** into the **external jugular** vein. The **anterior branch** drains the **facial vein** into the **interior jugular vein**.

MUSCLES OF THE HEAD AND NECK

It is essential that a dental hygienist know where the muscles of the head and neck are located, as this helps to locate other structures during a patient exam. There are three main parts to the muscle:

- The **origin** (or head) of muscle attaches to the least movable portion of the bone or stationary bone.

- The **belly** is the fleshy contractile part between the origin and insertion.

- The **insertion** is where muscle attaches to the movable portion of the bone or where the action takes place.

Tendons connect muscle to bone. Each muscle performs a specific action. **Ligaments** attach bone to bone.

Facial Muscles

The epicranial or occipitofrontalis muscle consists of two frontal bellies and two occipital bellies. The occipital bellies originate at the occipital bone and insert into the galea apo-neurotica. The frontal bellies originate from the galea and insert into the epidermis of the nose and eyebrow. They merge at the epicranial aponeurosis, the intermediate tendon connecting the frontalis and occipitalis muscles. Their action is to elevate the eyebrow and forehead.

The orbicularis oculi muscle originates from the frontal process of the maxilla and the nasal process of the frontal bone as it encircles the eye. It inserts circumferentially around the orbit and is innervated by the facial nerve (VII). Its action is to close the eyelid. Blood supply comes from the ophthalmic artery.

The **corrugator supercilium** in the eye region **originates** from the **frontal bone** just above the nose and **inserts** into the skin of the medial sector of the **eyebrow**. It **acts** to draw the **eyebrow medially and downward**. It is supplied by the **facial nerve** (VII) and **ophthalmic artery**.

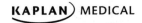

If the buccinator muscle is not working properly, food can get trapped in the cheek or vestibule. It is also pierced by Stenson's duct of the parotid gland.

The **buccinator** muscle composes the anterior section of the cheek. It **originates** from the **posterior alveolar** processes of both the **mandible** and **maxilla** as well as the **pterygomandibular raphe**. It **inserts** into orbicularis oris at the **angle** of the mouth. It **compresses** or **flattens** the cheek and is **innervated** by the **facial nerve** (VII). Blood is supplied by the **facial artery**. It **acts** in conjunction with the muscles of mastication to **retract the angle** of the mouth maintaining food on the chewing surfaces of teeth during mastication.

The **orbicularis oris originates** from the median portion of the **maxilla** and by an inferior bundle from the **mandible**. It **inserts** to **surround the mouth** in the **skin** and **mucous membranes**. Its **action** is to **close** and **pucker or purse** the lips. It is innervated by the **facial nerve** (VII) and blood is supplied by the **facial artery**.

The **risorius originates** from the **platysma** and the fascia of the **masseter** muscle. It **inserts** at the orbicularis oris at the **angle** of the mouth and is **innervated** by the facial nerve (VII) and facial artery. It acts to **draw the angle of the mouth laterally to widen the mouth into a smile**.

The **zygomaticus major** muscle **originates** at the **anterior** segment of the **zygoma** and **inserts** into the muscles at the **angle of the mouth**. It is **innervated** by the **facial nerve** (VII) with blood being supplied by the **facial artery**. It acts to **draw** the **upper lip superiorly** and **laterally** into a smile.

The **zygomaticus minor** muscle **originates** at the **posterior** segment of the **zygoma** and inserts into the orbicularis oris of the upper lip. It is **innervated** by the facial nerve (VII). Blood is supplied by the **facial artery**. It acts to draw the **upper lip upward and outward**.

The **levator labii superioris** muscle **originates** from the **maxilla** inferior to the infraorbital foramen. It **inserts** into the orbicularis oris of the **upper lip** and is **innervated** by the **facial nerve** (VII). The facial artery supplies blood. It acts to **elevate the upper lip**. The **levator labii superioris alaeque nasi** muscle originates at the nasal process of the **maxilla** and **inserts** into the wing of the **nose** and orbicularis oris of the **upper lip**. It is **innervated** by the **facial nerve** (VII) with blood being supplied by the **facial artery**. It acts to **elevate the upper lip** and **nose** as if snorting.

The **levator anguli oris** muscle **originates** in the **maxilla** at the canine fossa and **inserts** into the orbicularis oris and skin at the **angle of the mouth**. It is **innervated** by the **facial nerve** (VII) with blood supplied by the **facial artery**. It acts to raise the angle of the mouth when **smiling**.

Depressor anguli oris muscle **originates** in the lower anterior border of the **mandible** and **inserts** into the other muscles of the **lower lip** near the angle of the mouth. It is **innervated** by the **facial nerve** (VII). The **facial artery** supplies blood. It acts to **depress the lower lip** at the angle.

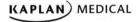

Depressor labii inferioris muscle **originates** at the lower anterior border of the **mandible** and **inserts** into the orbicularis oris muscles of the **lower lip**. It is **innervated** by the **facial nerve** (VII). The **facial artery** supplies blood. It acts to **depress the lower lip** downward and laterally.

The **mentalis** muscle **originates** in the **mandible** at the incisor fossa and **inserts** into the skin of the **chin** and acts to **elevate the chin**. It is innervated by the **facial nerve** (VII).

The **platysma** muscle **originates** from the superficial fascia of the deltoid and **pectoral muscles** as it passes over the clavicles upward and **inserts** into the lower border of the **mandible** and **facial muscles**. It is innervated by the **facial nerve** (VII). The **superficial arteries** supply the blood.

Muscles of Mastication

The buccinator muscle is *not* a true muscle of mastication, but it does aid in maintaining food between the teeth during chewing. If it is not working properly, then food may become trapped in the vestibule.

The **masseter** muscle is the largest and strongest of the muscles of mastication. It **originates** at several places of the **zygomatic arch**. The superficial origins are at the zygomatic process of the maxilla and the inferior border of the zygomatic arch. The other origins are at the inner and posterior, inferior borders of the zygomatic arch. It **inserts** superficially at the **lateral** surface of the **mandible**, and deeply at the **ramus** and coronoid process of the **mandible**. It is innervated by the **masseteric nerve** of the **trigeminal nerve** (V3). The **masseteric artery** supplies blood. The masseter muscle functions to **close or elevate** the mandible to centric occlusion.

The lateral pterygoid muscle has two heads. The **superior head of the lateral pterygoid** muscle **originates** from the greater wing of the **sphenoid bone** and **inserts** with the **articular disc** of the TMJ and anterior **condyle**. The **inferior head of the lateral pterygoid** muscle **originates** from the lateral pterygoid plate of the **sphenoid bone** and **inserts** at the anterior **condyle**. It is **innervated** by the **mandibular division** of the **trigeminal nerve** (V3) with blood being supplied by the **maxillary artery**. Its function is to **open** and **protrude** the mandible. If only one side is functioning, then the mandible will deviate away from the functioning side.

The **medial pterygoid** muscle **originates** at the medial surface of the pterygoid fossa of the **sphenoid bone**. It **inserts** at the medial surface of the **ramus** of the mandible. It is **innervated** by the **mandibular division** of the **trigeminal nerve** (V3). The **maxillary artery** supplies the blood. It functions to raise the jaw **by elevating** the mandible.

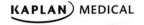

The **temporalis** muscle **originates** at the temporal fossa of the **temporal bone** and inserts at the **coronoid** process of the **mandible**. It is **innervated** by the **mandibular division** of the **trigeminal nerve** (V3). The **temporal artery** supplies the blood. It functions to **elevate** the jaw, but also **retracts** the mandible if only the posterior segment contracts.

Posterior Cervical Muscles

Important in a patient's extra-oral exam is the inspection of the trapezius and the sternocleidomastoid muscles, the posterior cervical muscles that support the head. The paired **trapezius** muscles join the shoulders with the head. This superficial, irregular, four-sided muscle extends from the skull to the lower thorax. It **originates** at the base of the skull at the **occipital bone** and from the **7th cervical to the 12th thoracic vertebrae**. The trapezius **inserts** at the lateral one third of the **clavicle** and **scapula**. The action that the trapezius performs is to shrug the shoulders. It is **innervated** by the **accessory nerve** (XI) and **third** and **fourth cervical nerves**. The **transverse cervical artery** supplies it with blood.

The **sternocleidomastoid muscle** (SCM) is an important muscle for palpating the lymph nodes of the head and neck. The SCM **originates** at the **medial portion of the clavicle and sternum**. It **inserts** at the **mastoid process** of the temporal bone. The **action** result of the SCM is as follows: If **both** muscles contract **simultaneously**, the neck will **flex the head forward**. If **one contracts**, it bends the **head in that direction**. The SCM is **innervated** by the **accessory nerve** (XI) with blood supplied by the **occipital artery** and **superior thyroid artery**.

Suprahyoid Neck Muscles

The **digastric** muscle has an anterior and posterior belly. The **anterior belly originates** from the **intermediate tendon** of the **hyoid bone** and **inserts** at the symphysis of the mandible. The **posterior belly originates** from the mastoid notch of the **temporal bone** and **inserts** at the **intermediate tendon** of the **hyoid bone**. The **inferior alveolar** division of the **trigeminal nerve** (V3) innervates the anterior belly while the **facial nerve** (VII) innervates the **posterior belly**. The **lingual** and **facial arteries** supply blood to the digastric muscle. It functions to **elevate** the **hyoid** when the mandible is fixed and **depresses the mandible** when the hyoid is fixed.

The **geniohyoid muscle originates** at the inferior mental spine or **genial tubercules** of the mandible and **inserts** into the **hyoid bone**. It functions to **raise the tongue** and **depress or open the mandible**. It is innervated by the **hypoglossal nerve** (XII). The lingual artery supplies the blood.

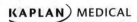

The **mylohyoid** muscle **originates** at the mylohyoid line on the inner surface of the **mandible** and **inserts** into the **hyoid bone**. It functions to **elevate the tongue and depress the mandible**. The **mylohyoid nerve** branch of the mandibular nerve from the **trigeminal nerve (V3) innervates** the mylohyoid muscle. The **lingual artery** supplies blood to it.

The **stylohyoid** muscle **originates** at the styloid process of the **temporal bone** and **inserts** into the body of the **hyoid bone**. It functions to **elevate** and **retract** the **hyoid bone** during swallowing. It is **innervated** by the **facial nerve** (VII) with blood being supplied by the **facial artery**.

Infrahyoid Neck Muscles

The inferior belly of the **omohyoid muscle** starts at the upper border of the scapula and attaches into the superior belly by a tendon. The superior belly of the omohyoid muscle, too, originates at that same tendon attachment of the inferior belly, and then inserts into the body of the hyoid bone. It is innervated by the ansa cervicalis (loop in the cervical plexus) with blood supplied by the thyroid artery. The omohyoid muscle functions to depress the hyoid bone.

The **sternohyoid** muscle originates at the first segment of the **sternum** and **inserts** into the body of the **hyoid bone**. It is innervated by the ansa cervicalis with blood supplied by the **thyroid artery**. It functions to **depress** the **larynx** and **hyoid bone**.

The **sternothyroid** muscle originates at the manubrium of the **sternum** and the first intercostal cartilage and **inserts** into the **thyroid cartilage**. It is innervated by the ansa cervicalis with blood supplied by the **thyroid artery**. Its purpose is to **draw** the **larynx downward** as it **depresses** the **thyroid cartilage**.

The **thyrohyoid** muscle **originates** at the **thyroid cartilage** and **inserts** into the body and greater horn of the **hyoid bone**. It is innervated by the first cervical spine nerve (C1) with blood supplied by the **thyroid artery**. It functions to **depress** the **hyoid bone** and **elevate** the **thyroid cartilage**.

Muscles of the Pharynx

Pharyngeal constrictors break into three groups: inferior, middle, and superior. The **inferior** constrictor **originates** at the **cricoid** and **thyroid cartilages**. The **middle** constrictors **originate** from the **greater horn** of the **hyoid bone**. The **superior** constrictor originates from the **hamulus** of the **medial pterygoid plate** and **pterygomandibular raphe**. They join together to **insert** as one into the **median pharyngeal raphe** at the **occipital** bone. These muscles are innervated by the **pharyngeal plexus** with blood being supplied by the **pharyngeal arteries**. The **superior** constrictor **narrows** the pharynx during **swallowing** while the **inferior** and **middle** constrictors move the food bolus along by **peristalsis**.

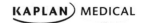

The **stylopharyngeus** muscle **originates** at the styloid process of the **temporal bone** and **inserts** into the **superior** and **middle constrictor muscles** of the pharyngeal wall. It is the *only* pharyngeal muscle to be innervated by the **glossopharyngeal nerve** (IX). The **pharyngeal arteries** supply blood. Its function is to **elevate** and **enlarge** the **pharynx** during swallowing.

Muscles of the Tongue

Ventral is underneath. Dorsal is on the top or toward the back. Think of the dorsal fin of a shark that you see skimming the top of water.

The **intrinsic** muscles **originate** and **insert within** the **tongue** itself and are named for their location within the tongue. They include both the inferior and superior longitudinal muscles as well as the transverse and vertical muscles. The **ventral, inferior longitudinal** muscle runs in a **longitudinal** or lengthwise direction from the **base of the tongue to the tip** of the tongue. The **dorsal, superior longitudinal** muscle also runs **longitudinally** or lengthwise from the **base to the tip** of the tongue.

The **transverse** muscle lies beneath the superior longitudinal muscle and **goes across** the tongue from the **median septum** to the **lateral borders** of the tongue. The **vertical** muscles travel vertically or from the dorsal (**top**) surface to the ventral (**bottom**) surface. These muscles are innervated by the **hypoglossal nerve (CN XII)** with blood being supplied by the **lingual artery.**

The **extrinsic** tongue muscles include genioglossus, hyoglossus, and styloglossus and are also supplied by the **lingual artery** and innervated by the **hypoglossal nerve.** Their names reveal their place of origin.

The **genioglossus** muscle originates at the **genial tubercules** (mental spine) of the mandible and **insert** into **hyoid bone** and **muscle fibers** of the tongue. It **protrudes** and **depresses** the tongue.

The **hyoglossus** muscle **originates** at the greater wing of the **hyoid** bone and inserts into the **sides** or **lateral borders** of the **tongue.** It functions to **depress** the tongue.

The **styloglossus** originates at the **styloid process** of the temporal bone and inserts at the **lateral borders** and **undersurface** of the tongue. It functions to **retract** the tongue.

Muscles of the Palate

The **levator veli palatini** muscle that lies mostly in the **soft palate originates** at **temporal bone** and medial rim of the **auditory tube.** It inserts at the **palatine aponeurosis** (fibers that pass into a tendon) at the midline of the palate. The LVP **is innervated** for **sensation** by the **pharyngeal** branch of the **vagus nerve** (X) and with **motor** function by the **accessory nerve** (XI). The **greater palatine artery** supplies blood. Its function is to **elevate** and **retract** the soft palate.

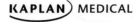

The **palatoglossus** muscle originates from the **soft palate**. It inserts in the posterolateral surface of the **tongue** forming part of the **palatoglossus arch**. The pharyngeal plexus innervates it with blood being supplied by the **greater palatine artery** and **ascending palatine arteries**. The palatoglossus works along with the extrinsic muscles of the tongue to **elevate** the back of the **tongue**.

The **palatopharyngeus** muscle originates at the **palatine aponeurosis** and inserts into the posterior border of the **thyroid cartilage**. It is innervated for sensory by the **vagus nerve** (X) from the **pharyngeal plexus** and motor by the **accessory nerve** (XI). Blood is supplied by the **greater palatine artery** and **ascending palatine arteries**.

The **tensor veli palatini** muscle originates at the **sphenoid bone** and **eustachian tube**. It then **loops** around the **pterygoid hamulus** to utilize it as a **pulley** before it **inserts** in the border of the **hard palate** at the palatine **aponeurosis**. The TVP is **innervated** by the **medial pterygoid nerve**. The **greater palatine artery** supplies the blood. Its function is to **tense** the **soft palate** which then opens the eustachian tube.

GLANDS OF THE HEAD AND NECK

Glands of the head and neck have two roles: First, to aid in digestion with the major and minor salivary glands (exocrine glands). Second, to strengthen the immune system to defend the body from invading pathogens (lymph nodes).

Major Salivary Glands

The **largest** salivary gland is the **parotid gland**. As an **encapsulated** gland, the parotid is located on the surface of the masseter muscle in the cheek. It sits behind the ramus of the mandible where it lies anteriorly and inferiorly to the ear. Its **serous fluid** provides only 25% of the total saliva volume.

This secretion passes out of the gland by way of **Stenson's duct**. It is innervated for the parasympathetic increased flow of saliva by the **glossopharyngeal nerve** (IX) and for afferent by the auriculotemporal branch of the **trigeminal nerve** (V). Lymph drainage occurs in the deep parotid lymph nodes.

The second largest salivary gland is the **submandibular gland**, also an **encapsulated** gland that lies in the submandibular fossa below the angle of the mandible. It produces 60 to 65% of the total saliva volume, that is **mixed secretions** of both serous and mucous fluids. Secretions pass out of this gland by way of **Wharton's duct**, which empties into the oral cavity at the sublingual caruncle or eminence on

Sublingual caruncles are the bilateral eminences on either side of the lingual frenum.

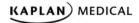

each side of the frenum of the tongue. It is innervated by the chorda tympani and submandibular ganglion of the **facial nerve** (VII). Lymph drainage occurs in the submandibular lymph nodes.

The **smallest** major salivary gland is the **sublingual gland**, which is **not encapsulated**. It lies in the sublingual fossa of the anterior floor of the mouth near the symphysis. It produces both serous and mucous or **mixed secretion** of about 10% of the total saliva volume. Secretions pass out of the gland by way of **Bartholin's duct**, and join Wharton's duct of the submandibular gland at the sublingual caruncle. The sublingual gland has the same innervation as the submandibular gland, that is the chorda tympani and submandibular ganglion of the **facial nerve** (VII). Lymph drainage also occurs in the submandibular lymph nodes.

Minor Salivary Glands

The **minor salivary glands** are too numerous to name and are located on the buccal mucosa, labial mucosa, lingual mucosa, and soft and lateral portions of the hard palate. They are exocrine glands that produce mixed or **mucous secretions**. Other minor salivary glands called **von Ebner's glands** are located alongside the circumvallate papillae of the tongue on the dorsal posterior surface. They secrete **serous saliva**.

Minor types of salivary glands are innervated by the **facial nerve** (VII). Their lymph drainage is dependent on their location.

Lymph Glands of the Head and Neck

The lymph system contains glands that play an important role in our immune system to defend the body from invading pathogens. It has the ability to quickly release lymphocytes into circulation to fight disease. This system also maintains a constant environment with fluid balance, returns excess interstitial fluid to blood, and aids in the absorption of lipids in the intestines. It is composed of lymph nodes and lymph vessels.

Lymph nodes are bean shaped clusters containing lymphocytes to fight invading pathogens. They have the ability to filter out invading organisms from lymph fluid. **Lymph vessels** are small tubules that run throughout the body carrying white blood cells to fight infection. **Lymph fluid** is a clear fluid that travels throughout the lymph system that contains the lymphocytes.

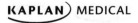

Tonsils

The tonsils are a part of the lymph system and contain a large amount of lymphoid tissue. Their job is to filter invading antigens whether bacterial or viral. The **tonsils drain into the superior deep cervical nodes.**

The **palatine tonsils** are prominent masses of lymphoid tissue located between anterior and posterior tonsillar pillars. The **lingual tonsils** are located at the base or pharyngeal aspect of the dorsal surface of the tongue. The **pharyngeal tonsils**— formerly know as the **adenoids**—are located on the posterior wall of the pharynx. The **tubal tonsils** are located near the pharyngeal opening of the eustachian tubes.

Lymphadenopathy is swollen, diseased lymph glands.

Lymph Nodes of the Head

The **facial lymph nodes** have many branches. All drain into the **submandibular lymph nodes.** The **malar lymph nodes** drain the malar or zygomatic areas in the infraorbital areas of the face. The **nasolabial lymph nodes**, located near the nose, drain its skin and mucous membranes. The **buccal lymph nodes**, located superficial to the buccinator muscle, drain that area. The **mandibular lymph nodes** lie anterior to the masseter muscle and drain the skin and mucous membranes in that area.

Deep parotid lymph nodes are deep lymph nodes of the head, located deep in the parotid gland. They drain the auditory tube, middle ear, and parotid gland, then into the superior deep cervical lymph nodes. **Retropharyngeal lymph nodes** are a deep lymph node of the head and are also located in the parotid gland area. They drain the nasal cavity, paranasal sinuses, palate, and pharynx. They then drain into the superior deep cervical nodes.

The **occipital lymph nodes** are located near the occipital artery and drain the posterior scalp and adjacent neck areas. They drain into the inferior deep cervical lymph nodes.

The **auricular lymph nodes** drain the anterior portion of the ear. Along with the retroauricular and superficial parotid lymph nodes, the auricular lymph nodes drain into the superior deep cervical nodes.

The **retroauricular lymph nodes** located near the mastoid process drain the posterior auricle or ear and adjacent scalp. The **superficial parotid lymph nodes** are located in the parotid region and drain the external ear and adjacent scalp.

Cervical Lymph Nodes

The **submental lymph nodes** are located at the midline of the chin superficial to the mylohyoid muscle. They drain the apex of the tongue, lower lip, and mandibular anterior mouth including incisors. They empty into the submandibular nodes or

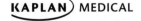

deep cervical nodes. The **submandibular lymph nodes** are located between the mandible and submandibular gland near the angle of the mandible. They drain the maxillary teeth, maxillary sinuses, mandibular canines and mandibular posterior teeth **except** for the mandibular third molars. They also drain the anterior nasal cavity, hard palate, the floor of the mouth, tongue, sublingual salivary gland, submandibular salivary gland, and cheek.

The **external jugular lymph nodes** are located alongside the external jugular vein and receive drainage from the anterior auricular node, retroauricular nodes, occipital nodes, and superficial parotid nodes.

The **anterior jugular lymph nodes** are located alongside the anterior jugular vein and receive drainage from the infrahyoid vicinity of the cervical area. The **superior deep cervical lymph nodes** are located lateral to the internal jugular vein, but beneath the sternocleidomastoid muscle, and drain the maxillary third molar area, posterior nasal cavity, posterior hard palate, soft palate, and base of the tongue.

The **inferior deep cervical lymph nodes** are also located lateral to the internal jugular vein and deeper beneath the sternocleidomastoid muscle. They drain the posterior scalp and base of the neck.

SINUSES

The paranasal sinuses are mucous-lined airspaces in the bones of the skull that communicate with the nasal cavity but whose function is not entirely understood. The paired **frontal sinuses** are located in the frontal bone superior to the orbit of the eye. They drain the middle nasal meatus.

The **largest** sinuses are the paired **maxillary sinuses** located in the maxilla. Superiorly they form the floor of the orbit, and medially they form the lateral wall of the nose. Due to their close proximity to the maxillary teeth, maxillary tooth symptoms may occur. They drain the middle meatus. The **ethmoid sinus** is situated on either side of the ethmoid bone and drain the superior meatus. The **sphenoid sinuses** are irregular cavities in the sphenoid bone and drain the superior nasal meatus.

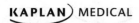

REVIEW QUESTIONS

1. In oral anatomy, which of the following dental terms describes the bone that forms a ridge over the maxillary canines?

    A. Canine fossa

    B. Canine eminence

    C. Infraorbital rim

    D. Palatine process

    E. Frontal process

2. Cranial nerves can have afferent or efferent functions. The hypoglossal nerve controls the efferent motor function of all the following tongue muscles EXCEPT:

    A. Genioglossus

    B. Styloglossus

    C. Palatoglossus

    D. Geniohyoidus

3. Which of the following cranial nerves innervates the muscles of facial expression?

    A. V

    B. VII

    C. X

    D. XI

    E. XII

4. The skull has many foramina but the maxillary division of the trigeminal nerve exits through which of the following?

    A. Magnum

    B. Spinosum

    C. Lacerum

    D. Ovale

    E. Rotundum

5. The muscle that originates in the medial side of the lateral pterygoid plate of the sphenoid bone and inserts in the pterygoid fovea of the mandible is the

    A. Buccinator

    B. Masseter

    C. Medial pterygoid

    D. Lateral pterygoid

    E. Levatur anguli oris

6. There are several cranial nerves that supply afferent and efferent stimulation to and from the eye. The cranial nerve responsible for constricting eye pupils is

    A. Optic nerve

    B. Occulomotor nerve

    C. Abducent nerve

    D. Trochlear nerve

7. A patient arrives with an abscess to tooth #1. An infection of the maxillary third molars area drains principally into which of the following lymph nodes?

    A. Retroauricular nodes

    B. Superior deep cervical

    C. Submandibular and facial nodes

    D. Submental nodes

    E. External jugular nodes

8. The hyoid bone articulates with which of the following?

    A. Second cervical vertebra

    B. Hyaline cartilage

    C. Ethmoid bone

    D. None of the above

9. Trigeminal neuralgia can be very painful. Which of the following nerves is affected by trigeminal neuralgia?

   A. Cranial nerve V

   B. Cranial nerve VI

   C. Cranial nerve VII

   D. Cranial nerve X

   E. Cranial nerve III

10. Of the 12 cranial nerves, which one is the longest nerve in the body?

    A. Trigeminal (V)

    B. Trochlear (IV)

    C. Spinal accessory (XI)

    D. Abducen (VI)

    E. Vagus (X)

11. The temporomandibular joint opens by translation of the condylar head as it depresses or elevates the mandible. It also works by rotation of the condyle and meniscus, as it allows the mandible to move forward or backward.

    A. Both statements are true.

    B. The first statement is true. The second statement is false because the condyle works by translation to depress or elevate the mandible.

    C. The first statement is false because rotation moves the mandible backward and forward. The second statement is true.

    D. Both statements are false because the condylar head uses rotation to depress and elevate the mandible. The joint also works by translation or gliding of the condyle and meniscus to protrude the mandible back and forth.

12. Cranial nerves can function as sensory, motor, or both. Which of the following cranial nerves is responsible for motor movement only of the tongue?

    A. Hypoglossal (XII)

    B. Glossopharyngeal (IX)

    C. Abducent (VI)

    D. Trigeminal (V)

    E. Facial (VII)

13. The bones of the skull have many foramina. Which of the following bones contains the foramen ovale, foramen rotundum, and superior orbital fissure?

    A. Vomer

    B. Occipital

    C. Sphenoid

    D. Ethmoid

    E. Temporal

14. Stenson's duct of the parotid gland passes through which of the following facial muscles?

    A. Masseter

    B. Medial pterygoid

    C. Lateral pterygoid

    D. Buccinator

15. The submandibular gland is an encapsulated gland that is innervated by the facial nerve (VII). It produces serous secretions that exit the gland by way of Bartholin's duct.

    A. Both statements are true.

    B. The first statement is true. The second statement is false because the duct is Wharton's duct with mixed secretions.

    C. The first statement is false because the gland is not encapsulated and nerve innervation is by the trigeminal nerve (V).

    D. Both statements are false. The submandibular gland is not encapsulated; it is innervated by the glossopharyngeal (IX) nerve, the secretions are mixed only and the duct is the duct of Rivinus.

16. The tongue can perform many functions. Which of the following tongue muscles retracts the tongue?

    A. Styloglossus
    B. Hyoglossus
    C. Genioglossus
    D. Palatoglossus
    E. None of the above

17. Many important arteries pass through the neck en route to supplying the head with oxygen. The artery that supplies blood to the brain is

    A. Facial artery
    B. Maxillary artery
    C. Temporal artery
    D. External carotid artery
    E. Internal carotid artery

18. The masseter muscle originates at _____ and inserts at _____.

    A. Zygomatic arch, lateral surface of the mandible at the ramus & coronoid process
    B. Medial surface of the pterygoid fossa of the sphenoid bone, ramus of the mandible
    C. Temporal fossa of the temporal bone, coronoid process of the mandible
    D. Posterior alveolar process of the mandible & maxilla, orbicularis oris at the angle of the mouth

19. Nerves are protected by

    A. Tunica intermedia
    B. Neurilemma
    C. Myelin sheath
    D. Dendrite

20. Which of the following is a kind of natural passageway other than a canal?

    A. Fossa
    B. Col
    C. Pedicle
    D. Meatus
    E. Placode

21. The V2 division of the maxillary nerve division includes all the following branches EXCEPT

    A. Greater palatine nerve
    B. Buccal nerve
    C. Middle superior alveolar nerve
    D. Infraorbital nerve
    E. Middle meningeal nerve

22. The orbicularis oculi muscle encircles which of the following structures?

    A. Mouth
    B. Ear
    C. Eye
    D. None of the above

23. Veins carry deoxygenated blood back to the heart. The internal jugular vein that exits the skull through the jugular foramen drains blood from all the following structures EXCEPT

    A. Pharynx
    B. Brain
    C. Facial area
    D. Palatal tonsils
    E. Exterior cranium

24. The lingual nerve conveys afferent sensation for all the following EXCEPT

    A. Floor of the mouth
    B. Anterior two thirds of the tongue
    C. Posterior one third of the tongue
    D. Mandibular lingual gingival surfaces

25. Nerve supply to the maxillary first molar includes all of the following nerves EXCEPT

    A. Middle superior alveolar
    B. Posterior superior alveolar
    C. Lesser palatine
    D. Greater palatine

KAPLAN) MEDICAL

ANSWER EXPLANATIONS

1. B

The bone that forms the ridge over the maxillary canines is the canine eminence.

A. The canine fossa is a depression in the bone.

C. The infraorbital rim is bone that forms the floor of the orbit by the zygoma and maxilla.

D. Palatine processes are the two palatal bones that fuse to form the anterior hard palate.

E. The frontal process articulates with the frontal bone and lacrimal bones in the maxilla.

2. C

The palatoglossus muscle is controlled by the vagus nerve (X).

3. B

The facial nerve (VII) innervates the muscles of facial expression.

A. V is the trigeminal nerve that innervates muscles of mastication.

C. X is the vagus nerve that innervates muscles of soft palate, pharynx, larynx.

D. XI is the accessory nerve that innervates the muscles of the trapezius, sternocleidomastoid, soft palate, and pharynx.

E. XII is the hypoglossal nerve that innervates muscles of the tongue for movement.

4. E

The maxillary division of the trigeminal nerve exits through the foramen rotundum.

A. The spinal cord exits through the foramen magnum, located in the occipital bone.

B. Meningeal vessels pass through the foramen spinosum, in the sphenoid bone.

D. The mandibular division of the trigeminal nerve passes through the foramen ovale.

5. D

The muscle referred to is the lateral pterygoid.

A. Buccinator originates on maxilla, mandible, and pterygomandibular raphe, inserts at the angle of the mouth.

B. Masseter originates at the zygomatic arch, inserts on the lateral surface of the angle of the mandible.

E. Levatur anguli oris originates at the maxillary canine fossa and inserts into the angle of the mouth.

6. A

The optic nerve constricts (and dilates) the pupil.

B. The occulomotor nerve controls eyeball movement with muscle contraction.

C. The abducent nerve supplies motor movement to the lateral eyeball.

D. The trochlear nerve supplies motor movement to one muscle of the eye.

7. B

An infection of the maxillary third molars area drains principally into the superior deep cervical nodes. These same nodes also drain the hard and soft palates, base of the tongue, and tissues of the trachea and thyroid.

A. Retroauricular nodes drain the ear and ear region.

C. Submandibular nodes drain maxillary molars and premolars and associated tissues but NOT the maxillary third molars.

D. Submental nodes drain the chin, lower lip, floor of the mouth, apex of the tongue, and mandibular incisors.

E. External jugular drains the retroauricular, anterior auricular, occipital, and superficial parotid nodes.

8. **D**

The hyoid bone does not articulate with any bones.

9. **A**

Trigeminal neuralgia affects cranial nerve V. This malady used to be called Tic Doloreux.

C. Cranial nerve VII is the facial nerve that can be affected by Bell's Palsy.

D. Cranial nerve X can be affected by a vasovagal response. It can cause a patient to have a syncopal episode when he passes out.

10. **E**

The longest nerve in the body is the vagus (X).

A. The trigeminal nerve (V) is the largest nerve.

B. The trochlear nerve (IV) is the smallest nerve.

11. **D**

Both statements are false. The condylar head uses rotation to depress and elevate the mandible. The joint also works by translation or gliding of the condyle and meniscus to protrude the mandible back and forth.

12. **A**

The hypoglossal (XII) nerve controls motor movement of the tongue.

B. The glossopharyngeal (IX) is responsible for sensory detection for the posterior $\frac{1}{3}$ of the tongue.

13. **C**

The sphenoid bone contains the foramina ovale, foramen rotundum, and superior orbital fissure.

A. The vomer bone is a single bone that has no muscle attachment and no foramina.

B. The occipital bone is the single most posterior bone that contains the foramen magnum for the spinal cord.

D. The ethmoid bone is a single midline bone that forms part of the wall of the orbit of the eye.

E. The temporal bone contains foramen lacerum for the carotid artery.

14. **D**

Stenson's duct of the parotid gland passes through the buccinator muscle.

15. **B**

The first statement is true. The second statement is false because the duct is Wharton's duct with mixed secretions.

16. **A**

The styloglossus muscle retracts the tongue.

B. Hyoglossus depresses the tongue.

C. Genioglossus depresses and protrudes the tongue.

D. Palatoglossus elevates the base of the tongue.

17. **E**

The internal carotid artery supplies blood to the brain.

A. The facial artery supplies the digastric muscles, mylohyoid, submandibular lymph nodes, submandibular salivary gland, lower and upper lips, and muscles of facial expression.

B. The maxillary artery supplies blood to the floor of the mouth and the mylohyoid muscle.

C. The temporal artery supplies blood to the parotid gland and the temporalis muscle.

D. The external carotid artery supplies the thyroid, tongue, floor of the mouth, mandible, face, palate, tonsils, submandibular gland, and nose.

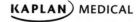
KAPLAN MEDICAL

18. A

The massester muscle originates at the zygomatic arch and inserts at the lateral surface of the mandible at the ramus and coronoid process.

B. The medial pterygoid muscle originates at the medial surface of the pterygoid fossa of the sphenoid bone and inserts at the ramus of the mandible.

C. The temporalis muscle originates at the temporal fossa of the temporal bone and inserts at the coronoid process of the mandible.

D. The buccinator muscle originates at the posterior alveolar process of the mandible and maxilla and inserts at the orbicularis oris at the angle of the mouth.

19. C

Nerves are protected by the myelin sheath.

A. Tunica intermedia is an inner layer of a blood vessel.

B. Neurilemma is the sheath covering the Schwann cell of a nerve.

D. Dendrites are projections from a nerve cell that transmit impulses to other nerves.

20. D

Other than a canal, a natural passageway is a meatus.

C. Pedicle is a narrow basal attachment on bone.

E. Placode is ectoderm involved with embryonic development of sensory organs.

21. B

Buccal nerve is the exception because it is a part of the V3 segment of the mandibular division of the trigeminal nerve.

22. C

The eye is surrounded by the obicularis oculi.

A. The mouth is surrounded by the obicularis oris.

B. The ear has two small skeletal muscles: the tensor tympani attaches to the malleus and the stapedius attaches to the stapes.

23. E

The exception is the exterior cranium, which is drained by the external jugular vein.

24. C

Posterior one third of the tongue afferent sensation is conveyed by the glossopharyngeal nerve.

25. C

The exception is the lesser palatine nerve, which conveys afferent sensation from the soft palate and palatine tonsil.

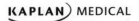

Chapter Five: **Dental Anatomy**

A dental hygienist needs to have good knowledge of the intraoral and extraoral structures of the head and neck. Oral tissue exams may reveal abnormal tissues, periodontal disease, nutritional needs, or any disorders upon which patient education and a treatment plan may be formulated.

NOMENCLATURE

Dental anatomy has its own set of nomenclature. It is essential that the dental hygienist be well-versed in all of these names, as they provide the basis for patient treatment.

- **Anatomical crown** is the whole crown from the cementoenamel junction (CEJ) to the cusp tip(s) whether or not it is fully erupted into the mouth.
- **Clinical crown** is the portion of the crown that is fully seen intraorally.
- **Abrasion** is tooth wear as a result of something other than teeth, such as biting on a pencil.
- **Attrition** is the wear from tooth to tooth contact.
- **Erosion** is wear from a chemical force such as lemon juice.
- **Line angle** stands for two surfaces on a tooth that converge such as the mesiobuccal surface or distolingual surface.
- **Point angle** is the convergence or meeting of three tooth surfaces such as mesiobucco-occlusal or distolabioincisal.

Abrasion is wear from another physical force.

Attrition = tooth to tooth wear.

Erosion is chemical wear.

TOOTH STRUCTURES

The tooth comprises different structures, with some components harder and thicker than others. Enamel, which covers the crown portion, is the hardest tissue contained in the body. Dentin makes up the bulk of the tooth structure, while cementum covers the root portion. Pulp conveys life and sensation to the tooth.

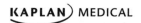
KAPLAN MEDICAL

Pulp

Pulp tissue is a soft, connective tissue derived from the dental papillae along with dentin. It is formed by the remnants of its surrounding tissues—namely, fibroblasts, and mesenchymal cells. These cells differentiate into the blood vessels and nerve tissue.

Pulp is the innermost tooth structure. The outer layer of pulp contains the odontoblastic layer, where dentin continues to grow throughout life. The **pulp chamber corresponds to the shape of the tooth.** Coronal pulp lies within the crown of a tooth. **Pulp horns extend up into cusp tips** of posterior teeth. Radicular pulp carries the nerve and blood supply from the apex of the root to the pulp chamber. The apical foramen at the apex of the tooth is where the nerve and blood supply enter into the pulp.

In the pulp, nerves diverge into small bundles that lose their myelin sheath before splitting into single axons (**subodontoblastic plexus** or **plexus of Raschkow**). These are the main fibers distributed to the pulp dentin border of the cell-free zone.

Pulp contains a cell-free zone and a cell-rich zone. The cell-free zone of Weil is located just inside the odontoblastic (subodontoblastic) layer and overlies the cell-rich zone. The cell-rich zone is a denser cellular region under the cell-free zone.

Pulp Abnormalities

Pulp can change throughout life due to the deposition of secondary and tertiary dentin. Occasionally, pulp will contain a pulp stone (lump of calcified tissue) called a **denticle. True denticles** form in the root during tooth formation and show traces of odontoblasts. **False denticles** do not show true dentin structure. Denticles can be attached, free floating, or embedded.

The purpose of pulp is to **provide nutrients** to the odontoblasts so that they can form dentin, to supply **sensory function**, and to supply **protective function** that allows for stimuli to generate secondary and reactive dentin.

Dentin

Dentin makes up the majority of the tissue tooth structure. It is derived from the neural crest cells that differentiate into the mesenchyme to then become the dental papillae. It is 70% inorganic, 18% organic, and 12% water.

Odontoblasts form dentin. **Odontoblasts** begin **dentinogenesis** by secreting **predentin** which is later mineralized into **dentin**. An **apposition** is the layer formation of the dentinal matrix. Like enamel, dentin consists of calcium hydroxyapatite crystals.

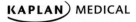

Odontoblasts start forming the dentin matrix at the DEJ as it develops inward toward the pulp. The first layer of dentin closest to the DEJ is called **mantle dentin**. It contains heavy and coarse collagen fibers called Korff's fibers. **Korff's fibers** extend from fibroblasts toward the inner enamel epithelium, forming bundles that make up the dentin matrix.

Circumpupal dentin makes up the remainder of the dentin. It is deposited as thin fibrils. **Primary dentin** is formed until the root is completely formed at the apex. **Secondary dentin** is more calcified, and forms in response to stimuli after the root is complete. It is black in color. Unlike enamel, dentin forms throughout life.

Secondary dentin is black.

Globular dentin is the completion of the crystalline fusion of dentin matrix. **Interglobular dentin** is dentin matrix that formed imperfectly between calcified globules under the DEJ. **Intertubular dentin** is found between the dentinal tubules; though highly mineralized, it is less mineralized than peritubular dentin.

Peritubular dentin is highly calcified dentin that surrounds the odontoblastic process. **Reactive, reparative, or tertiary dentin** is irregular, secondary dentin that forms in response to pathological stimuli.

Sclerotic or **transparent dentin** occurs when the dentinal tubules calcify to produce a translucency. **Tomes' granular layer** is dentin matrix that forms imperfect globules found under the CEJ. As dentin develops inward, the odontoblasts leave behind tiny tunnels called **odontoblastic processes**. These processes are live tissue called dentinal tubules, where fluid can pass in and out. It is believed that tooth sensitivity is transmitted in these tubules. In an S-shape, each tubule traverses the dentin from the DEJ to the pulp tissue. This S-shape can be primary or secondary.

The **primary S-shape curve** is a larger S and reflects the movement of crowded odontoblasts. The **secondary S-shape** curve is a smaller S, seen in the length of the enamel. Patients with higher tubule density have teeth that are more sensitive. **Imbrication lines of von Ebner** are dark incremental lines in mature dentin.

Dentin Abnormalities

Denticles are true denticles if they developed during root formation. They are round or ovoid in structure, and have dentinal tubules. False denticles develop during pulp degeneration and calcify into irregular masses that don't contain dentinal tubules or show true dentin in their structure. Denticles may be free-floating and surrounded by pulp tissue, or they may adhere to the pulp chamber.

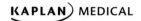

Enamel

Enamel is the hardest tissue substance in the body. It is 95% inorganic, 1% organic, and 4% water. It has a higher percentage of calcium hydroxyapatite than does dentin.

It takes 4 ameloblasts to form 1 enamel rod.

Enamel is generated by the **ameloblasts** of the **inner enamel epithelium** derived from **ectodermal tissue**. Ameloblasts are hexagonal, tall, columnar cells. During the apposition stage of enamel development, it takes four ameloblasts to form one enamel rod.

Tomes' process is the finger-like projection of the ameloblasts during the **secretory phase** of amelogenesis, when enamel matrix is deposited. Apposition begins at the incisal/occlusal surface with the secretory phase, and is followed by the **maturation stage**. Maturation occurs as enamel matrix mineralizes, when hydroxyapatite crystals are deposited.

Enamel rods or prisms that make up the crystalline structure of enamel are dictated by Tomes' process, which determines their shape. The head of an enamel rod is formed by one ameloblast that also contributes to the tail formed by the three other ameloblasts. The heads and tails of enamel rods are keyhole shaped. They are stacked in perpendicular rows that interlock at the keyhole-shaped head and tail. The tail of one enamel rod interlocks with the heads of two other rods.

Each enamel rod extends from the DEJ to the outer surface of the enamel; its length is dependent on its location. The meeting of dentin and enamel at the **DEJ** is a **scallop shape**, which allows for better adherence to each other.

The **lines or stripes of Retzius** are bands that indicate there may have been a gradual change in enamel production. The concentric rings resemble the rings of a tree. **Imbrication** lines that are raised surfaces and **perikymata** that are grooves are associated with the lines of Retzius.

The **bands** of **Hunter-Schreger** represent alternating light and dark bands in enamel. These run perpendicular from the DEJ, ending just before the surface of the enamel. They are curved lines running parallel to the surface as a result of the optical effects of light. **Enamel lamellae** are weakened areas of enamel that were not totally calcified. They extend from the DEJ to the surface of the enamel. **Enamel spindles** occur when dentin production by odontoblasts cross over into enamel before enamel has a chance to mature.

Enamel tufts are weakened areas of partially calcified enamel that extend from the DEJ to a short distance in the enamel. **Reduced enamel epithelium** (REE) occurs when the secretory phase of amelogenesis ceases and ameloblasts shrink from columnar to cuboidal cells to become a thin layer covering enamel. It includes ame-

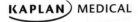

loblasts and stratum intermedium layers. The REE can become part of **Nasmyth's membrane** which can stain green on newly erupted teeth.

Enamel Abnormalities

Enamel hypocalcification describes a defect in the mineralization of formed enamel matrix. It is softer under-calcified enamel that is yellow–dark brown in color. **Enamel hypoplasia** is a deficient amount of enamel. It is harder in content but has a thinner matrix layer that is also yellow–dark brown. Enamel appears to be pitted. It is caused by trauma, high fever, or too much fluoride.

Enamel pearls form when the ameloblasts create an excess of enamel. They usually form at the CEJ of bifurcated teeth near furcations. **Mottled enamel** is caused by ingesting too much fluoride, whether from too much fluoridated water or too much prescription fluoride. The enamel formed becomes hypoplastic and appears white and chalky.

Cementum

Cementum is part of the periodontium. It is calcified connective tissue covering the root and is the mode of attachment to alveolar bone. It is 65% inorganic, 23% organic, and 12% water. It is derived from the dental sac which is derived from the mesenchyme. Cementum is produced by **cementoblasts**.

> Mesenchyme = Dental sac = PAC = **P**eriodontal ligament, **A**veolar bone, **C**ementum

The **shape of the root** is determined by **Hertwig's root sheath** which is generated from the **cervical loop** of the enamel organ. As Hertwig's root sheath grows apically to reach its entire length, it starts to disintegrate into the **epithelial rest of Malassez**. After the odontoblasts form root dentin, cementogenesis occurs when cells from the mesenchyme of the dental sac differentiate into cementoblasts. Cementoblasts deposit intrinsic collagen fibers that run parallel to the long axis of the tooth as well as **Sharpey's fibers** which insert at a 90-degree angle with the tooth. **Sharpey's fibers** are the mode of attachment for the periodontal ligament.

> Cementum (65% inorganic) is the dentinal tissue that most resembles bone, which is 60% inorganic.

Acellular cementum forms a thin layer more slowly over the coronal portion of the root and does not contain any embedded cementocytes. **Cellular cementum** is deposited at the apical portion of the tooth at a more rapid rate and in layers. Cellular cementum contains embedded cementocytes. Cellular cementum **forms throughout life** at the **apical third of the cementum where it is thickest**. It is thinnest at the cementoenamel junction (CEJ).

The CEJ can meet in three different ways. In most cases, the cementum overlaps the enamel. The other configurations are they meet end to end or the cementum falls shy of meeting the enamel, leaving a gap.

> The dental hygienist must be able to discern the CEJ and not mistake it for calculus.

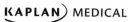

The root has the ability to **resorb** itself with occlusal force trauma or with orthodontic treatment but it also has the ability to redeposit cementum and repair itself.

Cementum Abnormalities

Cemental spurs found near the CEJ are excessive symmetrical masses of cementum. **Cementicles** are small abnormal calcified masses found in the periodontal ligament. They can be adherent to the cementum or free-floating in the periodontal ligament. **Hypercementosis or cemental hyperplasia** is the excessive buildup of secondary cementum on the root surface. It commonly occurs at the apical two thirds of the tooth.

PERMANENT DENTITION

Maxillary Arch

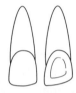

Maxillary Central Incisor

The **maxillary central incisor** is the most prominent tooth in the maxillary arch, and erupts at the age of 7 or 8. It is the largest anterior tooth mesiodistally. The two central incisors contact each other mesially at the incisal third, and then contact the lateral incisor at the middle and incisal thirds. Mamelons are present with eruption. The distoincisal contour is rounder than the mesioincisal. Its root shape is conical.

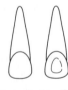

Maxillary Lateral Incisor

The maxillary lateral incisor's lingual groove may extend onto the root surface, making it harder to root plane. This tooth is the most likely tooth to have a lingual pit.

The **maxillary lateral incisor** usually resembles the central incisor but can also have many variations. It erupts at 8–9 years of age. The lingual fossa of the maxillary lateral is deeper with a more **prominent cingulum** than the maxillary central. This area may have a **lingual pit** or **lingual groove** that may extend onto the root. The mesial aspect meets the distal of the central incisor at the junction of the middle and incisal thirds. The distal aspect contacts the canine at the middle third. Its root shape is conical.

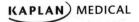

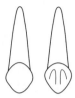

Maxillary Canine

The **maxillary canine** is the longest tooth in the mouth and has the longest root in the maxillary arch. It erupts at 11–12 years of age. It is considered the **cornerstone** of the mouth. It has a more prominent cingulum on the lingual aspect than the incisors with a mesial and lingual fossa separated by a lingual ridge. Its prominent cusp tip is centered with the root. The mesial aspect contacts the distal of the lateral incisor at the middle and incisal thirds. The distal aspect contacts the first premolar at the middle third. Its root shape is ovoid with a blunt apex.

The last succedaneous tooth to erupt is the maxillary canine.

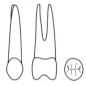

Maxillary First Premolar

The **maxillary first premolar** has two cusps with the buccal cusp being the larger. It erupts at 10–11 years of age. It has a very **prominent concavity** on the **mesial aspect** that is called a **development depression**. The distal aspect does not have a concavity. The hexagon-shaped occlusal surface has a buccal and lingual transverse ridge. The mesial aspect contacts the distal of the canine at the occlusal and middle thirds. The distal aspect contacts the mesial of the second bicuspid at the middle and occlusal thirds. It has a bifurcated root with two canals. If there is only one root present, there are still usually two canals.

A developmental depression or concavity on the maxillary first premolar can be mistaken for a carious lesion, as it is also an area that floss will not get into. It is more difficult to scale and root plane a concavity.

Maxillary Second Premolar

The **maxillary second premolar** resembles a first premolar except for the shape of the crown. It erupts at 10–12 years of age. It does not have a concavity on either the mesial or distal aspect. The occlusal aspect is rounder than the first premolar. The mesial aspect contacts the distal of the first premolar at the occlusal and middle thirds. The distal aspect contacts the first molar at the occlusal and middle thirds. The root is a single root and is elliptical.

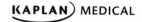

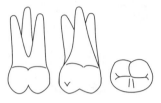

Maxillary First Molar

The **maxillary first molar** is the largest tooth in the maxillary arch. It is the first permanent tooth to erupt in the maxillary arch at 6 years of age. It has five developmental lobes: two on the buccal aspect and three on the lingual. The **fifth lobe** develops into the **cusp of Carabelli** on the mesiolingual cusp. The occlusal view is a rhomboid shape with an **oblique** ridge that is **uninterrupted by a central groove**. It is formed by the merger of the triangular ridge of the distobuccal cusp and the distal ridge of the mesiolingual cusp. The mesial aspect contacts the distal of the second premolar at the occlusal and middle thirds. The distal aspect contacts the second molar at the middle third. There are three roots, with the lingual root being the longest and largest. The mesiobuccal and distobuccal roots have more curvature.

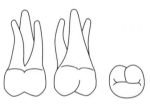

Maxillary Second Molar

The **maxillary second molar** is smaller than the first molar. It usually has four cusps on the occlusal surface although it can have three. It erupts at 12–13 years of age. The occlusal view is usually rhomboid but can occasionally be heart-shaped and is similar to the first molar. Its mesial aspect contacts the first molar more broadly because the mesial aspect is flatter. The distal aspect does not contact the third molar until it has erupted. It has three roots with the lingual root being the longest and the mesiobuccal and distobuccal roots not as curved as those of the first molar.

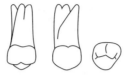

Maxillary Third Molar

The **maxillary third molar** has the **most anomalies** of all the permanent teeth.
It erupts at 18–25 years of age. The occlusal view is heart shaped unless this tooth
developed with a fourth cusp, in which case it would be rhomboid shape. The distolingual cusp is poorly developed. Its mesial aspect contacts the second molar at the
middle third. Its distal aspect does not have contact since it is the last molar. The
trifurcated roots are usually fused together.

Mandibular Dentition

Mandibular Central Incisor

The simplest teeth in the mouth, the **mandibular central incisors** are also the
smallest. They are very **symmetrical** and erupt at 6–7 years of age. They contact
each other mesially at the incisal thirds. The distal contacts the lateral incisor at the
incisal third. The root is oval-shaped.

Mandibular Lateral Incisor

The **mandibular lateral incisor** is larger than the central incisor with the mesial
being longer than the distal. It erupts at age 7–8. The tooth is twisted distally at the
cervical segment. The mesial aspect contacts the central incisor at the incisal third.
The distal aspect contacts the canine at the incisal third. Its root is oval-shaped.

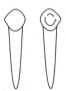

Mandibular Canine

The **mandibular canine** has the **longest root** in the **mandible**. It erupts at age 10–12. It is not as thick as the maxillary canine from the labial aspect to the lingual aspect, nor is the lingual fossa as pronounced. The mesial aspect contacts the lateral incisor at the mesioincisal edge. The distal aspect contacts the first premolar at the incisal third. The **root** has **developmental depressions** on the mesial and distal aspects and is more pointed than the maxillary incisor.

Mandibular First Premolar

The **mandibular first premolar** develops from four lobes and has a **nonoccluding, nonfunctioning lingual cusp**. It erupts at age 10–12. It resembles a mandibular canine. The occlusal surface has a **prominent buccal ridge**. The mesial aspect contacts the canine at the junction of the occlusal and middle thirds. The distal aspect contacts the second premolar at the junction of the occlusal and middle thirds. The root has proximal concavities.

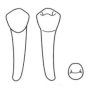

Mandibular Second Premolar

The **mandibular second premolar** can have **two** or **three cusps** with different occlusal configurations. It erupts at age 11–12. If it has **three cusps**, the mesial developmental groove and distal developmental groove converge to make a **Y** pattern with a central pit. If it has **two cusps,** then these same developmental grooves may converge into a **U** or **H** pattern. The mesial and distal contacts are at the middle and occlusal thirds.

U shape   H shape   Y shape

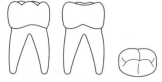

Mandibular First Molar

The **mandibular first molars** are the first molars to erupt at age 6–7. Each has **five cusps**: three buccal and two lingual. It is the largest tooth in the mandible. The buccal has two developmental grooves between the three cusps. The mesiobuccal groove separates the mesiobuccal and the distobuccal cusps. The distobuccal groove separates the distobuccal cusp and the distal cusp. The occlusal view is pentagonal in shape with a central pit, mesial pit, and distal pit from the convergence of the grooves. The developmental grooves are the central, mesiobuccal, distobuccal, and lingual grooves. The mesial and distal aspects contact their adjoining tooth at the juncture of the occlusal and middle thirds. It has two roots with the mesial root being longer than the distal root.

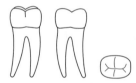

Mandibular Second Molar

The **mandibular second molar** has **four cusps**. It erupts at age 11–13. The four cusps are divided by a buccal groove that separates the mesiobuccal and distobuccal cusps and a lingual groove that separates the mesiolingual and distolingual cusps. The occlusal view is rectangular. The mesial and distal aspects contact their adjoining teeth at the juncture of the occlusal and middle thirds. The two roots are closer in proximity than the first molars and are distally inclined.

Pericoronitis can occur at the mandibular third molars if the **operculum** has not receded at the distal aspect of the crown.

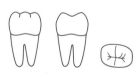

Mandibular Third Molar

The **mandibular third molar** can have four or five cusps. It erupts around age 17–21. The crown can vary in shape, with the occlusal view oval in shape. The two roots are short and poorly developed, and could be fused.

ERUPTION DATES

The last succedaneous tooth to erupt in the mouth is the maxillary canine. Remember that the permanent molars are not succedaneous teeth.

You may be asked on the exam about the **best time to place sealants**. We know it is when the 6-year molars and the 12-year molars erupt. Keep in mind that the question might ask you what grade in school the patient is in rather than how old he is. In that case, remember that kindergarten usually starts at age 5, so the **6-year** molars usually come in when the patient is in the **first grade**. If you cannot remember which grade is appropriate for the 12-year molars, start with kindergarten at age 5 and add up.

Eruption Dates: Deciduous Dentition

Tooth	Maxillary	Root Completion	Mandibular	Root Completion
Central incisor	8–12 months	1.5 yrs	6–10 months	1.5 yrs
Lateral incisor	9–13 months	2 yrs	10–16 months	1.5 yrs
Canine	16–22 months	3.25 yrs	17–23 months	3.25 yrs
First molar	13–19 months	2.5 yrs	14–18 months	2.25 yrs
Second molar	25–33 months	3 yrs	23–31 months	3 yrs

Eruption Dates: Permanent Dentition

Tooth	Maxillary	Root Completion	Mandibular	Root Completion
Central incisor	7–8 yrs	10 yrs	6–7 yrs	9 yrs
Lateral incisor	8–9 yrs	11 yrs	7–8 yrs	10 yrs
Canine	11–12 yrs	13–15 yrs	9–10 yrs	12–14 yrs
First premolar	10–11 yrs	12–13 yrs	10–12 yrs	12–13 yrs
Second premolar	10–12 yrs	12–14 yrs	11–12 yrs	13–14 yrs
First molar	6 yrs	9–10 yrs	6–7 yrs	9–10 yrs
Second molar	12 yrs	14–16 yrs	11–13 yrs	14–15 yrs
Third molar	17–21 yrs	18–25 yrs	17–21 yrs	18–25 yrs

DEVELOPMENTAL ABNORMALITIES

Amelogenesis imperfecta is a hereditary condition of enamel **hypoplasia** where there is a deficient amount of enamel. There are four types of amelogenesis imperfecta.

- **Type 1** is a deficiency in the quantity of enamel. Enamel could be thin in areas or missing with open contacts, or it could have vertical groves or furrows and could be pitted. It is usually yellow to brown in color. Radiographically, it appears absent or thin on cusp tips.

- In **Type 2**, the enamel is **hypocalcified** causing low mineralization of enamel. This hypomineralized enamel can fracture soon after the tooth erupts. It is yellow-orange to brown in color. Radiographically, it appears normal, with the enamel and dentin having a similar density, but the enamel appears more "moth-eaten."

- **Type 3** occurs when enamel is **hypomatured**—opaque and porous. The enamel is of normal thickness but is softer as a result of reduced mineral content, causing chipping or wearing of the tooth crown. The color can be opaque white at the occlusal third of the tooth to yellow-brown. Radiographically, the enamel appears to have the same density as dentin or has slightly reduced radiopacity than normal enamel.

- **Type 4** is related to **taurodontism**, with enamel that is **hypomatured** or **hypoplastic**. The enamel is thin or has pits on the facial surfaces and is white-yellow to brown. Radiographically, the enamel appears normal to slightly more radiopaque than dentin with large pulp chambers.

Anodontia represents missing teeth that never developed due to missing tooth germs.

Concresence is the fusion of two teeth at the root or cementum.

> Think of *concresence* being concrete or cement. Think of *cementum* being cemented to other cementum.

Dens in dente or **dens invaginatus** is the appearance of a tooth within a tooth. The tooth **infolds** or **invaginates** into itself as it is developing and a tooth-like structure appears in its canal. It is more commonly found in the maxillary incisors, especially the lateral incisors. **Dens evaginatus** is an accessory cusp typically found on mandibular premolars.

Dentogenesis imperfecta is a hereditary condition where there is a disturbance in the formation of dentin. The teeth appear to have an **opalescent blue gray** or **blue brown hue**.

Dilaceration is a sharp bend of a root from trauma.

Fusion is the **union** of **two separate teeth** usually from physical pressure. Radiographically, there are **two separate canals**.

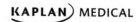

To determine whether you have fusion or gemination, count the number of crowns. If you have the correct number of teeth when counting the union of the two crowns, it is fusion. If you have more than the usual number, it's gemination.

Gemination is one tooth germ producing two united teeth that share one canal. (Think of Gemini, the astrological twins, for the twinning of teeth with gemination.) For fusion, you count the number of teeth—including the united crowns—as separate teeth. If you get the correct number of crowns, then you have a case of fusion. If you get more than the correct number of crowns, you have gemination.

Hutchinson's incisors are anterior notched, bell-shaped teeth caused by congenital syphilis, which creates disturbances during tooth formation. **Mulberry molars** are also caused by congenital syphilis, which can cause poor cusp development of the first molars.

Macrodontia are abnormally large teeth. **Microdontia** are abnormally small teeth and include peg teeth such as peg lateral incisors and third molars. Down syndrome patients have a small-tooth crown to root ratio.

Taurodontism occurs in larger teeth with the pulp horn extending further into the cusps, making them more prominent. The roots are shorter.

Tetracycline should not be prescribed to pregnant or nursing mothers, or to children whose teeth are still developing.

Tetracycline staining occurs if tetracycline is ingested while the teeth are still developing. The teeth are gray tan or yellow tan in color.

SUPPORTING STRUCTURES

The **periodontia** are the supporting structures of teeth. They consist of **alveolar bone**, **gingiva**, **periodontal ligament**, and **cementum**.

Bone

Alveolar bone and **basal bone** are part of the maxilla and mandible that surround and support each tooth. **Alveolar** bone forms over basal bone. It consists of both **trabecular bone** and **cortical bone**. **Cortical bone** is found covering the facial and lingual surfaces of teeth and is **not seen radiographically** since tooth structure blocks it out. It is, however, seen as a radiopaque line on the facial and lingual surfaces of an occlusal film.

Cortical bone is not seen radiographically. Trabecular bone is seen radiographically.

Trabecular bone is **cancellous** or **spongy bone** situated between the alveolar bone proper and cortical bone. It is **seen radiographically** at the interproximal surfaces on bitewings and periapicals as well as between the roots of multirooted teeth. Alveolar bone located between the roots of a tooth is called **interradicular septum**, while alveolar bone found between adjacent teeth is called **interdental septum**.

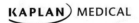

Alveolar bone also splits into **alveolar bone proper** which forms the **inner tooth socket** and **supporting alveolar bone** which **surrounds** and **supports alveolar bone proper**.

Alveolar bone proper, also called **cribriform plate**, is compact bone that is highly porous, allowing communication with cancellous bone. Radiographically, it is termed **lamina dura** which is seen as a **radiopaque** line outlining the root(s) of the tooth. The **alveolar crest** is the most cervical portion of the coronal bone. It is normally **1.5–2.0 mm** apical to the CEJ when the periodontium is healthy. Alveolar bone proper also contains **bundle bone** where **Sharpey's fibers** embed to support the periodontal ligament of the tooth.

Epithelial tissue termed **lamina propria** is not seen radiographically since it is connective tissue made up of **collagen fibers** and **elastic fibers** that are embedded into the basement membrane.

The bone of the maxilla and mandible is basal bone. **Basal bone** and **apical base** are synonymous terms for bone that is continuous with alveolar bone and plays an important role in orthodontic movement. Alveolar bone remodels more easily with orthodontic movement. With orthodontic movement, appliances such as bands, brackets, wires, headgear, retainers, and fixed or removable appliances apply pressure to the alveolar bone on one side of each tooth. This pressure **compresses** the periodontal ligament on that same side, causing the infiltration of osteoclasts to resorb or break down bone for the tooth to move in that direction. As the tooth moves, it leaves a vacant **tension** area of bone for osteoblasts to rebuild new bone.

Periodontal Ligament

The **periodontal ligament** attaches the cementum of teeth to the alveolar bone. It is organized fibrous tissue that transmits occlusal forces. The principal fibers that attach the periodontal ligament to bone and cementum are Sharpey's fibers which embed at a 90-degree angle into these supporting structures. The alveolodental ligaments include the alveolar crest fibers, apical fibers, horizontal fibers, interradicular fibers, and oblique fibers. The **alveolar crest fibers** extend from the cementum below the CEJ obliquely to the alveolar crest bone.

The **apical fiber** group extends from the cementum of the root tip the alveolar bone proper. The **horizontal fiber** group extends horizontally from cementum to alveolar bone. The **interradicular fiber** group extends from the cementum of one root to the cementum of another root of the same tooth. This group is on multi-rooted teeth only, and doesn't involve bone attachment.

The **oblique fibers** extend from alveolar bone to cementum in an apical direction. It is the **main mode of attachment** of the periodontal ligament. Other fibers include **transseptal fibers** that attach cementum to cementum as they connect tooth to tooth, gingival fibers that support the marginal gingival tissues, and circular fibers that circle the tooth to support the gingiva.

> The first bone lost in periodontal disease is alveolar crest bone.

> It is easy to mix up lamina dura (bone) seen radiographically with lamina propria (connective tissue), which is not seen radiographically.

> The alveolar crest fibers are the first fibers lost in periodontal disease.

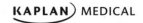

KAPLAN MEDICAL

Occlusion Evaluation

Occlusion is the relationship of the maxillary and mandibular arches to each other. Recognizing occlusal discrepancies is necessary to assess for orthodontic referrals and for assessment of occlusal trauma. **Ideal occlusion** occurs when all the teeth in the maxillary arch touch all the teeth in the mandibular arch. **Centric occlusion** is the usual or routine occlusion of the cusps of the maxillary teeth and mandibular teeth interdigitating maximally. **Centric relation** occurs when the condyles of the mandible are in the rearmost and uppermost location to the articular fossa of the temporomandibular joint.

Ideally, **centric occlusion** and **centric relation** should be **equal**. If the patient has a shifting or sliding of teeth when he squeezes them together, it is caused by **premature contacts**. The **working** (functioning) **side** is simply the side to which the mandible is moved—whether left or right—during mastication, for instance. The opposite side of lateral occlusion is the **balancing** (nonfunctioning) **side**. **Physiological rest** occurs when no teeth occlude.

> When a patient is in physiological rest, no teeth are touching.

Lateral occlusion is guided by the contact of the maxillary canine with the mandibular canine when the mandible is moved to the right or left side. **Canine rise** occurs when the canine cusps contact each other, and no other teeth occlude or contact each other. Canine rise does not occur in worn dentition, when the cusps are worn.

ANGLE'S CLASSIFICATION OF MALOCCLUSION

Angle's classification of malocclusion expresses what is not ideal with a patient's occlusion. It describes how the dentitions malocclude. There are three groups included within this classification.

Class I Malocclusion

Class I malocclusion is **neutrocclusion** where, ideally, the molar and canines intercuspate. Other discrepancies, however, do occur such as crossbites, crowding, open bite, protrusion, retrusion, or too much spacing caused by large jaws and small teeth.

Molars: The mesiobuccal cusp of the maxillary first molar occludes with the mesiobuccal groove of the mandibular first molar.

Canines: The maxillary canine occludes with the distal half of the mandibular canine and also the mesial half of the mandibular first premolar.

Profile: Mesognathic (old terminology) jaw has a **normal profile** with a relatively flat face.

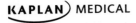

Class II Malocclusion

Class II malocclusion occurs when there is **distoclusion** of the dentition. Within this class, there are two subdivisions (Divisions I and II) that describe differences of the anterior relationship of the dentition.

Molars: The mesiobuccal cusp of the maxillary first molar occludes mesial to the mesiobuccal groove of the mandibular first molar.

Canines: The distal surface of the mandibular canine is distal to the mesial surface of the maxillary canine by at least the width of a premolar.

Class II Division I

Profile: Retrognathic (old terminology) jaw is **convex** with a protruded lip or recessive chin. The maxillary anterior teeth protrude more facially away from the mandibular anterior teeth.

Class II Division II

Profile: Mesognathic (old terminology) jaw has **normal profile** with a prominent chin. The overbite is extremely deep, and the maxillary central incisors are retruded or upright. Also, the maxillary lateral incisors may be tipped labially or overlap the centrals.

Class III Malocclusion

Class III malocclusion is considered to be mesioclusion.

Molars: The mesiobuccal cusp of the first maxillary molar occludes distal to the mesiobuccal groove of the mandibular first molar.

Canines: The distal of the mandibular canine is mesial to the mesial surface of the maxillary canine by at least half the width of a premolar.

Profile: Prognathic is the profile with a prominent mandible.

If all the mandibular anterior teeth are in cross-bite with the maxillary anterior teeth, the patient likely has a Class III malocclusion.

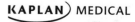

OCCLUSAL DISTURBANCES

Occlusal disturbances can occur from discrepancies of the interarch alignment, excessive wear, or tensional forces on the dentition.

- **Bruxism** is the grinding of teeth.

- **Crossbite** occurs when any of the maxillary teeth occlude more lingually with the mandibular teeth. It may also be defined as the anterior mandibular teeth occlude more facially when occluding with the maxillary teeth. This also includes the posterior mandibular teeth that occlude more buccally than the posterior maxillary teeth.

- **End to end (edge to edge)** occurs when the anterior maxillary incisal edges occlude with the mandibular incisal edges; there is neither overjet nor overbite. In posterior teeth, this occurs when the cusp tips meet cusp-to-cusp with no intercuspation.

- **Excessive overbite** occurs when the maxillary incisors occlude to overlap the mandibular incisors at their cervical third of the teeth. **Excessive overjet** occurs when the maxillary anterior teeth overjet the mandibular teeth by at least 3 mm.

- **Mesial drift** is the tendency of teeth to migrate toward the midline of the mouth over a long period of time.

- **Occlusal trauma** occurs when there has been progressive injury to the supporting structures of the teeth. It doesn't cause periodontal disease, though it can hasten an existing periodontal condition. With trauma, the PDL will widen.

- **Open bite** occurs when incisal or occlusal surfaces fail to contact each other and an open space develops.

A patient in her late teens who still has her mamelons has an open bite.

Vertical dimension is an estimated measurement of the lower one-third of the face, determined by the intervening space of the mandible and maxilla. With time, there can be a **loss in the vertical dimension** due to mechanical wear of attrition and loss of alveolar bone. In that case, the mouth appears to have a collapsed, shortened appearance.

TMJ

The **temporomandibular joint** allows for movement of the mandible. The condyle of the mandible articulates with the articular fossa and articular eminence of the temporal bone. A joint disc that is surrounded by a joint capsule is located between the condyle and temporal bone. It is a synovial joint filled with lubricating synovial fluid, so that the joint can move by rotation of the condylar heads and translation or gliding.

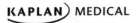

The sphenomandibular ligament helps to stabilize the jaw, while the lateral temporomandibular joint ligament prevents inferior and posterior displacement. Blood is supplied by the **external carotid artery** and it is innervated by the **trigeminal** (V) nerve.

ORAL MUCOSA

Oral mucosa is composed of **stratified squamous epithelium.** It is continuous with **lamina propria**, connective tissue made up of **collagen fibers** and **elastic fibers** that are embedded into the basement membrane. The basement membrane, located between the oral mucosa and connective tissue, is formed by the basal lamina of epithelial tissue and the reticular lamina of connective tissue.

There are three types of stratified squamous epithelium:

1. **Nonkeratinized epithelium** acts as a cushion against any tension. It includes the lining mucosa of the alveolar mucosa, buccal mucosa, cheeks, floor of the mouth, lips, soft palate, and ventral part of the tongue. It appears as a soft, moist surface. It includes the basal-cell, prickle-cell, and outmost nonkeratinized layers.

2. **Orthokeratinized epithelium** acts as a mechanical barrier. It includes attached gingiva, dorsal surface of the tongue, and hard palate. It is coral-pink in color and is highly vascular. It includes the basal-cell, prickle-cell, granular, and outmost keratinized layers.

3. **Parakeratinized epithelium** is located between nonkeratinized epithelium and orthokeratinized epithelium. It is found on the dorsum of the tongue and in attached gingiva. It is associated with the lingual papillae of the tongue. It includes the basal-cell, prickle-cell, and keratinized layers.

The **muccogingival junction** is a scalloped demarcation line between pink attached gingiva and red alveolar mucosa.

There are different types of gingival tissue within the oral cavity: attached gingiva, marginal gingiva, and interdental gingiva. **Attached gingiva** connects the periosteum of alveolar bone to cementum, and is separated from marginal gingiva by a **free gingival groove.**

Marginal gingiva is cuff-like, unattached tissue that surrounds the facial, lingual, and interproximal surfaces of teeth. The **gingival sulcus**—where the attachment of the marginal gingiva occurs—is lined with **nonkeratinized junctional epithelium**. It is attached to the tooth by hemidesmosomes. **Free gingiva** is the most coronal segment of marginal gingiva.

Interdental gingiva is the interproximal papillae of marginal gingiva that also lies coronal to alveolar bone. A concavity in the interdental gingiva is called a **col.**

Nonkeratinized junctional epithelium is attached to the tooth by hemidesmosomes.

The col is a concave depression in interproximal gingiva.

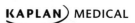

MUCOSAL TISSUES

There are three types of mucosal tissue: lining mucosa, masticatory mucosa, and specialized mucosa. **Alveolar mucosa** is **lining mucosa**. It is red–pink in color, and it is very glossy because its minor salivary glands give it a moist look. **Attached gingiva** is a **masticatory mucosa**. It is pink when healthy and adheres firmly to the periosteum of alveolar bone. **Buccal mucosa** is a **lining mucosa** of the inner cheek. This area will sometimes include Fordyce granules and linear alba. **Labial mucosa** is a **lining mucosa** of the inner upper lip. The vermillion border is the transition area of the epithelial tissue of the face and oral mucosa.

The **hard palate** is a **masticatory mucosa** that is pink in color, and it is glossy because its minor salivary glands give it a moist look. On the anterior portion of the hard palate are irregular firm ridges called rugae.

Soft palate is a **lining mucosa** that is deep pink in color and moist. The **ventral surface of tongue** and **floor of the mouth** are both **lining mucosa** that are red–pink in color and interspersed with superficial blue veins. Here the **lingual frenum** attaches the ventral surface of the tongue to the floor of the mouth. **Sublingual caruncle**, a round elevation on either side of the lingual frenum in the floor of the mouth, serves as the opening for Wharton's duct.

Mucobuccal fold is the "gutter" formed by the merging of the alveolar mucosa and the buccal mucosa.

TONGUE

The **tongue's dorsal** and **lateral surfaces** are both **masticatory** and **specialized mucosa**. Orthokeratinized masticatory mucosa lines the tongue's exterior surface, while lingual papillae that are both orthokeratinized and special parakeratinized mucosa are found on the dorsal and lateral surfaces.

<u>Fili</u>form papillae
<u>fill</u> in the spaces.

There are four types of papillae on the dorsum of the tongue: **Filiform papillae** are the most common, and are not involved in taste. They are cone-shaped papillae with a velvety appearance that **fill in the spaces** of the other lingual papillae.

Fungiform papillae have a **mushroom shape**, and appear as little red dots on the anterior two-thirds of the dorsum of the tongue. Their function is taste sensation.

Foliate papillae are **leaf-shaped** and are located on the posterior lateral borders of the tongue. Their function is taste sensation.

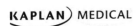

Circumvallate papillae or **vallate** papillae are mushroom-shaped papillae surrounded by a valley. They are located at the V-shaped groove (sulcus terminalis) at the most posterior segment of the anterior $\frac{2}{3}$ of the tongue. Their function is taste sensation.

The **lingual tonsils** are a collection of lymph follicles located at the base of the tongue. The **foramen cecum** of the tongue is a depression that is located at the sulcus terminalis. That is where the thyroid gland starts to develop before it migrates downward into the neck region.

> The foramen cecum is a depression in the tongue where the thyroid gland starts to develop.

Tongue Abnormalities

- **Bifid tongue** occurs at the anterior segment that divides it longitudinally by a fissure.

- **Black hairy tongue** is a brown–black color that occurs on the posterior dorsal surface of the tongue. The filiform papillae lengthen, don't slough off, and pick up pigments from food, tobacco, and bacteria. It takes on a furry appearance.

- **Fissured tongue** has deep crevices or grooves that radiate outward on the dorsal and lateral surfaces of the tongue. The fissures can collect food and, as a result, can attract candida albicans. It is seen in patients who have Down syndrome or Melkerson-Rosenthal syndrome.

- **Geographic tongue** (wandering rash or migratory glossitis) occurs when the filiform papillae experience modifications from parakeratinized epithelium that is darker red than the white-colored orthokeratinized epithelium. It takes on the appearance of a geographic map that keeps changing its topography.

- **Hairy leukoplakia** occurs on the lateral borders of the tongue with a white, shaggy appearance. It is seen in immune-compromised patients, such as those with HIV or Epstein Barr.

- **Median rhomboid glossitis** is a benign, asymptomatic lesion that occurs at the V-shaped groove (sulcus terminalis) and extends anteriorly. It is a rhomboid or oval area of red depapillation.

SALIVARY GLANDS

The salivary glands are **exocrine glands** with ducts that produce saliva. Saliva serves different purposes: it lubricates, cleanses, and acts as a buffer in the oral cavity. It also contains **salivary amylase** which begins **starch digestion** in the mouth.

> Starch digestion begins in the mouth with salivary amylase.

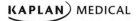

Besides helping with digestion, saliva contributes to the acquired pellicle where bacterial plaque adheres. Saliva also contains the minerals calcium and phosphorus, needed for supragingival calculus formation.

Saliva contains both serous (watery protein) and mucous (thick carbohydrate) secretions that are produced by secretory cells. Mucous epithelial cells produce mucous secretions, while serous epithelial cells produce serous secretions. Serous secretions are located in **acini**, clusters of cells that secrete fluid.

Small **minor salivary glands** are located in the buccal, labial, and lingual mucosa in addition to the soft and hard palates and floor of the mouth. They secrete mucous or mixed mucous serous fluids. Another minor salivary gland called **von Ebner's gland** secretes only serous fluid, and is found near the circumvallate papillae.

The **largest** salivary glands are the **parotid glands**. They are situated on the surface of the masseter muscle underneath the external auditory canal and to the rear of the ascending ramus of the mandible. The parotids produce **serous saliva**, which is about 25% of the combined saliva volume. **Stenson's duct** or the **parotid duct** passes through the buccinator muscle as it delivers saliva into the oral cavity on the buccal mucosa near the second maxillary molar. It is an encapsulated gland.

The **submandibular gland** is the second-largest gland, situated in the submandibular space below the angle of the mandible. The submandibular gland produces **mixed secretions** of serous and mucous saliva and delivers 60–65% of the combined saliva volume. **Wharton's duct** or the **submandibular duct** delivers saliva into the floor of the mouth at sublingual caruncle on either side of the lingual frenum. It is an encapsulated gland.

The **sublingual gland** is the **smallest** salivary gland, located at the sublingual fossa of the mandible which is anterior to the submandibular gland. The sublingual gland produces mixed secretions of some serous secretions, but mainly mucous secretions which are 10% of the combined saliva volume. Saliva exits the gland by way of small ducts called **ducts of Rivinus** and also by a larger duct called **Bartholin's duct** or **sublingual duct**. This gland is not encapsulated.

REVIEW QUESTIONS

1. Of the different types of epithelial tissue in the mouth, which one is a cuff-like, unattached tissue that surrounds all surfaces of a tooth?

   A. Col

   B. Marginal gingiva

   C. Interdental gingiva

   D. Attached gingiva

   E. Free gingiva

2. A 19-year-old Down syndrome patient who has a lisp is being seen in your office for the first time. You notice that he still has mamelons present on #8 and #9. What type of bite does he have?

   A. Crossbite with tongue thrust

   B. Crossbite with orofacial myofunctional

   C. Open bite with apraxia

   D. Open bite with tongue thrust

3. Salivary glands are exocrine glands with ducts. Which of the following ducts is not located on the floor of the mouth?

   A. Bartholin's duct

   B. Stenson's duct

   C. Wharton's duct

   D. Rivinus' duct

4. A variety of tooth anomalies can occur. What teeth other than the third molars are most likely to have anomalies?

   A. Mandibular 2nd premolar

   B. Mandibular 1st molar

   C. Mandibular 2nd molar

   D. Maxillary 1st premolar

   E. Mandibular lateral

5. Which of the following dental anomalies is associated with a tooth that appears to have two crowns merged together but radiographically shares one canal?

   A. Fusion

   B. Concresence

   C. Gemination

   D. Dilaceration

   E. Dens in dente

6. What structure is found on both anterior and posterior permanent teeth?

   A. Oblique ridges

   B. Supplemental groove

   C. Transverse ridges

   D. Cingula

   E. Marginal ridges

7. Which anterior tooth is more likely to have a bifurcated root?

   A. Maxillary lateral incisor

   B. Maxillary canine

   C. Mandibular lateral incisor

   D. Mandibular central incisor

   E. Mandibular canine

8. How many erupted premolars will a 9-year-old child have?

   A. 2

   B. 4

   C. 8

   D. None

9. Hydroxyapatite is found in

   A. Enamel
   B. Bone
   C. Calculus
   D. Dentin
   E. All of the above

10. Which artery—an extension of the external carotid artery—supplies the mandibular teeth with blood?

    A. Maxillary
    B. Facial
    C. Labial
    D. Lingual
    E. Mylohyoid artery

11. Lingual fossa are depressions typically located on the lingual surfaces of which teeth?

    A. Maxillary premolars
    B. Anterior teeth
    C. Mandibular molars
    D. Mandibular premolars
    E. Maxillary molars

12. What anterior tooth is most likely to have a lingual pit that can become carious?

    A. Mandibular central
    B. Mandibular lateral
    C. Maxillary central
    D. Maxillary lateral

13. Foramina allow for the passage of nerves and blood vessels. The mental foramen is located nearest to the

    A. Mandibular first molar
    B. Mandibular second premolar
    C. Mandibular canine
    D. Mandibular lateral incisor
    E. Mandibular first molar

14. If the buccal groove of the mandibular first molar is distal to the mesiobuccal cusp of the maxillary first molar by at least the width of a premolar, what type of occlusion would the patient have? The patient also has retrognathic profile with anterior teeth that protrude.

    A. Class I
    B. Class II, Division I
    C. Class II, Division II
    D. Class III

15. Each part of a tooth has a specific function. The primary function of dental pulp is to

    A. Complete root formation
    B. Protect the periodontal ligament
    C. Allow lymphocytes to enter
    D. Form dentin
    E. Form denticles

16. The papillae of the tongue have many functions. Which type of papillae are most numerous on the human tongue?

    A. Foliate
    B. Circumvillate
    C. Fungiform
    D. Filiform

17. Homeostasis allows a tooth to continue forming cementum throughout life. Where on the root portion of the tooth is the thickest layer of cementum?

    A. Apical third
    B. Middle third
    C. Coronal third
    D. None of the above

18. Which of the following premolars is most likely to have three cusps?

    A. Maxillary first
    B. Maxillary second
    C. Mandibular first
    D. Mandibular second

19. A tooth infolding into itself as it develops is called

    A. Enamel pearl
    B. Hutchinson's incisors
    C. Dens evaginatus
    D. Gemination
    E. Dens invaginatus

20. Sharpey's fibers of the periodontal ligament embed into what type of bone?

    A. Alveolar bone
    B. Bundle bone
    C. Trabecular bone
    D. Cortical bone
    E. Cancellous bone

21. When the condyles of the mandible are in the rearmost and uppermost location to the articular fossa of the temporomandibular joint, it indicates what type of occlusion?

    A. Centric occlusion
    B. Centric relation
    C. Lateral occlusion
    D. Ideal occlusion

22. Of the following types of amelogenesis imperfecta, which is related to taurodontism and has enamel that is yellow–brown in color?

    A. Type I amelogenesis imperfecta
    B. Type II amelogenesis imperfecta
    C. Type III amelogenesis imperfecta
    D. Type IV amelogenesis imperfecta

23. Which tongue abnormality is characterized by papillae that alter themselves from parakeratinized epithelium of dark-red areas to orthokeratinized epithelium that is white in color?

    A. Fissured tongue
    B. Geographic tongue
    C. Median rhomboid glossitis
    D. Hairy leukoplakia
    E. Hairy tongue

24. There are different types of mucosal tissue in the oral cavity, but the muccogingival junction separates the

    A. Marginal gingiva and free gingiva
    B. Parakeratinized tissue and orthokeratinized tissue
    C. Stratified squamous epithelium and lamina propia
    D. Pink attached gingiva and red alveolar mucosa

25. The maxillary right molar is lingual to the mandibular right molar, and the maxillary left molar is buccal to the mandibular left molar. What type of occlusion do you have?

    A. Crossbite on the left side with normal occlusion on the ride side
    B. Crossbite on the right side with normal occlusion on the left side
    C. Freeway space
    D. Incisal guidance
    E. End to end occlusion

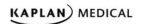

ANSWER EXPLANATIONS

1. B

Marginal gingiva is a cuff-like, unattached tissue surrounding all surfaces of a tooth.

A. Col is a depression on the interdental papillae of anterior teeth.

C. Interdental gingiva doesn't surround the tooth on all surfaces.

D. Attached gingiva adheres firmly to the periosteum of alveolar bone.

E. Free gingiva is the most coronal segment of marginal gingiva.

2. D

A 19-year-old Down syndrome patient who still has mamelons present on #8 and #9 has an open bite. The tongue thrust causes the lisp and open bite, which is why the mamelons are not worn even at this age. The most common type of lisp is caused by tongue thrusting.

C. Apraxia is a motor disorder when a patient cannot complete complex coordinated movement. The patient's mouth and tongue muscles don't process the brain's signal to make the correct sounds for words.

3. B

The Stenson's duct is not located on the floor of the mouth. As a duct of the parotid gland, it empties alongside the maxillary second molars.

A. Bartholin's duct empties on the floor of the mouth and serves the sublingual gland.

C. Wharton's duct empties on the floor of the mouth and serves the submaxillary gland.

D. Rivinus' duct is a small duct that serves the sublingual gland.

4. A

Other than the third molars, the mandibular second premolars tend to have anomalies; they can have anondontia, either unilateral or bilateral.

5. C

Gemination appears to have two crowns merged together. It occurs from one tooth bud.

A. Fusion occurs with two separate tooth buds each having a separate canal.

B. Concresence occurs with crowding when the cementum only of the root adhere together. Think of cementum as cement or concrete = concrescence.

D. Dilaceration is a bent root.

E. Dens in dente or dens invaginatus is a tooth within a tooth. The tooth infolds or invaginates into itself as it develops.

6. E

Marginal ridges are found on posterior and anterior teeth. They are raised borders on the mesiolingual and distolingual surfaces.

A. Oblique ridges are found on the occlusal surfaces of posterior teeth.

B. Supplemental grooves are secondary grooves found on the lingual surfaces of anterior teeth.

C. Transverse ridges join two triangular ridges across the occlusal surface of posterior teeth.

D. Cingula are located at the cervical one-third of the anterior teeth.

7. E

Mandibular canines are the anterior teeth most likely to have bifurcated roots. Very rarely, bifurcated roots can develop with the mandibular lateral or central incisors. The maxillary lateral incisors and canines can have dilacerations as anomalies.

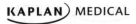

8. D

A 9-year old will have no erupted premolars. The maxillary first premolars erupt around age 10–11. The maxillary second premolar and mandibular first premolar erupt around age 10-12. The mandibular second premolars erupt around age 11-12.

9. E

Hydroxyapatite is a calcium phosphorus compound found in bone, enamel, dentin, cementum, and even in calculus.

10. A

The inferior alveolar branch of the maxillary artery supplies blood to the mandibular teeth. It also supplies the floor of the mouth.

B. The facial artery supplies blood to palate and related muscles, tonsils, submandibular salivary glands and lymph nodes, lower and upper lips, and some muscles of facial expression.

C. The labial artery is a branch of the facial artery and supplies blood to the lips.

D. The lingual artery supplies blood to hyoid bone, including the suprahyoid muscles and the floor of the mouth.

E. The mylohyoid artery supplies blood to the inner mandible, the floor of the mouth, and the mylohyoid muscle.

11. B

Lingual fossae are shallow-wide depressions that border the cingulum on anterior teeth only. Some contain a pit.

12. D

The maxillary lateral incisor is most likely to have a lingual pit. That is because it is a deeper lingual fossa that has a more pronounced narrow cingulum, separated by a more pronounced lingual groove than the maxillary central. This lingual groove can extend onto the root and occurs more often here than on the maxillary central.

A. The mandibular central incisor has a very smooth lingual surface with a barely noticeable lingual fossa.

B. The mandibular lateral incisor has a more pronounced lingual fossa with a small cingulum than the mandibular central, and lingual pits are rare.

C. The maxillary central incisor has a lingual groove between the lingual fossa and cingulum is present, but not as pronounced as on the lateral incisor.

13. B

The mental foramen is located near the mandibular second premolar and is often mistaken for an abscess. There are no foramina near the other teeth.

14. B

This scenario is Class II, Division I. In this case, the patient also has retrognathic profile with anterior teeth that protrude.

A. Class I is neutrocclusion with the mesiobuccal cusp of the maxillary first molar, aligning with the buccal groove of the mandibular first molar.

C. Class II, Division II occurs when the buccal groove of the mandibular first molar is distal to the mesiobuccal cusp of the maxillary first molar by at least the width of the premolar, the profile mesognathic with one or more of the anterior teeth retruded.

D. Class III has a prominent mandible with a prognathic profile. The mesiobuccal cusp of the maxillary first molar occludes distally to the buccal groove of the mandibular first molar.

15. D

The main function of dental pulp is to form dentin in response to stimuli, such as carious lesion, trauma, etc.

A. Root formation is taken care of by Hertwig's sheath.

B. The periodontal ligament is exterior to the pulp and not a pulp function.

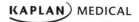

C. While lymphocytes are important to protect the tooth from invading antigens, this is not the most important function of the pulp.

E. Denticles are round or ovoid structures that have dentinal tubules in the dentin.

16. D

The most numerous papillae are the filiform papillae, which "fill in" all the spaces not taken up by the other papillae.

A. Foliate, whose function is taste, are leaf-shaped papillae located on the posterior lateral borders of the tongue.

B. Circumvillate, whose function is taste, are mushroom-shaped papillae surrounded by a valley in the V-shaped groove (sulcus terminalis) at the base of the tongue.

C. Fungiform are little red dots on the anterior two-thirds of the dorsum of the tongue.

17. A

The root portion of the tooth with the thickest layer of cementum is the apical third. It is 100–150 μm thick.

B. The middle third has acellular cementum that does not increase once formed.

C. The coronal third has a thin layer of cementum, around 10 μm thick.

18. D

The mandibular second premolars are most likely to have (two or) three cusps. With three cusps, the occlusal surface will have a Y configuration that lacks a transverse ridge. With two cusps, their occlusal surface will have an H or U configuration which has a transverse ridge. The maxillary first, maxillary second, and mandibular first premolars will typically have two cusps, all exhibiting a transverse ridge.

19. E

A tooth infolding into itself as it develops is dens invaginatus (or dens in dente). During development, the tooth infolds into itself, producing the appearance of a tooth within a tooth. This typically occurs in the lateral incisors.

A. Enamel pearl typically occurs on the molars at the CEJ, when the ameloblasts produce excess enamel.

B. Hutchinson's incisors are notched incisal surfaces that occur congenitally from syphilis.

C. Dens evaginatus is an accessory cusp typically found on mandibular premolars.

D. Gemination occurs when a single tooth tries to divide into two teeth but does not progress to full division.

20. B

Sharpey's fibers of the periodontal ligament embed into bundle bone adjacent to the PDL. It is so named because it contains numerous Sharpey's fibers.

A. Alveolar bone that lines the alveolus is cancellous bone, with Sharpey's fibers forming bundle bone.

C. Trabecular bone is cancellous or spongy bone located between the alveolar bone proper and cortical bone.

D. Cortical bone is located on the facial and lingual surfaces of teeth.

E. Cancellous bone is trabecular bone.

21. B

This type of occlusion is called centric relation.

A. Centric occlusion is the habitual occlusion of the cusps of the maxillary teeth and mandibular teeth interdigitating maximally.

C. Lateral occlusion occurs with the contact of the maxillary canine with the mandibular canine when the mandible is moved to the right side or left.

D. Ideal occlusion occurs when all the teeth in the maxillary arch touch all the teeth in the mandibular arch.

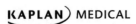

22. D

Type IV amelogenesis imperfecta causes taurodontism with hypomatured or hypoplastic enamel and teeth that are white-yellow to crown in color.

A. Type I results in is a deficiency in the quantity of enamel (thin in areas or missing). There may be vertical grooves, furrows, or pitting. The teeth are usually yellow to brown in color.

B. Type II results in hypocalcified enamel causing low mineralization and fragile enamel. The teeth are yellow orange to brown in color.

C. Type III results in hypomatured enamel that is opaque, porous, and of normal thickness, though it is softer because of the reduced enamel mineral content The color can be opaque white to yellow–brown at the occlusal third of the tooth.

23. B

In geographic tongue, papillae alter themselves from parakeratinized epithelium of dark red areas to orthokeratinized epithelium that is white in color.

A. Fissured tongue features deep crevices or grooves on the dorsal and lateral surfaces of the tongue.

C. Median rhomboid glossitis features a rhomboid or oval area of red depapillation.

D. Hairy leukoplakia features the lateral borders of the tongue as a white, shaggy appearance.

E. Hairy tongue is brown–black in color, and occurs on the posterior dorsal surface of the tongue when filiform papillae lengthen but don't slough off.

24. D

The mucogingival junction separates the pink attached gingiva and red alveolar mucosa.

A. Marginal gingiva is cuff-like, unattached tissue that surrounds the facial, lingual, and interproximal surfaces of teeth. Free gingiva is the most coronal segment of marginal gingiva.

B. Parakeratinized epithelium is found between nonkeratinized epithelium and orthokeratinized epithelium, and is located on the dorsum of the tongue and attached gingiva. It includes the basal-cell, prickle-cell, and keratinized layers. Orthokeratinized tissue is a coral–pink mechanical barrier found in attached gingiva, dorsal surface of the tongue, and hard palate. It includes the basal-cell, prickle-cell, granular, and outermost keratinized layers.

C. Oral mucosa is comprised of stratified squamous epithelium that is continuous with lamina propria, connective tissue made up of collagen fibers and elastic fibers.

25. B

When the maxillary right molar is lingual to the mandibular right molar, and the maxillary left molar is buccal to the mandibular left molar, the result is crossbite on the right side with normal occlusion on the left side.

C. Freeway space occurs when there is no occlusal contact during physiologic rest.

D. Incisal guidance is an anterior tooth term that has to do with protrusion guided by the incisors.

E. End to end occlusion occurs when the anterior maxillary incisal edges occlude with the mandibular incisal edges with no overjet or overbite.

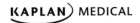

Chapter Six: **Microbiology**

It is believed that over 500 species of microorganisms reside in the oral cavity, though only 200 or so have been identified. As such, this places dental hygienists at risk to develop disease. It is especially important in this case for hygienists to have a thorough understanding of the transmittal of disease. Microbiology is the study of **algae, bacteria, fungi, prions, protists, protozoa,** and **viruses.**

Cells can be divided into two extensive groups: eukaryotes and prokaryotes. **Eukaryotes** are unicellular structures that contain a nucleus. They include **algae, protozoa,** and **fungi.** Eukaryotes divide by **mitosis**; the chromosomes arrange themselves into **mitotic spindles** just before cell division occurs.

Prokaryotes are unicellular or multicellular. **Bacteria** fall into this category. Less complex than eukaryotes, prokaryote cells contain a singular circular chromosome that has a genetic "blueprint." This chromosome **lacks a nuclear membrane** but is attached to the cell membrane.

These types of cells divide by **binary fission** and so no mitotic spindle appears before division. Bacteria have different basic shapes: **cocci** (round), **bacilli** (rod), **spirilli** (spiral shaped), spirochetes (cork-screw spiral), and vibrios (comma shape).

Bacterial Arrangements

Diplo-	Arranged in pairs
Strepto-	Arranged in chains
Tetrad-	Arranged in squares
Staphylo-	Arranged in clumps or sheets

Viruses are unique **symmetrical** microorganisms that feed off other cells. They are **unable to produce outside of a living host cell** and contain a limited amount of DNA or RNA for replication. As such, they must use the host cell to reproduce.

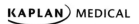

There are over 80 virus families, with many subfamilies in each. The biggest viruses are only as big as the smallest bacteria. Moreover, they have a less complex structure than bacteria.

GRAM STAINING

Gram staining helps to differentiate microorganisms in the diagnosis and treatment of an infection. Bacteria have differences in the **peptidoglycan** contained in their cell walls. **Gram-positive** bacteria are the denser of the two types, with about five times as much peptidoglycan than **gram-negative** bacteria. Gram-negative bacteria have walls that contain 1–3 layers and that affects the way they stain. The size and type of the cell wall can also account for the virulence of the bacteria and its susceptibility to antibiotics.

Gram positive-bacteria have a strong affinity for violet gram stain and remain **purple** when rinsed with alcohol. **Gram-negative bacteria** have a low affinity for violet gram stain and appear **pink to red** in color when rinsed with by alcohol.

MICROBIAL GROWTH AND ENVIRONMENTS

Bacteria replicate by binary division as two new cells are replicated from one parent cell. The **lag phase** occurs when the cells begin to **grow in size** but have not yet divided. The **log phase** occurs when binary fission of the cell takes place. The **stationary phase** occurs when the rate of cell growth equals the rate of cell death. The **decline phase** occurs when all the nutrients are depleted and the cells die off.

Penicillin inhibits bacterial growth during cell wall synthesis of the multiplication stage or log phase.

Lag phase	Cell grows in size but do not divide
Log phase	Binary fission takes place as cell replicates
Stationary phase	Rate of cell growth = Rate of cell death
Decline phase	Nutrients are depleted resulting in cell death

Different bacteria require different environments to survive. **Obligate aerobes** can survive only in oxygenated environments. **Obligate anaerobes** cannot survive in oxygen environments. **Facultative anaerobes** can survive in either state. **Microaerophiles** require lower than normal amounts of oxygen for growth. **Aerotolerant** bacteria are not inhibited by oxygen but do not usually use oxygen to transform energy.

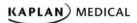

Viruses obtain nutrients and materials from cells to replicate themselves. They attach to the cell wall during **the initiation stage** to penetrate the cell by injecting their DNA or RNA. The virus then takes over the cell's production during the replication stage, producing hundreds of new virus particles. These new virus particles then go in search of new host cells.

Fungal organisms have two basic structures of yeast or mold form. **Yeasts** are unicellular spheres while **molds** are multicellular threadlike tubes. **Fungi** reproduce sexually or asexually by forming spores, by fission or budding, or by fragmentation from a parent cell (mycelium).

Protozoa are unicellular eukaryotic microorganisms that can cause disease. They reproduce asexually by budding (pinching off from the parent cell), schizogony (multiple fission), or fission (one cell splits into two). Protozoa form protective cysts to survive harsh environments.

BARRIERS TO DISEASE

Portals of entry to the body include skin, eyes, oral cavity, respiratory tract, gastrointestinal tract, genitourinary tract, and circulatory system. These systems all help to prevent microorganisms from entering into the body. Some of these systems also contain non-threatening microbial flora or specialized bacteria that are actually beneficial to our systems. A woman who takes an antibiotic for an extended time could develop a yeast infection, because the antibiotic affects the normal bacteria flora.

Infections that occur suddenly are **acute**, while those that slowly develop are **chronic**. Some antigens are more **virulent** or invasive than others. At times, when the body isn't up to fighting off microorganisms, **opportunistic infections** take over. Should there be a breach in one of these systems, the body has a way of taking care of the invading microorganisms often through the production of antibodies.

Fever

Bacteria have an optimal temperature at which they thrive and multiply. In fact, it is the same as a human's **ideal** body **temperature: 37° C.** As bacteria multiply in this ideal environment, they may release **exotoxins** (in particular, gram negative bacteria), which in turn cause macrophages to release endogenous pyrogens. These pyrogens act on the hypothalamus, causing it to reset the "thermostat" and create **fever** in the body. When the fever becomes too high, the bacteria cannot survive.

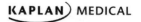

Blood Cells

Neutrophils or polymorphonuclear (PMN) leukocytes are the phagocytes that act against invading pathogens when microorganisms invade. **Neutrophils** are involved with **acute** inflammation. **Eosinophils** that are involved in allergic responses secrete chemical mediators that cause bronchoconstriction. They also fight parasitic infections. **Basophils** play an important role along with mast cells in inflammatory and allergic responses when they release histamine along with mast cells. **Mast cells** get involved when an allergen releases IgE to stimulate mast cells into action, releasing histamine.

Monocytes become large **macrophages** when they leave the capillaries and are involved in **chronic** inflammation. **Lymphocytes** produce **T cells** or **T lymphocytes** and **B cells** or **B leukocytes. T cells** are involved with **cell-mediated immune response. B cells** can produce **antibodies** with **humoral immunity.**

Immune Response

Immunoglobulins are **antibodies** produced by **B cells** after an antigen is introduced into the body. There are five subdivisions of immunoglobulins that play a major role in the body's defense mechanism. These immunoglobulins include:

- **Immunoglobulin A** or **IgA** lines the **body surfaces** to protect microorganisms from entering the body's natural cavities. It is found in tears, saliva, the respiratory tract, the gastrointestinal tract, reproductive tract, and urinary tract.

- **Immunoglobulin D** or **IgD** is present in small amounts but is a major factor on the surface of B cells. It may recognize antigens.

- **Immunoglobulin E** or **IgE** is involved with immediate hypersensitivity or **anaphylactic** reactions. It is chiefly bound to basophils and mast cells.

- **Immunoglobulin G** or **IgG** is also known as gamma globulin and is the **most common antibody.** It functions to **aggregate or clump microorganisms together** and then **opsonise** them. It is the only immunoglobulin that **can cross over the placenta** from the mother to the baby.

- **Immunoglobulin M** or **IgM** stimulates the production of IgG and is **produced first** in the immune response. It binds to an antigen cell surface to **lyse** that cell. It is a larger immunoglobulin with heavier molecular weight.

Once antigen stimulation has been introduced in the body, four types of hypersensitivities can occur:

- **Type I** hypersensitivity is the **most serious type** of reaction. It involves **anaphylaxis** that can be life-threatening. This hypersensitivity involves the IgE antibody. **Urticaria** or **hives** may be seen in this type of reaction, as can asthma.

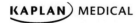

- **Type II** hypersensitivity (or cytotoxic hypersensitivity) is an **antibody–antigen reaction** that can affect organs and tissues. **IgG** and **IgM** are the antibodies involved. here. This type of reaction can occur from Rh factor with incompatibility from mother to baby. It may also occur if there is blood transfusion incompatibility.

- **Type III** occurs when soluble **antigen–antibody complexes accumulate**. These complexes are normally removed by the liver, but in this case, they inundate the body—and often build up in joints, epidermis, blood vessels, lungs, and kidneys. After some time, **arthus** (inflammation) reactions such as **serum sickness** or **rheumatoid arthritis** can occur. IgG is largely involved with this reaction though some IgM may be present.

- **Type IV** is a cell-mediated hypersensitivity that does not involve antibodies. It is a delayed reaction that is mediated by T cells. Symptoms that may ensue are **skin rash, eczema, ulcers,** or **dermatitis**. Reaction to PPD (TB test) is a Type IV reaction.

DISEASE TRANSMISSION AND IMMUNITY

The **lymphatic system** transports lymphocytes to fight off microorganisms and returns fluids back into circulation once extraneous microbes have been filtered out. It also generates responses with our immune system.

Lymphocytes are matured in one of two ways: **T cells,** or **T lymphocytes** cells, are matured in the **thymus,** while **B cells** or **B lymphocyte cells** are matured in the **bone marrow.** Some B cells coat the antigen with antibodies by **opsonization,** which acts like a meat tenderizer on microbes and makes it easier for macrophages to ingest them.

Macrophages and lymphocytes move back and forth into lymph nodes and then back into blood. **Lymphocytes,** when activated, produce glycoprotein-like cytokines termed **lymphokines. Macrophages** produced from monocytes produce **monokines.** These types of cytokines initiate the immune response.

Humoral immunity occurs when the B cells release antibodies that interact with bacteria, toxins, and viruses. The **B cell binds** to the **antigen** and then **engulfs** it until the antigen becomes fragments. Some **B cells** have memory to **produce antibodies** against a future encounter with the same antigen. T cells orchestrate the immune system against the invading microbe. First the **T helper cells activate the B cells** while **T suppressor cells regulate the whole immune response. Cytotoxic T cells** kill the antigens. They can also activate the scavenger macrophages.

Cell-mediated immunity deals mostly with viruses that invade host cells where they **conceal themselves** away from the immune system that wants to make anti-

Humoral immunity produces antibodies with B cells. Cell mediated immunity does not produce antibodies with T cells.

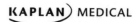

bodies for these antigens. This system is most effective against viruses, but does defend the body against fungi, protozoa, and bacteria. The T-cells stimulate macrophages and create antigen-specific cytotoxic T-cells. Cell mediated immunity does NOT produce antibodies.

Acquired immunity can be either naturally acquired or artificially acquired. Both may be active or passive.

- **Naturally active acquired immunity** occurs when the person becomes infected with an antigen and the body naturally produces antibodies against it. An example of this is the flu. Once you have had that particular strain of the flu, your body has built up antibodies against it. That does not mean you will not ever get the flu again, because there are many types of flus.

- **Naturally passive acquired immunity** occurs when antibodies produced by one individual are passed on to another individual such as Rh antibodies from a mother to her baby.

- **Artificially active acquired immunity** occurs with a **vaccination of antigen that is in an artificially safe form.** The vaccination antigen aids the body's ability to produce antibodies against it. The body produces **long-term B cell memory cells** or antibodies. An example would be the measles, mumps, and rubella vaccine (MMR). Recombinant Hepatitis B vaccine is also included here.

- **Artificially passive acquired immunity** occurs with a vaccination of an **immunoglobulin** or serum that has antibodies incorporated into it. This is a **short-term** immunization. An example would include the hepatitis B vaccination of HBIG.

Inflammation

Inflammation is an inherent part of the immune system. Classic signs of inflammation are **heat** (calor), **redness** (rubor), **swelling** (tumor), and **pain** (dolor). When an injury occurs, the immune system launches a host of white blood cells into the trauma or insult area where microbes or toxins may enter. **Mast cells** release **histamine** there to **vasodilate** the blood vessels and allow for the maximum number of white blood cells to enter into the injury. This causes the redness and increased temperature.

Neutrophils (PMN) arrive quickly to the scene of an acute infection. Monocytes are more numerous at the scene of a chronic infection.

Endothelial cells then flatten and thin out, allowing leukocytes to squeeze through and cause swelling. The **first** leukocytes for early response are the **neutrophils** (PMN), who migrate to the perimeter of the injury (margination). Neutrophils lyse or breakdown bacterial cells. Macrophages follow the neutrophils to become phagocytes, which ingest microorganisms and debris. As leukocytes accumulate along with dead cells, they form pus.

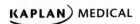

TRANSMISSIBLE DISEASES

Disease is easily transmissible in a dental office. It can occur through contact on surfaces or equipment, or in sprays and aerosols. Prevention of disease transmission through standard precautions is a vital role of the dental hygienist.

Chicken Pox

Chicken pox is a highly contagious disease that is caused by the **varicella zoster** virus which is a member of the herpes family. Incubation period is 2–3 weeks, though it can remain dormant in the dorsal root ganglia.

Mode of Transmission: Droplet respiratory secretions to a susceptible person

Signs & Symptom: Low grade fever, malaise, loss of appetite, rash with cloudy vesicles or scabs.

Vaccination: Varicella vaccine (chicken pox)

Common Cold

The **common cold** is caused by over 200 viruses, including the **coronavirus, rhinovirus,** and **adenovirus** families. Mild infections may be the result of **parainfluenza viruses** and **respiratory syncytial viruses** (RSV).

Mode of Transmission: Airborne droplets; direct contact with secretions

Signs & Symptom: Low grade fever, malaise, runny nose, sneezing, coughing.

Vaccination: None

Conjunctivitis

Conjunctivitis is an **inflammation** of the **conjunctiva** of the **eye.** It may be generated by contaminated hands or towels, eye make-up, or extended-wear contact lenses.

Mode of Transmission: Bacterial sources come from the person's own skin or respiratory tract or from someone else with bacterial conjunctivitis. Viral sources can be from the common cold. It may also result from allergies or irritations, such as extended-wear contact lenses. Viral conjunctivitis spreads rapidly.

Signs & Symptoms: "Pink eye"; itching; redness; sensitivity to light; discharge from the eye.

Vaccination: None

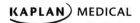

Cytomegalovirus

The **cytomegalovirus (CMV)** is a member of the herpes family that often affects adults over 40, but can be transmitted to a baby before birth. It can remain dormant in the body for an extended period of time, so much so that people are often infected and don't realize it.

Mode of Transmission: Sexually transmitted; mother to baby when nursing; blood; urine; transplanted organs. Hand-washing after touching bodily fluids is a must to prevent transmission.

Signs & Symptoms: In **mother to baby prenatal**: liver and spleen enlargement, which can be fatal; visual impairment; hearing loss; mental retardation. In **adults**: same symptoms as infectious mononucleosis, but the test result for mono is negative: fatigue; swollen glands; fever; enlarged spleen; loss of appetite; sore throat. May also include symptoms for hepatitis, but the test result for hepatitis is negative.

Vaccination: None

Erythema Infectiosum (Fifth Disease)

Erythema infectiosum or **Fifth Disease** is caused by the **parvovirus B19**. The patient is infectious before the appearance of a rash 4–14 days after exposure. Symptoms last 5–10 days.

Mode of Transmission: Direct contact or respiratory droplets

Signs & Symptoms: "Slapped cheek" appearance; itchiness; red lacy rash on trunks & limbs; fever; malaise.

Vaccination: None

Hepatitis

Hyperbilirubinemia
Hyper = too much
Bilirubin = bile pigmentation from the breakdown of old erythrocytes
Emia = in the blood

Hepatitis is an **inflammation** of the **liver** caused by invasion of an antigen or pathogen. There are several types of hepatitis: A, B, C, D, E, G, with Hepatitis F being unconfirmed.

Both **Hepatitis A** and **Hepatitis B** occur in stages. The **first stage**—the **prodromal** or early onset of symptoms stage—is called **preicteric,** which stands for "pre-jaundice." The **second stage** is **icteric**—or affected by jaundice. **Jaundice** is the build-up of bilirubin in the blood when the diseased liver cannot remove the dead red blood cells.

Hepatitis A

Hepatitis A is caused by the **hepatitis A virus (HAV).** It is a member of the picornaviridae family having its own genus *Hepatovirus*. Incubation period is 15–50 days.

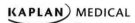

There is usually no chronic effect, though some necrosis of the liver may result. (This situation, however, is not as likely as in Hepatitis B, C, and D.) The patient becomes immune after being infected.

Mode of Transmission: Oral-fecal route from feces in drinking-water; unclean hands after using the lavatory. Sometimes found in day-care centers, when children do not wash their hands after bathroom use.

Signs & Symptoms: In **preicteric** phase: little or no cytopathology or change in cells; nausea; vomiting, fatigue; malaise; loss of appetite; joint pain; fever; dark urine; weight loss. In **icteric** phase: liver damage; jaundice; pale stools; liver enlargement; upper right quadrant pain. In **convalescent** phase: complete recovery, though symptoms may persist for 1–3 months.

Vaccine: **Havrix** vaccination in 2 doses; second dose follows the first by 6–12 months

Hepatitis B

Hepatitis B is caused by the **hepatitis B virus (HBV)**. It is a member of the DNA hepadnavirus family. The hepatitis B virion may also be called **Dane particle**. Incubation period is 45–160 days. Chronic liver disease afterward may have a mortality rate of 15–25%. HBV can survive on surfaces for up to one week. Some individuals remain in a **carrier state** of Hepatitis B, never fully recovering, and harbor the virus for life.

Modes of Transmission: Unprotected sex; needle-sharing; health care worker's exposure to sharps, mother to baby during birth; unsterile tattoo-needle use. In dental operatories, primarily bloodborne.

Signs & Symptoms: In **preicteric** phase: nausea; vomiting; lethargy; loss of appetite; joint pain; fever; sore throat; weight loss. In **icteric** phase: jaundice; dark urine; pale stools; liver enlargement; upper-right-quadrant pain. In **convalescent** phase: general malaise and fatigue for months until symptoms subside.

Vaccine: **Recombivax** or **Engerix-B** vaccine is given to adults in 3 doses; second dose follows the first by 1 month, and the third dose follows that by 6 months.

Hepatitis C

Hepatitis C occurs with the hepatitis C virus or HCV, a member of the flaviviridae family of viruses. About 70% of the time, the disease results in chronic liver disease; in those cases, the mortality rate is 1—5%. Hepatitis C is the leading cause of liver transplants. It is believed that the hepatitis C virus makes an error during replication to become mutated. There are 6 different genotypes, depending upon the region of the world where it is based. At one time, this disease was known as **non-A** and **non-B** hepatitis.

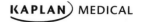

Mode of Transmission: Needle-sharing among IV drug users; tattooing, acupuncture; razor sharing; sexual transmission (rare); mother to baby (rare).

Signs & Symptoms: In **preiceric** phase: few **(vague)** symptoms, with most people unaware that they are infected. In **icteric** phase: jaundice (very rarely). In **convalescent** phase: chronic hepatitis C (sometimes).

Vaccination: None

Hepatitis D

Hepatitis D is also called the delta virus or hepatitis D virus (HDV). This virus needs the hepatitis B virus in order to replicate, so it is found in those who are co-infected with hepatitis B. It is said to be a **superinfection**, because 70–90% of individuals will develop a chronic delta infection. Incubation period is 2 weeks–6 months.

Mode of Transmission: IV drug use; sexual transmission (rare); mother to baby (rare).

Signs & Symptoms: Identical to an acute hepatitis B infection but even more severe

Vaccination: Recombivax vaccine for hepatitis B

Hepatitis E

Hepatitis E is caused by the hepatitis E virus (HEV). It occurs mostly in young to middle-age adults who live in developing nations with poor sewage and drainage. Incubation period is 15–60 days.

Mode of Transmission: Oral–fecal route in countries where there is poor sewage. When it rains heavily, the sewage spills out into the community's drinking water.

Signs & Symptoms: Similar to all the other types of hepatitis but also includes arthralgia, diarrhea, and hives. Symptoms may be abrupt but may disappear with jaundice.

Vaccination: None

Hepatitis G

Hepatitis G is an acute disease caused by the **hepatitis G virus (HGV)** belonging to the flaviviridae family. A chronic infection occurs in 90–100% of infected people, with symptoms lasting up to 9 years.

Mode of Transmission: IV drug users sharing needles, frequently seen with hepatitis C, transfusion recipients.

Signs & Symptoms: Clinical manifestations are very limited at this time.

Vaccination: None

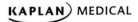

Herpes

Herpes simplex I and Herpes simplex II are similar though they differ in location. They can both be brought on by fever, stress, hormonal changes, or sun exposure.

Herpes simplex I (HSV I) is found on the lips or face. Some people experience outbreaks more often than others. It is believed that one-third of genital herpes cases are the result of HSV I contact.

Herpes simplex I

Mode of Transmission: Fluid from vesicle during kissing; sexual contact; sharing of utensils; direct contact with saliva or secretions

Signs & Symptoms: Clear, fluid-like blister or cold sore on lips or facial area. With acute gingivostomatitis in children: fever, pain on eating or drinking; lymphadenopathy; ulcers on the tongue; buccal mucosa and palate; dehydration due to inability to eat and drink fluid. Incubation period is 2–12 days.

Vaccination: None

Herpes simplex II

Mode of Transmission: Sexual transmission in the genital area; direct contact with saliva/secretions

Signs & Symptoms: Sores in the genital area.

Vaccination: None

Herpetic Whitlow

Herpetic whitlow is the result of the herpes simplex virus that occurs on the finger as a weeping wound.

Mode of Transmission: Direct contact with saliva or secretions

Signs & Symptoms: **Weeping wound** on the finger with erythema and soreness.

Vaccination: None

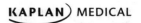

Immunodeficiency Disease AIDS/HIV

Immunodeficiency disease occurs when the immune system is compromised and cannot identify—or destroy—invading pathogens. As we know, viruses need a host cell to reproduce off of, since they cannot replicate on their own. They penetrate the cell, inject their DNA or RNA, and take over during the replication stage of that cell. *Hundreds* of new virus particles are produced as a result, and those new viruses go on to look for more cells to mooch off of.

HIV or human immunodeficiency virus occurs when the **HIV virus mooches** off its favorite **T lymphocyte cells**, called **CD4 helper cells**. These cells are important in defending our bodies from invading pathogens. If the CD4 count drops too low, the body cannot protect itself.

HIV affects the CD4 to CD8 ratio that defends the body. The CD8 supressor cells (killer cells) increase proportionately with infections when the CD4 cells decrease. The lower the ratio, the more damage has been done.

A healthier individual will have one or two CD4 cells for every CD8 cell, but an HIV+ patient will have a much greater CD8 count than CD4 count.

In a healthy individual, the CD4 count is 450–1,200 cell μL. If the **CD4 count is <200 cell μL**, then there is severe damage to the immune system with HIV. **AIDS** will result in the later phase of HIV infection. The immune system deteriorates, making the individual more vulnerable and unable to fight off opportunistic infections. Incubation period is 3 months–12 years.

Category 1	CD4 T lymphocytes greater than 500 cell μL	Asymptomatic HIV
Category 2	CD4 T lymphocytes 200–499 cell μL	HIV (pre-AIDS)
Category 3	CD4 T lymphocytes less than 200 cell μL	AIDS

Mode of Transmission: Unprotected sex, needle sharing, mother to baby

The test for HIV/AIDS is the ELISA test followed by the western blot test.

Signs & Symptoms: In **early HIV**: flu-like symptoms; possible fever, chills, and rashes. In **later HIV**: sore throat; oral candidiasis; lymphadenopathy; fever; lethargy; headache; diarrhea; vaginal yeast infections; night sweats; weight loss. In **AIDS**: opportunistic infections such as oral candidiasis, pneumonias, Kaposi's sarcoma, herpes, tuberculosis, hairy leukoplakia, lymphoma, periodontal disease, and weight loss

Vaccination: None, though a preventive vaccine is being developed for HIV-negative patients, and a therapeutic vaccine for HIV-positive patients

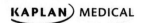

Infectious Mononucleosis

Infectious mononucleosis is caused by the **Epstein-Barr virus** (EBV), a member of the **herpes** virus family, and is a dormant infection for life. It primarily affects lymphoid tissue. It occurs primarily in adolescents and young adults but can occur in immune-compromised individuals as well. Mononucleosis is known as "kissing disease," since it is transmitted orally by direct contact of kissing or sharing glasses. Incubation period is 4–6 weeks, with symptoms rarely lasting more than 4 months,

Mode of Transmission: Direct contact of the Epstein-Barr virus that is present in saliva

Signs & Symptoms: Enlarged spleen, lymphadenopathy, lethargy, fever, chills, and sore throat.

Vaccination: None

Influenza

Influenza is an RNA-Orthomyxoviridae virus that occurs worldwide in three sub-types. **Influenza A** can spread from humans to animals and vice versa, creating new strains that most people are not immune to. Major changes in mutations of influenza A are called antigenic shifts. These shifts produce new strains that can be conveyed freely from person to person. **Influenza B** viruses are transmitted freely from human to human. **Influenza C** produces mild respiratory symptoms that do not result in epidemics. Incubation period is 1–5 days.

Mode of Transmission: Inspiration of droplets from someone coughing or sneezing; the touching of fluids from an infected person

Signs & Symptoms: Body aches, nausea, vomiting, diarrhea, runny nose, sore throat, cough, lethargy, fever and/or headache.

Vaccination: Developed yearly in response to new strains

Legionnaires Disease

Legionnaires disease is in a category of its own with **Legionella** bacteria. It was first discovered in the 1970s during an outbreak at a convention of the American Legion. *Legionella* are present in soil, water, and air conditioning units. An individual with this disease should get early diagnosis and treatment since severe legionnaires disease has a mortality rate of 30–50%. Incubation period is 1–18 days.

Mode of Transmission: Bacteria aerosols of inspired air with *Legionella pneumophila*

Signs & Symptoms: Radiographs confirming pneumonia; diarrhea and confusion.

Vaccination: None

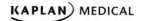

Measles, German (Rubella)

German measles is caused by the **rubella** virus of the rubivirus genus of the Togaviridae family of viruses. It highly contagious. If a woman contracts rubella when pregnant, severe birth defects may occur. With vaccines, rubella has been nearly eliminated in the United States. Incubation period is 2–3 weeks.

Mode of Transmission: Nasal secretions, airborne droplets, direct contact

Signs & Symptoms: Fever, malaise, lymphadenopathy, erythematous maculopapular rash for 2–3 days.

Vaccination: Inactivated rubella virus contained in the MMR vaccine

Measles (Rubeola)

Measles occurs when one is infected with the **rubeola** virus, a highly contagious disease that is a member of the paramyxoviridae family. One symptom of measles is **Koplik's spots**, small red spots with blue-white centers that tend to appear in the buccal mucosa. Koplik's spots appear after the fever, but before the appearance of a rash.

Mode of Transmission: Airborne droplets, direct contact

Signs & Symptoms: Erythematous maculopapular rash, fever, lymphadenopathy, cough, Koplik's spots.

Vaccination: Inactivated virus of MMR (measles, mumps, and rubella)

Mumps

Mumps is the result of an infection in the parotid gland. Also called parotiditis, mumps is a highly contagious disease that can affect the central nervous system causing meningitis. It is a member of the paramyxoviridae family. **Orchitis** results in sterility of post-pubertal males with mumps. Incubation period is 12–25 days.

Mode of Transmission: Airborne droplets, direct contact

Signs & Symptoms: Fever, swollen parotid gland, malaise.

Vaccination: Inactivated virus of MMR (measles, mumps and rubella)

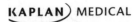

Pertussis

Whooping cough is an acute, highly contagious disease caused by *Bordetella pertussis* bacteria. It occurs in early childhood. Incubation period is usually 7–10 days, though it can be anywhere from 4–21 days. After the incubation period comes the **catarrhal stage**, during which time the bacteria attach to the cilia of the respiratory tract. This causes a runny nose, for instance, to have a more watery mucous. One or two weeks later, the **paroxysmal stage** occurs, when the mucous becomes thicker and the patient coughs spasmodically to clear the tracheobronchial tract. After the spasmodic cough, the patient makes a long inspiratory effort that makes a "whooping" sound. This stage can last from 1–6 weeks and requires a long convalescent period.

Mode of Transmission: Inhalation of *B. pertussis* droplets; direct contact with secretions

Signs & Symptoms: Initially low-grade fever; sneezing; symptoms of a common cold followed by spasmodic cough with high-pitched whoop; vomiting.

Vaccination: Purified, inactivated *B. pertussis* cells that are part of the triple vaccine DPT

Pneumonia

Pneumonia can be caused by bacteria or by viral, fungal, or bacteria-like organisms that are mycoplasma-like. Pneumonia that affects one lobe or segment of the lung is called lobar pneumonia. Pneumonia that affects the lung bilaterally is called bronchopneumonia. Aspiration pneumonia occurs if vomit or chemicals are inhaled into the lungs, or if **dental plaque** is inhaled, which occurs in hospitalized and chronically institutionalized adults, especially those with preexisting conditions such as seizures that predispose them to aspiration. Some of the more common microorganisms include *Chlamydia pneumoniae, Haemophilus influenzae, Streptococcus pneumoniae, Mycoplasma pneumoniae*, respiratory syncytial viruses in children, and human parainfluenza viruses. Incubation period varies with the type of microorganism.

Mode of Transmission: Inhalation of droplets from an infected person; person to person contact; person to contaminated-surface contact

Signs & Symptoms: Fever; dyspnea; tachycardia; chills; wheezes; rhonchi; rales; malaise; productive sputum with color; headache.

Vaccination: Hib vaccine for *Haemophilus influenzae* and pneumoncoccal vaccine for *S. pneumoniae*.

Aspiration pneumonia can occur in the elderly from the aspiration of bacterial plaque.

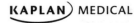

Prions

The CDC has brought to light microorganisms called **transmissible spongiform encephalopathies**—or **prions**—that are associated with **Mad Cow Disease**. Prions produce small holes in the brain, making it look like Swiss cheese. There is no evidence of cross-contamination by contact or by air from one person to another, nor has there been any occurrence of prions in the dental setting. They have, however, shown a unique resistance to routine decontamination techniques.

The CDC is concerned with **Creutzfeldt-Jakob disease (CJD)**, one type of transmissible spongiform encephalopathy in dentistry. The risk of cross-contamination when treating a patient with CJD is extremely low, but special precautions might be suggested during treatment of such an individual. CJD occurs on average around age 67, and death usually occurs within a year.

Variant CJDs have surfaced recently outside of North America: nvCJD and vCJD. These forms occur in much younger individuals, with age 29 as the average mean when death occurs. Slightly different symptoms have a longer duration from the beginning until death.

Mode of Transmission: Unknown for transmissible spongiform encephalopathies

Signs & Symptoms: In **CJD**: change in personality; depression; failing memory; unsteady gait at first. Then: mental deterioration; insomnia; myoclonus (involuntary muscle contractions); nystagmus (rapid involuntary eye movement); confusion; blindness. Late-stage symptoms: inability to speak or move; severe mental impairment; coma. In **vCJD**: psychiatric disturbances; behavioral changes; uncoordinated muscle movement; loss of peripheral sensation.

Vaccination: None

Rheumatic Fever

Rheumatic fever is the result of a group A ß-hemolytic streptococcal bacteria pharyngeal infection—strep throat. If the heart is affected with this infection, an acute valvulitis occurs that can thicken, fuse, or destroy the valves. If this occurs, the valve will not completely close or completely open.

Mode of Transmission: Direct contact with secretions or respiratory droplets

Signs & Symptoms: Joint swelling and pain, skin rash, abdominal discomfort, fever, malaise.

Vaccination: None

Paget's Disease

Paget's disease also known as **osteitis deformans** is a chronic, painful bone disease in which bone is destroyed and then replaced with distorted, fragile bone. It can result in bone fractures, bone deformation, and arthritis. It is of unknown etiology and may possibly be genetic. It occurs more often after age 40. Mild cases may be asymptomatic. Most cases have a good prognosis if treated early.

Mode of Transmission: Unknown etiology

Signs & Symptoms: Bone pain, joint damage leading to osteoarthritis, hearing loss, tendency to form kidney stones, tooth loss, sarcoma, bone deformity, fractures occurs easily, headaches, and vision loss.w

Vaccination: None

Scarlet Fever

Scarlet fever is a result of a **group A ß-hemolytic streptococcal bacterial** infection that primarily affects children. It accompanies a strep throat infection which could lead to rheumatic fever. Scarlet fever affects the skin, tongue, and throat.

Mode of Transmission: Direct contact with secretions or respiratory droplets

Signs & Symptoms: Strawberry-red tongue; rash; lymphadenopathy; headache; fever; sore throat.

Vaccination: None

Shingles

Shingles is caused by the **herpes zoster virus** (reactivation of the chicken pox virus) which is in the same family as chicken pox. It lies dormant in the dorsal root ganglia until stimulated by illness, stress, weakened immunity, or trauma.

Mode of Transmission: Reactivation of the varicella zoster (primary infection causing chicken pox) that lies dormant in the dorsal root or cervical ganglia

Signs & Symptoms: Fever; itching; tingling; burning on one side of the body that becomes a red rash. The rash can become vesicles that last 2–3 weeks.

Vaccination: None

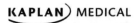

Staphylococci Infections

Staphylococcus aureus and *Staphylococcus epidermis* are part of our normal bacteria flora that reside intraorally, around the nares, and on our skin. Both are spread by direct contact from hands. The CDC has stressed the importance of hand-washing among health personnel largely as a result of these infections. Intact skin is stressed because constant washing of hands can result in long-term damage. Moisturizing prevents dry, cracked hands, which are an entryway for microorganisms. Hands that have damage are more likely to harbor pathogens such as *S. aureus*, *S. hominis*, and a vast number of other species.

S. aureus has become especially resistant to antibiotics including *methicillin* and other penicillins and antibiotics. This bacteria can cause many suppurative lesions. *S. epidermis* can result in endocarditis, bacteremias, and wound infection.

Mode of Transmission: Direct contact with saliva and other secretions

Signs & Symptoms: Suppurative lesions such as furuncle (boil), an infection of the hair follicle; carbuncles (several furuncles together); impetigo; septicemias; toxic shock syndrome.

Vaccination: None

Streptococcus Pharyngitis

Strep throat or pharyngitis is caused by *Streptococcus pyogenes* bacteria. Should it become serious, it can go on to become scarlet or rheumatic fever. It is easily treatable with antibiotics.

Mode of Transmission: Airborne droplets; direct contact with secretions

Signs & Symptoms: Sore, red throat; fever, malaise; lymphadenopathy; exudate on the tonsils.

Vaccination: None

Syphilis

Intraoral defects from congenital syphilis can result in Mulberry molars or Hutchinson's incisors.

Syphilis is a sexually transmitted disease caused by the *Treponema pallidum* bacteria. It can result in congenital defects intraorally, such as **Mulberry molars** or **Hutchinson's incisors** when *T. pallidum* crosses the placenta. It can also result in mental retardation if a newborn is not properly treated at birth. Some babies are born without symptoms. Incubation period is 10 days–3 months.

Mode of Transmission: Sexual contact with lesion on mucous membranes or skin

Signs & Symptoms: Stage 1: small, round **nodule (chancre)** on the lip, tongue, or sex organs, with few other symptoms. It heals in 1–5 weeks with no remnants. **Stage 2 (6–8 weeks after exposure):** Painless **mucous patches intraorally**; non-

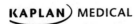

itching rash; lymphadenopathy; fever; malaise; headache; weight loss. **Stage 3: gummas** (soft tumors containing dead, swollen fibrous tissue) intraorally on the tongue or palate, though possibly on the skin, bones, or internal organs. At this stage, damage occurs to body organs such as the brain, heart, etc. that results in uncoordinated muscle movement, paralysis, blindness, dementia, joint pain, damage to blood vessels, and possibly death.

Vaccination: None

Stage	Intraoral symptom	Other symptoms
Primary	Chancre	Usually asymptomatic
Secondary	Mucous patches	Rash, lymphadenopathy, fever, malaise, headaches, weight loss, fatigue
Tertiary	Gumma	Body organ damage resulting in uncoordinated movements, paralysis, blindness, dementia, joint pain, possibly death

Tetanus

Tetanus is an acute disease that occurs when **Clostridium tetani** enters the body through a wound. Tetanus can be fatal. The toxin produced by these spore-forming bacilli attaches to the central nervous system, hindering neurotransmitters from being released. This results in prolonged muscle contraction through motor impulses that are triggered so rapidly that the muscles are not allowed a chance to relax. Should this occur, laryngospasm could result, making it difficult for the individual to breathe. Incubation period is 3–21 days.

Mode of Transmission: Entrance of *C. tetani* into a wound

Signs & Symptoms: Muscle-stiffness in jaw (lockjaw or **trismus**); headache. Then, general muscle rigidity; painful convulsions.

Vaccination: Tetanus immune globulin, DPT vaccine

Tuberculosis

Mycobacterium tuberculosis are bacilli encapsulated by a thick, waxy coat. This coat protects these bacilli from sunlight or chemical exposure, rendering them hard to kill. TB has been found in archeological dig sites where there is no sun exposure. It can also remain airborne up to 8 hours, and can survive on surfaces in wet or dried sputum up to 6 weeks. Not everyone who is exposed to this aerosol and inhales it becomes infected. It resides in the alveoli, where, in some people, it can start to multiply, causing infection or creating a latent infection. A **latent infection** occurs when the macrophages of the body stop the bacteria from multiplying and become inactive. They can reactivate at a later time but in most cases, do not. When tested, this person will have a positive TB test and will be asymptomatic.

The test for TB is the Mantoux PPD test or purified protein derivative. A new complete blood test is called QuantiFERON-TB test (QFT).

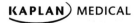

Mode of Transmission: Droplet inhalation

Signs & Symptoms: Fever; weight loss; night sweats; persistent cough with or without blood; lethargy; chills.

Vaccination: None

ORAL MICROFLORA

When a baby is born, its mouth is sterile, and microorganisms quickly develop within hours of birth. Within the first month, identifiable bacteria include *Lactobacillus*, *Neisseria*, *Staphylococcus*, *Streptococcus*, and *Veillonella*. When teeth erupt, even more microorganisms appear, such as *S. mutans*, *S. salivarius*, and *S. sanguis* along with the following spirochetes: *Actinomyces*, *Bacteroides*, *Fusobacterium*, *Norcardia*, *Veillonella*.

Bacteria amass themselves in different locales: buccal mucosa, tooth surfaces, gingiva, crevicular sulcus, dorsum of the tongue, and appliances.

Tongue

The tongue is an ideal environment for many species of microorganisms to live. A fissured tongue, especially, can harbor many bacteria.

One microorganism that is intraorally **exclusive** to the tongue is ***Stomatococcus mucilaginosus***. Other microorganisms include *S. mitis*, *S. oralis*, and *S. salivarius*. Bacteria in smaller numbers would include *Haemophilus* and *Veillonella* along with *A. naeslundii*.

The **buccal mucosa** microflora consists largely of *Haemophilus sp* and *Streptococcus sp.*, along with *S. mitis*, *S. oralis*, and *S. sanguis*. *S. vestibularis* is located in the vestibule.

Saliva

Saliva is a buffer of serous and mucous secretions from the parotid, sublingual, and submaxillary exocrine glands that aids in starch digestion with salivary amylase. Saliva also moisturizes food to aid in swallowing and cleanses teeth with its natural flow. Saliva does not have it very own resident microflora but obtains microorganisms from all of its surrounding tissues.

Tooth Surfaces

Each tooth surface has different microorganisms that predominate on each of the different surfaces. Pits and fissures primarily contain *A. naeslundii* and *S. mutans*. Interproximal surfaces contain *S. sanguinis*, *A. israelii*, *A. naeslundii*, *Prevotella* sp., *Streptococcus* sp., and *Veillonella* sp.

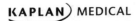

Caries Formation

The **normal pH** of plaque is **6.75–7.0.** When eating food, the pH of the oral cavity is lowered to a critical **pH range of 4.5–5.5** with the **intake of sugar.** This is when **decalcification of the enamel** surface can begin. For the **root portion** that is covered with cementum and is not as hard as enamel, the pH at which decalcification starts is **6.0–6.7.** Streptococci species **initiate** carious lesions in the mouth by converting fructose into lactic acid, in particular, *S. mutans.* **Lactobacilli** are found in large numbers in **deep carious lesions.**

Carious Lesions

Location	pH (Normal pH 6.75–7.0)	Microbe responsible
Pits & fissures	4.5–5.5	*S. mutans*
Smooth surfaces	4.5–5.5	*S. mutans*
Root	6.0–6.7	*A. viscosus, A. naeslundii*
Dentin	Below 5	*Lactobacillus* sp., *A. naeslundii*

Biofilm Microflora and Formation

An **acquired pellicle** is a tenacious film of salivary glycoprotein that attaches to hydroxyapatite. This pellicle is one manner in which biofilm can attach itself. Microorganisms found in the acquired pellicle include *Streptococcus sanguis, Streptococcus mutans*, and *Actinomyces viscosus.*

Plaque is a non-mineralized, organized, mixed microbial **biofilm.** It is made up of 80% water and 20% solids. Bacterial biofilm starts to colonize with *S. mitis, S. oralis*, and *S. sanguis*, using the acquired pellicle as a means of attachment. Once attached, these cells start to replicate; they spread into a **corn-cob** configuration. As biofilm matures, more microbes appear: *A. naeslundii* predominates along with *S. sanguis* and *S. mutans* as other species enter in such as *A. israelii, Bacteroides, Capnocytophaga* spirochetes, *Treponema* spirochetes, and *Veillonella.* Tertiary microorganisms such as *Prevotella intermedia* and *Porphyromonas gingivali* start to enter, causing gingival inflammation. Supragingival biofilm elongates into subgingival plaque.

Time	Stage	Type	Gram +/–	Microbes
Day 1–2	Colonizing	Aerobic	+	*S. mutans, S. sanguis*, streptococci
Day 2–4	Multiplication	Aerobic	+	Rods, filaments
Day 4–7	Starts to mature	Aerobic & Anaerobic	+ / –	Rods filaments, fusobacteria
Day 7–14	Maturation	Anaerobic	–	Vibrios, spirochetes
Day 14–21		Anaerobic	–	Vibrios, spirochetes, cocci, filaments

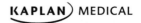

Calculus Formation

Calculus forms by **depositing minerals** into plaque. After biofilm forms on the acquired pellicle, **saliva** provides **calcium** and **phosphorus** to supragingival biofilm, causing mineralization of supragingival calculus. **Subgingival** plaque obtains its minerals from **gingival crevicular fluid** to form subgingival calculus. **Biofilm mineralization** occurs within **24–72 hours** of forming on a tooth surface.

Some individuals have a higher incidence of calculus than others. Factors that contribute to this are elevated salivary pH, elevated salivary calcium and phosphorus salts, higher lipid and protein concentrates in saliva, and lower levels of parotid pyrophosphate. Calculus harbors the bacteria that cause gingival disease.

PERIODONTAL DISEASE MICROFLORA

Gingival disease and **periodontal disease** are separate categories that affect everyone at some point in time. The leading offender of periodontal disease is plaque but other factors may enter into the disease process such as genetics, systemic conditions, medications, anxiety, and smoking.

Gingival Diseases

Gingivitis is a **reversible disease** whose symptoms include inflamed, swollen gingival tissues that bleed easily. This condition may be improved with proper dental prophylaxis and with correct home-care.

Plaque-induced gingivitis can occur both with or without local contributing factors, such as an overhanging filling or calculus. **Systemic conditions** that can contribute to plaque-induced gingivitis include diabetes, blood dyscrasias, and malnutrition. **Hormonal changes,** with the onset of puberty, menstruation, pregnancy, or lactation can cause it as well.

Non-plaque induced gingival lesions may be genetic in origin or may be caused by a variety of other factors: **bacteria, viruses, fungi, systemic conditions, injury,** or **foreign objects.**

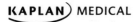

Periodontal Diseases

Periodontal diseases are **not reversible** since **bone is lost** in the disease process and cannot grow back. With these diseases, **recession** can occur because of the loss of connective tissue. The severity of the disease depends on its progression in **pocket formation** and **bone loss**. Periodontal disease can be **localized** or **generalized chronic periodontitis**, but it may also be localized or generalized **aggressive** periodontitis, which occurs in younger individuals.

Periodontitis may also be associated with **systemic conditions or disease**. Necrotizing periodontitis includes **necrotizing ulcerative gingivitis (NUG)** and **necrotizing ulcerative periodontitis (NUP)**. The periodontium can develop a **periodontal abscess**, and an endodontic lesion can also produce a periodontitis.

Deformities in the periodontium can create localized areas of periodontal disease as well. This will be discussed further in chapter 8 along with surgical and non-surgical procedures.

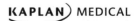

Main Bacteria with Associated Gingival and Periodontal Oral Diseases

Bacteria	Gram +/—	Disease	
Actinobacillus actinomycetemcomitans	—	Aggressive periodontitis* Necrotizing Ulcerative Periodontitis	Facultative anaerobe rod
Actinomyces israelii	+	Gingivitis*	Anaerobe rod
Actinomyces naeslundii	+	Gingivitis*	Facultative anaerobe rod
Bacteroides forsythus †	—	Chronic periodontitis	Anaerobe rod
Borrelia vincentii	—	Necrotizing Ulcerative Periodontitis	Anaerobe spirochete
Campylobacter rectus	—	Chronic periodontitis	Microaerophilic rod
Campylobacter spp.	—	Gingivitis	Microaerophilic rod
Candida albicans		Candidiasis*	Fungus
Capnocytophaga sputigena	—	Aggressive periodontitis	Anaerobe rod
Eikenella corrodens	—	Aggressive periodontitis	Microaerophilic coccobacilli
Eubacterium spp.	+	Chronic periodontitis Gingivitis Necrotizing Ulcerative Periodontitis*	Anaerobe rod
Fusobacterium nucleatum	—	Chronic periodontitis Gingivitis Necrotizing Ulcerative Periodontitis*	Anaerobe rod
Haemophilus actinomycetemcomitans	—	Necrotizing Ulcerative Periodontitis*	Facultative anaerobe coccobacilli
Lactobacillus spp.	+	Gingivitis	Microaerophilic rod
Porphyromonas gingivalis	—	Chronic periodontitis Necrotizing Ulcerative Periodontitis*	Anaerobe rod
Prevotella intermedia	—	Chronic periodontitis Gingivitis Necrotizing Ulcerative Gingivitis*	Anaerobe rod
Prevotella oralis	—	Chronic periodontitis	Anaerobe rod
Streptococcus anginosus	+	Gingivitis	Anaerobe cocci
Streptococcus mitis	+	Gingivitis	Anaerobe cocci
Treponema spp.	—	Chronic periodontitis Gingivitis	Anaerobe spirochete
Veillonella parvula	—	Gingivitis	Anaerobe cocci
Wolinella spp.	—	Gingivitis	Anaerobe flagella

† Bacteroides genus is in the process of undergoing a reclassification

* Designates the predominant microorganisms associated with this disease

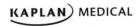

REVIEW QUESTIONS

1. Viruses need a host cell in which to replicate. In which of the following cells does the HIV virus prefer to replicate itself?

   A. CD4 helper cell

   B. CD8 supressor cell

   C. CD8 killer cells

   D. T lymphocytes

   E. B lymphocytes

2. Your patient presents with a periodontal abscess that started last night. Which type of blood cell is the body's first line of defense with a new infection?

   A. Monocytes

   B. Eosinophils

   C. Neutrophils

   D. Mast cells

   E. Platelets

3. Which of the following microorganisms is *not* normally found in the acquired pellicle?

   A. *Streptococcus sanguis*

   B. *Streptococcus anginosus*

   C. *Actinomyces viscosus*

   D. *Streptococcus mutans*

4. The oral cavity normally has a pH of 6.75–7.0. What pH is necessary for root caries to begin formation?

   A. 4.5–5.5

   B. Below 5.0

   C. 6.0–6.7

   D. 3.0–4.0

5. As plaque starts to mineralize on the tooth surface, streptococci begin to stack up. Microscopically, they take on what type of appearance?

   A. Granules

   B. Chains

   C. Corn-cob

   D. Scaffold

   E. Grainy

6. Syphilis is a sexually transmitted disease that is caused by which of the microorganisms?

   A. *Borrelia burgdorferi*

   B. *Haemophilus ducreyi*

   C. *Neisseria gonorrhea*

   D. *Treponema carateum*

   E. *Treponema pallidum*

7. All the following microorganisms are involved with aggressive periodontitis EXCEPT

   A. *Actinobacillus actinomycetemcomitans*

   B. *Eikenella corrodens*

   C. *Veillonella parvula*

   D. *Capnocytophaga sputigena*

8. The virus associated with severe acute respiratory syndrome (SARS) is

   A. Rhinovirus

   B. Coronavirus

   C. Cytomegalovirus

   D. Adenovirus

   E. Picornaviridae

9. The phase of hepatitis that involves liver damage and jaundice is

   A. Preicteric
   B. Icteric
   C. Convalescent
   D. Carrier state

10. Which of the following pathogens resides exclusively on the tongue?

    A. *Capnocytophaga sputigena*
    B. *Streptococcus sanguis*
    C. *Porphyromonas gingivalis*
    D. *Actinomyces naeslundii*
    E. *Stomatococcus mucilaginosus*

11. Which of the following terms renders bacteria easier to digest?

    A. Lysis
    B. Opsonization
    C. Phagocytosis
    D. Interferons

12. Penicillin has the ability to inhibit bacterial growth. During which of the following phases of microbial growth does this occur?

    A. Lag phase
    B. Log phase
    C. Stationary phase
    D. Decline phase

13. Which of the following immunoglobulins triggers the production of IgG?

    A. IgA
    B. IgD
    C. IgE
    D. IgM

14. Hepatitis spread by the oral–fecal route is

    A. Hepatitis B
    B. Hepatitis C
    C. Hepatitis D
    D. Hepatitis E
    E. Hepatitis G

15. Which of the following microorganisms is associated with Creutzfeldt-Jakob disease (CJD)?

    A. Protists
    B. Prions
    C. Pseudomonads
    D. Proteus
    E. Plasmodium

16. Syphilis has three different stages. An oral sign and symptom of the third stage is

    A. Mucous patches
    B. Chancre
    C. Gummas
    D. Gules
    E. Gonococcal glossitis

17. Vaccinations prevent the spread of disease. Which of the following diseases has a vaccination that produces artificially acquired passive immunity?

    A. Measles, mumps, and rubella (MMR)
    B. Polio
    C. Hepatitis B Immunoglobulin (HBIG)
    D. Pertussis
    E. None of the above

18. Streptococcal infections can cause a variety of infections. Which of the following streptococcal groups is responsible for rheumatic fever?

    A. Group A beta-hemolytic streptococcal bacteria
    B. Group B streptococci
    C. Group C streptococci
    D. Group B beta-hemolytic streptococci

19. The microorganism that can stay airborne for up to 8 hours is

    A. Haemophilus influenzae
    B. HIV
    C. Mycobacterium tuberculosis
    D. Staphylococcus aureus
    E. Hepatitis B

20. The most severe hypersensitivity is

    A. Type I hypersensitivity
    B. Type II hypersensitivity
    C. Type III hypersensitivity
    D. Type IV hypersensitivity

21. The maturation of plaque occurs at

    A. 1–2 days
    B. 2–7 days
    C. 7–14 days
    D. 14–21 days

22. The formation of the pellicle depends on

    A. Thin homogenous acellular layer
    B. Colonization of bacteria
    C. Glucans
    D. Endotoxins
    E. Biofilm

23. Which of the following diseases can cross the placenta and cause birth defects?

    A. Rubeola
    B. Rubella
    C. Varicella zoster
    D. Pertussis

24. Which of the following microorganisms is responsible for inflicting a dental hygienist with herpetic whitlow?

    A. HBV
    B. HCV
    C. HGV
    D. HIV
    E. HSV

25. Shingles is caused by a latent virus that lays dormant in the dorsal root ganglia. Which of the following microorganisms is responsible for shingles?

    A. Herpes zoster
    B. Varicella zoster
    C. Rubella
    D. Rubeola
    E. Herpes simplex

ANSWER EXPLANATIONS

1. A

CD4 helper cells are the cells that the HIV virus normally infects.

B. CD8 supressor cells try to fight off the virus so their number increases when the body is invaded by a pathogen.

C. CD8 killer cells are exactly the same as CD8 suppressor cells.

D. T lymphocytes includes both the CD4 helper cells and the CD8 supressor cells.

E. B lymphocytes produce antibodies.

2. C

Neutrophils act first against the invading pathogen as it enters the body with acute inflammation.

A. Monocytes are involved with chronic infection.

B. Eosinophils are involved in allergic responses.

D. Mast cells are also involved with allergic response with the release of histamine.

E. Platelet cells aid in blood clotting.

3. B

Streptococcus anginosus is NOT normally found in the acquired pellicle but is found in gingivitis.

Streptococcus sanguis, *Actinomyces viscosus*, and *Streptococcus mutans* are found in the acquired pellicle.

4. C

6.0–6.7 is the pH for root caries to begin

A. 4.5–5.5 is the pH for pits and fissure caries and smooth surfaces.

B. Below 5.0 is the pH for dentinal caries.

D. 3.0–4.0 is much too acidic for the mouth.

5. C

Corn-cob appearance is how streptococci look microscopically.

A. Granules appear in cells.

B. The prefix for chains of bacteria is *strepto*.

D. Scaffold appearance is how fimbriae or filamentous proteins on the surface of bacterial cells look.

E. Grainy appearance is how cells look.

6. E

Syphilis is caused by *Treponema pallidum*

A. *Borrelia burgdorferi* is the microorganism responsible for Lyme disease.

B. *Haemophilus ducreyi* is the microorganism responsible for chancroid.

C. *Neisseria gonorrhea* is the microorganism responsible for gonorrhea.

D. *Treponema carateum* is the microorganism responsible for pinta which is a skin infection where papules form then erupt, leaving red to blue-black spots.

7. C

Veillonella parvula is seen more in gingivitis

A. *Actinobacillus actinomycetemcomitans* is involved with aggressive periodontitis.

B. *Eikenella corrodens* are involved with aggressive periodontitis.

D. *Capnocytophaga sputigena* is involved with aggressive periodontitis.

8. B

Coronavirus is associated with SARS.

A. *Rhinovirus* is associated with the common cold.

C. *Cytomegalovirus* is a herpes member and has similar symptoms to mononucleosis.

D. *Adenovirus* is associated with the common cold.

E. Picornaviridae is associated with the polio virus, rhinovirus, and hepatitis A virus.

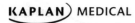

9. B

In the icteric phase of hepatitis, jaundice appears and liver damage occurs.

A. Preicteric phase occurs before the appearance of jaundice.

C. Convalescent phase occurs after the active infection.

D. Carrier state occurs when someone never fully recovers.

10. E

Stomatococcus mucilaginosus resides exclusively on the tongue.

A. *Capnocytophaga sputigena* is a microorganism involved in aggressive periodontitis.

B. *Streptococcus sanguis* is found in the acquired pellicle and plaque.

C. *Porphyromonas gingivalis* are found in various periodontal diseases.

D. *Actinomyces naeslundii* is found on tooth surfaces.

11. B

Opsonization renders bacteria easier to digest.

A. Lysis is the disintegration of bacteria.

C. Phagocytosis is the packman that gobbles up the bacteria.

D. Interferons interfere with viral replication.

12. B

Log phase occurs with the binary fission of the cell during mitosis. That is when bacteria are susceptible to penicillin.

A. Lag phase occurs when the cell grows in size but has not yet divided.

C. Stationary phase is cell growth where the rate of cell division equals the rate of cell death.

D. Decline phase occurs when the nutrients are depleted and the cells die off.

13. D

IgM is the most numerous immunoglobulin that triggers IgG.

A. IgA lines the body surfaces to protect from entering the body's natural cavities.

B. IgD may recognize antigens.

C. IgE is involved with immediate hypersensitivity or anaphylactic reactions.

14. D

Hepatitis E is found in impoverished countries with poor sewage and drainage problems. It is spread by the oral–fecal route.

A. Hepatitis B transmits through unprotected sex, needle sharing, sharps exposure of health care workers, mother to baby during birth, or unsterile tattoo needles.

E. Hepatitis G is spread through needle sharing when the HGV virus is present.

15. B

Prions—also called transmissible spongiform encephalopathies—are associated with Mad Cow Disease and Creutzfeldt-Jakob disease (CJD).

C. Pseudomonads are a group of bacteria responsible for wound infections.

D. Proteus is a species of bacteria in the enterobacterium genus that is responsible for UTI infections.

E. Plasmodium spp are associated with malaria.

16. C

Gummas occur in third stage of syphilis.

A. Mucous patches occur in the second stage of syphilis.

B. Chancre occur in the first stage of syphilis.

D. Gules is a red color that was included here as a distractor.

E. Gonococcal glossitis occurs with gonorrhea.

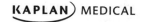

17. C

HBIG produces artificially acquired passive immunity. For its use, individuals need a booster shot.

A. MMR vaccine produces artificially acquired active immunity.

B. Polio vaccine produces artificially acquired active immunity.

D. Pertussis vaccine produces artificially acquired active immunity for whooping cough.

18. A

Group A ß-hemolytic streptococcal bacteria are responsible for rheumatic fever.

B. Group B streptococci can cause meningitis in newborn babies.

C. Group C streptococci can cause throat, ear, and eye infections.

D. Group B ß-hemolytic streptococci can cause pharyngitis.

19. C

Mycobacterium tuberculosis is the microorganism that can remain airborne for up to 8 hours.

A. *Haemophilus influenzae* is a fragile virus.

B. HIV is a fragile virus that cannot survive for very long without a host.

D. *Staphylococcus aureus* can cause suppurative lesions on epidermis and is not an airborne infection.

E. Hepatitis B can live on surfaces up to 1 week.

20. A

Type I hypersensitivity is the most serious type of reaction. It involves anaphylaxis, which can be life threatening.

B. Type II involves an antibody-antigen reaction. IgG and IgM are the antibodies involved here. An example would be Rh- mother to baby.

C. Type III involves the accumulation of soluble antigen-antibody complexes involving inflammation.

D. Type IV is a delayed type cell-mediated hypersensitivity, like a positive PPD test.

21. C

7–14 days is when plaque matures.

A. 1–2 days is when it is colonizing.

B. 2–7 days is when it starts to replicate.

D. 14–21 days is older plaque.

22. A

The formation of a pellicle depends on a thin homogenous acellular layer.

D. Endotoxins are produced by the bacteria but do not influence the adherence of the pellicle.

23. B

Rubella can cross the placenta and cause birth defects.

24. E

HSV infects fingers with herpetic whitlow.

A. HBV causes hepatitis B.

B. HCV causes hepatitis C.

C. HGV causes hepatitis G.

25. A

Herpes zoster causes shingles.

B. *Varicella zoster* causes chicken pox but lies dormant to become Herpes Zoster that produces shingles.

D. Rubeola causes regular measles.

E. Herpes can lay dormant in the trigeminal ganglia.

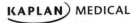

Chapter Seven:
Infection Control and Sterilization

Dental professionals work in an environment that puts them at risk for many pathogens, particularly airborne and bloodborne pathogens. The CDC, ADA, and OSHA (Occupational Safety & Health Administration) consider dental personnel especially at risk for hepatitis B, cytomegalovirus, tuberculosis, herpes, and influenza.

INFECTION CONTROL

In 2003, the CDC altered the guidelines to reduce the risk of transmission of all pathogens in the dental office. **Standard precautions** were replaced with universal precautions. Modifications were made for hand washing, quality of the dental waterline, boiled water advisories, surface disinfectants, flash cycles, and pre-procedural mouth rinsing.

The CDC has found that **pre-procedural mouth rinses** have not been proven to cross-contaminate the patient with dental personnel. However, these rinses can reduce the number of microorganisms that are generated in aerosols during dental procedures.

Every patient is to be treated with standard precautions regardless of his infection status. **All body fluids except sweat** are considered to be a contamination source. Blood—whether or not it is seen—should be considered present in all body fluids except sweat.

The different **modes of transmission** for infection in the dental setting include the following. The chain of infection includes a susceptible host, a pathogen, and a portal of entry.

- **Direct contact** from person to person
- **Indirect contact** from person to a contaminated object or surface
- Inhalation of **air** or **droplets**

Getting a patient's current medical history before treatment is crucial so that any potential exposure can be established. Of course, not every infected patient fully discloses her medical history, so the dental hygienist can work only with what information she has been given.

Other modes of transmission are vectors (ticks, mosquitoes, fleas), vehicles (water, food, airborne), and contact.

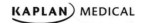

Protective Equipment

In order to prevent exposure of potentially harmful agents, **OSHA** dictates that employers must supply **personnel protective equipment (PPE)** to dental professionals. This equipment includes eyewear, face masks, outerwear, and gloves.

Eyewear

Eyewear includes safety goggles/glasses, the employee's own prescription glasses with proper top and side shields, and face shields. With these items, conjunctivitis will not occur since microorganisms will not be able to enter through mucous membranes. Wearing eyewear also prevents injury from debris or chemicals. Patients should also be given eyewear if treatment is going to produce chemical or flying debris.

Face Masks

While a face shield protects the eyes, a face mask goes even further: It prevents a hygienist from inhaling droplets and airborne microorganisms. The **mask** protects the mucous membranes of the nose and mouth from being contaminated by spatter and from the inhalation of airborne droplets. There are many types of masks that are filtration-efficient and fluid-resistant, including dome masks, tie-on masks, elastic masks, and ear-loop masks. A new mask should be worn for each patient. Proper fit is important to ensure that droplets from aerosols are effectively kept out.

Outerwear

Outer protective clothing prevents contamination of the dental hygienist's clothing and skin. It also prevents cross-contamination from taking place once the hygienist is outside the office. As per OSHA regulations, an employer must provide disposable garments or reusable outer garments that can be laundered. Laundering by the employer may be done in the office or at a laundry service. The garments should have long sleeves with fitted cuffs and a high neck at the collar. Outer protective clothing should be changed daily and immediately if soiled or moistened.

Gloves

Gloves provide an important barrier while treating the dental patient. It has been proven that there has been cross-contamination by ungloved dental personnel. Ambidextrous **latex** gloves are the most widely used in dentistry.

Utility gloves or **nitrile gloves** can be used when cleaning or handling contaminated instruments, when disinfecting surfaces, or when handling chemicals such as developer, fixer, ultrasonic solutions, or denture solutions. When necessary, **clear plastic overgloves** may be worn on top of regular treatment gloves to write on a chart, touch radiographs, or touch cabinets. **Sterile surgical gloves** and **sterile water** should be used during any surgical procedure.

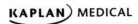

Hygienists should wear **non-latex** hypoallergenic **vinyl** or **nitrile gloves** if they or the patient has a latex allergy. Employees should be familiar with the signs and symptoms of latex allergies or hypersensitivities.

Hand washing prevents the transmission to patients of microorganisms that are part of the normal skin flora residing in our hands, such as **staphylococcus aureus** and **staphylococcus epidermis**. The CDC and ADA recommend washing hands with an antimicrobial soap at the beginning of the day, before gloving, **after** glove removal, and before leaving the building.

There has been much discussion about the importance of having **intact skin** on a dental professional's hands. Dental personnel are advised to wash their hands frequently and also to keep them moist with lotion, because frequent washing will dry them out. Alcohol-based waterless gels are a good alternative However, **petro-leum-based creams** are **not recommended** while working, since they break down latex gloves.

IMMUNIZATION

OSHA requires that employers offer immunization to new dental personnel not previously immunized for hepatitis B. This must be done **within the first 10 days of employment**. For those over age 20, this would involve **three injections**: the second immunization is administered one month after the first, and the third is administered six months after the first. Should the employee refuse the immunization, documentation of that refusal will remain in the employee's confidential medical file.

EXPOSURE PLAN

Parenteral injury or exposure to non-intact skin, eyes, mucous membranes, or the mouth should all be treated as **potentially infectious**. Should there be an **exposure** in the office, OSHA requires employers to offer an immediate confidential medical evaluation. After the individual has received immediate **first aid**, he would then **report** the incident to the employer, who then provides a **medical evaluation**. Documentation of the exposure, the incident, and the source shall be placed in the employee's confidential medical file.

The employer must request **permission** from the **source** to be tested for **HBV** and **HIV**, and also to allow disclosure of the test results to the exposed employee. **Counseling** should be made available to the exposed employee.

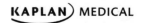

STERILIZATION AND DISINFECTION

Sterilization kills all forms of microbial life. **Disinfection** kills some pathogenic microorganisms, though not all microbial forms. Disinfectants kill different microorganisms according to their different levels effectiveness.

High-level disinfectants kill most microorganisms but not all bacterial spores. **Intermediate-level disinfectants** are tuberculocidal and eradicate mycobacterium and most viruses. **Low-level disinfectants** eradicate some bacteria, fungi, and viruses. Acceptable liquid chemical disinfectant solutions include glutaraldehyde, peracetic acid, and hydrogen peroxide, but some are toxic. Glutaraldehydes also are a skin irritant.

The **steam autoclave** kills all life forms; therefore, it sterilizes. The steam autoclave uses high heat and pressure to denature and coagulate microbes. The steam autoclave sterilizes when the temperature reaches **121° C** or **250° F** at **15 lbs. of pressure** for **15–30 minutes**.

Although NOT recommended, when sterilizing a heavier load of instruments, the load must be run for twice the amount of time.

The newer **statims** are able to run a load of instruments for **6–9 minutes**, depending on the model. Rather than heating the entire chamber as with an autoclave, the steam is injected into the cassette. The temperature is **135° C** at **32 lbs. of pressure**. This allows for a more rapid heating and cooling, which reduces instruments' heat exposure.

The colored indicator on the autoclave bag or striped indicator on the strip of tape does NOT indicate sterility. It indicates that the autoclave or statim has reached the proper temperature.

A **flash cycle** is an **unwrapped cycle** that should be used only in an **emergency situation**. Since the instrument is not wrapped, there is no way to maintain sterility and should be used only during a surgical procedure when an instrument may have become contaminated. The instrument should be transported aseptically to the operatory to maintain sterility once sterilized.

Dry heat sterilization cooks like an oven to oxidize cell parts. Sterilization occurs when the temperature has been at **160° C** or **320° F** for two hours, or **170° C** or **340° F** for one hour. The advantage of dry heat is that it does not corrode instruments the way a steam autoclave does.

Chemical vapor with heat sterilization destroys microbes and viruses but is not widely used in dentistry; the **chemicals** needed for sterilization are very expensive. Because of the chemicals, **adequate ventilation** is needed. Sterilization is achieved when the temperature reaches **127–132° C** or **260–270° F** for 20 minutes at 20-40 pounds of pressure.

Along with paper and cloth, meltable plastics may be sterilized by ethylene-oxide gas.

Ethylene oxide is a **gas** that is toxic to all microorganisms. It is utilized more in hospitals than in dental settings. Paper, meltable plastics, and cloth as well as instruments may be sterilized for a much longer period of time of **10-16 hours** and at a much lower temperature of **25° C** or **75° F**. Instruments such as plastic and rubber need to be **aerated for 24 hours afterward**.

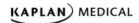

Biological verification of sterilization should be performed weekly on all the previous mentioned modes of sterilization. For the **steam autoclave** and **chemical vapor** sterilizer, the **Bacillus (Geobacillus) stearothermophilus** spore strips monitor the efficacy of sterilization. For **dry heat** and **ethylene oxide**, the **bacillus subtilis** spore strips monitor the efficacy of sterilization.

Sterilization of Critical, Semi-Critical, & Non-Critical Items

Instruments that must be disinfected or sterilized can be divided into three categories: critical, semi-critical, and non-critical. **Critical items** such as scalpels and bone chisels must be heat-sterilized or placed in a high-level disinfectant for a set amount of time. A high-level disinfectant, such as glutaraldehyde or hydrogen peroxide, will destroy most spores as well as bacteria, fungi, and viruses.

Semi-critical items such as mirrors and amalgam carriers that **contact mucous membranes** should be heat-sterilized or placed in high-level disinfectant. **Non-critical items** such as counters, floors, and pens can be disinfected with low-level disinfectants.

Some chemicals can disinfect in a short period (10–30 minutes), but require longer periods (6–10 hours) for full sterilization to occur.

Sterilization of the Patient Treatment Area

The patient treatment area should be kept clean and disinfected with a **spray–wipe–spray** technique: Spray the surface once—that **cleans** the surface. Then, spray the surface a second time—that **disinfects** the surface. Make sure to leave the spray for the full length of time recommended by the manufacturer. Acceptable surface disinfectants are chlorine, iodophors, phenols, and sodium bromide. **Plastic bags** (to cover chairs, tube heads, headrests, and bracket tables) and **plastic barriers** (to cover overhead light handles and radiograph-exposure buttons) help prevent cross-contaminants from entering crevices.

Disinfection of the Dental Lab

Personnel protective equipment should also be utilized when working in the dental laboratory. Materials to be transported to the dental laboratory should be cleaned of any blood or debris and be properly disinfected according to the manufacturer's recommendation for the particular material used. Items like rag wheels can be heat-sterilized.

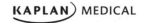

Sterilization of Dental Waterlines

In 2003, the CDC issued a new acceptable level of biofilm in a dental waterline: from 500 colony-forming units (CFU/mL) to 200. This level is more consistent with the level found in drinking water. At this new level, flushing the waterline at the beginning and end of the day is not necessary.

For any device connected to the dental waterlines, hygienists are advised to discharge water for 20–30 seconds between patients.

Management of Waste

Most items disposed of from the dental office are considered to be general medical waste. Only about 1 or 2% is considered regulated medical waste. **General medical waste** includes lightly saturated gauze, environmental barriers, gloves, gowns, and masks. **Regulated medical waste** includes a blood- or saliva-saturated gauze pad (heavily saturated), extracted teeth, surgically removed hard and soft tissues, and contaminated sharps.

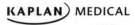

REVIEW QUESTIONS

1. In the sterilization bag for instruments, the indicator-strip turns color in the autoclave when

    A. the instruments are sterile.

    B. the instruments have been in the sterilizer for the proper amount of time, but are not necessarily sterile.

    C. the proper temperature has been achieved, but the instruments are not necessarily sterile.

    D. there is a faulty bag.

    E. it is touched by epidermal tissue.

2. Which of the following groups of microorganisms is the hardest to kill?

    A. Viruses

    B. Bacteria

    C. Fungi

    D. Protozoa

    E. Spores

3. Though they can irritate tissues, most glutaraldehydes can sterilize instruments in _____ amount of time.

    A. 30 minutes

    B. 4 hours

    C. 8 hours

    D. 10 hours

4. The tuberculosis spore has a wax coating for protection, and can stay airborne for

    A. 30 minutes

    B. 2 hours

    C. 6 hours

    D. 8 hours

5. As per standard precautions, all bodily fluids except one of the following should be considered potentially infectious for HBV, HIV, and other blood-borne pathogens. Which one is this EXCEPTION?

    A. Blood

    B. Sweat

    C. Saliva

    D. Excretions

    E. Lesions

6. The ultrasonic scaler produces an aerosol spray that is contraindicated for use on all the following people EXCEPT

    A. A patient with newly erupted teeth

    B. Down syndrome patient

    C. Hepatitis patient

    D. Respiratory infection

    E. A patient with an unshielded pacemaker

7. Sterilization is defined as

    A. The removal of bacteria, viruses, and some spores

    B. The inhibition of bacterial growth

    C. The removal of all life forms.

    D. The removal of viruses and protozoa

    E. The static effect of microbial growth

8. Sterilization is achieved by all of the following EXCEPT

    A. Dry heat at 170° C (350° F), 60 min.

    B. Autoclave at 90° C (200° F), 15–20 lbs. pressure, 15 min.

    C. Chemical vapor at 134° C (273° F), 20–40 lbs. pressure, 20 min.

    D. Ethylene oxide 25° C (75° F), 10–16 hrs.

    E. Statim at 135° C at 32 lbs. of pressure, 6–9 min.

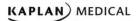

9. Once sterilized instruments are removed from a cold-sterilizing solution, which of the following statements is true?

    A. They can be stored in a disinfected drawer and still be considered sterile.

    B. They should be placed in a sterilization bag.

    C. Rinsing is not necessary to maintain sterility.

    D. Sterility cannot be monitored once they have come out of the solution.

10. You have just treated someone suspected of having hepatitis B. Which of the following surface disinfectants could be used to clean the treatment area?

    A. Quaternary ammonium compound

    B. Isopropyl alcohol

    C. Phenolic compounds

    D. Sodium hypochlorite 1:500

11. With so many surface disinfectants to choose from, which one of the following disinfectants stains surfaces?

    A. Isopropyl alcohol

    B. Iodophors

    C. Glutaraldehydes

    D. Sodium bromide

    E. Synthetic phenols

12. Which of the following uses a vector—a mode of transmission for a microorganism to enter the body?

    A. Salmonella

    B. Tuberculosis

    C. Contact with a contaminated surface

    D. East Nile virus

13. Regulated medical waste includes all the following EXCEPT

    A. Gauze saturated with blood

    B. Extracted teeth

    C. Soft tissues

    D. Sharps

    E. Gloves

14. All of the following are critical items that need to be heat-sterilized EXCEPT

    A. Mouth mirrors

    B. Scalpel handles

    C. Curets

    D. Surgical burs

15. One disadvantage in using ethylene oxide to sterilize instruments is that

    A. it dulls instruments.

    B. instruments can corrode.

    C. sterilized rubber and plastic need to be aerated for 24 hours afterward.

    D. it uses a very high temperature and can burn cloth.

16. Water should be discharged from ultrasonic scalers for ___ between patients.

    A. 20–30 seconds

    B. 1–2 minutes

    C. 2–3 minutes

    D. It is not necessary at all

17. The biological verification of sterilization for glutaraldehydes is the

    A. Bacillus stearothermophilus
    B. Bacillus subtilis
    C. There is no biological verification for glutaraldehydes
    D. All of the above

18. Which of the following bactericidal agents is effective against ALL known organisms?

    A. Boiling water for 20 minutes
    B. 70% ethyl alcohol
    C. Ethylene oxide
    D. 70% isopropyl alcohol
    E. Quarternary compounds

19. Of the following microorganisms or groups found in waterlines, which one is the CDC most concerned about?

    A. Bacteroides
    B. Mycobacterium
    C. Streptococci
    D. Staphylococci
    E. Biofilm

20. Which of the following chemical agents are EPA-registered for surface disinfecting?

    A. Sodium hypochlorite, iodophors, synthetic phenols
    B. Quaternary ammonium compounds, iodophors, alcohol
    C. Glutaraldehydes, quaternary ammonium compounds, sodium hypochlorite
    D. Alcohol, sodium hypochlorite, glutaraldehydes

21. Of the following microorganisms, which is the most fragile to disinfecting?

    A. AIDS/HIV
    B. Hepatitis virus
    C. Rhinovirus
    D. Coxsackie virus
    E. Mycobacterium tuberculosis

22. Bacteria like to grow at the same optimal temperature as human beings. That temperature is

    A. 25°C
    B. 37°C
    C. 48°C
    D. 55°C
    E. 98.7°C

23. A Boil Water Advisory has been issued in your area. You would not use the tap water for which of the following?

    A. Dental line
    B. Washing hands
    C. Water for the patient's rinsing
    D. All of the above.

24. Hepatitis B can survive on an inanimate surface for up to

    A. 1 hour
    B. 8 hours
    C. 1 week
    D. 1 month
    E. Indefinitely

25. When disinfecting a surface, the first spray wipe of the spray–wipe cycle is meant to:

    A. Totally disinfect the surface
    B. Be the cleansing portion of disinfecting
    C. Sterilize the surface
    D. None of the above

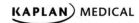

ANSWER EXPLANATIONS

1. C

The indicator-strip turns color in the autoclave when the proper temperature is achieved, but is not necessarily sterile. Sterility may not have been achieved if the proper pressure and temperature were not maintained for the full length of time.

2. E

Spores are most resistant to sterilization. This why we use the bacillus stearothermophilus and bacillus subtilis spore strips; they are biological indicators when testing for sterility.

A. Viruses are very fragile and need a host to live off of.

B. Bacteria can be resistant to some disinfectants but most are destroyed.

C. Fungi are fragile and can be easily destroyed with intermediate- or high-level disinfectants.

D. Protozoa are fragile and can be easily destroyed with intermediate- or high-level disinfectants.

3. D

Glutaraldehydes can sterilize instruments in 10 hours.

A. 30 minutes will simply disinfect the instruments.

4. D

Tuberculosis can stay airborne for up to 8 hours.

5. B

All bodily fluids should be considered potentially infectious for HBV, HIV, and other blood-borne pathogens EXCEPT sweat.

6. B

An ultrasonic scaler is safe to use on a Down syndrome patient who does not have an infectious disease.

A. Newly erupted teeth with their large pulp chambers can be overheated despite the spray for cooling.

7. C

Sterilization is defined as the removal of all life forms.

A. The removal of bacteria, viruses, and some spores is called disinfection.

B. The inhibition of bacterial growth is defined as bacteriostatic which inhibits bacterial growth.

D. The removal of viruses and protozoa represents disinfection.

E. The static effect of microbial growth indicates that the microbial growth is inhibited but they are not killed.

8. B

The autoclave as described in this question would not achieve sterilization. It should be at 121° C (250° F), 15 to 20 lbs. pressure, 15–20 min.

9. D

Sterility cannot be monitored once they have come out of the solution.

A. Storing them in a disinfected drawer still keeps them exposed to air and anybody's hands reaching into that drawer.

B. Placing instruments in an unsterilized bag does not maintain sterility.

C. Rinsing is necessary since most solutions can cause skin irritations.

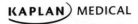

10. C

The surface disinfectants that should be used to clean the treatment area are phenolic compounds.

D. Sodium hypochlorite 1:500 is considered a low-level disinfectant only.

11. B

The disinfectants that stain surfaces are iodophors which contain iodine.

12. D

A vector has to do with entomology or insects carrying a pathogen. A mosquito carrying East Nile virus would be one example.

A. Salmonella is transmitted by a vehicle. In this case, it is a food pathogen.

B. Tuberculosis is transmitted by a vehicle. In this case, it is airborne and inhaled.

C. Contact with a surface is just that—contact by cross-contamination.

13. E

Regulated medical waste does not include gloves.

14. A

Mouth mirrors are semi-critical items, though they still need to be sterilized.

15. C

One disadvantage in using ethylene oxide for sterilization is that rubber and plastic need to be aerated for 24 hours afterward.

16. A

20–30 seconds is recommended for water discharge between patients.

17. C

There is no biological verification for **glutaraldehydes.** When instruments are taken out of the solution, there is no way to monitor sterility.

18. C

Ethylene oxide is effective against ALL known organisms. It is a carcinogen, however, so the instruments must be aerated afterward.

B. 70% ethyl alcohol is not sporicidal.

D. 70% isopropyl alcohol is not sporicidal.

E. Quaternary compounds are not acceptable for use by the ADA or CDC.

19. E

The CDC is most concerned about biofilm. Biofilm contains all of the microorganisms listed in the other answer choices, along with many other organisms.

A. Bacteroides are in biofilm.

B. Mycobacterium is in biofilm.

C. Streptococci are in biofilm.

D. Staphylococci are in biofilm.

20. A

The chemical agents that are EPA registered for surface disinfecting include sodium hypochlorite, iodophors, and synthetic phenols. The EPA assigns a hospital registered number for each surface disinfectant.

B. Quaternary compounds and isopropyl alcohol are not acceptable surface disinfectants according to the ADA or CDC.

21. A

The most fragile microorganisms to disinfecting are HIV/AIDS viruses, which need a host to survive.

22. B

Bacteria like to grow at the same optimal temperature of human beings which is 37° C.

23. D

In the case of a Boil Water Advisory, you would not use the dental waterline, wash hands, or have the patient rinse. Once the advisory was lifted, you would call the local waterworks plant to find out how to disinfect the waterlines.

24. D

Hepatitis B can survive on an inanimate surface for one month.

25. B

When disinfecting a surface, the first spray-wipe of the spray-wipe cycle is meant to clean only. It is the second spray—when left for the appropriate amount of time—that disinfects the surface.

A. To totally disinfect the surface, the second spray should stay on the surface as long as the manufacturer has recommended.

C. Surfaces cannot be sterilized, only disinfected.

Chapter Eight: **Periodontics**

It is estimated that about one-third of adult Americans have either localized or generalized periodontal disease. It is the action of the bacteria growth within the sulcus and exaggerated host response that breaks down the gingiva and adjacent tissues, creating bleeding and eventually a periodontal pocket if left untreated. Out of the over 500 different microorganisms that reside in the oral cavity, a relatively small amount proliferate in the periodontal pocket. These bacteria affect the connective tissue and cause epithelial tissue to migrate apically as the disease process destroys bone along the way.

GINGIVAL HEALTH

The oral cavity is the gateway to the body. Healthy gingiva aid in keeping the body healthy. Recent studies have shown that unhealthy oral tissues can contribute to coronary artery disease (which can lead to heart attacks or strokes), diabetes, arthritis, or even to premature, low birth weight babies. Maintaining healthy oral tissues is key to prevention.

Periodontium

The **periodontium** that supports teeth is composed of the gingiva, periodontal ligament, cementum and alveolar bone. The gingiva is made up the **keratinized oral epithelium** that is exposed in the mouth, the **non-keratinized sulcular epithelium** in the gingival sulcus, and the **non-keratinized junctional epithelium** that attaches gingiva to the tooth surface.

Marginal gingiva surrounds the coronal portion of the tooth. The **interdental gingival** are the papillae that fill the embrasures between teeth. A gingival groove is a slight depression in the marginal gingiva; it exists in approximately in 25–40% of patients.

The gingiva adjoins the oral mucosa at the **mucogingival junction**. The definitive line between the two tissues alters the firmly attached gingiva into relaxed motile mucosa.

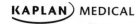

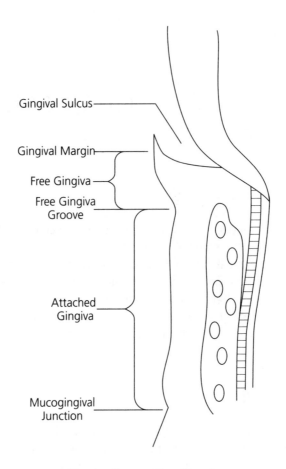

Gingival Sulcus

Gingival Margin

Free Gingiva

Free Gingiva Groove

Attached Gingiva

Mucogingival Junction

Gingiva Supporting Structures

Gingiva: Healthy Versus Diseased

	Healthy	Diseased
Color	Pink/coral pink-brown for dark pigmented individuals	Red, erythematous, blue-red, purple-red from capillary proliferation
Texture	Smooth margins with stippled attached gingiva	Loss of stippling, shiny as epithelial tissue thins
Consistency	Firm, resilient	Soft, friable, increased edema in acute
Contour	Pointed, knife-like	Blunted, absent, edematous, edema in acute

Attached Gingiva

Attached gingiva measures the bottom of the sulcus to the mucogingival junction. Loss of attachment tells us how much periodontal disease has progressed. Periodontal disease affects the apical migration of attached gingiva.

Having attached gingiva is also important for successful dental implants because gingival attachment levels on the implants need to coincide with the periodontal attachments on the adjacent teeth.

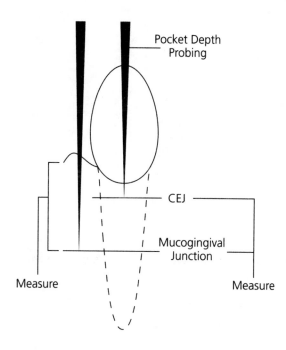

Measuring the Attached Gingiva

- The first measurement is the CEJ to the mucogingival line
- The second measurement is the CEJ to the base of the pocket
- Subtract the second measurement from the first to find the amount of attached gingiva

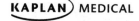

Clinical-Attachment Level (CAL)

Clinical-attachment level (CAL) is a measurement of the distance between the CEJ and the base of the pocket. Maintaining clinical-attachment levels aids in reducing or eliminating pocket depths as well as inflammation and infection. There are two ways to measure CAL: with and without recession.

Measuring CAL

- With **no recession**, one pocket depth measurement is recorded.

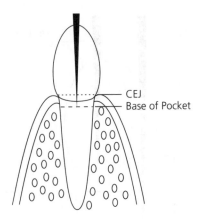

- With **recession**, two measurements are taken and added together.

Measure the pocket depth
+ Measure the amount of recession

Clinical-attachment level (CAL)

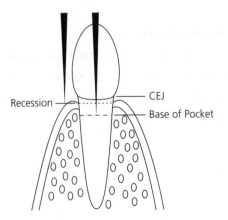

Gingival Fiber Groups

Gingival fibers are connective tissues that are comprised mostly of type I **collagen fibers, the most abundant collagen fiber in the human body**. These collagen fibers found in the lamina propria serve to withstand the forces of mastication and hold healthy gingival tissue firmly to the tooth. Apical migration of gingival tissue indicates disease and a loss of attachment of gingival fibers.

Primary Gingival Fiber Groups

Fiber group	Connection	Function
Dentogingival	Cementum to free gingiva and attached gingiva	Gingival support
Alveologingival	Periosteum of bone to attached gingiva	Attaches gingiva to bone
Dentoperiosteal	Cementum at CEJ to alveolar crest	Anchors teeth
Circular	Surrounds coronal portion to alveolar crest	Supports free gingiva
Transeptal	Interdental space to cementum	Maintains associations with other teeth

Secondary Gingival Fiber Groups

Fiber group	Connection	Function
Periostogingival	Periosteum to alveolar bone	Attaches gingiva to bone
Interpapillary	Coronal segment to transeptal bundles	Support papillary gingiva
Transgingival	Coronal segment to CEJ	Supports marginal gingiva
Intercircular	Distal, facial, and lingual of one tooth to adjacent tooth and mesial of next adjacent tooth	Sustains dental arch
Semicircular	Mesial to distal of same tooth	Supports free gingiva
Intergingival	Mesiodistal connective tissue to gingival epithelium	Supports attached gingiva

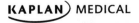

BONE

Bone surrounds and supports teeth. The **alveolar bone proper** is the bone surrounding the root that is lined by cribriform plate. **Compact bone** is comprised of cortical plates on the facial and lingual aspects of a tooth. **Cancellous bone** fills in bone between the cortical bone and the alveolar bone. **Bundle bone** is the means of attachment for the periodontal ligament. **Lamina dura** is a radiographic term defining the thin radiopaque line of bone surrounding the root. **Alveolar crest bone** is at the coronal rim of alveolar bone and is the **first bone lost in periodontal disease**.

> The first bone to be lost in periodontal disease is alveolar crest bone.

Dehiscence and fenestration are two **nonpathogenic bone modifications** that can occur. **Dehiscence**, bone resorption in the absence of disease, can occur on the facial surfaces of teeth with labially inclined teeth. **Fenestrations** are openings or windows into the bone.

PERIODONTAL LIGAMENT

> The first periodontal ligaments to be lost in periodontal disease are alveolar crest fibers.

The periodontal ligament is the connective tissue that connects the tooth to alveolar bone. Collagen fibers attach to bone and cementum in different directions by Sharpey's fibers.

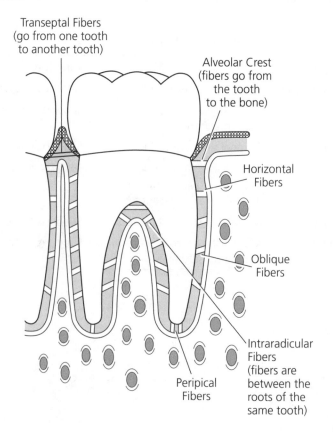

Transseptal Fibers (go from one tooth to another tooth)

Alveolar Crest (fibers go from the tooth to the bone)

Horizontal Fibers

Oblique Fibers

Intraradicular Fibers (fibers are between the roots of the same tooth)

Peripical Fibers

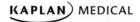

Following are the types of fibers, attachment modes, and functions.

Periodontal Fibers and Their Function

Fiber Name	Attachment Mode	Function
Alveolar crest	Connects cementum to alveolar crest bone	Oppose lateral forces and counter coronal thrust of other ligaments
Horizontal	Connects horizontally cementum to alveolar bone	Resists tilting and rotational forces and counter coronal thrust of other ligaments
Oblique	Connects obliquely from occlusal aspect apically to alveolar bone	Main mode of attachment, counter vertical mastication forces
Apical	Radiates apically from cementum to alveolar bone	Resist extrusion
Interradicular	Connect cementum to cementum in furcations of multirooted teeth	
Transeptal	Connect cementum to cementum of an adjacent tooth	Undergo reconstruction with bone loss from periodontal disease

Interradicular fibers are found only on multirooted teeth.

CEMENTUM

Cementum covers the root of the tooth. Sharpey's fibers from the periodontal ligament attach to both alveolar bone and cementum to hold the tooth into the bone. Cementum can be classified by the presence or absence of cells, the source of organic matrix, or by both classifications.

Cellular cementum contains cementocytes (cementum cells), while **acellular** cementum does not. **Cellular cementum** forms new cementum at the apical one-third of the tooth throughout the life of the tooth, while **acellular** cementum is located over the dentin on about two-thirds of the root.

Cementum contains different types of fibers. **Extrinsic fiber cementum** derives it fibers from the implantation of Sharpey's fibers into cementum by the periodontal ligament. Since these fibers are not generated within cementum itself but come from an outside source (the fibroblasts of the periodontal ligament), they are called extrinsic. Horizontal periodontal ligament fibers implant into cementum horizontally, oblique periodontal ligament fibers implant into cementum in the same oblique

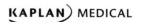

direction, etc. These fibers primarily cover the two-thirds of acellular cementum overlaying the roots—hence the name **acellular extrinsic fiber cementum**.

Intrinsic fiber cementum fibers are produced by the cementoblasts of cementum. They extend parallel to the root surface. These fibers are found primarily at the apical two-thirds of the tooth—hence the name **cellular intrinsic fiber cementum**. **Mixed-fiber cementum** contains intrinsic and extrinsic fibers.

Collagen fibrils or fibrillar cementum is found in extrinsic, intrinsic, and mixed fiber cementum. However, **afibrillar cementum** contains only a scant amount of fibers that sometimes extend into the enamel of a tooth at the cementoenamel junction (CEJ).

The four classifications of cementum are as follows:

- Type I: Acellular, afibrillar cementum is coronal cementum
- Type II: Acellular, extrinsic fiber cementum; part of Sharpey's fibers and continuous with the periodontal ligament to make up the bulk of the matrix
- Type III: Cellular, intrinsic fiber cementum; contains cementocytes in locations where cementum repair is occurring
- Type IV: Cellular, mixed-fiber cementum; located at the apical third and in furcations

INFLAMMATION PROCESS

Neutrophils or polymorphonuclear leukocytes are more numerous with acute infections. Monocytes are more numerous with chronic infections.

As microbes enter into a periodontal pocket, the host tries to wall off the invading antigens. This sets off an inflammatory response, which then causes clinical, histological, and radiographic changes in the tissues. As the antigens or microbes enter into tissue, they let off a chemical or "smell." The specialized mobile cells called **neutrophils or PMNs** (polymorphonuclear leukocytes) recognize the chemicals produced by the microbes and migrate toward their "smell." The movement of a cell or organism in reaction to a chemical stimulus or "smell" is called **chemotaxis**. This response then induces a change in the internal environment, causing more cells to migrate to the site. The PMNs release lysozymes to destroy bacteria, but this ultimately leads to the death of the PMNs.

Macrophages and **lymphocytes** are also chemotactically attracted to the area of invading pathogens. **Lymphocytes** recognize specific antigens or microbes producing antibodies, and retain them in their memory in order to react to them specifically with any future invasions. **Macrophages** are scavenger cells that perform phagocytosis to ingest or engulf microbes.

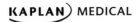

Physiologic incidence of inflammation includes:

- Immediate brief vasoconstriction (mast cells isolate antigen)
- Vasodilation increases blood flow to the area to bring in more blood cells
- Margination (adherence) of polymorphonuclear leukocytes (PMNs) to vascular endothelium
- Lymphocytes enter with specific antibodies to take care of specific antigens but rely on the monocytes to tell them which antibodies are needed
- Monocytes become phagocytes to engulf the microbes; monocytes are also more numerous with chronic infection
- Exudate (pus) forms
- As inflammation subsides, capillaries become fibrin clots
- Fibroblasts produce new connective tissue to replace the fibrin as the clot dissolves

Inflammation results in pain, redness, swelling (edema), and heat at the localized site. **Redness** occurs from the proliferation of blood to the area. **Swelling** occurs from the release of histamine, bradykinin, and serotonin by damaged tissues. The release of these chemicals causes blood vessels to leak fluids into the injury site. As leukocytes enter the inflamed connective tissue, increased metabolic activity by the leukocytes generates **heat** to the area. **Pain** results from the direct action on nerve endings by chemical agents released by the inflammatory process.

GINGIVAL AND PERIODONTAL POCKET FORMATION

A **gingival pocket** is generated by **enlarged gingiva without the apical migration** of junctional epithelium. The gingival pocket is formed by the coronal enlargement of gingival tissue. The base of the sulcus is at the enamel level.

A **periodontal pocket** is generated when there is **apical migration of the junctional epithelium**, as periodontal ligament detachment and bone loss occur. Alveolar crest fibers and bone are first affected. The base of the pocket is at the cementum level.

Suprabony pockets that involve **horizontal bone loss** are located coronal to alveolar crest bone. **Intrabony** or **infrabony** pockets are located apical to alveolar crest bone. Intrabony pockets may be involved with horizontal and/or vertical bone loss.

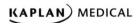

BONY DEFECTS

Periodontal disease causes loss of bone and osseous deformities. Infrabony or intrabony defects are classified by the number of walls that remain in the defect.

A **one-wall defect** occurs interdentally with only one surface remaining—whether the proximal, facial, or lingual surface. This defect has the **worst prognosis**.

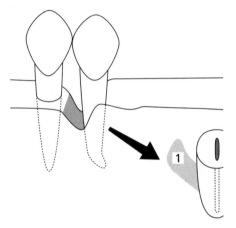

A **two-wall defect** is the most common defect. Two walls remain interproximally on either the facial and proximal surface (lingual cortical plate is destroyed) or the lingual and proximal surface (facial cortical plate is destroyed).

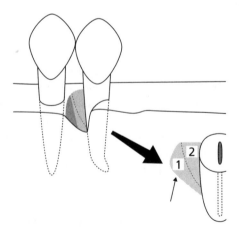

A **three-wall defect** has facial, lingual, and proximal bony surface still intact. This defect has the **best prognosis**.

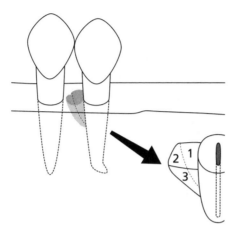

GINGIVAL DISEASE

The evolution of oral disease relies on the amount of microbes in bacterial plaque, risk factors, and the response by the host to the disease. Risk factors that enter into the progression of disease include genetic predisposition, tobacco usage, stress, inadequate nutrition, systemic diseases, aging, hormonal influences, chronic alcoholism, and side effects from prescription drugs.

Dental Biofilm

Dental biofilm contains microorganisms that reside in groups of microcolonies surrounded by an enveloping matrix. The matrix generates fluid channels for communication by allowing chemical signals between the colonies and for the flow of nutrients, oxygen, and waste. The chemical signals instigate bacteria to generate enzymes and proteins that are harmful to dental tissues. Gram-positive cocci and rods initially are present with the onset of gingivitis along with *Actinomyces* species. As gingivitis progresses, there is a higher number of gram-negative anaerobic *Fusobacterium*, *P. intermedia*, and spirochetes.

Gingivitis

Gingivitis is the first stage of periodontal disease. It presents with red, swollen gingiva that bleeds easily. There are changes in the color, texture, consistency, and contour of the gingiva, and there is also the presence of bleeding and/or exudate. Gingivitis is **reversible**; there is **no loss of attachment** of collagen fibers from cementum and **no apical migration** of a pocket.

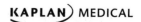

Classification of gingival disease by the American Academy of Periodontology includes plaque- and non-plaque-induced disease. **Plaque-induced disease** is the result of inadequate oral hygiene and includes the following:

- Plaque-induced gingivitis
- Gingivitis associated with systemic conditions
- Side effect of medication with gingival disease
- Nutritional deficiency gingivitis

Non-plaque induced disease may include:

- Bacterial gingival diseases
- Viral gingival diseases
- Fungal gingival diseases
- Genetic lesions
- Systemic disorder gingivitis
- Traumatic lesions
- Foreign body reactions

Plaque-Induced Gingivitis

Plaque-induced gingivitis presents initially with inflammation due to a proliferation of blood vessels, edema, clear gingival fluid that becomes white or yellow from exudate, loss of stippling causing the tissue to become shiny, bleeding upon probing, and loss of fibroblasts in connective tissue. As gingivitis progresses to an established phase, an increase of destruction of connective tissue collagen generates thickened junctional epithelium that begins to extend apically. Also the gingival margin migrates coronally from edema that increases pocket depth. The redness increases with some possible blue–red areas from venous congestion.

Gingivitis associated **with systemic conditions** such as the hormonal influences of puberty, menstrual cycle and pregnancy, diabetes mellitus, or blood dyscrasias such as leukemia modifies how the immune system responds to the disease process.

Hormonal increases in females during pregnancy, lactation, puberty, or menstruation exacerbates gingival inflammation due to a proliferation of subgingival bacteria when there is poor plaque control. During pregnancy especially, the gingiva initally bleeds mildly but can advance to a dark-red hyperlasia or pregnancy tumor.

With diabetes, the body is not able to respond to acute inflammation as well due to a lack of PMNs. Diabetics have a slower healing response.

Acute leukemia is a blood disorder of an overabundance of abnormal white blood cells which shows a pronounced inflammatory reaction to the biofilm.

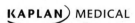

Many **medications** cause oral side effects, such as xerostomia or gingival hyperplasia. Phenytoin (for seizures), cyclosporines (anti-rejection drugs), and nifedipine or verapamil (calcium channel blockers) all cause gingival hyperplasia, which in turn causes the gingiva to become more fibrotic. Fibroblasts generate more dense connective tissues, and that in turn, causes an overgrowth of tissue that enlarges gingival contour. The result is an increase in plaque retention.

Nutritional deficiency gingivitis alters the body's response to the disease process. An example is vitamin C that is so very necessary for connective tissue to remain healthy. Lack of vitamin C, folic acid, and zinc may increase the permeability of gingival tissue, rendering a patient more susceptible to bacterial plaque.

Treatment for plaque-induced gingivitis includes plaque control with thorough oral hygiene instructions and regular dental visits.

Non-Plaque-Induced Gingivitis

Bacterial gingival diseases such as streptococcal infections are more common in the throat and oral tissues, but the *Treponema pallidum* of sexually transmitted disease can have oral manifestations in the mouth.

Viral gingival diseases such as herpes virus infections as a primary herpetic gingivostomatitis, recurrent oral herpes, or varicella zoster infections may look similar to plaque-induced gingivitis. Primary herpes is a highly contagious viral infection that presents as secondary oral lesions of cold sores or fever blisters.

Primary herpetic gingivostomatitis is a viral herpes infection with similar signs and symptoms as necrotizing ulcerative gingivitis (NUG). Primary herpetic gingivostomatitis symptoms include fever, malaise, and vesicles on the gingiva, or oral mucosa that can coalesce into large ulcers.

Fungal gingival diseases such as candida infections of generalized candidiasis, linear gingival erythema, or histoplasmosis may occur in patients who are immune-compromised. Many fungal infections are opportunistic infections, such as oral candidiasis. Patients who have worn a prosthesis for a very long time and whose immune system is deficient may present with an erythematous outline of the prosthesis from a candida infection. **Oral candidiasis** is an opportunistic fungal infection that presents as linear gingival erythema or severe redness with white patches that when rubbed off leave an ulcerated area.

Genetic lesions such as gingival fibromatosis are a generalized fibrous enlargement of gingival tissue. The overgrown tissue is a benign, slowly progressive, fibrous enlargement of maxillary and mandibular keratinized gingiva.

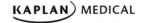

Systemic disorder gingivitis can occur from mucocutaneous disorders or allergic reactions. **Mucocutaneous disorders** may include lichen planus, lupus erythematous, pemphigoid, pemphigus vulgaris, or the side effects of medications.

- **Lichen planus** is a chronic disease that manifests intraorally as an asymptomatic or erosive lichen planus of the gingival mucosa. With lichen planus, diffuse, erythematous areas may be interspersed with white striae or keratotic lines termed Wickham's striae.

- **Mucous membrane or cicatricial pemphigoid** is an autoimmune disease. A patient's antibodies become altered, causing the body to attack the fibrous attachment of the skin and underlying connective tissues. Oral lesions manifest as small or large, clear-fluid blisters that break easily, resulting in a flat, white ulcer encircled by a thin, red line.

- **Pemphigus vulgaris** is an autoimmune disease associated with desmosomes and a positive Nikolsky's sign. Pemphigus occurs first in the mouth, and then throughout the entire body with flaccid, easily-broken blisters.

- **Desquamative gingivitis** can be an early clinical sign of a serious systemic disease such as cicatricial pemphigoid or pemphigus vulgaris. Gingival tissue sloughs off, leaving a raw, red area.

Nikolsky's sign is a test to show the loss of contact of desmosomes. It occurs when the pressure of the finger causes the formation of a bulla, or the pressure of the finger near a bulla causes extension of the bulla.

Systemic disorder gingivitis can also occur from allergic reactions, perhaps in dental material such as nickel or mercury or in a reaction to mouthwash. **Desquamative gingivitis** can also be a result of an allergic reaction.

Traumatic lesions can be caused by many things: chemical injury (holding an aspirin by an aching tooth); physical injury (abrasion from hard, crusty bread); thermal injury (hot pizza); accidental injury; or iatrogenic injury (acid etch on gingival tissue).

Foreign body reactions can result from something lodged underneath gingival tissue—a popcorn husk, for instance, or a broken toothpick interproximally. The gingiva reacts by creating a lesion to wall off the foreign object.

PERIODONTAL DISEASE

One-third of American adults have some sort of localized or generalized periodontal disease. Periodontal disease can cause the loss of perfectly healthy teeth. Early tooth loss without replacement can cause occlusal discrepancies leading to more tooth loss. Maintaining healthy tissues prevents tooth loss.

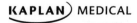

Periodontitis

Periodontitis is advanced periodontal disease where bone loss has occured. Collagen fibers detach pathologically from cementum, causing irreversible bone loss and the apical migration of junctional epithelium.

Bacteria involved in **chronic periodontitis** include *Porphyromonas gingivalis* (a major periodontal pathogen), *P. intermedia, Bacteroides forsythus, Actinobacillus actinomycetemcomitans, Fusobacterium nucleatum, Eikenella corrodens, Campylobacter rectus*, and Treponema spp. **Refractory chronic periodontitis** includes *P. gingivalis, P. intermedia, B. forsythus, A. actinomycetemcomitans, F. nucleatum,* and *C. rectus*.

Necrotizing ulcerative periodontitis (NUP) bacteria include *A. actinomycetemcomitans, F. nucleatum,* Eubacterium spp, *B. vincentii, C. albicans, P. gingivalis,* and *P. intermedia*. **Aggressive periodontitis** microbes include *P. gingivalis, P. intermedia, A. actinomycetemcomitans,* and *E. corrodens*.

Classification of diseases and conditions by the American Academy of Periodontology of periodontal diseases include:

- Chronic periodontitis localized or generalized
- Aggressive periodontitis localized or generalized
- Periodontitis as a manifestation of systemic diseases
- Necrotizing periodontal diseases
- Abscesses of the periodontium
- Periodontitis associated with endodontic lesions
- Developmental or acquired deformities and conditions

Chronic Periodontitis

Chronic periodontitis is the most common type of periodontal disease. Bone is slowly resorbed or destroyed as the disease progresses, causing loss of attachment of collagen fibers. Periodontitis will alternate between periods of heightened activity with loss of attachment and periods of inactivity. The severity depends on the amount of plaque and calculus deposits, the patient's resistance to disease, and the patient's ability to control the disease. The disease may be localized or generalized.

The most reliable way to confirm that a patient's periodontal disease has progressed is to measure clinical attachment level (CAL).

Periodontitis may also be sub-classified as slight, moderate, or severe.

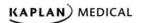

Sub-Classifications of Periodontal Disease

Type	Soft Tissue Characteristics	Bone Loss	Mobility	Pocket Depths
I. Gingivitis	Slight red inflammation with slight bleeding	None, no furcation	<0.5	1–3 mm
II. Slight chronic periodontitis	Red inflammation into alveolar crest with slight to moderate bleeding	Early loss of crestal bone, some horizontal loss	0.5–1	4–5 mm
III. Moderate chronic periodontitis	Red inflammation with recession with moderate bleeding	30–50% bone loss, furcation involvement on multirooted teeth, horizontal with some vertical	1–2	5–7 mm
IV. Advanced chronic periodontitis	Red-purple/red-blue inflammation with severe recession and severe bleeding	>50% bone loss, severe destruction into the furcation of multi-rooted teeth, horizontal and vertical	2–3	>7 mm
V. Aggressive periodontitis	Red inflammation with moderate to severe bleeding	Rapid with aggressive periodontitis	Varies	Possibly lose 1 mm/yr

Aggressive Periodontitis

Aggressive periodontitis can also be localized or generalized but has sub-classifications as well. Early onset periodontitis includes periodontitis found in patients younger than age 30. It includes juvenile periodontitis (both localized and generalized), prepubertal periodontitis, and rapid progressive periodontitis.

Juvenile periodontitis (JP) results in rapid loss of attachment and bone destruction that is often localized to first permanent molars and permanent incisors. Gingival tissues may appear completely normal, with very little plaque present. Inflammation, bleeding, and **heavy plaque accumulation** are *not* present.

Diagnosis depends heavily on periodontal probing and radiographs that show localized, deep (vertical) bone loss. Treatment includes scaling and root planing, good oral home care, and antibiotic therapy.

Prepubertal periodontitis is a low prevalence pathology of less than 1%. It is characterized by severe gingival inflammation, rapid bone loss, mobility, and early loss of deciduous teeth. These patients typically have defective polymorphonuclear leukocytes, and are susceptible to the infections of others. Prepubertal periodontitis can be associated with systemic illnesses such as Papillon-Lefèvre syndrome. It responds poorly to routine treatment, though antibiotic therapy may slow progression.

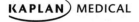

Rapid progressive periodontitis occurs in young adults ago 20–30. It causes severe inflammation, rapid bone loss, tooth loss, and connective tissue loss. Bone loss occurs in a very short period of time—weeks or months—with the patient possibly losing his teeth within a year of onset. Early detection with radiographs and periodontal pocket-depth probing is essential.

HIV-associated periodontitis is a particularly virulent, rapidly progressing form of periodontitis. It resembles acute necrotizing ulcerative gingivitis. Patients may lose 9–12 mm of attachment in as little as 6 months. Treatment includes good oral home care, subgingival scalings, antibiotic therapy (tetracycline), and periodontal surgery if indicated.

Periodontitis as a Manifestation of Systemic Disease

Periodontitis as a manifestation of systemic diseases includes hematological disorders, genetic disorders, and not otherwise specified disorders.

Hematological disorders include acquired neutropenia and leukemia. **Neutropenia** is a lower-than-normal neutrophils count (PMN-count) in blood, rendering the host more susceptible to infection. Neutropenia can be inherited, but it can also be acquired after a viral infection or chemotherapy. Neutrophils are necessary to fight infection.

Leukemia is a cancer of the blood that produces an overabundance of abnormal white blood cells. There are four types of leukemia: acute or chronic lymphocytic leukemia, and acute or chronic myelogenous leukemia. Lymphocytes are important for making antibodies, while myelocytes produce neutrophils. These white blood cells are needed to fight off periodontal disease or any infection.

Genetic disorders with periodontitis will be discussed separately here.

- **Neutropenia** was discussed under hematological disorders.

- **Down syndrome** patients have an early onset of *P. gingivalis* bacteria which increases with age, increasing their risk for periodontal disease.

- **Leukocyte adhesion deficiency** (LAD) is a genetic leukocyte disorder that causes patients to be vulnerable to life-threatening infections.

- **Papillon-Lefèvre syndrome** is a genetic disorder whose characteristics include hyperkeratosis of palms and soles, and susceptibility to periodontitis at a very early age, which affects the primary dentition.

- **Chediak-Higashi syndrome** is genetic disorder of the immune system. It is characterized by chronic infection, decreased pigmentation in skin and eyes, neurological disease, and early death.

- **Histiocytosis syndrome** includes Langerhans histiocytosis that can be genetic or of unknown etiology, resulting in unifocal or multifocal granulomatous lesions.

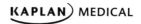

- **Glycogen storage disease** is a genetic deficiency that prevents the body from properly metabolizing or breaking down glycogen. This causes the body to store abnormal amounts of glycogen.

- **Infantile genetic agranulocytosis** is genetic disorder in children who lack neutrophils needed to fight infection.

- **Cohen syndrome** is a genetic disorder characterized by head malformations, eye abnormalities, diminished muscle tone (hypotonia), obesity, abnormally narrow hands and feet, long fingers and toes, and/or mental retardation.

- **Ehlers–Danlos syndrome** (Types IV and VIII) is genetic in origin and is primarily a dermatological and joint disorder. Some ED patients are susceptible to aneurysms, mitral valve prolapse, and periodontitis.

- **Hypophosphatasia** causes defective calcification of bones in infants and children.

Necrotizing Periodontal Diseases

Necrotizing periodontal diseases include necrotizing ulcerative gingivitis and necrotizing ulcerative periodontitis. **Necrotizing ulcerative gingivitis** (NUG) can be an acute or chronic infection that presents with punched-out papillae covered by a white or gray pseudomembrane; redness; swelling; pain; and a distinctive necrotic, fetid odor. Stress, poor diet, smoking, and viral infections predispose a person to this illness. Treatment includes a complete debridement, rinsing with equal amounts of hydrogen peroxide and warm water, and oral hygiene instructions.

Necrotizing periodontitis (NUP) shares many of the clinical characteristics of NUG though there is more loss of clinical attachment and destruction of alveolar bone. It can occur in patients who have had single or multiple episodes of NUG, HIV-infected patients, or those with systemic immune deficiencies.

Abscesses of the Periodontium

Abscesses of the periodontium include gingival abscess, periodontal abscesses, and pericoronal abscesses. Gingival abscesses are superficial and not involved in deep tissues. They present as shiny raised areas. An endodontic or periapical abscess can come after a pulpal infection, causing necrosis of pulp tissue. It may be difficult to differentiate from a periodontal abscess.

Periodontal abscesses occur on VITAL teeth.

Periodontal abscesses occur in the vicinity of **vital teeth.** They are inflamed, deep-tissue lesions and may present as a suppurative lesion. An acute periodontal abscess occurs when bacteria invade an occluded periodontal pocket, resulting in an inflamed, painful, elevated round mass that may present with exudate (pus). Chronic periodontal abscesses are very similar to acute abscesses but are not painful, because the exudate is able to drain.

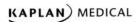

Developmental or Acquired Deformities and Conditions

Developmental or acquired deformities and conditions alter susceptibility to periodontal disease. These deformities and conditions might be tooth anomalies, mucogingival deformities surrounding teeth, mucogingival deformities in edentulous patients, or occlusal trauma (see below).

OCCLUSAL TRAUMA

Heavy occlusal forces can damage the teeth, the periodontium, the muscles, or the temporomandibular joint (TMJ). Traumatic occlusion can cause teeth to become sensitive, become mobile from widening of the periodontal ligament, create sore muscles, or produce TMJ dysfunction. In addition, they contribute to a more rapid spread of inflammation apically and to more bone loss with periodontal disease.

–Trauma does NOT cause periodontal disease

–Inflammation aggravates trauma

- **Arthralgia**: Joint pain

- **Bruxism**: Grinding of teeth, usually nocturnal

- **Clenching**: Heavy clamping of teeth, usually from stress or activity

- **Clicking** of the TMJ: Occurs when the meniscus is anteriorly displaced

- **Crepitation**: Bone grating against bone

- **Fremitus**: Tooth vibration as the teeth occlude

- **Myalgia**: Muscle pain

- **Occlusal trauma:** Causes periodontal tissue injury due to recurring excessive occlusal forces

  - Primary trauma is excessive force exerted on a tooth with normal bone support

  - Secondary trauma is excessive force exerted on a tooth with bone loss and inadequate bone support

- **Prematurities**: Isolated occlusal contacts that occur before the correct occlusion, causing a deflection of mandibular movement

- **Spasms**: Involuntary muscle contractions

- **Trismus**: Tonic contraction of the muscles of mastication

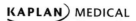

FURCATION AND MOBILITY CLASSIFICATIONS

Furcation involvement and tooth mobility indicate bone loss of the supporting structures of teeth.

Furcation Involvement

Grade	Involvement
I	Early involvement, probe just into the notch or V; no intraradicular bone loss
II	Moderate involvement, probe just enters into furcation; some loss of interradicular bone
III	Severe involvement, probe enters root to opposite side; complete loss of interradicular bone
IV	Severe involvement, through and through visible furcation; complete loss of interradicular bone

Tooth Mobility

Class	Involvement
+	Very slight mobility
I	Slight mobility of about 1 mm buccolingually
II	Moderate mobility of about 2 mm buccolingually
III	Severe mobility of 3 mm in all directions and tooth is compressible

PERIODONTAL PROBES

Periodontal probes are smooth, round instruments that have markings to measure pocket-depth and furcation involvement. These measurements are used to evaluate periodontal health. The **Nabor's probe** is the preferred probe for measuring **furcations**.

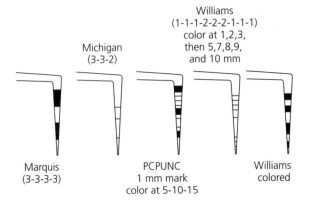

Marquis
(3-3-3-3)

Michigan
(3-3-2)

Williams
(1-1-1-2-2-2-1-1-1)
color at 1,2,3,
then 5,7,8,9,
and 10 mm

PCPUNC
1 mm mark
color at 5-10-15

Williams
colored

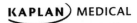

SOFT-TISSUE MANAGEMENT AND ROOT DEBRIDEMENT

Patient therapy begins with a thorough periodontal exam, along with an oral hygiene review for controling the biofilm on a daily basis. After the patient's condition has been assessed, a treatment plan is formulated. Nonsurgical therapy would include scaling and root debridement—procedures that remove all hard and soft deposits as well as the biofilm from the root and coronal surfaces. In addition, removing a thin layer of diseased cementum will render a healthy root surface. (Incidentally, a thin layer of diseased pocket epithelium may be removed at the same time during **incidental curettage**.) Debridement of the root surface can be done with curets and/or an ultrasonic scaler with the water spray flushing away debris, calculus, and blood so that the root surface can be seen more easily.

For patients with moderate or advanced periodontal disease, scaling and root debridement may be the initial therapy, with re-evaluation in 6 weeks. Conventional therapy can entail 1–4 appointments of scaling and debridement by quadrant.

According to the American Academy of General Dentistry, the new theory is to debride the deepest pockets first, then follow up with a series of root debridement therapy appointments. At these successive appointments, after a quadrant debridement is completed, pockets should be re-evaluated for antibiotic therapy. At this same appointment, antibiotic therapy should be administered into pockets of 5.0–6.0 mm.

Additional quadrant debridement should be accomplished at 2-week intervals with the same antibiotic treatments of 5.0–6.0 mm pockets. Six weeks after the last appointment, another re-evaluation of pockets is made. At that time, the patient is evaluated for further localized pocket debridement with placement of antibiotics, referral to a periodontist, or follow-up periodontal prophylaxis.

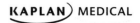

Treatment Options Adapted from the American Academy of General Dentistry†*

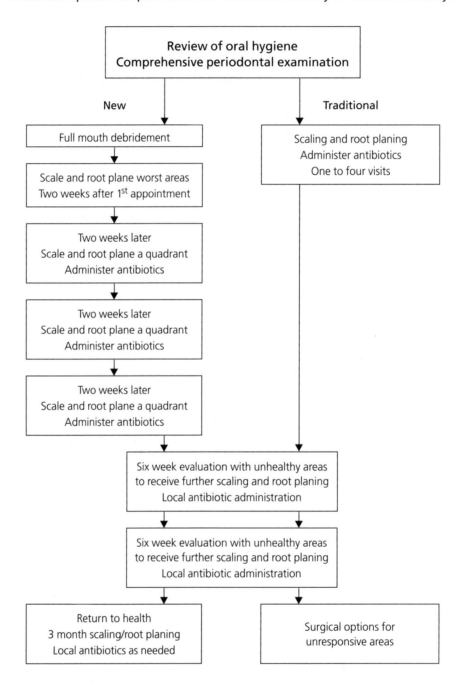

† For treatment of adult periodontal disease, adapted from the Academy of General Dentistry

* For advanced chronic periodontal disease or aggressive periodontitis, occlusal equilibration
  (if necessary) and bacterial culturing are performed on the first visit along with a dual referral
  to a periodontist. A third option for the second 6th week evaluation would be to reculture the
  bacteria, start systemic antibiotics if indicated, and Periostat.

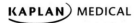

SITE-SPECIFIC THERAPY

Site-specific therapy is designed to reduce the amount of microorganisms residing in the periodontal pocket, with either chlorhexidine (Periochip) or antibiotics such as tetracycline (Actisite), minocycline (Arestin), or doxycycline (Atridox, Periostat). Chlorhexidine (Periochip) disrupts the bacterial cell wall in order to gain entry into the cell, causing cell lysis.

The following antibiotics suppress the multiplication of bacterial growth:

- **Tetracycline (Actisite)** is a cord impregnated with tetracycline that must be removed 7–10 days after therapeutic treatment. It is a bacteriostatic that inhibits protein synthesis. Its concentration is remarkably higher than systemic tetracycline.

- **Doxycycline (Atridox)** slowly releases doxycycline for about 1 week. Administered subginivally 42.5mg for 21 days. It also inhibits protein synthesis, interfering with messenger RNA and transfer RNA. Administered subgingivally 43.5 mg for 21 days.

- **Doxycycline (Periostat)** suppresses increased levels of tissue-destroying collagenase enzymes produced by bacteria. These unwanted enzymes destroy the collagen of connective tissue. It is 20 mg tablet taken orally twice daily.

- **Minocycline (Arestin)** is a bacteriostatic agent that inhibits protein synthesis of bacterial cells. It works over a two-week period.

SURGICAL INTERVENTION

After initial therapy, the patient is reevaluated for any surgical intervention to correct refractory areas. Surgery allows for better access to root surface areas, furcations, infrabony pockets, and bone defects. Pocket elimination gives the patient better access for plaque control.

Excisional surgery that rapidly eliminates excessive tissues is called gingivectomy. Gingivoplasty, another type of excisional surgery, reshapes gingival tissues.

Periodontal flap surgery is an **incisional surgery** that exposes the underlying bone for modification, removes diseased epithelial, granulation, and connective tissue, and exposes the root surface so that residual calculus can be removed. This surgery may include open flap curettage, reverse bevel flap surgery, modified Kirkland flap procedure, Widman surgery, and/or modified Widman surgery.

Mucogingival surgery corrects mucogingival defects where the diseased pocket has extended beyond the mucogingival junction, creating an area of no attached gingiva.

Osseous surgery corrects bony defects by resculpturing the bone. This procedure reshapes the alveolar process to attain a more physiologic form.

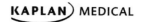

Bone grafts stimulate regeneration of bone in defects. These would include an **autograft** (bone taken from the patient); **allograft** (cadaver bone); **xenograft** (bone from another species such as a cow or pig); and **alloplast** (synthetic bone).

Guided-tissue regeneration regenerates bone by placing a barrier membrane between the periodontal flap and alveolar bone of a defect. By doing so, this stimulates bone growth. This type of regeneration may also be used in conjunction with bone replacement grafts.

A **root hemisection** is the **removal of half the tooth**—both crown and root. A **root resection** is the **removal of one root** on a multirooted tooth with the crown still intact. In both cases, the tooth will require endodontic treatment.

Pedicle soft tissue graft can be elevated from an edentulous ridge, adjacent teeth, or from existing gingival tissue on the same tooth and can be moved laterally or coronally.

Free soft tissue graft utilizes a donor site (i.e., palate) to create gingiva over a deficient site.

> The tissue in the mouth that most resembles gingival tissue is the palate, which explains why that tissue is used on free gingival grafts.

IMPLANT SURGERY

Dental implants can be utilized for crowns, as a bridge abutment, or to support dentures. Dental implants osseointegrate into bone. Dorland's medical dictionary defines **osseointegration** as the "direct anchorage of an implant by the formation of bony tissue around it without growth of fibrous tissue at the bone-implant interface."

Titanium is the metal of choice for dental implants. Implants are coated with oxygen and titanium oxide before implantation into bone. Research has found that a nontoxic, noncorrosive ceramic coating makes an ideal coating material for titanium.

Endosseous implants are screw-shaped, cylindrical, or bladed implants that serve as an anchor for a crown or bridge. The procedure—originally done in two steps of first placing the implant into bone and then covering it with gingiva to heal for 3 months—has now become a one-step procedure if preferred. The one-step implant is exposed above the gingiva after placement into bone.

Subperiosteal implants are custom-fabricated to the patient and fit over the bone and under the periosteum. These implants can fit the whole arch or can be unilateral. In a two-step procedure for this type of implant, the tissue is flapped open to expose bone for making an impression of the area. The implant is then custom-fabricated and placed during a second surgical procedure. A one-step procedure utilizes computer tomography to custom-fabricate the framework which is then placed in only one surgical procedure.

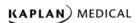

Transosteal implants are not as widely used due to the success of the osseointegrated implants. This implant (referred to as a staple implant) is placed into alveolar bone and the cortical plates, and stabilized with a metal plate at the inferior border of the mandible. Retaining posts for overdentures protrude into the oral cavity.

Peri-implantitis is an infection around an implant due to a change in the microbial growth within an implant pocket. Symptoms may include bleeding upon probing, pocket formation, exudate, redness and edema, and/or bone loss.

Maintaining the implant with good oral hygiene, regular dental care, and yearly radiographs ensures success. In the dental office, plastic curets are safe and will not scratch the titanium surface. Air abrasive powders, coarse prophylaxis pastes, metal instruments, and steel sonic and ultrasonic tips should be avoided.

The best way to check for implant failure is with yearly radiographs. If a prosthesis is loose, it may not be the implant itself but rather the prosthesis.

SUTURES

Sutures are a material used to close tissues following surgical procedures to promote primary intention healing. Sutures may be absorbable such as surgical or chromic gut or be non-absorbable such as silk or synthetic materials. Sutures typically are removed 7–14 days after periodontal surgery. Epithelial healing occurs in about 7 days, with osseous healing and recontouring taking place in 4–6 months.

PERIODONTAL DRESSINGS

Periodontal dressings are placed to hold flaps securely to teeth and aid in patient comfort. The preferred type of toothbrushing method to be used with periodontal pack is **Charter's method** which places the bristle of the brush at a 45° to the occlusal surface.

SURGICAL HEALING PROCESS

First intention healing occurs when the edges of the wound are close together as a clot forms to act like a scaffolding. The clot is replaced by granulation tissue as capillaries migrate into the wound site. Fibroblasts produce collagen fibers, healing the wound in about 2 weeks.

With **second intention healing**, the edges of the wound are not within close proximity. The wound heals from the base and outer borders inward one cell layer at a time. An example of this would be a donor site from the palate for a free gingival graft.

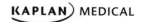

AMERICAN ACADEMY OF PERIODONTOLOGY CLASSIFICATIONS

Gingivitis

I. Gingival Diseases

    A. Dental plaque-induced gingival diseases

        1. Gingivitis associated with dental plaque only

            a. without other local contributing factors

            b. with local contributing factors (See VIII A)

        2. Gingival diseases modified by systemic factors

            a. associated with the endocrine system

                1) puberty-associated gingivitis

                2) menstrual cycle-associated gingivitis

                3) pregnancy-associated

                    a) gingivitis

                    b) pyogenic granuloma

                4) diabetes mellitus-associated gingivitis

            b. associated with blood dyscrasias

                1) leukemia-associated gingivitis

                2) other

        3. Gingival diseases modified by medications

            a. drug-influenced gingival diseases

                1) drug-influenced gingival enlargements

                2) drug-influenced gingivitis

                    a) oral contraceptive-associated gingivitis

                    b) other

        4. Gingival diseases modified by malnutrition

            a. ascorbic acid-deficiency gingivitis

            b. other

    B. Non-plaque-induced gingival lesions

        1. Gingival diseases of specific bacterial origin

            a. Neisseria gonorrhea-associated lesions

            b. Treponema pallidum-associated lesions

            c. streptococcal species-associated lesions

            d. other

        2. Gingival diseases of viral origin

            a. herpes virus infections

                1) primary herpetic gingivostomatitis

                2) recurrent oral herpes

                3) varicella-zoster infections

            b. other

        3. Gingival diseases of fungal origin

            a. Candida-species infections

                1) generalized gingival candidosis

            b. linear gingival erythema

            c. histoplasmosis

            d. other

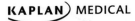

4. Gingival lesions of genetic origin
    a. hereditary gingival fibromatosis
    b. other
5. Gingival manifestations of systemic conditions
    a. mucocutaneous disorders
        1) lichen planus
        2) pemphigoid
        3) pemphigus vulgaris
        4) erythema multiforme
        5) lupus erythematous
        6) drug-induced
        7) other
    b. allergic reactions
        1) dental restorative materials
            a) mercury
            b) nickel
            c) acrylic
            d) other
        2) reactions attributable to
            a) toothpastes/dentifrices
            b) mouthrinses/mouthwashes
            c) chewing gum additives
            d) foods and additives
        3) other
6. Traumatic lesions (factitious, iatrogenic, accidental)
    a. chemical injury
    b. physical injury
    c. thermal injury
7. Foreign body reactions
8. Not otherwise specified (NOS)

Periodontitis

II. Chronic Periodontitis†
    A. Localized
    B. Generalized
III. Aggressive Periodontitis†
    A. Localized
    B. Generalized
IV. Periodontitis as a Manifestation of Systemic Diseases
    A. Associated with hematological disorders
        1. Acquired neutropenia
        2. Leukemias
        3. Other
    B. Associated with genetic disorders
        1. Familial and cyclic neutropenia
        2. Down syndrome
        3. Leukocyte adhesion deficiency syndromes
        4. Papillon-Lefèvre syndrome
        5. Chediak-Higashi syndrome

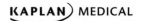

6. Histiocytosis syndromes

7. Glycogen storage disease

8. Infantile genetic agranulocytosis

9. Cohen syndrome

10. Ehlers-Danlos syndrome (Types IV and VIII)

11. Hypophosphatasia

12. Other

   C. Not otherwise specified (NOS)

V. Necrotizing Periodontal Diseases

   A. Necrotizing ulcerative gingivitis (NUG)

   B. Necrotizing ulcerative periodontitis (NUP)

VI. Abscesses of the Periodontium

   A. Gingival abscess

   B. Periodontal abscess

   C. Pericoronal abscess

VII. Periodontitis Associated With Endodontic Lesions

   A. Combined periodontic-endodontic lesions

VIII. Developmental or Acquired Deformities and Conditions

   A. Localized tooth-related factors that modify or predispose to plaque-induced gingival diseases/periodontitis

     1. Tooth anatomic factors

     2. Dental restorations/appliances

     3. Root fractures

     4. Cervical root resorption and cemental tears

   B. Mucogingival deformities and conditions around teeth

     1. Gingival/soft tissue recession

       a. facial or lingual surfaces

       b. interproximal (papillary)

     2. Lack of keratinized gingiva

     3. Decreased vestibular depth

     4. Aberrant frenum/muscle position

     5. Gingival excess

       a. pseudopocket

       b. inconsistent gingival margin

       c. excessive gingival display

       d. gingival enlargement (See I.A.3. and I.B.4.)

     6. Abnormal color

   C. Mucogingival deformities and conditions on edentulous ridges

     1. Vertical and/or horizontal ridge deficiency

     2. Lack of gingiva/keratinized tissue

     3. Gingival/soft tissue enlargement

     4. Aberrant frenum/muscle position

     5. Decreased vestibular depth

     6. Abnormal color

   D. Occlusal trauma

     1. Primary occlusal trauma

     2. Secondary occlusal trauma

AAP, www.perio.org, 1999

REVIEW QUESTIONS

1. The thin radiopaque bone that follows the outline of the root of a tooth in a radiograph is called

   A. Cortical bone
   B. Lamina propria
   C. Lamina dura
   D. Cancellous bone
   E. Bundle bone

2. What is the average distance of alveolar crestal bone to the cementoenamel junction?

   A. 0.5–1.0 mm
   B. 1.0–1.5 mm
   C. 1.5–2.0 mm
   D. 2.0–2.5 mm
   E. 2.5–3.0 mm

3. Periodontal disease destroys exisiting structures. The very first bone to be lost in the periodontal disease process is

   A. Alveolar crest bone
   B. Alveolar bone proper
   C. Cortical bone
   D. Cancellous bone

4. Interproximally between the facial and lingual surfaces of gingiva, there is a slight depression in the tissue. This depression is called

   A. Mucogingival junction
   B. Sulcus
   C. Free gingival groove
   D. Col
   E. Embrasure

5. A patient has presented at the office with a chief complaint of bleeding gums and a fetid odor. Upon examination, you see gray necrotic gingiva with punched-out papillae. This patient most likely has

   A. Primary herpetic gingivostomatitis
   B. Gingivitis
   C. Necrotizing ulcerative gingivitis
   D. Gingival hyperplasia

6. The microorganism most often associated with endocrine-influenced gingivitis is

   A. *P. gingivalis*
   B. *E. corrodens*
   C. *P. intermedia*
   D. *B. forsythus*
   E. *F. nucleatum*

7. Localized risk factors that can contribute to periodontal disease include

   A. Open contacts that can trap food debris easier contributing to the disease
   B. Overhanging fillings that can trap plaque and debris to contribute to disease
   C. Occlusal discrepancies that cause stress on the periodontal ligament to widen it, contributing to disease.
   D. Furcation involvements that will be a place for bacteria to convene and contribute to disease
   E. All of the above

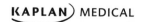

8. A periodontal pack is placed to keep the tissue in place after periodontal surgery. Which of the following toothbrushing methods is used with periodontal dressings?

    A. Bass
    B. Modified Bass
    C. Stillman
    D. Roll method
    E. Charter's

9. In question 8, it was mentioned that the periodontal pack keeps the tissue in place after periodontal surgery. Periodontal dressings help to

    A. Maintain blood clot
    B. Inhibit food impaction into the site
    C. Protect the wound
    D. Increase patient comfort
    E. All of the above

10. Periodontal dressing should be removed __ days after surgery.

    A. 4
    B. 6
    C. 7
    D. 14

11. Which of the following systemic diseases would put a patient at greater risk for periodontal disease?

    A. Sjogren's syndrome
    B. Down syndrome
    C. Papillon-LeFèvre Syndrome
    D. Uncontrolled diabetes
    E. All of the above

12. Which of the following systemic antibiotics would be useful in treating a 12-year-old for juvenile periodontal disease?

    A. Penicillin
    B. Tetracycline
    C. Diflucan
    D. Decadron
    E. Zovirax

13. Gingival hyperplasia can be drug induced. Which of the following heart medications can cause gingival hyperplasia?

    A. Furosemide
    B. Digoxin
    C. Cyclosporin
    D. Nifedipine
    E. Lidocaine

14. Which of the following periodontal treatments best removes endotoxins from the root surfaces?

    A. Scaling
    B. Oral irrigation
    C. Root debridement
    D. Chlorhexidine

15. Gingival disease can manifest itself in many ways. The first sign of gingival disease is

    A. Loss of attachment
    B. Recession
    C. Bleeding
    D. Purulence
    E. Swelling

16. A true pocket is differentiated from a pseudopocket by which of the following?

    A. Gingival inflammation and edema that swell the tissue

    B. Apical movement of the epithelial attachment

    C. Gingival proliferation in a coronal direction

    D. None of the above

17. Which of the following gingival diseases has characteristics similar to NUG?

    A. Desquamative gingivitis

    B. Pregnancy gingivitis

    C. Linear gingival erythema

    D. Lichen planus

    E. Scorbutic gingivitis

18. How is primary herpetic gingivostomatitis different from most other gingival disease?

    A. It is a localized disease.

    B. It is bacterial in origin.

    C. It is an adult disease.

    D. It is not plaque-induced.

19. Your 4-month recare patient admits to not performing his daily oral hygiene lately because of a tight work schedule. Which of the following signs would tell you that this patient's periodontal disease has progressed?

    A. Bleeding upon probing

    B. Increased tooth mobility

    C. Edematous gingival tissue

    D. Loss of attachment

    E. Change in gingival color

20. Implants can fail due to peri-implantitis. When evaluating an implant for failure, the best criterion is

    A. Checking the mobility

    B. Checking pocket depth

    C. Yearly radiographs

    D. Suppurative lesions

21. The oral cavity has many types of epithelial tissues—both keratinized and nonkeratinized. Of the following oral tissues, which is the most similar to gingival tissue?

    A. Buccal mucosa

    B. Palatal

    C. Tongue

    D. Vestibule

22. Which of the following can happen to gingival tissue in a patient with refractory periodontitis?

    A. There can be rapid loss of attachment even after intensive therapy.

    B. It will occur at only one tooth.

    C. It is caused by *P gingivalis*.

    D. Systemic diseases such as diabetes mellitus decrease the patient's chances for refractory periodontitis.

    E. It occurs from poor plaque control.

23. Your periodontal maintenance patient has returned for his 3-month recare appointment. The best way to test for tooth mobility is

    A. With two fingers

    B. With a finger and a blunt end of an instrument

    C. With the working ends of two curets

    D. With the blunt ends of two instruments

    E. All of the above

24. Which of the following agents delivers minocycline into a gingival pocket?

    A. Periochip

    B. Periostat

    C. Atridox

    D. Arestin

25. A bone graft that has been derived from cadaver bone is called

    A. Autograft

    B. Xenograft

    C. Allograft

    D. Alloplast

ANSWER EXPLANATIONS

1. C

The lamina dura follows the outline of the root of a tooth on a radiograph.

A. Cortical bone is on the facial and lingual surfaces, so it isn't seen radiographically.

B. Lamina propria is highly vascular tissue between the basement membrane and epithelial lining.

E. Bundle bone is adjacent to alveolar bone and contains Sharpey's fibers.

2. C

The average distance of alveolar crestal bone to the cementoenamel junction is 1.5–2.0 mm.

3. A

The first bone to be lost in the periodontal disease process is alveolar crest bone.

4. D

The depression between the facial and lingual surfaces of gingiva is called the col.

A. Mucogingival junction is a definitive line at the juncture of attached gingiva and alveolar mucosa.

B. Sulcus is the collar of tissue around the neck of the tooth.

C. Free gingival groove is a groove that separates the marginal gingiva and attached gingiva. It isn't seen in every individual.

E. Embrasure is the interproximal space formed by the curvatures of adjacent teeth.

5. C

A patient with a chief complaint of bleeding gum, a fetid odor, and gray, necrotic punched-out papillae has necrotizing ulcerative gingivitis.

A. Primary herpetic gingivostomatitis is seen in children and adolescents. Symptoms are similar to NUG, but there is more general malaise and fever.

B. Gingivitis would not be this severe.

D. Gingival hyperplasia is an overabundance of gingival tissue.

6. A

The microorganism most often associated with endocrine-influenced gingivitis is *P. gingivalis*. *E. corrodens, P. intermedia, B. forsythus,* and *F. nucleatum* are all present in gingivitis but *P. gingivalis* is the most predominant.

7. E

All of the choices listed are localized risk factors that can contribute to periodontal disease. Open contacts can trap food debris easily, contributing to disease. Overhanging fillings will trap plaque and debris. Occlusal discrepancies will cause stress on the periodontal ligament and widen it. Furcation involvements will invite bacteria to convene.

8. E

The toothbrushing method used with periodontal dressings is Charter's, which is used at a 45° to the occlusal surface.

9. E

Periodontal dressings help to accomplish all of the answer choices.

10. C

Periodontal dressing should be removed 7 days after surgery.

11. E

All of the answer choices would put patients at a greater risk for periodontal disease.

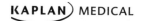

12. B

Tetracycline would be useful in treating juvenile periodontal disease. It has a longer half-life in gingival crevicular fluid. At this point, all of the teeth are fully formed.

A. Penicillin is used for NUG, pericoronitis, periapical and periodontal abscesses.

C. Diflucan treats oral candidiasis.

D. Decadron treats lichen planus.

E. Zovirax treats primary herpes.

13. D

Nifedipine, a heart medication, can cause gingival hyperplasia.

A. Furosemide is a loop diuretic.

B. Digoxin is a cardiac glycoside that increases heart contractions.

C. Cyclosporin is not a heart medication but it does cause gingival hyperplasia.

E. Lidocaine treats dysrhythmias.

14. C

Root debridement best removes endotoxins from the root surfaces.

A. Scaling will remove plaque, calculus, and stains.

B. Oral irrigation has superficial benefits only.

D. Chlorhexidine will not penetrate into deep pockets.

15. C

The first sign of gingival disease is bleeding from the proliferation of capillaries. This allows blood cells to get to the site to fight off the invading pathogens.

A. Loss of attachment shows that the disease is progressing.

B. Recession is also a more advanced sign.

D. Purulence is pus from advanced periodontal disease.

E. Swelling is from edema in the area, after the capillaries bring in the blood cells to fight off the disease.

16. C

A true pocket is differentiated from a pseudopocket by gingival migration in a coronal direction.

A. Gingival inflammation and edema swell the tissue but this is not the best answer.

B. Apical movement of the epithelial attachment is a true pocket.

17. C

The gingival disease that has similar characteristics to NUG is linear gingival erythema.

A. Desquamative gingivitis is a lesion that when rubbed with a 2X2 sloughs off leaving a red inflamed area.

B. Pregnancy gingivitis is not similar.

D. Lichen planus is a benign chronic disease.

E. Scorbutic gingivitis is due to a lack of vitamin C and affects connective tissues.

18. D

Unlike most gingival disease, primary herpetic gingivostomatitis is not plaque-induced.

A. It is not a localized disease—it is systemic.

B. It is not bacterial—it is viral.

C. It is not an adult disease—it is a disease that children and adolescents get.

19. D

Loss of attachment would tell you that your 4-month recare patient's periodontal disease has progressed.

A. Bleeding upon probing is an early sign.

B. Increased tooth mobility indicates more bone loss but this isn't the best answer.

C. Edematous gingival tissue would not be a true sign of disease progression.

E. Change in gingival color is an indication but is not the best answer.

20. C

Yearly radiographs would be the best way to evaluate for implant failure. This would allow you to observe the bone loss by counting its level at the threads.

A. By checking the mobility of the implant, you may find that the prosthesis and not the implant is loose.

B. Checking pocket depth is done with a plastic probe but it is not the best determining factor.

D. Suppurative lesions are advanced peri-implantitis.

21. B

The oral tissue most similar to gingival tissue is palatal tissue, which explains why this tissue is used as a donor site for a free gingival graft.

22. A

A patient with refractory periodontitis can experience rapid loss of attachment, even after intensive therapy.

B. It can occur at one or many teeth.

C. It is caused by several microbes.

D. Systemic diseases increase a patient's chances for refractory periodontitis.

E. This does not happen from poor plaque control. It can happen even with the most meticulous plaque control.

23. D

The best way to test for tooth mobility is with the blunt ends of two instruments.

24. D

The agent that delivers minocycline into a gingival pocket is Arestin.

A. Periochip delivers chlorhexidine.

B. Periostat delivers doxycycline.

C. Atridox delivers doxycycline.

25. C

Allograft comes from cadaver bone.

A. Autograft is from the person himself.

B. Xenograft is from another species such as a cow.

D. Alloplasts are synthetic bone.

Chapter Nine: **Radiology**

Dental radiographs are a critical diagnostic tool. They can help to detect teeth conditions and/or abnormalities, check supporting structures, and monitor changes in a patient's health.

The dental hygienist plays an important role in exposing, developing, and mounting radiographs. Knowing how to properly perform these duties is essential, not only for the safe use of ionizing radiation, but also for the appropriate development of the patient's treatment plan.

> The ADA recommends that radiographs be taken on an individual basis, as per a patient's dental needs.

HISTORY OF RADIOLOGY

Radiographs were first discovered in 1895, when Wilhelm Roentgen was exploring the properties of the Hittorf–Crookes cathode ray tube. The cathode ray tube was a partially evacuated tube with an anode and a cathode at both ends. When high voltage electricity was passed from the anode to the cathode, Roentgen observed a fluorescent glow on a barium platinocyanide-coated screen across the room. When he shrouded the tube in a heavy black box, he could still see the greenish fluorescent light on the platinocyanide-coated screen.

After passing the radiation through several objects, Roentgen decided to use his own hand. As he did, he saw that the bones in his hand projected onto a fluorescent screen.

RADIATION PHYSICS

Electromagnetic radiation comes in varying levels of energy, wavelengths, and frequencies, which determine if the rays are visible or invisible. Electromagnetic radiation occurs in visible light or invisible infrared rays, ultraviolet rays, and x-rays.

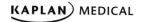

In x-rays, there are varying wavelengths (length of wave) and frequencies (how many times the wave appears from point *x* to point *y*) that determine if the x-ray penetrates an object. X-rays that penetrate more effectively have a shorter wavelength with a high frequency rate. Less penetrating x-rays will have low frequency with longer wavelengths.

Radiation wavelengths

Longer wavelength / Less frequent occurrence = Less penetrating x-rays

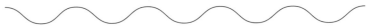

Shorter wavelength / More frequent occurrence = More penetrating x-rays

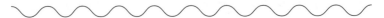

Particulate radiation contains bundles of energy that consist of particles and waves of electromagnetic radiation. These bundles, called x-ray photons, move at the speed of light. As photons interact with electrons in the x-ray tube head, they remove the electrons from atoms. This produces the negative or positive imbalanced ions of **ionizing radiation**.

Bremsstrahlung or **braking radiation** is the sudden deceleration a negatively charged electron experiences when it passes near a positive nucleus, becoming attracted to it.

RADIOLOGICAL EFFECTS

X-ray photons interact with the patient's tissues, and may be absorbed or scattered. Some photons are **attenuated** or **absorbed** by the patient, resulting in **radiopaque** areas on the radiographic films. Other photons exit the patient, and are exposed on radiographic films as **radiolucent** areas.

Absorbed x-ray photons can have biological effects. Ionizing radiation can alter the DNA of the nucleus of a cell, causing a disturbance with cell division or mitosis. This results in future tissue mutations.

Direct Interaction with Molecules

Classic scatter radiation, also called **coherent** or **Thompson effect**, occurs when a low-energy x-ray photon that is unable to eject an electron from an atom excites the electron instead. That photon fails to survive, though the excited electron produces a new photon to be ejected from the atom.

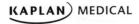

Characteristic radiation or **photoelectric effect** occurs when a high-speed photon ejects a tightly bound inner orbit electron from an atom. This causes an outer orbit electron to drop down into the space left empty by the ejected electron. This action **emits energy**. The electron that was originally ejected from the inner orbit is called a recoil electron.

Compton effect is the result of a high-energy photon ejecting a loosely bound outer orbit electron after the two collide. In this case, **energy is absorbed**.

Incidental Interaction with Molecules

When X-ray photons intermingle with water and oxygen of biological molecules or human tissue, the result is **free radicals**. Free radicals have a high likelihood of interacting with human biological tissue and of causing damage to the biological cells.

Tissue Sensitivity

High	Moderate	Low
Lymphocytes	Developing bone & cartilage	Mature bone & cartilage
Bone marrow	Connective tissue	Salivary glands
Reproductive cells	Small vasculature	Thyroid glands in adults
Thyroid glands in children		Kidneys
Intestines		Liver
Endocrine glands		Muscles
Skin		Nerve tissue
Oral mucosa		

Each column is listed from higher sensitivity to lower sensitivity

OPERATOR AND PATIENT PROTECTION

When exposing and developing radiographs, standard ADA and CDC precautions must be taken. It is advised that plastic barriers be placed over the x-ray tube head unit and exposure switch. Post exposure, the unit and switches should be decontaminated as per guidelines.

Dental personnel should wear protective equipment as per OSHA guidelines. That would include gloves, a mask, and protective eyewear. Overgloves may also be used with sterile technique during exposure.

A lead apron with a thyroid collar should be placed over the patient to protect her reproductive organs and thyroid gland.

The lead in the apron should be 0.25 mm thick.

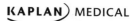

During film exposure, the clinician should remain behind a lead barrier. Should this not be possible, however, she should make sure to cover any exposed anatomy with a lead apron 0.25 mm thick. The safest area in which to stand is within 90–135 degrees at the side of the patient and away from the primary beam.

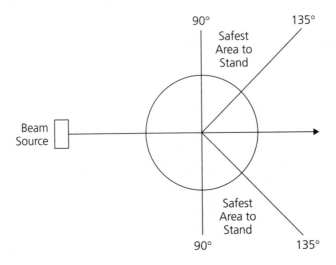

Distance also raises the level of safety, with at least 6 feet of distance from the direction of the beam being best. Dental personnel should wear film badges to monitor their occupational exposure.

The **maximum permissible dose (MPD)** that dental personnel should receive takes into account the whole anatomy to prevent genetic alterations. For dental personnel, that dose is 5.0 rem (.05 Sv) per year. For the general public, it is 0.5 per year.

The **maximum accumulated exposure** takes age into account. The formula for this uses the 5 rem per year dose along with the patient's age (N) minus the first 18 years when she was not a dental hygienist. The formula is:

5 (N – 18) R

MPD does *not* use the age-based formula.

The **maximum permissible dose (MPD)** per year for any dental hygienist **no matter what age** is **5 rem** per year.

RADIOLOGICAL MEASUREMENTS

Radiation is accumulated by repeated exposures. **Lethal dose** is the amount of radiation absorbed that would cause biological death. **LD 50/30** is the amount of radiation that causes biological death in 50% of a population in 30 days. **Latent period** is the period from the time of exposure to the actual occurrence of a biological effect from radiation.

There are two ways to measure radiation. The first way uses traditional units including **Roentgen (R), rads** (radiation **a**bsorbed **d**ose), and **rems** (**r**oentgen-**e**quivalent-**man**). The second way, adopted in 1985, uses the international system (SI), which is calculated in coulombs per kilogram. This system includes **Gray, Sievert,** and **coulombs/kg.**

Radiation Amounts

Traditional Measurement	SI Measurement	Corresponding Measurements	What Is Measured
Rad	Gray	100 rad = 1 Gy	Absorbed radiation
Rem	Sievert	100 rems = 1 Sv	Dose equivalence or cause of biological effects
Roentgen	Coulomb per kilogram (C/kg)	1 R = 2.58×10^{-4} C/kg	Dose or energy absorbed per unit mass of tissue

THE X-RAY UNIT

An x-ray machine is able to produce radiation through electricity. The x-ray tube contains a protective housing which has a lead lined-casing and an anode and cathode. It is surrounded by an oil bath that serves as the cooling system for the tube head.

The **cathode** contains the **filament** that produces electrons. **Thermionic emission** occurs when the heated filament "boils off" electrons in a cloud which surrounds the filament. The cathode is controlled by milliamperage, which, when turned up, "boils off" more electrons. The molybdenum focusing cup of the cathode directs the beam of electrons toward the target of the anode.

1% of electrons are converted into radiographic electrons, while 99% are converted to heat.

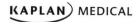

KAPLAN MEDICAL

Schematic drawing of the tube head

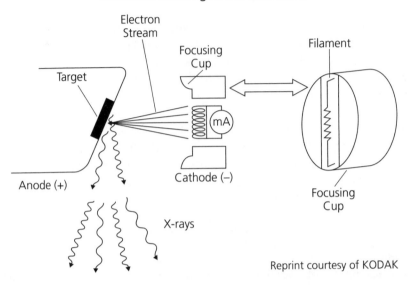

Reprint courtesy of KODAK

C− → A+

To remember whether the cathode and anode are positive or negative, and in which direction the electrons travel, think about wanting a grade of C- to go to an A+.

When the high-voltage circuit is concluded, an electrical potential difference develops. This draws the "boiled off" electrons toward the positive anode.

The **anode** contains a **focal spot** on the **tungsten target** that is inundated with electrons from the cathode. Due to tungsten's high atomic number, it has the ability to generate excess x-rays. A copper stem surrounding the target rapidly absorbs the heat that is generated by the tungsten target.

The beam is then directed toward the filter with an aperture. The filter prevents lower energy x-rays from getting to the patient. Regulations state that the **aluminum filter** must be **1.5 mm** for x-ray exposure **below 70kVp**, and **2.5 mm** for x-ray **exposure greater than 70kVp**.

Collimation utilizes lead diaphragms to restrict the size of the beam. It does so through a round or rectangular aperture (opening) of the **position indication device (PID)** or **beam indication device (BID)**.

The BID or PID has a **circular** or **rectangular** shape, **lead lined** tube head extension. *Federal law regulates* that the size of the beam be *no larger* than the following:

Circular tube heads: $2\frac{3}{4}$" (7 cm) in diameter

Rectangular tube heads: $1\frac{3}{8}$" by $1\frac{3}{4}$" (3.5 × 4.4 cm)

PID or BID length: **8"** (20 cm), **12"** (30 cm), or **16"** (40 cm)

DIGITAL RADIOGRAPHY

In the future, dental radiography will see more and more computer-based electronic dental imaging. It is **charge-coupled devices (CCD)** that receive the image onto a computer monitor.

Three types of dental imaging will be discussed here.

- **Direct digital imaging** utilizes a wired sensor that is placed like a regular radiographic film in the oral cavity. When the sensor is exposed to radiation, it transmits an electronic image to the computer monitor, where it is stored. Software allows for the image to be enhanced. The image isn't a film but rather a hard copy that may be printed on paper.

- **Indirect digital imaging** scans and digitizes a radiographic film onto the monitor. This method uses a CCD camera to scan in the radiograph.

- **Storage phosphor imager** utilizes a reusable imaging plate that is coated with phosphor. The phosphor plate is very much like a radiographic film that captures an image on the plate. The plate is placed onto a laser scanner that transfers the image to the computer monitor. Since the plate is reusable, it can be recycled: Place the imaging plates face down under a white light to erase the latent image.

RADIOGRAPHIC QUALITY

An ampere is a unit of electrical current. X-ray cathode units operate on a smaller amount of electricity than most other appliances, so they are measured in **milliamperes**. The cathode controls the milliamperage (mA). Turning up the mA is similar to turning up the burner on a stove; more electrons are boiled off. **Milliamperage** controls the **quantity** of radiation (number of Xrays).

The work capacity of an x-ray unit is measured in volts or **kilovolt** peak (**kVp**). kVp generates a potential difference of electricity as x-rays are created by the cathode and anode. It controls the **quality** of radiation.

Dental x-rays are black, white, and shades of gray. Where **more radiation** is absorbed onto the film during exposure of soft tissue, for instance, **more film emulsions are exposed** to the radiation. These areas become **black** in color and are called **radiolucent**.

When **less radiation** reaches a radiographic film (perhaps because a harder substance such as an amalgam filling prevents penetration), **less** or **no film emulsions are exposed**. These **white** areas are called **radiopaque**.

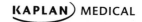

Contrast is the variation in **shades of gray** or **densities** that appear on a radiographic film. Contrast depends on bone thickness and other structures of the patient, film speed, processing, and kVp used.

Density refers to **darkness** on a film; it is dependent on the amount of radiation absorbed. Density is controlled by source-to-film distance, quantity of mA, quality of kVp, film speed and processing, and use of intensifying screens.

High contrast =
Decreased kVp penetrates less

↓ kVp ⟋△⟍ ↑ contrast

Low contrast =
Increased kVp penetrates more

↑ kVp ⟍△⟋ ↓ contrast

Increased kilovoltage results in **shorter** and **more frequent wavelengths**, generating more of the useful x-rays. Kilovoltage controls the contrast on the radiographic film. Decreased kilovolt peak yields high contrast, while increased kilovolt peak yields low contrast.

Decreasing the kilovolt peak to **65–70 kVp** allows for more contrast of **black and white**. This helps in examining the radiographs for **caries**.

Increasing the kilovolt peak to **75–90 kVp** allows for a better contrast of **shades of gray**. This helps in assessing radiographs for **bone levels**.

kVp Adjustments

Low kVp = high contrast

High kVp = low contrast

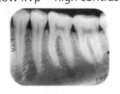 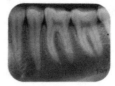

Reprint courtesy of Eastman KODAK

Exposure time of radiographs is measured in **impulses** of **60 impulses per second**. Impulses can change when mA is adjusted to preserve the same density. For instance:

If the density of a radiographic film is 1.5 with a mA of 16, and the impulses are 5 at a kVp of 75, how many impulses are required for radiograph with the same density with a mA of 8 and a kVp of 75?

In this question, the **density** and **kVp** remained the **same**, so they are not a factor.

$$\frac{\text{old mA} \times \text{old impulse}}{\text{New mA}} = \text{New impulse} \quad \text{or} \quad \frac{16\,\text{mA} \times 5\,\text{impulse}}{8\,\text{mA}} = 10\,\text{impulses}$$

RADIOGRAPHIC FILM

A radiographic film is coated on both sides with a green gelatin called an emulsion. The emulsion is made up of silver halide crystals (silver bromide and silver iodide), which are suspended in a Jell-O-like gelatin material. Exposure to radiation allows the crystals to store the radiation, producing a latent image on film once processed.

The speed of the film reacts to the radiation exposure time, producing an image. Film speed depends on the size of the silver halide crystals: High-speed film requires less radiation exposure. Film speeds range from A to F, but typically most dental radiographic films are D and E speed. **E-speed film** needs about **50% less** exposure time than D-speed film.

Film size varies by number:

Number 0: Children

Number 1: Mixed dentition

Number 2: Adult dentitions, both periapicals and bitewings

Number 3: Long bitewings

Number 4: Occlusal films

Extraoral films such as **panoramic film** come in two sizes: **5" × 12"** or **6" × 12"**. Cephalometric films are **8" × 10"**.

The **panoramic radiograph** lacks definition of detail and should be used in conjunction with periapicals x-rays. It is useful for an edentulous patient, when checking for pathology, for a patient with a strong gag reflex, and when performing orthodontics.

Panoramic film is placed in a cassette and is housed between two **intensifying screens**. The screens are made up of a **phosphor layer** that **converts** the **energy of x-rays into light**. That in turn **exposes** the panoramic film. This process reduces the amount of radiation needed to expose the film, but it also causes some loss of detail.

RADIOGRAPHIC TECHNIQUES

It is important that the film be set at the correct angle, so that it can be properly exposed. If it is not set correctly, retakes of the film—and further radiation exposure to the patient—are required. Proper angulation also allows for accurate assessment and diagnosis.

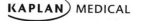

Bisecting technique uses geometry to determine the angulation of the x-ray tube head. The radiographic film touches the incisal or occlusal edge of the tooth, and the remainder of the film is angled away from the tooth. An **imaginary line** is drawn down the **long axis** of the tooth, with another **imaginary line bisecting** the imaginary line of the tooth and the angle of the film. The central ray of the tube head is directed perpendicular to the bisecting angle.

Bisecting Technique

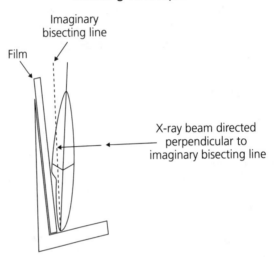

Imaginary bisecting line

Film

X-ray beam directed perpendicular to imaginary bisecting line

Parallel technique minimizes distortion by placing the radiographic film at the same angulation as the long axis of the tooth. The central ray of the tube head is then directed perpendicular to both the tooth and the angle of the radiograph, which are both at the same angle.

Parallel Technique

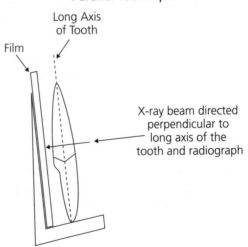

Long Axis of Tooth

Film

X-ray beam directed perpendicular to long axis of the tooth and radiograph

With **horizontal** angulation, it is important to direct the rays directly through the interproximal areas of the teeth being radiographed, so that overlapping and superimposition of teeth are prevented.

Horizontal angulation

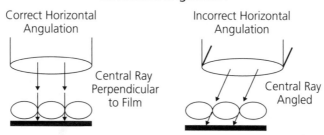

Correct Horizontal Angulation — Central Ray Perpendicular to Film

Incorrect Horizontal Angulation — Central Ray Angled

In order to obtain radiographs that are not **foreshortened** with **too much angulation** or that are **elongated** with **not enough vertical angle**, **vertical angulation** is important. Too much or too little angulation may cut off the root tips or the crowns.

Vertical Angulation

Not enough vertical angle

Cuts off root tip or elongates

Too much vertical angle

Foreshortens or cuts off crowns

Cuts off crown   Foreshortens

The **buccal object rule** or **SLOB rule** (**S**ame on **L**ingual, **O**pposite on **B**uccal) is used to locate whether some pathology or an object is on the buccal or lingual aspect of a tooth. The first film is taken normally, while the second is taken either horizontally or vertically at a different angle. If the tube is moved mesially by 20° and the object moves mesially, then it is on the same side or <u>s</u>ame <u>l</u>ingual. If the film was still taken 20° to the mesial but the object moved more distally, it is on the opposite side or <u>o</u>pposite <u>b</u>uccal.

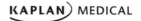

The image that appears on the radiographic film is a **shadow** of the teeth and their periodontium. The resulting "shadow" may be thought of as an eclipse of the moon with earth. As earth blocks the sun's rays, a **darker shadow** appears where the moon cannot be seen, the **umbra**. The **partial shadow** at the edge of the eclipse shadow is the **penumbra**.

Umbra and Penumbra

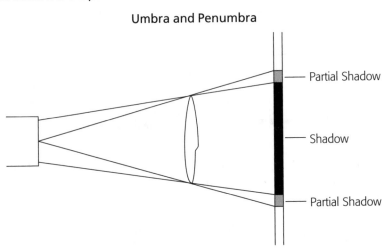

Partial Shadow

Shadow

Partial Shadow

Different things affect the shadow of the teeth on the radiograph. A **smaller focal spot** from the target of the anode **produces a larger amount of parallel photons** that then **reduce the penumbra** or partial shadow. This yields a **much sharper image**.

Object-to-film distance (OFD) refers to the distance between the radiograph and the tooth. **Source-to-film distance** (SFD) refers to the distance between the radiograph and the x-ray tube head or BID or PID. The BID and PID are more commonly found in 8", 12" and 16" lengths.

A **shorter object-to-film distance** yields a **sharper image** and **reduces magnification** of the object being filmed. **Increasing** the **source-to-film distance** (SFD) also **reduces magnification.**

INVERSE SQUARE LAW

The **inverse square law** is a physics term having to do with distance. In this case, **the source-to-film distance** (SFD) is where the inverse square law applies.

When the distance changes with a shorter or longer PID, the intensity of the central beam changes. If the **source-to-film distance** becomes farther away, the central ray **widens** or **becomes larger**, causing it to become **less potent**. An **increase in exposure** time is needed to maintain a sharper image.

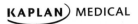

The opposite is true if the distance becomes shorter. If the **source-to-film distance** becomes closer, the central ray **narrows** or **becomes smaller** and thus becomes **more potent**. A **decrease in exposure** time is needed to maintain a sharper image.

$$\frac{\text{Old Intensity}}{\text{New Intensity}} = \frac{(\text{New distance})^2}{(\text{Old distance})^2}$$

To make this easier, first take the amount of distance that changed, whether halved or doubled. Square either the $\frac{1}{2}$ distance $[(\frac{1}{2})^2]$, which equals $\frac{1}{4}$, or the doubled distance $[(2)^2]$, which equals 4. Now multiply that result by the amount of time used for the original exposure.

If the **distance** is **doubled**, the distance is twice as far away and a greater amount of exposure time is needed. So twice the distance squared or 2^2 times the original exposure time is needed for exposure, resulting in a longer exposure time.

If the **distance** is **cut in half** $(\frac{1}{2})$, **less exposure time** is needed. With the inverse square law, you would take the square of one half the distance or $(\frac{1}{2})^2$. One half squared is one quarter $(\frac{1}{4})$, which is then multiplied by the original time, resulting in a smaller fraction of time.

Let's say that the source-to-film distance is 16" at 2 seconds. What would be the new amount of exposure time if the source-to-film distance were 8"?

In this case, the distance is **halved** from 16" to 8", so you would multiply the original time to be changed by $\frac{1}{4}$.

The distance was cut in half so $(\frac{1}{2})^2 = \frac{1}{4}$, so 2 seconds $\times \frac{1}{4} = \frac{1}{2}$ or 0.5 seconds.

Here's another example. If the source-to-film distance is 8" at 0.3 seconds, what would be the new amount of exposure time if the source-to-film distance were 16"?

The distance was doubled so $(2)^2 = 4$, so 0.3 seconds $\times 4 = 1.2$ seconds.

In this example, the distance is **doubled** from 8" to 16". You would multiply the time to be changed by **4**. Other distances may not involve doubling or halving the distance. For example:

If the source-to-film distance is 6" at 1.5 seconds, what would be the new amount of exposure time if the source-to-film distance were 1"?

The distance was cut by one-sixth so $(\frac{1}{6})^2 = \frac{1}{36}$. So 1.5 seconds $\times \frac{1}{36} = 0.04$ seconds.

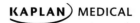

RADIOLOGICAL LANDMARKS

The teeth themselves distinguish how radiographs are mounted. The dot on the radiograph helps us to identify the right side from the left, but we also use landmarks to identify different things. Some landmarks are radiolucent (dark), while others are radiopaque (white).

Anatomical Landmarks

Zygomatic arch · Eye Orbit · Maxillary sinus · Nasal septum · Coronoid process · Mandibular notch · Condyle · Angle of mandible · Inferior border of mandible · Mandibular canal · Genial tubercles · Mental foramen · External oblique ridge

Maxillary Radiolucent Landmarks

Incisive foramen: Where the nasopalatine nerve and artery enter is a radiolucency located between the maxillary incisors.

Median palatine suture: A radiolucent line between the maxillary incisors. It is the juncture of the two palatal shelves.

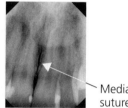

Median palatine
suture (radiolucent)

Maxillary sinus: A radiolucent area delineated by a radiopaque area extending from the vicinity of the maxillary canine posteriorly.

Maxillary Radiopaque

Inverted Y: A radiopacity at the juncture of the anterior sinus with the floor of the nasal fossa. Inverted Y created by the juncture of the anterior maxillary sinus and the floor the nasal fossa.

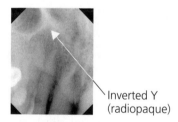

Inverted Y
(radiopaque)

Nasal septum: A radiopaque area located between the central incisors that divides the nasal cavity into two parts.

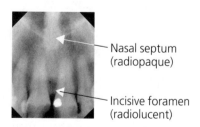

Nasal septum
(radiopaque)

Incisive foramen
(radiolucent)

Zygomatic arch: A radiopaque area seen on posterior radiographs where the temporal process of the zygomatic bone joins the zygomatic process of the temporal bone.

Maxillary tuberosity: A radiopaque area at the most posterior end of the maxilla.

Styloid process: A posterior radiopaque area that is an extension of the temporal bone. It serves to attach muscles and ligaments.

Hamular process: A radiopaque area that is a thin, curved line of the medial pterygoid plate.

Lateral pterygoid plate: A radiopaque area that is a flattened appendage of the sphenoid bone.

Palatal tori: Radiopaque areas of extra-bony growth in the palate.

Mandibular Radiolucent Landmarks

Mandibular canal: A horizontal radiolucent area through which the inferior alveolar nerve and corresponding vessels travel to exit the mandible. They do this by way of the mental foramen.

Mental foramen: A radiolucent area is located in the area of the mandibular second premolar. It is where the mental nerve exits.

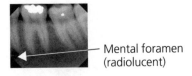

Mental foramen
(radiolucent)

Lingual foramen: An anterior radiolucency located in the middle of the genial tubercles. It serves as an exit for blood vessels and nerves.

Mandibular Radiopaque Landmarks

Genial tubercles: A radiopaque area at the anterior center of the mandible. They serve as a mode of attachment for muscles.

Interior oblique ridge: A radiopaque area on the interior surface of the mandible that is the mode of attachment for the mylohyoid muscles.

Exterior oblique ridge: A radiopaque area inferior to the coronoid notch that joins the ramus to the body of the mandible.

Inferior border of the mandible: An inferior radiopaque area of the mandible with thick cortical bone.

Mandibular tori: Radiopaque areas on the lingual surfaces of the mandible where extra bony growth occurred.

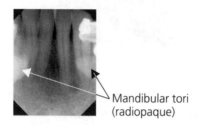

Mandibular tori
(radiopaque)

INTERPRETATION

Dental radiographs are exposed and developed in order to evaluate a patient's dentition. The teeth are evaluated for disturbances of the hard structures. The periodontium is evaluated for disease and bone loss. Dental radiographs are also beneficial for assessing pathology or injuries. A diagnosis is not determined with radiographs alone but by also considering the visual exam and patient's symptoms.

Bitewing radiographs are taken to detect early caries.

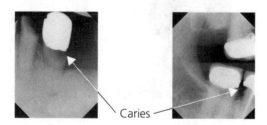

Caries

Radiographs also help to identify **iatrogenic abnormalities,** such as an overhanging or amalgam filling that has fallen into soft tissue.

Iatrogenic errors

Overhang filling on #12 D   Amalgam filling in soft tissue

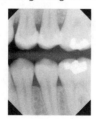
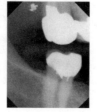

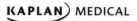

Periapical abscess is also a pathology that needs to be diagnosed and assessed for treatment.

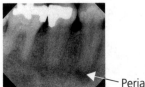

Periapical abscess

Another thing that is looked at routinely is bone levels and loss of bone. This helps to assess the patient's need for periodontal treatment in the prevention of further bone loss.

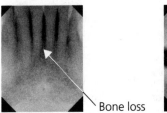

Bone loss   Bone loss

Spicules of calculus aid in assessing the type of periodontal treatment a patient is to receive.

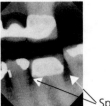

Spicules of calculus

With respect to checking **dental implants for bone loss**, it is best to check yearly with radiographs. An implant may be loose because the prosthesis is loose and not the implant itself.

Implants

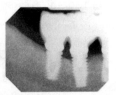

THE DARKROOM

Standard precautionary care should be taken when developing exposed radiographs. The film packet should be wiped with an EPA-registered disinfectant as it is removed, and then released into a receptacle such as a cup.

Contaminated film should be opened with a sterile technique. The film should not be touched before it is dropped onto a barrier surface. As soon as all packets are opened and dropped onto a barrier surface, the gloves may be removed. The radiographic film can then be placed into the developing solution or automatic processor.

Automatic processors are a series of rollers that are more costly than developing solution, but the processing time is shorter with them. The results are more dependable, as well, and they require less space. With the use of a daylight box, a darkroom is not required.

The manual dip tank method—where films are placed on racks—is reliable, though the processing time is longer. For that, a darkroom is required, along with tanks for the developer, water, and fixer. Also required are a thermometer, timer, and racks or hangers.

Temperature and time must be maintained in order to achieve good results. For manual processing, the temperature should be 68°F for 5 minutes or 72°F for 4 minutes. For automatic processing, the temperature will be higher and is monitored by an internal thermometer.

The **developing solution** is a combination of hydroquinone and elon. **Hydroquinone** (producing **contrast**) changes the latent image in the **silver halide crystals** to **black metallic silver**. The **elon** (generating **detail**) produces **gray tones** of the latent image. Sodium carbonate or potassium hydroxide softens and swells the emulsion to provide an access for hydroquinone and elon to contact the silver bromide crystals. Sodium sulfite is the preservative that reduces oxidation to prolong the effective ability of the solution. Potassium bromide and potassium iodide are restrainers that reduce the action potential of the solution.

The **fixer neutralizes** and **stops** the developing action. Ammonium or sodium thiosulfate is the fixing agent that eliminates unexposed, underdeveloped silver halide crystals of the emulsion or gelatin. The acidifier of either acetic acid or sulfuric acid neutralizes the developing solution to inhibit its action. Sodium sulfite is the preservative that reduces oxidation to maintain the chemical balance of the solution. The hardener of aluminum chloride or aluminum sulfide also shrinks the emulsion.

The **darkroom light** is a safelight with a red filter, set **4 feet** above the working surface. The bulb should be **15 watts** or less. The room needs to be at least **16 square feet** in size.

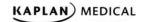

TECHNICAL AND OPERATOR ERRORS

Errors do occur but knowing how to correct them so that they can be prevented in the future is essential. Prevention is done through correct angulation, film exposure, and processing.

Technical Errors

Temperature: If the temperature is **too warm**, the radiograph will be **overdeveloped** and **dark** in color. If it is **not warm enough**, the radiograph will be **underdeveloped** and **too light**. The corrective measure is to monitor temperature.

Temperature Errors

Underdeveloped =
Temperature too low

Overdeveloped =
Temperature too high

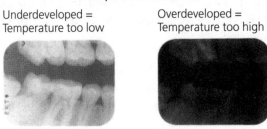

Reprint courtesy of Eastman KODAK

Splashing: If **developer** splashes onto the radiograph prior to developing, it will result in a **dark** spot. If **fixer** splashes onto the radiograph, it is a **white or lighter** spot.

Splash

Fixer splash

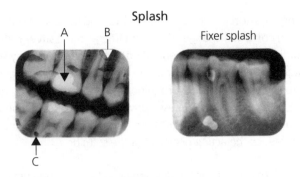

Reprint courtesy of Eastman KODAK

Developer splash = Dark
Fixer splash = Light or white

A – dark emulsions from another radiograph
B – emulsion not developed due to contact with side of tank or another film
C – developer splash on film prior to processing

Wrong exposure: If a radiograph comes out **clear** with nothing on it, then the film was **not exposed**. If a radiograph is **completely black**, it was **exposed to light**.

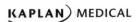

Film fog: Film fog may be due to old chemical solutions, improper safelight, out-of-date film, or improper storage near a radiation source.

Green film: A green film indicates that the film was not fixed enough.

Operator Errors

Overlap: Overlap occurs from **incorrect horizontal angulation.** The corrective measure would be to make sure the central beam is directed perpendicular to the film through the interproximal surfaces.

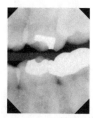

Blurred image: A blurred image results if the **patient moves** during film exposure. The corrective measure is to instruct the patient to not move.

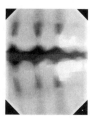

Interference with the central beam: The cord from the digital sensor appeared on this film because it was in the way of the central beam. The corrective measure would be to make sure all equipment is out of the way of the central beam.

Digital radiograph cord in picture

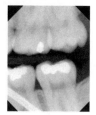

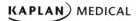

Foreshorten = too steep

Elongation = not enough angle

Vertical angulation errors: Vertical angulation errors include **foreshortening** from **too much** or **too steep** angulation while **elongation** occurs from **not enough** angulation. The corrective measures to take are with adjusting the vertical angulation.

Foreshortened

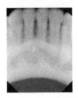

Double exposure: When the same film has been exposed twice, double exposure results. The corrective measure would be to use fresh film for every exposure.

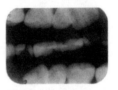

Reprint courtesy of Eastman KODAK

Static electricity: When film is removed hastily from its package and the surrounding air is very dry, static electricity results. Tree-like branches show up on the film. The corrective measure would be to remove film slowly during less humid conditions.

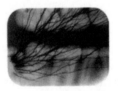

Reprint courtesy of Eastman KODAK

Black streak: When a film is **bent**, the precise location of the bend shows up as a black streak.

Bent film

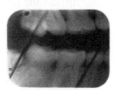

Reprint courtesy of Eastman KODAK

Scratch: A scratch shows up as a **white** area on the film. The emulsion has been scratched off prior to development.

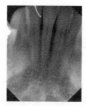

Cone cut: Incorrect horizontal angulation causes cone cut. The corrective measure is to ensure that the dental beam is directly perpendicular to the center of the radiograph.

Round cone cut   **Rectangular cone cut**

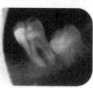 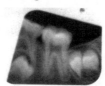

Reprint courtesy of Eastman KODAK

Improper film placement: This can occur from improper positioning or from backward placement as seen below.

Improper film placement (backward)

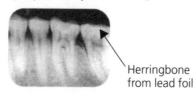

Herringbone from lead foil

Reprint courtesy of Eastman KODAK

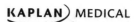

REVIEW QUESTIONS

Scenario for Questions 1–5

A 42-year-old male has presented to the practice today as a new patient. He states that his upper right 1st and 2nd bicuspids seem to be getting darker in color, but the teeth themselves don't have any symptoms. He has not had a dental cleaning in several years since he is new to the area and has not "gotten around to finding a dentist." Office protocol calls for radiographs for each new patient, but this patient states that he doesn't like radiation since he has read about dental radiation exposure. Upon examination, you find #4 and #5 gray in color with no apparent lesions or restorations. The periodontal exam reveals 4–6 mm posterior pockets with detectable subgingival calculus, generalized bleeding, and moderate stain. After explaining further the need for radiographs to diagnose the discoloration of #4 and #5 and to better assess his periodontal condition, the patient consents to the digital radiographs.

1. What is the best radiographic survey to take on this patient?

   A. Full mouth radiographs with horizontal bitewings

   B. Full mouth radiographs with vertical bitewings

   C. Vertical bitewings and a periapical of #4 and #5

   D. Horizontal bitewings and a periapical of #4 and #5

   E. Vertical bitewings and a panoramic survey

2. According to the ADA, how often should radiographs be taken?

   A. Every 6 months

   B. Once a year

   C. Once every 2 years

   D. Based upon the patient's individual health needs

3. You inspect the periapical radiograph of #4 and #5. There seems to be a radiolucent larger-than-normal pulp chamber on #4, and a radiolucency of the pulp chamber of #5 that extends almost to the distal surface. This lesion is most likely

   A. Internal resorption

   B. Dentinal caries

   C. Radicular cyst

   D. Residual cyst

   E. Dentigerous cyst

4. Based upon the patient's pocket depth readings, what kind of bone loss might be seen radiographically?

   A. Generalized horizontal bone loss

   B. Generalized vertical bone loss

   C. Generalized vertical and horizontal bone loss

   D. Localized vertical bone loss

5. Based upon the patient's statement of not liking radiation of any sort, what might you say to allay his fears?

   A. You get more radiation in the sun every day than you do from dental radiation.

   B. Digital radiography today offers less exposure than ever before.

   C. All of the articles he has read are completely false.

   D. The newer, faster film speed requires less radiation.

   E. The lead apron and thyroid collar will protect him.

6. Radiographs were discovered by a man who put his hand in the path of electrical current. The man who saw his bones on the screen was

   A. Exner
   B. Crookes
   C. Jennings
   D. Edison
   E. Roentgen

7. A 40-year-old dental hygienist has been working in the profession for 20 years. The maximum permissible dose per year for this hygienist would be

   A. 0.5 rem
   B. 5.0 rem
   C. 100 rem
   D. 800 rem

8. The Department of Health and Human Services of the FDA requires that the x-ray beam be limited to 2.5 mm by the aluminum filter for greater than 70 kVp. For less than 70 kVp, the beam should be limited to

   A. 1.0 mm
   B. 1.5 mm
   C. 1.75 mm
   D. 2.75 mm

9. When changing from a beam indication device (BID) of 6" with an exposure time of 0.5 seconds to a BID of 12", the new exposure time would be

   A. 1.0 seconds
   B. 1.5 seconds
   C. 2.0 seconds
   D. 2.5 seconds
   E. 4.0 seconds

10. When modifying a BID from 6" at 2 seconds to a 1" BID, the new exposure time would be

    A. 0.05 seconds
    B. 0.1 seconds
    C. 0.2 seconds
    D. 0.3 seconds
    E. 0.5 seconds

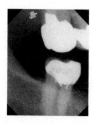

11. The radiopaque area distal to #2 is

    A. An amalgam tattoo
    B. Part of an amalgam filling
    C. Calculus
    D. Static bone cyst

12. All of the radiographs that you just developed are dark and you can barely see the image of the teeth. This processing error is due to

    A. Light exposure
    B. Fixer splash
    C. The temperature is too high.
    D. Milliamperage was decreased.

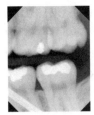

13. What is the technical error on this radiograph?

    A. The XCP was placed improperly.

    B. The film was scratched.

    C. The film was bent.

    D. The digital sensor cord was exposed.

    E. The patient's eyeglasses.

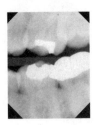

14. What is the technical error on this radiograph?

    A. Incorrect vertical angulation

    B. Incorrect horizontal angulation

    C. Incorrect film placement

    D. Incorrect film holder

    E. Incorrect positioning of the patient

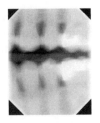

15. What is the technical error on this film?

    A. Solutions were too warm

    B. Solutions were too cool

    C. The patient moved

    D. Film was double exposed

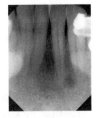

16. What is the bilateral radiopacity found near the apices of the canines?

    A. Amalgam fillings

    B. Odontoma

    C. Chondroma

    D. Mandibular tori

    E. Osteoma

17. Which of the following structures is radiopaque?

    A. Nutrient canals

    B. Median palatine suture

    C. Inverted Y

    D. Submandibular fossa

18. Which of the following structures is radiolucent?

    A. Genial tubercles

    B. External oblique ridge

    C. Hamular process

    D. Nasal septum

    E. Submandibular fossa

19. Streaks appear across the full series of radiographs that you just developed. This processing error is from

    A. Film fog

    B. Dirty rollers

    C. Developer splash

    D. Fixer splash

20. The ideal time and temperature for manual processing of radiographs is 72° F for 4 minutes. For automatic processing, it is 83° F for 5 minutes.

    A. Both statements are true.

    B. The first statement is true. The second statement is false because the temperature should be 68° F for 4 minutes.

    C. The first statement is false because the temperature should be 68° F for 5 minutes. The second statement is true.

    D. Both statements are false because the manual and the automatic processors should both be 68° F for 5 minutes.

21. The cell in the adult body most sensitive to radiation exposure is

    A. Lens of the eye

    B. Liver

    C. Small blood vessels

    D. Small lymphocytes

    E. Thyroid gland

22. Which of the following errors would look like black tree branches?

    A. Scratch

    B. Bent film

    C. Static electricity

    D. Air bubble

23. Panoramic x-rays need less radiation due to the _____ of the cassette.

    A. Metal back protection

    B. Film emulsion

    C. Intensifying screen

    D. Focal trough

    E. Patient position

24. Which of the following is found in both the developing and fixing solutions of dental radiographs?

    A. Sodium sulfite

    B. Acetic acid

    C. Sodium carbonate

    D. Ammonium sulfate

25. Collimation refers to

    A. Film speed

    B. The x-ray tube head

    C. Focusing cup

    D. The lead disk

ANSWER EXPLANATIONS

1. B

Full mouth radiographs with vertical bitewings would be best in this case.

C. Vertical bitewings are needed to check bone levels but a periapical of #4 and #5 would not be sufficient for a complete diagnosis.

D. Horizontal bitewings could provide only a limited survey of the bone levels, and a periapical of #4 and #5 would not be sufficient for a complete diagnosis.

E. Vertical bitewings are needed but a panoramic survey would lack detail for a complete diagnosis.

2. D

The ADA recommmends that radiographs be taken based upon the patient's individual health needs.

3. A

The lesion is most likely internal resorption.

B. Dentinal caries extend from outside the pulp inward.

C. Radicular cyst is at the apex of a tooth.

D. Residual cysts occur in the bone after an extraction.

E. Dentigerous cysts occur in the third molar areas.

4. C

Based upon the patient's pocket depth readings, you would probably see generalized vertical and horizontal bone loss.

5. B

You would tell him that digital radiography today offers less exposure than ever before.

A. People do get more radiation in the sun than from dental xrays, but this would not allay his fears.

C. Articles he may have read could have skewed some minor statistics to look factual. Patients who have a phobia about xrays will seek out information in favor of their argument.

D. Newer, faster film speed does require less radiation but this office uses digital imagery.

6. E

Roentgen discovered the radiograph when he put his hand in the path of an electrical current that went from a shrouded, highly evacuated glass tube to a screen.

A. Exner was a physicist to whom Roentgen sent a copy of the x-rays.

B. Crookes discovered the cathode ray tubes that Roentgen used.

C. Jennings also exposed a radiograph in the same year as Roentgen but claimed he discovered them first.

D. Edison followed up with Roentgen's discovery by allowing people to see their bones.

7. B

For a 40-year-old dental hygienist who has been working for 20 years, the maximum permissible dose per year is 5.0 rem.

8. B.

For less than 70 kVp, the radiation beam going through the aluminum filter should be limited to 1.5 mm.

9. C

Going to a BID of 12" from a 6" BID doubles the distance. The inverse square law states that when doubling (2) the distance, the square of 2 equals 4, so $0.5 \times 4 = 2.0$ seconds.

10. A

Changing from a 6" BID to a 1" BID decreases the distance by one-sixth. The inverse square law states that $(\frac{1}{6})^2 = \frac{1}{36}$ times the old time of 2 seconds equals 0.05 seconds.

11. **B**

The radiopaque area distal to #2 is part of an amalgam filling.

A. An amalgam tattoo is a soft tissue lesion that this radiopacity may manifest as a blue–gray area.

C. Calculus is not as radiopaque as this object.

D. Static bone cyst is radiolucent.

12. **C**

If all of the radiographs are dark and tooth images are barely visible, the temperature while processing was too high.

A. Light exposure is totally dark and you would not observe the teeth.

B. Fixer splash turns out as a light spot on the radiograph.

D. Decreasing milliamperage lightens the film.

13. **D**

This technical error on this radiograph is exposure of the digital sensor cord.

A. Improper placement of the XCP would appear more radiopaque.

14. **B**

The technical error here is incorrect horizontal angulation

15. **C**

The technical error here is that the patient moved.

16. **D**

The bilateral radiopacity is mandibular tori.

A. Amalgam fillings are more radiopaque and located in tooth crowns, not apices.

B. Odontoma are irregular tooth-like structures and these masses are regular.

C. Chondroma is an irregular radiolucency and this radiograph is radiopaque.

E. Osteoma are not typically found in the maxilla or mandible.

17. **C**

An inverted Y is a radiopaque oral structure; it is the juncture of the anterior wall of the nasal floor and the wall of the sinus. Nutrient canals, median palatine suture, and submandibular fossa are all radiolucent.

18. **E**

A submandibular fossa is radiolucent, located at the posterior mandible. Genial tubercles, external oblique ridge, hamular process, and the nasal septum are all radiopaque.

19. **B**

Streaks across all of the radiographs are the result of dirty rollers.

A. Film fog from an unsafe darkroom light would not result in streaks.

C. Developer splash would be droplet-shaped dark spots.

D. Fixer splash would be droplet-shaped light spots.

20. **A**

Both statements are true. Manual processing of radiographs requires 72° F for 4 minutes. Automatic processing requires 83° F for 5 minutes.

21. **D**

The small lymphocytes are most sensitive to radiation exposure. In order of most sensitive to least sensitive: small lymphocytes, lens of the eye, small blood vessels, thyroid, and the liver.

22. **C**

The appearance of black tree brances would indicate static electricity.

A. A scratch is white.

B. Bent film would appear as a dark line.

D. An air bubble would appear as a white spot.

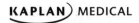

23. **C**

Panoramic x-rays need less radiation because of the intensifying screen in the cassette.

24. **A**

Sodium sulfite is found in both solutions as a preservative.

B. Acetic acid is the acidifier of fixing solution.

C. Sodium carbonate is found in developing solution. It swells and softens the emulsions.

D. Ammonium sulfate is found in fixer. It shrinks and hardens the emulsions.

25. **D**

Collimation is the lead disk that shapes and directs the beam.

C. Focusing cup is in the cathode and directs the beam to the anode.

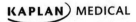

Chapter Ten: **Pathology**

Recognition of disease or pathology is an important role of the dental hygienist for early detection and treatment. Pathology can result from an inflammatory response, neoplasm, dysplasia, or an environmental influence—or it can be developmental in origin. Etiology is the study of the agents that cause disease. The diagnosis process includes clinical presentation, radiographic and histological differentiation, surgical treatment, and therapeutic treatment.

ORAL PATHOLOGY

A **cyst** can be defined as an epithelial-lined benign pathologic tissue within bone or in soft tissues. A **neoplasm** or **tumor** is an aberrant growth of new tissue that appears as an abnormal mass, swelling, or enlargement. It can metastasize to other sites but it can also be benign. Malignant neoplasms display a higher level of anaplasia (loss of cell differentiation and orientation) with qualities of metastases than do benign neoplasms.

Pathology can also occur from **chemicals** such as aspirin burns, from **physical forces** such as toothbrush abrasion, from **thermal forces** such as a hot coffee burn, or from **iatrogenic** causes, such as acid etch on gingiva.

Oral Cysts and Tumors

A **cyst** is an abnormal sac lined with epithelial tissue that contains a semisolid material or a liquid. A **tumor** is an uncontrolled and progressive atypical growth of abnormal cells.

Cyst Origins

Oral pathology can occur from origins of normal tissue, such as odontogenic tissue that gives rise to radicular cysts, residual cysts, glandular odontogenic cysts, or odontogenic keratocysts.

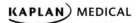

Cyst	Etiology	Tissue Origin
Radicular or periapical	Inflammatory	Rests of Malassez
Residual	Inflammatory after extraction	Rests of Malassez
Paradental	Inflammatory	Odontogenic epithelium
Follicular or dentigerous	Developmental	Reduced enamel epithelium
Odontogenic keratocyst	Developmental	Dental lamina
Glandular odontogenic	Developmental	Dental lamina
Gingival	Developmental	Dental lamina

Type of radicular cysts

Apical radicular cyst

Originates from

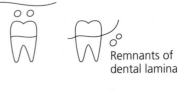

Rests of Malassez

Remnants of Hertwig's Sheath

Types of keratocyst and gingival cysts

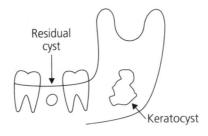

Residual cyst

Keratocyst

Originates from

Remnants of dental lamina

Types of follicular cysts

 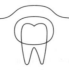

Dentigerous   Eruption

Originates from

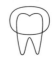

Reduced enamel epithelium

Non-odontogenic cysts do not originate from dental tissue such as nasopalatine duct cyst or nasolabial cyst.

Nasopalatine duct cyst ↗ ↖ Nasolabial cyst

■ **Ameloblastic Fibroma**

A mixed tumor of two embryonic tissues of the epithelium and connective tissues of the mesenchyme. These **benign and expansible** lesions are found **predominantly over unerupted molars.**

- **Etiology**: Epithelial and mesenchymal fragments of the enamel organ

- **Originates**: Odontogenic epithelium and connective tissue

- **Clinical presentation**: Solid, soft tissue mass that produces swelling

- **Radiographic appearance**: Uniocular or multiocular radiolucency

- **Treatment**: Block excision

■ **Ameloblastoma**

An epithelial disturbance that arises from dental lamina, Hertwig's sheath, or enamel organ. It can occur in the maxilla or mandible of both males and females. An ameloblastoma is an aggressive disturbance that is slow-growing, persistent, and hard to eradicate.

- **Etiology**: Unknown

- **Originates**: Arises from dental lamina, Hertwig's sheath, or enamel organ

- **Clinical presentation**: Initially an asymptomatic slow-growing swelling that can become painful

- **Radiographic appearance**: Soap bubble radiolucency

- **Treatment**: Aggressive surgery with wide free margins

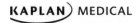

■ **Aneurysmal Bone Cyst**

Not a true cyst, it can occur anywhere in the skeleton. About 50% of cases occur in long bones. Orally, it occurs most often in the mandible. It develops rapidly as a tumor-like swelling or ballooning-out of bone from venous engorgement and bone resorption. Palpation or auscultation with a stethoscope of the lesion reveals a pulse. It can arise from a pre-existing condition such as tumor.

- **Etiology**: Unknown
- **Originates**: Unknown
- **Clinical presentation**: May be asymptomatic with radiographic finding or an expanding, rapidly destructive lesion
- **Radiographic appearance**: Radiolucent cyst, honeycomb, moth-eaten, or soap bubble appearance
- **Treatment**: Careful surgical excision with precautions for severe bleeding

■ **Cementoblastoma**

A true neoplasm that is benign and associated most often with the mandibular first molar. It is never found on anterior teeth. Cementoblasts form a large mass of cementum-like tissue at the tooth apex of vital teeth. This slow-growing tumor can cause bone expansion, unlike a cementoma.

- **Etiology**: Unknown
- **Originates**: Odontogenic tissue
- **Clinical presentation**: Asymptomatic, found radiographically
- **Radiographic appearance**: Radiopaque mass at the tooth apex surrounded by a thin radiolucent rim
- **Treatment**: Tooth extraction with attached calcified mass along with enucleation of the site

■ **Cementoma**

Not considered to be a true neoplasm, cementoma lesions appear to arise from the teeth but in fact arise within bone. This may occur as a reactive lesion from periodontal ligament irritation. It is most commonly found at the apices of the mandibular incisors. During the initial years, it is slow-growing on vital teeth as a radiolucency on radiographs. Later, it is a cementum-osseous mass becoming predominant on radiographs.

> Radiographic appearance changes:
> 1st   radiolucent
> 2nd radiopaque specks
> 3rd   circumscribed dense radiopacity

- **Etiology**: Unknown

- **Originates**: Periodontal ligament

- **Clinical presentation**: Asymptomatic, slow-growing lesion seen radiographically

- **Radiographic appearance**: First appears radiolucent, simulating a periapical granuloma, abscess, or cyst. Then appears as radiopaque specks. Finally, appears as mixed radiolucent and radiopaque change with the opaque portion predominant

- **Treatment**: None necessary

■ **Cherubism**

An autosomal dominant intraosseus fibrous swelling of the jaws. It occurs more often in the mandible than the maxilla, as a bilateral, symmetrical enlargement of alveolar ridge. It appears around age 3 or 4, and progresses to the late teens. It may regress in early adulthood.

- **Etiology**: Inherited

- **Originates**: Bone

- **Clinical presentation**: Chubby cheeks

- **Radiographic appearance**: Uniocular or multiocular bilateral expansive radiolucencies

- **Treatment**: Aesthetic and orthodontic considerations for proper function.

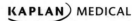

- **Dentigerous or Follicular Cyst**

  The **most common follicular cyst**, it forms around the crown of a developing tooth. It usually surrounds the crown of an unerupted mandibular third molar, maxillary canine, or maxillary third molar. Though usually small, it can become large and move other teeth.

  - **Etiology**: Developmental

  - **Originates**: Enamel epithelium after tooth is formed

  - **Clinical presentation**: Asymptomatic, found in areas of unerupted teeth (typically mandibular third molars, maxillary third molars, and maxillary canines)

  - **Radiographic appearance**: Solid, well-defined unilocular cyst surrounding the crown

  - **Treatment**: Enucleation and curettage

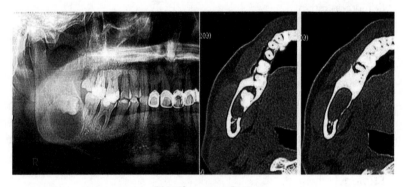

Dentigerous Cyst

Contributed by Dr. Akitoshi Katsumata Asahi University

- **Giant Cell Granuloma—Peripheral**

A dusky purple, sessile, or pedunculated, smooth-surfaced, dome-shaped papule or nodule. It is usually located on the anterior jaws at the gingival or alveolar process, but may appear at the crest of ridge of edentulous patient. Peripheral refers to tissue that covers bone; in this case, gingival tissue covers the bone.

- **Etiology**: Unknown

- **Originates**: Gingival mucosa

- **Clinical presentation**: Well-circumscribed lesion confined to the alveolar and gingival mucosa caused by local irritation or trauma

- **Radiographic appearance**: A radiolucent cuffing-out of the alveolar bone that underlies granuloma

- **Treatment**: Excision

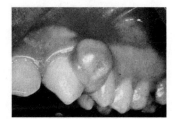

Peripheral Giant Cell Granuloma

Contributed by Dr. Michael Finkelstein, DDS College of Dentistry, University of Iowa

- **Giant Cell Reparative Granuloma**

An unusual, non-neoplastic fibrous lesion affecting the maxillary and mandibular bones and sinonasal cavity. This slow-growing lesion tends not to recur after surgical treatment.

- **Etiology**: Unknown; possible from injury

- **Originates**: Possible reactive response to intraosseous hemorrhage

- **Clinical presentation**: Clinical symptoms are nonspecific but may include bulge, pain, and local swelling. This lesion is indistinguishable from the brown tumor seen in hyperparathyroidism.

- **Radiographic appearance**: Radiolucent with a bubble-like appearance; is usually well-delineated and may contain calcifications

- **Treatment**: Excision or curettage. Over 60% of cases occur in the mandible at the midline of the anterior segment.

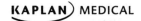

■ **Gingival Cyst**

A slow-growing lesion that develops in the interdental papillae. In adults, it often develops in the mandibular premolar-canine area as a painless swelling with normal gingival color. It is more common in newborns, however, and is usually called Epstein's Pearl or Bohn's Nodules. For infants, there is no treatment indicated.

- **Etiology**: Developmental

- **Originates**: Epithelial rests of the dental lamina

- **Clinical presentation**: Vesicular or bullous lesions that look like lateral periodontal cysts

- **Radiographic appearance**: Circumscribed radiolucency

- **Treatment**: Conservative surgical excision

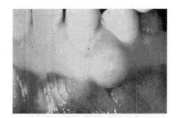

Gingival Cyst

Contributed by Dr. Michael Finkelstein, DDS College of Dentistry, University of Iowa

■ **Globulomaxillary Cyst**

The globulomaxillary cyst appears as a "pear-shaped" radiolucency on radiographs.

A maxillary bone cyst located in the globulomaxillary fissure between the lateral incisor and cuspid (both vital teeth). It appears as a pear-shaped radiolucency between the maxillary lateral incisor and cuspid.

- **Etiology**: Unknown

- **Originates**: Unknown; possibly from epithelial rests

- **Clinical presentation**: Asymptomatic, found radiographically

- **Radiographic appearance**: Radiolucent pear shape

- **Treatment**: Enucleation of cystic sac

■ **Lateral Periodontal Cyst**

A slow-growing odontogenic cyst that forms along the lateral root on **vital teeth**. It is found on the mandibular cuspids or premolars but may also occur on the maxillary anterior teeth.

- **Etiology**: Developmental

- **Origin**: Rests of the dental lamina

- **Clinical presentation**: Acute, painful, or chronic asymptomatic cyst usually on vital teeth

- **Radiographic appearance**: Radiolucent, uniocular, round shape that is well-circumscribed

- **Treatment**: Curettage or enucleation with no extractions

Periapical cysts occur on non-vital teeth.

Periodontal cysts usually occur on vital teeth.

■ **Median Palatal Cyst**

An uncommon inclusion cyst that appears posterior to the incisive canal at the maxillary midline of the hard palate. It occurs more posterior than a nasopalatine duct cyst.

- **Etiology**: Developmental

- **Originates**: Epithelial remnants

- **Clinical presentation**: Small lesions are not apparent with clinical intraoral examination, but large lesions raise the palatal mucosa

- **Radiographic appearance**: Well-circumscribed radiolucency at the midline of hard palate

- **Treatment**: Surgical excision

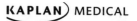

■ **Myxoma, Odontogenic**

A benign, infiltrative odontogenic lesion that is difficult to distinguish from an amelo-blastoma. This slow-growing, expansive lesion is invasive and destructive.

- **Etiology**: Unknown

- **Originates**: Dental papillae

- **Clinical presentation**: Painless, slow jaw enlargement

- **Radiographic appearance**: Not distinctive but similar in appearance to an amelo-blastoma as a soap bubble or honeycomb multiocular radiolucency

- **Treatment**: Wide, surgical block excision

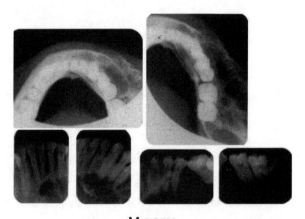

Myxoma

Contributed by Dr. Akitoshi Katsumata Asahi University

■ **Nasolabial Cyst**

A unilateral, soft-tissue swelling that occurs at the junction of the lateral nasal and maxil-lary processes. It is an asymptomatic lesion that is not detected with routine radiographs.

- **Etiology**: Unknown

- **Originates**: Epithelial remnants

- **Clinical presentation**: Swelling of the upper lip due to a swelling at the mucobuccal fold

- **Radiographic appearance**: Not seen radiographically, unless there is an injection of a radiopaque dye to define the cyst outline

- **Treatment**: Conservative excision

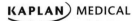

■ **Nasopalatine Duct Cyst**

A non-odontogenic, **heart-shaped cyst** located within the nasopalatine canal. In embryonic development, a "nasopalatine duct" had once connected the oral and nasal cavities, but underwent a progressive degeneration with the fusion of facial processes and the maxilla. Pulp-testing of the incisors will reveal vital teeth, but the roots may become divergent.

- **Etiology**: Developmental

- **Originates**: Degenerated nasopalatine duct site

- **Clinical presentation**: Cyst on the incisive papillae of the anterior hard palate, translucent or bluish- colored, dome-shaped swelling

- **Radiographic appearance**: Ovoid or round radiolucency located in the midline of the maxilla that appears heart-shaped due to the superimposition of the nasal spine

- **Treatment**: Enucleation

■ **Nevoid Basal Cell Carcinoma (Gorlin Syndrome)**

Autosomal dominant syndrome that includes multiple odontogenic keratocysts. Abnormalities include skin with early onset basal cell carcinoma, mental retardation, medulloblastomas, and skeletal anomalies.

- **Etiology**: Inherited

- **Originates**: Multiple occurrences

- **Clinical presentation**: Skin lesions, craniofacial abnormalities, central nervous systems disorders such as mental retardation or schizophrenia

- **Radiographic appearance**: Calcification of the falx cerebri (two folds of dura mater separating the hemispheres of the brain) with the presence of odontogenic keratocysts

- **Treatment**: Treatment of each abnormality independently

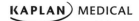

■ **Odontogenic Cyst, Calcifying (Gorlin Cyst)**

An uncommon, well-circumscribed, solid lesion derived from odontogenic epithelium that produces epithelial eosinic ghost cells and spherical calcifications. It may be an isolated lesion or alongside other lesions. This cyst—also termed Gorlin cyst—should not be confused with Gorlins syndrome, associated with odontogenic keratocysts.

- **Etiology**: Developmental

- **Originates**: Odontogenic epithelium

- **Clinical presentation**: Painless enlargement of the maxilla or mandible in the canine-incisal area

- **Radiographic appearance**: Well-circumscribed uniocular radiolucency with specks of vague radiopacities

- **Treatment**: Surgical excision

■ **Odontogenic Cyst, Glandular**

A very rare cyst that occurs in the anterior mandible and can reach such an impressive size that would require jaw resection. It is called *glandular odontogenic cyst* because the epithelial tissue creates small duct-like spaces that make it look glandular. It is also called a sialo-odontogenic cyst.

- **Etiology**: Developmental

- **Originates**: Dental lamina

- **Clinical presentation**: Painless swelling with localized destruction

- **Radiographic appearance**: Uniocular or multiocular radiolucency with scalloped borders

- **Treatment**: Surgical excision and curettage

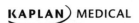

- ### Odontogenic Keratocyst

Developed from the remnants of the dental lamina, a very aggressive cyst that is hard to remove. It is not easily detected when it is a small unilocular radiolucency, and is more often detected radiographically as a large multilocular radiolucency. At that point, it has a soap-bubble appearance similar to that of an ameloblastoma radiograph.

- **Etiology**: Developmental

- **Origin**: Dental lamina

- **Clinical presentation**: Wide range of appearances since it mimics other lesions

- **Radiographic appearance**: Soap-bubble radiolucency similar to an ameloblastoma.

- **Treatment**: Surgical enucleation, but there is a high chance of recurrence

- ### Odontoma, Complex

A cyst that forms over unerupted teeth. Initially, it resembles an ameloblastic fibroma, but differentiates one step further into the tooth structures of enamel, dentin, pulp, and cementum. A complex odontoma produces poorly differentiated enamel, dentin and cementum, though not quite enough to create a recognizable tooth. It occurs most often in the mandibular molar area.

- **Etiology**: Developmental

- **Originates**: Odontogenic epithelium

- **Clinical presentation**: Unerupted tooth

- **Radiographic appearance**: Irregular calcified radiopaque mass surrounded by radiolucent band

- **Treatment**: Surgical excision or monitor radiographically

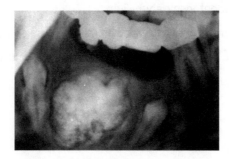

Odontoma

Contributed by Dr. Akitoshi Katsumata Asahi University

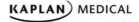

- **Odontoma, Compound**

A large mass of differentiated enamel dentin and cementum, but radiographically appears as masses of small misshapen teeth. This irregular, calcified lesion occurs most often in the anterior maxilla.

- **Etiology**: Developmental

- **Originates**: Odontogenic epithelium

- **Clinical presentation**: Unerupted tooth

- **Radiographic appearance**: Irregular radiopaque calcified mass surrounded by radiolucent band

- **Treatment**: Surgical excision or monitor radiographically

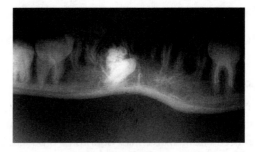

Compound Odontoma

Contributed by Dr. Akitoshi Katsumata Asahi University

- **Paradental Cyst**

Usually associated with the crown of a tooth—especially a partially erupted mandibular third molar—this is an inflammatory response usually found on the **distal or facial aspect of a vital erupting mandibular third molar.**

- **Etiology**: Inflammatory response

- **Originates**: Odontogenic epithelium

- **Clinical presentation**: Gingival inflammation of an erupting tooth

- **Radiographic appearance**: Well-circumscribed radiolucency

- **Treatment**: Surgical enucleation and extraction of associated tooth

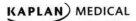

■ **Periapical Abscess (or Granuloma)**

An acute or chronic inflammation of tissues at the apex of a tooth, resulting in a collection of pus after a pulpal infection. The result of a carious lesion or injury, it causes pulp necrosis that creates a periapical granuloma.

- **Etiology**: Carious lesions or deep restorations
- **Originates**: Epithelial rests of Malassez
- **Clinical presentation**: Tooth sensitivity or fistula
- **Radiographic appearance**: Well-demarcated circular radiolucency at the tooth apex
- **Treatment**: Root canal, apicoectomy, or extraction

■ **Periapical Cyst (Radicular Cyst)**

An odontogenic cyst that is caused by caries, trauma, or pulpitis. It is a slow-growing, fluid-filled epithelial sac. The epithelium undergoes necrosis due to a lack of blood supply, causing the granuloma to become a cyst. These cysts are not usually clinically detectable and **occur on non-vital teeth.**

- **Etiology**: Developmental
- **Originates**: Epithelial rests of Malassez
- **Clinical presentation**: Asymptomatic
- **Radiographic appearance**: Well-demarcated, unilocular periapical radiolucency
- **Treatment**: Root canal, apicoectomy, or extraction

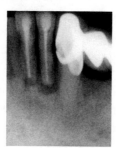

Periapical cyst

■ **Pleomorphic Adenoma**

A tumor of the salivary glands, also known as a benign mixed tumor. The gland most affected is the parotid gland (90%) but minor salivary glands are affected as well. The palate is the most common site for minor salivary glands that become pleomorphic adenomas. In very rare occurrences, they may become malignant.

- **Etiology**: Unknown
- **Originates**: Epithelium of displaced or aberrant salivary tissue
- **Clinical presentation**: Painless, slow-growing, firm mass
- **Radiographic appearance**: Asymptomatic, not seen radiographically
- **Treatment**: Surgical excision

■ **Primordial Cyst**

An odontogenic cyst that arises from primordial epithelium of a dental follicle. It is associated with a missing tooth since a tooth never developed in that location. Tooth formation was never completed since the follicle underwent cystic degeneration. These cysts are typically located in the mandibular third molar area.

- **Etiology**: Neoplastic
- **Originates**: Primordial epithelium
- **Clinical presentation**: Asymptomatic, found radiographically
- **Radiographic appearance**: Radiolucency in the alveolar process that is not associated with a tooth
- **Treatment**: Enucleation and curettage

■ **Residual Cyst**

A cyst that may form after a tooth is extracted if the periapical cyst wasn't removed at the same time. It may also form if debris entered into the socket during extraction. It is an odontogenic cyst, since it arises from tissues that were involved in odontogenesis.

- **Etiology**: Extraction site
- **Origin**: Rests of Malessez
- **Clinical presentation**: Asymptomatic, found radiographically
- **Radiographic appearance**: Radiolucency that is well demarcated
- **Treatment**: Excision

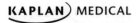

■ **Simple Bone Cyst**

A fluid-filled cavity that usually occurs in young patients. About 50% of cases result after a history of trauma. Many theories of the etiology abound; the most accepted being a lesion that stems from an intramedullary hemorrhage caused by trauma. It is theorized that the blood clot fails to totally organize but then goes on to degenerate, leaving behind an empty bone cavity. Edema then occurs in the space, causing resorption of trabecular bone. This space weakens bone, leaving it very fragile.

- **Etiology**: Unknown; possibly from trauma

- **Originates**: Bone

- **Clinical presentation**: Asymptomatic, found radiographically

- **Radiographic appearance**: Radiolucency that scallops around the root of the teeth

- **Treatment**: Surgical exploration; this causes the cavity to fill with blood, which usually causes the lesion to heal

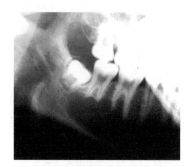

Simple Bone Cyst

Contributed by Dr. Akitoshi Katsumata Asahi University

■ **Stafne Bone Cyst (Static Bone Cyst)**

An unusual form of aberrant salivary gland tissue found within or adjacent to the lingual bone surface of the mandible. It is thought to be a congenital defect rather than a pathological defect, located in the posterior mandible.

- **Etiology**: Unknown

- **Originates**: Salivary gland tissue

- **Clinical presentation**: Asymptomatic, found radiographically

- **Radiographic appearance**: Well-circumscribed radiolucency within the bone

- **Treatment**: None required

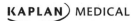

Hard Tissue Lesions

Hard tissue lesions can occur as normal benign lesions. Some are caused by metabolic disturbances or are genetic in origin.

Benign Bone Abnormalities

- **Exostosis** is a benign, bony protuberance that occurs on the facial bone of the mandible or maxilla or as **torus palatinus** at the midline hard palate. It also occurs as **torus mandibularis** on the lingual of surface of the mandible.

  - **Etiology**: Inherited
  - **Clinical presentation**: Hard benign protuberances that are nodular, lobular, or smooth
  - **Radiographic appearance**: Radiopaque
  - **Treatment**: None

- **Macrognathia** is a larger-than-normal jaw. It can be caused by acromegaly, the increased and unregulated growth-hormone (GH) production that causes enlarged hands, feet, and jaws.

  - **Etiology**: Inherited or acromegaly
  - **Clinical presentation**: Abnormally large jaws
  - **Treatment**: Orthodontia

- **Micrognathia** is an abnormally small jaw that is often associated with Pierre Robin syndrome, a condition present at birth. There is usually a cleft at the soft palate, causing the tongue to fall back and downward (glossoptosis).

  - **Etiology**: Inherited
  - **Clinical presentation**: Abnormally small jaw
  - **Treatment**: Orthodontia

Peripheral Lesions

- A **ranula** is the blockage of a salivary gland by a stone, typically in Wharton's duct in the floor of mouth. The blocked duct can rupture or sever. A **plunging ranula** forms by mucus extravastion from a blocked sublingual gland, causing swelling of the neck.

  > Ranula comes from the Latin word *rana* meaning "frog"; thus, the frog's belly appearance of the floor of the mouth from a ranula.

  - **Etiology**: Blockage by a sialolith
  - **Originates**: Salivary gland
  - **Clinical presentation**: Bluish, round, smooth bulge in the floor of the mouth that has a frog's belly appearance
  - **Radiographic appearance**: Radiopaque stone in salivary duct
  - **Treatment**: Surgical excision

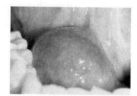

Ranula

Contributed by Dr. Michael Finkelstein, DDS College of Dentistry, University of Iowa

- A **sialolith** is a salivary stone or calculus produced in the salivary glands from mineral salts. It can be observed radiographically. It is commonly found in the submandibular gland or its duct.

  - **Etiology**: Unknown
  - **Clinical presentation**: Not seen
  - **Radiographic appearance**: Radiopaque stone in soft tissue
  - **Treatment**: Medical management with hydration, antibiotics, massage, warm compresses, or surgical excision

Tooth Abnormalities—Environmental

- **Abrasion** is the wearing-away of teeth due to an abnormal mechanical process (pathological)—perhaps holding a metal nail in the mouth or opening a bobby pin with one's teeth.

- **Attrition** is the wearing-away of teeth due to physiological forces of tooth-to-tooth wear.

- **Bruxism** is the abnormal occlusal wear due to grinding of teeth.

- **Erosion** is the loss of tooth structure due to chemical forces—perhaps acid if one sucks on lemons, or stomach acids if someone with bulimia nervosa purges. It typically appears on the lingual or buccal surfaces.

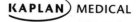

KAPLAN) MEDICAL

Tooth Abnormalities—Developmental

- **Amelogenesis imperfecta** is the genetic malfunction of the tooth germ that produces partial or completely missing enamel. Radiographically, the enamel is absent.

  - **Etiology**: Inherited

  - **Clinical presentation**: See table below and earlier in chapter for the different types of amelogenesis imperfecta

Types of Amelogenesis Imperfecta

Type	Clinical Presentation	Enamel	Radiographic Presentation	Genetics
Type I Hypoplastic	Small to normal size teeth. Color varies from normal to opaque white – yellow brown	Varies from thin and smooth to normal thickness with grooves, furrows, and/or pits	Enamel has normal to slightly reduced contrast/thin	Autosomal dominant, recessive
Type II Hypomaturation	Creamy opaque to marked yellow/brown. Soft and rough with dental sensitivity	Normal thickness with enamel that chips and abrades easily	Enamel has contrast similar to or greater than dentin, unerupted crowns have normal morphology	Autosomal dominant, recessive
Type III Hypocalcified	Opaque white to yellow-brown. Soft, rough enamel surface, dental sensitivity, and open bite common; heavy calculus formation common	Normal thickness with enamel that often chips and abrades easily	Enamel has contrast similar to or less than dentin, unerupted crowns have normal morphology	Autosomal dominant, recessive
Type IV Hypomaturation or hypoplastic associated with taurodontism	White/Yellow- brown. Mottled, teeth can appear small and lack proximal contact	Reduced, hypomineralized areas and pits	Enamel contrast normal to slightly greater than dentin, large pulp chambers	Autosomal dominant

Adapted from http://www.dent.unc.edu/research/defects/pages/aitypes.htm

- **Concrescence** is the union of two roots **after root formation is complete**. **Cementum** of one tooth **cements to cementum** of another tooth.

  - **Etiology**: Trauma

  - **Clinical presentation**: Merged roots radiographically

- **Dens evaginatus** is an extra or accessory cusp or an abnormal tooth shape as a tubercle projecting from the palatal or buccal surfaces (talon cusp).

  - **Etiology**: Developmental

  - **Clinical presentation**: An extra cusp or nodule on the palatal or buccal surfaces

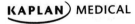

- **Dens in dente** or **dens invaginatus** is the appearance of a tooth within a tooth. As the tooth develops, it folds into itself, forming a small tooth-like shape within the pulp chamber.

  - **Etiology**: Increased localized forces

  - **Clinical presentation**: Not seen clinically, but is seen radiographically. It occurs more often in maxillary lateral incisors.

- **Dentogenesis imperfecta** is the abnormal development of dentin that is an autosomal dominant trait. It sometimes occurs along with osteogenesis imperfecta. Radiographically, the teeth will have short, blunted roots with obliterated pulp chambers.

  - **Etiology**: Inherited

  - **Clinical presentation**: **Opalescent**, translucent **gray–bluish brown**, bell-shaped teeth.

- **Dilaceration** is a sharply bent or curved root caused by trauma as the root is forming.

  - **Etiology**: Trauma during root formation

  - **Clinical presentation**: Not seen clinically, but is seen radiographically as a bent root.

- **Enamel hypocalcification** is a **defect in mineralization** of formed matrix. The enamel is softer underneath calcified enamel and is yellow–dark brown in color.

  - **Etiology**: Dental fluorosis, genetics

  - **Clinical presentation**: Yellow–dark brown enamel that is softer and underneath calcified enamel

- **Enamel hypoplasia** occurs when there is a deficient amount of enamel. The enamel is harder in context but thinner in quantity.

  - **Etiology**: Local, systemic, or genetic factors

  - **Clinical presentation**: Enamel appears pitted and is yellow–dark brown in color.

> A deficiency in quality is enamel hypocalcification. A deficiency in quantity is enamel hypoplasia.

- **Enamel pearls** occur when the ameloblasts formed too much enamel.

  - **Etiology**: Unknown

  - **Clinical presentation**: Excess enamel on root surfaces near CEJ and furcation of maxillary molars

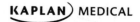

- **Fusion** occurs when two separate tooth germs merge together during tooth formation, and the **dentin becomes confluent.**
  - **Etiology:** Trauma
  - **Clinical presentation:** Radiographically, there are two separate canals. Clinically, there is the correct number of teeth in the dentition.

- **Gemination** is a single tooth that germinated into the formation of two teeth. Think of Siamese twins with gemination.
  - **Etiology:** Unknown
  - **Clinical presentation:** Radiographically, there is one shared root or canal. Clinically, counting the teeth reveals an extra tooth when the merged crowns are counted separately.

- **Incomplete root formation** is not pathology but is an open area at the root apex that is still forming the root.
  - **Etiology:** Root formation
  - **Clinical presentation:** Radiographically an open end on a root

Soft Tissue

First, let's review some basic terms:

- A **bulla** is an elevated lesion containing serous fluid.
- A **carbuncle** is a necrotizing skin infection made up of a cluster of boils (furuncles).
- **Carcinoma in situ** is a severe dysplasia that involves only the cells where it began. It is an uncontrolled growth of abnormal cells that has not spread or metastasized to nearby tissues.
- A **caruncle or caruncula** is a small, fleshy eminence that can be normal or abnormal.
- **Dysplasia** is the abnormal development and alteration of size, shape, and organization in adult cells.

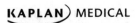

- **Fordyce granules** are normal aberrant sebaceous glands.

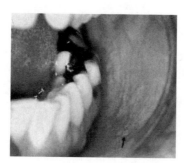

Fordyce Granules

Contributed by Dr. Michael Finkelstein, DDS College of Dentistry, University of Iowa

- A **furuncle** is a boil or painful skin nodule that has a circumscribed area of inflammation.

- A **macule** is a skin patch that is flat and altered in color.

- **Metaplasia** is the transformation of adult cells in a tissue to another form that is not normal for that type of tissue; in other words, a change in cells from a normal to an abnormal state.

- **Metastasis** is the migration of cells within the body from one organ (or part) to another organ (or part).

- **Nikolsky's sign** is the separation of the outer layer of the epidermis from the basal layer. This can be seen when spraying air from an air-water syringe onto abnormal epidermal tissue. With the blast of air pressure, a blister is created.

- A **nodule** is a small knot or node that is a minute collection of tissue.

- A **papule** is a small, solid, superficial elevation of skin that is circumscribed.

- **Pedunculated** refers to a **stalk-like base** of aberrant tissue that looks like a mushroom stem.

- **Sessile** refers to a **broad base** of aberrant or abnormal tissue.

- An **ulcer** is an acute or chronic lesion that is an inflammatory response. Epithelial tissue is destroyed along with underlying tissue.

- A **vesicle** is a circumscribed superficial elevation containing a clear fluid; if it ruptures, it can leave a superficial ulcer.

- **Xerostomia** is dry mouth due to insufficient saliva production. Many things can cause it, including chemotherapy, aging, salivary gland shrinkage, medication, or radiation treatment. Patients with xerostomia are at increased risk for oral candidiasis.

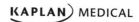

Soft Tissue Lesions

Soft tissue lesions can occur in a range of colors and locations within the oral cavity.

- **Amalgam tattoo** occurs when a particle of amalgam-filling embeds in mucosa, leaving a blue-gray tattoo.
  - **Etiology**: Amalgam filling
  - **Clinical presentation**: Blue–gray area on soft tissue near an amalgam filling
  - **Treatment**: None; benign

- **Angular cheilitis** is a red inflammation at the corners of the mouth, which results in cracks at the corners.
  - **Etiology**: Candida albicans or denture irritations
  - **Clinical presentation**: Red cracks at the corners of the mouth
  - **Treatment**: Antifungal ointments

- **Ankyloglossia** occurs when the lingual frenum is short, so the floor of mouth is fused with the tongue.
  - **Etiology**: Unknown
  - **Clinical presentation**: Short lingual frenum
  - **Treatment**: Frenulectomy

- A **cellulitis** is a diffuse-spreading inflammation of deep subcutaneous tissue, and sometimes muscle, that is not circumscribed.
  - **Etiology**: Bacteria, especially *Staphylococcus aureus*
  - **Clinical presentation**: The lesion is warm, tender, red, and not well-circumscribed. There may also be malaise, fever, and chills with regional lymphadenopathy.
  - **Treatment**: Oral antibiotics for mild cases; for more severe disease, intravenous antibiotics

- **Epulis fissuratum** is a slow-growing irritation from the flange of an ill-fitting denture or partial. The affected area is inflamed with a soft, flabby, erythematous tissue growth. One or more elongated rolls appear parallel to the border of the prosthesis.

  - **Etiology**: Irritation from denture or partial

  - **Clinical presentation**: Hyperplastic mucosa at the border of the denture flange. The lesions occur more frequently on the facial aspect of the denture, with rare occurrences on the lingual surface.

  - **Treatment**: Surgical excision

- A **fibroma** is a firm, smooth, round or ovoid, well-defined pink, pale projection that is asymptomatic.

  - **Etiology**: Irritation or trauma

  - **Clinical presentation**: Asymptomatic, firm nodule located on the buccal mucosa, gingiva, floor of mouth, palate, tongue, or lips

  - **Treatment**: For irritative fibromas, complete excision

- A **fissured tongue** is characterized by deep grooves on the dorsum area of the tongue. It is seen in Down syndrome patients. Infrequently, it is associated with benign migratory glossitis.

  - **Etiology**: Unknown

  - **Clinical presentation**: Deep grooves on the tongue that are asymptomatic

  - **Treatment**: None

- **Fordyce granules** are aberrant sebaceous glands located on the lips and buccal mucosa. Ricelike, they appear as white or yellow–white asymptomatic papules.

  - **Etiology**: Developmental

  - **Clinical presentation**: Yellow, multiple raised spots

  - **Treatment**: None

- A **hematoma** is a collection of blood caused by trauma. Hematomas can appear anywhere on the body to male and females of any age. They are not seen radiographically. An **eruption hematoma** surrounds a tooth that has erupted through bone, but not through soft tissue.

  - **Etiology**: Trauma
  - **Originates**: Reduced-enamel epithelium
  - **Treatment**: None

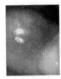

Eruption Hematoma

- A **lipoma** is a rare, non-metastic, yellow, fatty tumor that can be seen in multiples. Clinically, it can be sessile or pedunculated base, and soft to palpation. It can appear on the floor of mouth, tongue, buccal mucosa, or mucobuccal fold.

  - **Etiology**: Unknown
  - **Originates**: Mature fat cells
  - **Treatment**: Surgical excision

- **Lymphoma** is cancer of the lymph system. When lymph cells grow rapidly and randomly, they create too many cells and form into tumors. Hodgkin's disease and non-Hodgkin's lymphoma are two types of lymphomas. In HIV patients especially, aggressive B-cell lymphomas will be erythematous, purplish in color with a boggy consistency, but then may ulcerate and become necrotic. Oral lymphomas may appear on the palate, tongue, or gingiva. The vast majority of non-Hodgkin's lymphoma occurs in those infected with HIV or Epstein-Barr virus.

  - **Etiology**: Unknown
  - **Originates**: Lymph nodes
  - **Treatment**: Chemotherapy and radiation

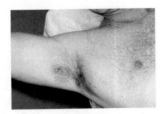

Lymphoma

Dr. Michael Finkelstein, DDS College of Dentistry, University of Iowa

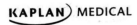

- A **mucocele** is a minor salivary gland that has become obstructed. It is a well-circumscribed, translucent or bluish vesicle most **commonly located on the lower lip.** Other locations of these minor salivary glands include the tongue, buccal mucosa, and palate.

  - **Etiology:** Gland obstruction or injury to minor salivary gland duct

  - **Originates:** Minor salivary glands

  - **Treatment:** Excision

- A **nevus** is a circumscribed, raised area of gray–white pigmentation (mole).

  - **Etiology:** Inherited

  - **Clinical presentation:** Thickened gray–white mucosa, usually located on the gingiva, buccal mucosa, lips, palate, or tongue

  - **Treatment:** None

- **Petechiae** are minute, round, purplish-red spots on palate that are the inflamed orifices of mucous glands. They are caused by an intradermal or submucous hemorrhage.

  - **Etiology:** Trauma, infection, nutritional deficiencies, medication reaction

  - **Clinical presentation:** Round, pinpoint-sized, flat dots whose color varies from red to blue or purple. With time, they disappear.

  - **Treatment:** Treat the underlying cause, but with trauma, it heals on its own

- A **papilloma** is pedunculated, stratified squamous epithelium arranged in papillary projections. Intraorally, it has a gray, white, or pink cauliflower-like surface, and is **slow-growing.**

  - **Etiology:** Human papilloma virus (HPV) infection

  - **Clinical presentation:** Pink, cauliflower-like surface found on the soft palate, tongue, labial or buccal mucosa

  - **Treatment:** Excision

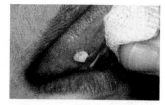

Papilloma

Contributed by Dr. Michael Finkelstein, DDS College of Dentistry, University of Iowa

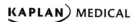

- **Verruca vulgaris** or wart is **faster-growing** than a papilloma. It can form multiple lesions on the lips, tongue, or mucosa.

  - **Etiology**: Human papillomavirus (HPV)

  - **Clinical presentation**: Painless, pedunculated papules or nodules with white, pointed (verruciform) surface projections

  - **Treatment**: Excision

- **Wickham's striae** are narrow, white mesh, or lacy lines associated with lichen planus

  - **Etiology**: Associated with lichen planus, which has an unknown etiology

  - **Clinical presentation**: Grayish dots or meshy lines on the surface of the papules of lichen planus

  - **Treatment**: No known cure for oral lichen planus. Symptoms may be relieved with topical corticosteroid creams and antihistamine drugs.

Vesicular Lesions and Viruses

A vesicular lesion is a fluid-filled layer of epithelial tissue, caused by a microbial infection such as a virus, an autoimmune disease, or genetics.

- **Aphthous ulcers major** are larger, longer-lasting, and more frequently occurring than aphthous ulcers minor. They can occur individually or in groups, and may take 10-40 days to heal, leaving a scar. They can occur on the oral mucosa, tongue, or palate, and are 1 cm or so in diameter or even larger.

  - **Etiology**: Possibly inherited, hypersensitivity reaction, tissue trauma

  - **Clinical presentation**: Round or ovoid white center surrounded by red halo with edematous tissue.

  - **Treatment**: Identify predisposing factors such as food allergies; topical steroids, chlorhexidine gluconate to relieve pain, or topical tetracycline

- **Aphthous ulcers minor** are small, round or ovoid lesions 2–4 mm in diameter. They can be located on the buccal or labial mucosa, tongue, soft palate, or pharynx. Contributing factors include nutritional deficiency, psychological (stress, anxiety), hormonal imbalance (pregnancy, menstrual), or allergy (asthma, hay fever, drug allergy). They may also occur during illnesses such as Crohn's disease or HIV.

  - **Etiology**: Possibly inherited, hypersensitivity reaction, tissue trauma

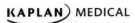

- **Clinical presentation**: Oval or round lesion with an ulcer floor that is initially yellow, then takes on a gray hue surrounded by an erythematous halo and some edema

- **Treatment**: Identify predisposing factors such as food allergies; topical steroids, chlorhexidine gluconate to relieve pain, or topical tetracycline.

■ **Epidermis bullosa** is an inherited or acquired disease of the skin and mucous membranes that forms blisters within the basement membrane. There are over 25 subtypes of this disease, ranging from mild to severe or fatal (from fluid loss and infection of open wounds).

- **Etiology**: Acquired disease or inherited as either autosomal dominant or recessive.

- **Clinical presentation**: Blisters of the skin and oral mucosa—especially mucous membrane blisters—that break open easily, leaving a flat, painless reddish ulcer bed with no inflammatory halo. Oral manifestations may include occasional bullae, gingival erythema, tenderness, and recession.

- **Treatment**: None, except to avoid trauma, replace lost body fluids, and treat with antibiotics if infection exists. In the dental office, **pad the chair for patient comfort and use topical anesthesia where needed.**

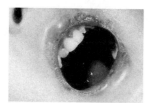 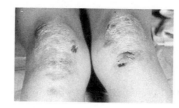

Epidermis bullosa

Contributed by Dr. Michael Finkelstein, DDS College of Dentistry, University of Iowa

■ **Erythema multiforme** or **Stevens-Johnson syndrome** is an allergic or hypersensitive reaction to medications, infections, or illness. This disorder damages the dermal blood vessels and then the skin tissues, in the form of macules, papules, or nodules that ulcerate and bleed.

Bullae of erythema multiforme resemble a bull's-eye target.

- **Etiology**: Unknown

- **Clinical presentation**: Macules, papules, or nodules with vesicles and bullae on the arms, hands, legs, feet, lips, or buccal mucosa. The center of the lesion is surrounded by gray and red concentric rings that resemble a bull's-eye target.

- **Treatment**: Control the underlying causes and treat symptoms with moist compresses, antihistamines, and topical anesthestics

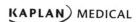

- **Hand, foot, and mouth disease** is an acute viral illness that results in vesicular eruptions in the mouth but can also involve the hands, feet, buttocks, and/or genitalia. It is a mild, self-limited illness that resolves in 7–10 days, and is moderately contagious.

  - **Etiology**: Coxsackie virus by the oral–fecal route

  - **Clinical presentation**: Macular lesions that become vesicles appear on the buccal mucosa, tongue, or hard palate. The lesions are superficial erosions surrounded by an erythematous halo. Flat, small blisters may also appear on the hands and feet.

  - **Treatment**: Pain-relief medication, topical anesthesia, antihistamines

- **Herpangina** is a coxsackie viral throat infection that results in red **football-shaped vesicles**. It is characterized by fever, malaise, and sore throat.

  - **Etiology**: Coxsackie virus by oral–fecal route

  - **Clinical presentation**: Vesicles or ulcerations with an erythematous margin on the tonsils, uvula, pharynx, and soft palate.

  - **Treatment**: Aspirin/acetaminophen, bed rest, hydration, topical analgesics

- **Herpes labialis** (cold sores) are large ulcers on the lips at the junction of the vermilion border and the skin. These ulcers can be hemorrhagic and are sometimes covered by a yellowish pseudomembrane. Risk factors include sun exposure, trauma, stress, and hormonal influences.

  - **Etiology**: Recurrent herpes simplex

  - **Clinical presentation**: Coalescing vesicles on the lips that rupture, causing ulcerations surrounded by an erythematous halo. May be covered by a yellowish pseudomembrane.

  - **Treatment**: Topical anesthetics, anti-viral drugs (Acyclovir)

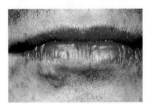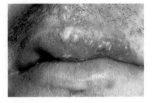

Herpes

Contributed by Dr. Michael Finkelstein, DDS College of Dentistry, University of Iowa

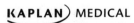

- **Herpes zoster** (shingles) is the reactivation of the varicella zoster virus of chicken pox that has lodged itself in the dorsal ganglia, where it remains latent for life. Herpes zoster is seen in patients with inadequate immune mechanisms, such as HIV or AIDS patients. Clusters of vesicles can cause severe pain.

  - **Etiology**: Varicella zoster virus (VZV)

  - **Clinical presentation**: Scattered skin lesions of vesicles and bullae marked by pruritus (itching) and pain associated with the vesicles. Intraoral vesicles occur at the earlier stages of the infection.

  - **Treatment**: Acyclovir, pain medication, topical anesthesia

- **Herpetic whitlow** is an intense, painful infection involving one or more fingers. The virus enters through a break in skin then invades the dermis and subcutaneous tissue.

  - **Etiology**: Approximately 60% from herpes simplex virus 1 (HSV1) and about 40% from herpes simplex 2 (HSV-2)

  - **Clinical presentation**: Pain and burning of the infected digit followed by erythema and edema. Groups of vesicles then form on an erythematous base These vesicles may ulcerate and rupture, expelling a clear fluid that creates a "weeping" wound.

  - **Treatment**: Symptom relief, Acyclovir

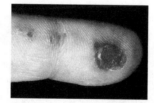

Herpetic Whitlow

Contributed by Dr. Michael Finkelstein, DDS College of Dentistry, University of Iowa

- **Mucosal pemphigoid** or **cicatricial pemphigoid** is a chronic autoimmune disease of the mucosal membranes and/or skin that is characterized by bullous lesions that rupture. These lesions are found most often on the oral mucosa and conjunctiva. Other areas include the esophagus, trachea, and genitalia.

  - **Etiology**: Autoimmune disease

  - **Clinical presentation**: Bullae that recur in the same area but most commonly the eyes and mucosa. The vast majority, with oral involvement, result in desquamative or erosive gingivitis.

  - **Treatment**: Topical steroids, oral corticosteroids, antibiotic therapy

- **Pemphigus vulgaris** is a severe, progressive autoimmune disease that affects the oral mucosa and skin. It is characterized by large bullae that collapse. Pain interferes with nutritional intake, causing fluid loss. Antibodies from the body's immune system interfere with the skin's normal function so skin cells no longer stick together. **Nikolsky's sign** is found with this disease.

  - **Etiology**: Relapsing autoimmune disease

  - **Clinical presentation**: Large skin and mucosal flaccid bullae that rupture. In the oral cavity, ragged sloughing occurs over a superficial ulcer.

  - **Treatment**: No cure but symptoms alleviated with corticosteroid therapy and antibiotic

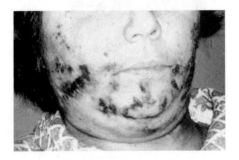

Pemphigus

Contributed by Dr. Michael Finkelstein, DDS College of Dentistry, University of Iowa

Red Lesions

- **Erythroplakia** occurs mostly in patients over 60 years of age as a rare, non-elevated, velvety red patch or lesion on the oral mucosa of the floor of the mouth, ventral surface of the tongue, or the soft palate. This chronic red patch has a high predisposition for becoming cancerous; it cannot be attributed to traumatic, vascular or inflammatory causes. Tobacco (smoking or chewing) and alcohol may increase the risk of erythroplakia. Erythroplakia is also associated with Bowen's disease, a form of squamous cell carcinoma.

  - **Etiology**: Unclear but risk factors include tobacco, alcohol, and betel quid

  - **Clinical presentation**: An asymptomatic, velvety red macule on the mucosal surface of the floor of mouth, tongue, and palate.

  - **Treatment**: Excision

- A **hemangioma** is an atypical dense proliferation of blood vessels that occurs on the skin or in internal organs. If the collection of vessels is on the surface, it is considered to be a superficial or "strawberry" hemangioma, but if it occurs deeper into the skin, it is considered a cavernous hemangioma.

  - **Etiology**: Congenital or trauma

  - **Clinical presentation**: Deep red or red-purple raised skin lesion or a massive raised tumor of blood vessels

  - **Treatment**: Typically none for superficial, but for cavernous, laser therapy, oral steroids and injectable steroids may be considered.

- **Pyogenic granuloma**, sometimes termed pregnancy tumor (increased estrogen), is a rapidly growing, benign vesicular lesion that is a response to injury or a chronic irritant. It can be found in males or females of any age.

  - **Etiology**: Unclear but local irritation or trauma contributes

  - **Clinical presentation**: Sessile or pedunculated, smooth firm nodules that are bright red or dusky red in color. These lesions are well circumscribed and dome shaped.

  - **Treatment**: Cauterize or surgical excision to remove the irritant

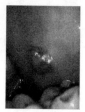

Pyogenic granuloma

White Lesions

- **Angular cheilitis** is an inflammation of the commissures or corner of the mouth. This lesion is often found in older patients and patients with dentures suffering from denture stomatitis. The odds of developing stomatitis and angular cheilitis are three times as great in denture wearers.

  - **Etiology**: A mixed infection of *C. albicans*, staph, and strep that occurs following a break in the skin

  - **Clinical presentation**: Red, eroded, fissured lesions that can be unilateral or bilateral at the corner of the mouth.

  - **Treatment**: Topical or antifungal steroids

- **Candidiasis** is an opportunistic infectious condition caused by a *Candida* fungus that includes eight different species of fungi with *Candida albicans* being the most common. Candidiasis affects the skin and mucous membranes in many different ways. The most common form is **pseudomembranous candidiasis** which is an easily removable, elevated, white, soft, creamy plaque that leaves a red ulcerated or eroded area at the base. **Chronic hyperplastic candidiasis** is an asymptomatic white plaque or papules that do not wipe off and are typically located on the anterior buccal mucosa and lateral and dorsal surfaces of the tongue. **Atropic erythematous candidiasis** is a chronic form found typically under dentures or on the mucous membranes or dorsum of the tongue as a smooth, velvety, red, flat lesion. **Median rhomboid glossitis** is discussed under tongue lesions. **Oral thrush** or moniliasis is a form of candidiasis that is found in children; it presents itself as creamy white curd-like ("cottage cheese") appearance that can be brushed away, leaving an ulcerated red area.

  - **Etiology**: *Candida albicans*

  - **Clinical presentation**: Discussed above with each type

  - **Treatment**: Topical or systemic antifungals

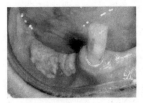
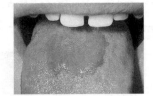

Candidosis   Median Rhomboid Glossitis

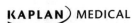

- A **chemical burn** that is seen intraorally is an aspirin burn by patient who places an aspirin in his mouth next to a painful tooth.

  - **Etiology**: Aspirin

  - **Clinical presentation**: White, irregular patches with raw, red tissues that bleed after necrotic tissue sloughs off

  - **Treatment**: Treat original condition that patient finds painful

- **Hyperkeratosis** is a benign, thickened keratin layer of organized connective tissue that occurs from a constant low-grade irritation such as cheek biting.

  - **Etiology**: Localized chronic irritation

  - **Clinical presentation**: Rough flat or raised area that is whitish or paler than normal anywhere in the oral cavity

  - **Treatment**: Typically none, but excision when indicated

- **Leukoplakia** is a whiter than normal coloration of tissue that is a dysplasia of the mucous membranes. Studies have shown that leukoplakia has the potential to be a premalignancy and that certain clinical features can be strong predictors of future risk.

  - **Etiology**: Tobacco usage, alcohol

  - **Clinical presentation**: A white patch that varies from flat and smooth to a translucent corrugated gray-white area that resembles elephant skin.

  - **Treatment**: Biopsy and monitor for changes

- **Lichen planus** is a benign asymptomatic white lesion that is a chronic disorder. It is an autoimmune mucositis that does not blister or ulcerate and is seen in adults but is extremely rare in children.

  - **Etiology**: Unknown, with contributing factors of stress or drugs

  - **Clinical presentation**: Raised lacy white lines known as **Wickham striae** appear on erythematous tissue. These lesions may be found on the buccal mucosa, buccal vestibule, tongue, and gingiva.

  - **Treatment**: Topical steroids

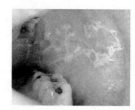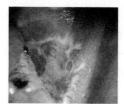

LichenPlanus
Contributed by Dr. Michael Finkelstein, DDS College of Dentistry, University of Iowa

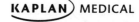

- **Nicotine stomatitis** is a diffuse gray or white change in the palate and/or buccal mucosa that is found in heavy smokers. The hyperkeratotic tissue becomes riddled with multiple small nodules with reddened centers.

  - **Etiology**: Tobacco usage

  - **Clinical presentation**: Elevated papules with red centers on a diffuse gray or white hard palate

  - **Treatment**: Smoking cessation

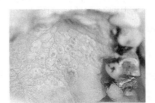

Nicotinic stomatitis

Contributed by Dr. Michael Finkelstein, DDS College of Dentistry, University of Iowa

- **Squamous cell carcinoma** is a malignant neoplasm of stratified epithelial tissue that occurs the majority of the time on the lower lip but may also be found intraorally on the tongue, floor of the mouth, soft palate, or buccal mucosa. Risk factors include alcohol and/or tobacco usage as well as sun exposure, immunosuppression, or genetics.

  - **Etiology**: Unknown

  - **Clinical presentation**: Firm crusted or scaly area of the skin with a red, inflamed base that may be a cone shaped nodule or flat growth

  - **Treatment**: Excision, chemotherapy, radiation

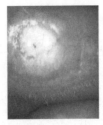

Squamous cell carcinoma

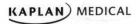

Tongue Abnormalities

- **Geographic tongue**, also called migratory glossitis or wandering rash, is a benign condition of the tongue that gives it a map-like appearance. Fungiform papillae can be observed as red mushroom like projections while filiform papillae become missing creating "bald" areas.

  - **Etiology**: Unknown

  - **Clinical presentation**: Red "bald" areas of missing filiform papillae that change daily.

  - **Treatment**: Typically none, but corticosteroids for discomfort

- **Hairy leukoplakia** is an unusual form of leukoplakia that is seen only in HIV patients and is **located on the lateral borders of the tongue**. This virally induced lesion is self-limiting, with no known potential for malignant transformation, but it is a sign of AIDS.

  - **Etiology**: Epstein-Barr virus may play a role in its pathogenicity

  - **Clinical presentation**: Fuzzy (hairy) white patches on the lateral borders of the tongue

  - **Treatment**: Typically none

- **Hairy tongue** is a discolored irritation of the keratinized elongated filiform papillae on the dorsum of the tongue that results in a hairy appearance.

  - **Etiology**: Unknown

  - **Clinical presentation**: Black, brown, or yellow thick "hairs" on the dorsum of the tongue at the midline

  - **Treatment**: Brush and/or use a tongue scraper

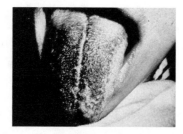

Hairy tongue

Contributed by Dr. Michael Finkelstein,
DDS College of Dentistry, University of Iowa

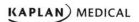

- **Median rhomboid glossitis** is a rhomboid or ovoid loss of filiform papillae anterior to circumvallate papillae at the midline of the dorsum of the tongue.

  - **Etiology**: *C. albicans*

  - **Clinical presentation**: Rhomboid or ovoid red, flat area of denuded filiform papillae at the midline dorsum of the tongue.

  - **Treatment**: Topical or systemic antifungal medications

BLOOD DYSCRASIAS

When speaking about blood components, *factor* represents the chemical makeup of a structure or its mechanism of action in the blood. **Factor VIII** is a **glycoprotein antihemophilic factor** that binds with von Willebrand factor to aid in clotting. **Factor IX** is a **plasma thromboplastin component** involved with intrinsic blood coagulation that activates Factor X or Stuart factor. **Stuart factor** is involved with **intrinsic and extrinsic blood coagulation**.

- **Von Willebrand factor** is a protein in blood that **mediates platelet cohesiveness** when endothelium is injured and also **maintains Factor VIII levels** in blood.

- **Prothrombin deficiency** is an acquired or a rare inherited autosomal recessive disorder that lacks Factor II. Prothrombin is one of the approximately 15 clotting proteins that prevents hemorrhaging. Vitamin K controls formation of coagulation Factor II.

- Hemophilia A and B are genetic blood disorders inherited by males. An X-linked recessive gene is carried by females who may pass it on to males. **Hemophilia A** patients lack the Factor VIII glycoprotein antihemophilic factor. **Hemophilia B** patients lack the Factor IX plasma thromboplastin component. **Hemophilia C** patients lack the Factor XI plasma thromboplastin antecedent.

- **Von Willebrand disease** is a hereditary bleeding disorder that can affect both **men and women**. Von Willebrand factor is a **protein released by the lining of blood vessels** that allows for platelets to adhere to each other. This same factor also transports the protein Factor VIII for clotting. With von Willebrand disease, the factor is either deficient or defective and occurs in about 1% of the population. The disease is usually so mild that it can go undiagnosed.

  There are three types of von Willebrand disease: Type 1 has low levels of Factor VIII. Type 2 is a defect in the function of the von Willebrand factor. Type 2A is less efficient at holding platelets together, while Type 2B adheres platelets together in the bloodstream rather than at the injury site. Type 2N is a rare form

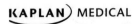

that is sometimes mistaken for hemophilia A. In this case, 2N von Willebrand factor does not bind to Factor VIII, creating a low level of Factor VIII which mimics hemophilia A. Type 3 is very rare, but is seen when the von Willebrand factor is totally absent or extremely low.

Patients with hemophilia may be treated normally in a dental office for routine prophylaxis/exams and do not need to have their factor levels raised. The factor does not necessarily need to be administered for routine restorative work or local infiltration anesthesia. If nerve block anesthesia, dental extractions, or deep scaling and root planing are to be performed, factor levels need to be raised— by 50% for hemophilia A and by 40% for hemophilia B.

Hemophilia A levels are increased by a slow intravenous infusion of pure preparation Factor VIII concentrate. Hemophilia B level are increased by a slow intravenous infusion of pure preparation Factor IX concentrate.

Anti-fibrinolytic agents may be used along with Factor VIII infusion for invasive dentistry but anti-fibrinolytics are not recommended along with Factor IX concentrate.

- **Leukemia** is a cancer of the blood that produces an overabundance of abnormal white blood cells. Since the cells are abnormal and cannot perform the normal duties of white blood cells, they accumulate in the body. There are four types of leukemia: acute or chronic lymphocytic leukemia and acute or chronic myelogenous leukemia. Lymphocytes are involved with the immune system by producing antibodies against specific antigens. Myelocytes produce neutrophils, which are the first line of defense in acute infection.

GENERAL PATHOLOGY

Pathology is the study of structural and functional changes in tissues that can affect body organs. Pathologic conditions may occur with disease, causing a change in tissues and their performance.

- **Acromegaly**: A slow-onset hormonal disorder of the pituitary gland that produces excess growth hormone (GH). Over 90% of acromegaly patients have excess GH due to a benign tumor of the pituitary gland. Hands and feet become enlarged, and gradual changes in facial features occur, such as an increase in spacing of the teeth, lower jaw protrusion, and nasal bone enlargement. Bone overgrowth often leads to arthritis. As tissue thickens, trapped nerves can cause problems such as carpal tunnel syndrome.

  - **Treatment**: Reduce growth hormone levels, remove tumor from pituitary gland

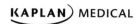

- **Bowen's disease**: A form of squamous cell carcinoma that looks like a bright red or pink scaly patch on a sun-damaged area of the skin. Regarded by some doctors as a pre-cancer that invades intraepithelial tissues, Bowen's is considered to be squamous cell carcinoma in-situ. If it invades the basement membrane, however, it can be lethal.

  - **Treatment**: Surgical excision, chemotherapy creams

- **Cleidocranial dysplasia**: A congenital disorder of bone formation and delayed closing of the skull sutures, sometimes into adulthood. *Cleido* refers to the clavicles or collarbones, while *cranial* refers to the skull. The clavicles may be absent or incompletely formed, so the child can touch or nearly touch his shoulders together. Head and neck anomalies include a highly arched palate, cleft palate, delayed tooth eruption, crown abnormalities, short roots that lack acellular cementum, supernumerary teeth, and over-retained deciduous teeth.

  - **Treatment**: Orthodontic treatment

- **Craniofacial dystosis**: A genetic disorder that results in midfacial depression, hypertelorism (wide-spaced eyes), exophthalmos (bulging eyes), external strabismus, parrot-beaked nose, short upper lip, hypoplastic maxilla, and prognathism.

  - **Treatment**: Corrective plastic surgery and eye surgery to prevent proptosis (forward displacement of the eyeball), which causes blindness

- **Glycogen storage disease** (GSD): A genetic disorder resulting from a shortage of enzymes that form or release glycogen. Glycogen is stored in the liver so that it can be used to release glucose during exercise and/or between meals. Low blood sugar can be life-threatening.

  - **Treatment**: Avoidance of low blood sugar and the intake of cornstarch between meals and through a feeding tube while sleeping at night

- **Mandibulofacial dystosis**: A genetic disorder caused by malformations of the first and second brachial arches in utero. It results in ear and facial malformations, such as the malformation of facial bones, micrognathia, cleft palate, and malformed ears with hearing loss.

  - **Treatment**: Ear reconstruction, orthognathic surgery, orthodontic corrections

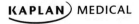

- **Marfan's syndrome**: An inherited connective-tissue disorder that occurs when defective connective tissue doesn't act normally. Since connective tissue is located throughout the body, it can affect many body systems including the skeleton, eyes, heart and blood vessels, nervous system, skin, and lungs. Patients with this syndrome are typically tall and lanky, and are **prone to aortic dissection (aneurysm)**. Dentally, they have narrow jaws and vaulted palates that can create dental and orthodontic problems.

  - **Treatment**: None, though body systems should be monitored carefully; an echocardiogram to monitor the aorta

- **Multiple myeloma**: An incurable but treatable cancer of plasma cells interrupting the bone marrow and immune system function. This hematological cancer is the second most prevalent cancer after non-Hodgkin's lymphoma. Since the early stages have no symptoms, this cancer is often discovered during a routine blood test. As the abnormal plasma cells multiply in the bone marrow, they erode the bone. Repeated episodes of bone resorption are followed by attempts by the body to repair the bone, resulting in weakened deformed bones. There are few symptoms, though most patients experience aching bones that worsen at night, joint pain swelling and stiffness, and nerve pressure such as sciatica.

  - **Treatment**: Radiation therapy, chemotherapy, stem cell transplant. Bisphosphonates and calcitonin to prevent bone loss.

- **Papillon-Lefèvre syndrome**: A rare, **autosomal-recessive disorder** characterized by **palmoplantar keratoderma** (dry, scaly patches on the palms and soles) and rapid progressive **periodontitis**. Early periodontitis results in the premature loss of deciduous teeth by age 5, and loss of the permanent teeth by about age 17 if left untreated. Other symptoms may include frequent pus-producing (pyogenic) skin infections, nail abnormalities, and excessive perspiration.

  - **Treatment**: Periodontal scaling and adjunctive systemic antibiotics

- **Peutz-Jegher syndrome**: A rare autosomal-dominant inherited condition. It causes gastrointestinal polyps to develop along the length of the bowel and mucocutaneous pigmentation of abnormal brown coloration of the lips, skin, and mouth, often looking like freckles.

  - **Treatment**: None, but routine colonoscopy to monitor polyps

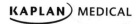

- **Pierre Robin syndrome**: A birth defect that causes a smaller-than-normal lower jaw (micrognathia), cleft palate, and **tongue "balling up"** in back of mouth. The lower jaw develops slowly in the first few months of fetal life, but catches up in the first year after birth. This growth discrepancy results in a more posterior placement of the tongue, which in turn causes choking episodes, and feeding and breathing difficulties. Symptoms abate as the jaw discrepancy catches up.

  - **Treatment**: Place infant face down, so that the tongue cannot "ball up" in the back of the throat

- **Sjogren's syndrome**: A chronic disorder when white blood cells reject the moisture glands (tear and salivary glands), causing dry eyes and dry mouth. The kidneys, GI tract, blood vessels, lung, liver, pancreas, and central nervous system may also be affected. Patients may also experience debilitating fatigue and joint pain. This disease may co-exist with other diseases, such as rheumatoid arthritis, systemic lupus, scleroderma, and polymyositis.

  - **Treatment**: OTC artificial tear and saliva substitutes

- **Syphilis**: A disease spread through sexual contact or from an infected mother to her unborn child by the *T. pallidum* bacterium. Syphilis can result in serious mental retardation or physical problems. Dentally, it can result in Hutchinson's incisors and mulberry molars. There are **three stages** to this disease: **primary stage**, when a **chancre** (macule) appears 10 days to 3 months after the infection; **secondary stage**, when a skin rash and **mucous patches** appear 3–6 weeks after the chancre disappears; and the **tertiary stage**, which occurs years later and causes **gumma**, damage to the heart, eyes, brain, nervous system, bones, or joints. Patients may also develop mental illness and blindness.

  - **Treatment**: Provide early treatment with penicillin or other antibiotic.

- **Von Recklinghausen disease** (or neurofibromatosis): An autosomal dominant disease characterized by disordered growth of ectodermal tissues. Numerous neurofibromas and **café-au-lait spots** form on the skin. Oral neurofibromas that present as a submucosal, non-tender, discrete mass may be a single lesion or the manifestation of Von Recklinghausen disease.

  - **Treatment**: For single neurofibromas, surgical excision; for multiple fibromas, surgical excision for functional and cosmetic reasons

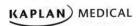

REVIEW QUESTIONS

1. A common benign, soft-tissue lesion in the oral cavity is

   A. Fibroma

   B. Verruca vulgaris

   C. Papilloma

   D. Herpetic whitlow

   E. Hemangioma

2. Which of the following conditions includes supernumerary teeth that would be a concern for orthodontic treatment?

   A. Cherubism

   B. Cleidocranial dysplasia

   C. Cleidofacial dystosis

   D. Cretinism

3. The *Treponema pallidum* bacterium causes

   A. Shingles

   B. Measles

   C. Syphilis

   D. Gonorrhea

   E. Lyme disease

4. Intraorally, the most common tumor involving the salivary glands is

   A. Odontoma

   B. Nasopalatine duct cyst

   C. Giant cell reparative granuloma

   D. Lipoma

   E. Pleomorphic adenoma

5. Xerostomia is dry mouth that is caused by which of the following conditions?

   A. Pierre Robin syndrome

   B. Bowen's Disease

   C. Papillon-Lefèvre syndrome

   D. Sjogren's syndrome

6. Which of the following systemic conditions is an auto-immune disease that affects the skin and mucous membranes in adults over 30?

   A. Paget's disease

   B. Pemphigus vulgaris

   C. Scleroderma

   D. Lupus erythematosus

   E. Myasthenia gravis

7. Referring to question 6, the use of Nikolsky's sign or test would indicate a separation of

   A. Epithelial attachment

   B. Attached gingival

   C. Desmosomes

   D. Hemidesmosomes

   E. Retina

8. A patient presents with a "little bump on his inside cheek that keeps going up and down." Upon inspection, you find a round 0.5 cm raised, circumscribed vesicle on the buccal mucosa that is firm and movable on palpation. This lesion is most likely a(n)

   A. Irritative fibroma

   B. Papilloma

   C. Hemangioma

   D. Lipoma

   E. Mucocele

9. The lesion described in question 8 is most commonly found on the

   A. Tongue

   B. Buccal mucosa

   C. Lower lip

   D. Palate

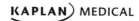

10. Oral candidiasis is present in most oral cavities. What group of pathogens is responsible for this opportunistic infection?

    A. Bacteria
    B. Viruses
    C. Fungi
    D. Protozoa
    E. Amoeba

11. Which of the following conditions would appear as a frog-belly-like lesion on the floor of the mouth?

    A. Sialolith
    B. Sialadenoma
    C. Sialosis
    D. Ranula
    E. Ranine

12. A dentigerous cyst is a tooth-associated lesion affixed to the root of a tooth and arises from which of the following?

    A. Reduced-enamel epithelium
    B. Remnant of the dental lamina
    C. Rest of Malessez
    D. Odontogenic epithelium

13. A patient presents to the office with several intra-oral lesions on the palate that he states seem to be getting larger and are migrating toward each other. This migration of the lesions is called

    A. Confluence
    B. Confrication
    C. Conidium
    D. Confabulation

14. Squamous cell carcinoma is often found on the lower lip, but the most common intraoral site is the

    A. Buccal mucosa
    B. Floor of the mouth
    C. Lateral border of tongue
    D. Vestibule
    E. Soft palate

15. Lymphoma—cancer of the lymph system—occurs when lymph cells grow rapidly and randomly create too many tumor-growing cells. Where in the oral cavity are lymphomas most frequently located?

    A. Tonsils and nasopharynx
    B. Nasopharynx and maxillary sinus
    C. Buccal mucosa and parotid gland
    D. Floor of mouth and tongue

16. Your patient has come in for a 6-month recare and you notice a small butterfly lesion on her nose. She states that the lesion appeared about 5 months ago, then disappeared for a while, and just recently returned. This lesion might be due to

    A. Erythema multiforme
    B. Steven's-Johnson syndrome
    C. Lupus erythematosus
    D. Cicatricial pemphigoid
    E. Behçet's syndrome

17. Lyme disease is spread through the vector of a deer tick. A frequent continuing symptom of Lyme disease is

    A. Irregular heart beat
    B. Erythematous rash
    C. Polyarthritis
    D. Flu-like symptoms

18. Your patient has presented to the office today with a boil or painful skin nodule that has a circumscribed area of inflammation. This lesion is a

    A. Macule
    B. Carbuncle
    C. Furuncle
    D. Caruncle
    E. Bulla

19. A white–gray, painless, wrinkled lesion that looks like elephant skin and is found in patients who chew tobacco is called

    A. Lichen planus
    B. Candidiasis
    C. Leukoplakia
    D. Hyperkeratosis

20. Hairy leukoplakia is a lesion found most often in which of the following patients?

    A. Down syndrome
    B. Paget's disease
    C. Kwashiorkor
    D. Crohn's disease
    E. AIDS

21. Megaloblastic or pernicious anemia occurs due to a lack of intrinsic factor in the stomach and is found in which of the following groups of individuals?

    A. Homeless
    B. Alcoholics
    C. Vegetarians
    D. Obese people
    E. Patients on fad diets

22. Sickle cell anemia is a genetic chronic blood dyscrasia found primarily in which of the following populations?

    A. Mediterranean
    B. African-Americans
    C. Chinese
    D. Consanguinity

23. Eyes that seem to be bulging out is termed exophthalmous and is due to a hormonal imbalance from which of the following conditions?

    A. Hyperthyroidism
    B. Hypothyroidism
    C. Hypercortisolism
    D. Hypocortisolism
    E. Hypoparathyroidism

24. Which one of the following cysts appears radiographically as a pear-shaped radiolucency?

    A. Nasopalatine duct cyst
    B. Dentigerous cyst
    C. Globulomaxillary cyst
    D. Odontoma
    E. Primordial cyst

25. Which of the following conditions is not an abnormality?

    A. Fordyce granules
    B. Amalgam tattoo
    C. Nevus
    D. Petechiae

ANSWER EXPLANATIONS

1. A

Fibromas occur frequently in the oral cavity.

B. Verruca vulgaris is a fast-growing wart.

C. Papilloma is a slow-growing cauliflower-like lesion.

D. Herpetic whitlow is an HSV infection of the finger and not an oral lesion.

E. Hemangioma is a proliferation of capillaries.

2. B

Cleidocranial dysplasia causes supernumerary teeth that would be a concern for orthodontic treatment.

A. Cherubism is bilateral enlarged mandible or maxilla that is genetic in origin.

C. Cleidofacial dystosis is a genetic disorder which results in midfacial depression, hypertelorism, exophthalmos, external strabismus, parrot-beaked nose, short upper lip, hypoplastic maxilla, and prognathism.

3. C

Syphilis is caused by the *Treponema pallidum* bacterium.

B. Measles is caused by the rubeola virus.

D. Gonorrhea is caused by gonococcus.

E. Lyme disease is caused by *B. burgdorfi*.

4. E

Intraorally, the most common tumor involved in the salivary glands is pleomorphic adenoma.

A. An odontoma is a hard-tissue lesion where a tooth failed to erupt and created a calcified mass instead.

B. A nasopalatine duct cyst is in the nasal midline and not involved with salivary glands.

C. A giant-cell reparative granuloma is a hard-tissue lesion that occurs at the anterior midline.

D. A lipoma is a fatty benign tumor.

5. D

Xerostomia is dry mouth that can be caused by Sjogren's syndrome, a chronic disorder where the white blood cells of the immune system reject the moisture glands (such as the salivary glands).

A. Pierre Robin syndrome is a birth defect that causes a smaller lower jaw, cleft palate, and the tongue to "ball up" in back of mouth.

B. Bowen's Disease is a form of squamous cell carcinoma that presents itself as a bright red or pink scaly patch found on sun-damaged areas of the skin.

C. Papillon-Lefèvre syndrome is a rare, autosomal disorder in which there is a development of dry scaly patches on the skin of the palms and the soles and rapid progressive periodontitis.

6. B

Pemphigus vulgaris is a severe auto-immune disease that affects skin and mucous membranes in adults over 30. It affects the oral mucosa, skin, and desmosomes.

A. Paget's disease is a bone disease that destroys bone and then replaces it with abnormal, fragile bone.

C. Scleroderma is an autoimmune disease that means hardening of the skin and connective tissues. It occurs when the skin loses its elasticity.

D. Lupus erythematosus is an autoimmune disease that causes inflammation and damage to the joints, skin, kidneys, heart, lungs, blood vessels, and brain.

E. Myasthenia gravis is an autoimmune disease affecting the neuromuscular system with periods of voluntary muscle weakness.

7. C

The use of an air-water syringe to produce Nikolsky's sign indicates a separation of desmosomes, since like cells lose contact with each other.

A. The epithelial attachment is where the junctional epithelium attaches to the tooth surface.

B. Attached gingiva is gingiva that is attached to alveolar bone and cementum.

D. Hemidesmosomes bind cells to a noncellular contact, such as the epithelial attachment to a tooth.

8. E

A firm, raised, circumscribed "bump" on the cheek that continues to "go up and down" is a mucocele.

A. Irritative fibroma is caused by an irritation—generally cheek-biting—but it does not go up and down.

B. Papilloma is cauliflower-like, rather than round and red.

C. A hemangioma can be congenital or developmental, and is a proliferation of capillaries that do not go up and down.

D. Lipoma is a benign, fatty lesion that is yellowish in color.

9. C

The lesion described in questions #8 is most typically found on the lower lip.

10. C

Oral candidiasis is an opportunistic infections that is fungal in origin.

11. D

A ranula is a frog-belly-like lesion that is found in the floor of the mouth. It is a retentive cyst that can obstruct the ducts of the submandibular or sublingual glands, causing a slowly enlarging, painless, deep burrowing mucocele on the floor of the mouth.

A. A sialolith is a salivary stone that can become a ranula if it travels in the duct.

B. A sialadenoma is a benign tumor of the salivary glands.

C. Sialosis is the flow of saliva.

E. Ranine pertains to a frog.

12. A

A dentigerous cyst arises from the reduced-enamel epithelium.

B. Remnants of the dental lamina can give rise to odontogenic keratocysts, glandular odontogenic or gingival cysts.

C. Rests of Malessez give rise to radicular or periapical and residual cysts.

D. Odontogenic epithelium gives rise to paradental cysts.

13. A

Intraoral lesions that migrate toward each other and merge as one larger lesion are called confluent. Another way to describe them would be to say they coalesce.

B. Confrication is the rubbing of a drug to the consistency of a powder.

C. Conidium is an asexual fungal spore that is deciduous.

D. Confabulation is the unconscious filling in of gaps in memory with fabricated facts and experiences.

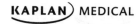

14. C

Squamous cell carcinomas are mostly found on the lower lip, but another common site is the lateral border of tongue. That happens in 25–40% of the cases.

A. Buccal mucosa accounts for 10% of the lesions.

B. The floor of the mouth accounts for 20% of the lesions.

E. The soft palate accounts for 10–20% of the lesions.

15. A

Intraoral lymphomas are most frequently located on the tonsils and nasopharynx.

16. C

A small butterfly lesion on the nose that can disappear and then return is caused by lupus erythematosus, a systemic condition.

A. Erythema multiforme is of unknown etiology and affects the mucous membranes with macular or bulbous eruption resembling bull's-eye targets.

B. Steven's-Johnson syndrome affects the skin with severe numerous lesions, the oral mucosa with bullae that rupture.

D. Cicatricial pemphigoid is an autoimmune disease that affects the mucous membranes and gingiva.

E. Behçet's syndrome is a multisystem disorder causing recurrent oral and/or genital ulcerations.

17. C

Lyme disease is caused by the *B. burgdorferi* bacteria carried by ticks, and causes continuing polyarthritis.

A. In lyme disease, an irregular heartbeat occurs at 1–3 weeks.

B. In lyme disease, an erythematous rash appears about 1 week after being infected.

D. Flu-like symptoms occur with early onset of the disease.

18. C

A furuncle is a boil or painful skin nodule that has a circumscribed area of inflammation.

A. A macule is a flattened skin patch that is altered in color.

B. A carbuncle is a necrotizing skin infection made up of a cluster of boils (furuncles).

D. A caruncle or caruncula is a small, fleshy eminence that can be normal or abnormal.

E. A bulla is an elevated lesion containing serous fluid.

19. C

Leukoplakia is a white–gray, painless, wrinkled lesion that resembles elephant skin and is seen in tobacco-chewers.

A. Lichen planus can be a benign, painless lesion that has white lacy-lines called Wickham's striae.

B. Candidiasis is a white, creamy plaque found in the buccal mucosa, and occurs as an opportunistic fungal infection.

D. Hyperkeratosis is a white, benign lesion caused by a low-grade irritation.

20. E

Hairy leukoplakia is a lesion found most often in patients with AIDS.

21. B

Megaloblastic or pernicious anemia occurs due to a lack of intrinsic factor in the stomach and is found in alcoholics. The stomach is unable to absorb vitamin B12 due to the lack of instrinsic factor.

22. B

Sickle-cell anemia is a genetic, chronic blood dyscrasia found primarily in African-Americans.

A. People of Mediterranean descent often suffer from thalassemia.

C. People of Chinese descent can have benzene-linked blood disorders.

D. Consanguinity describes a state of being related by blood or descended from a common ancestor.

23. A

Exophthalmus or bulging eyes is caused by a hormonal imbalance of hyperthyroidism.

B. Hypothyroidism causes cretinism in children and myxedema in adults.

C. Hypercortisolism causes moon-face, buffalo-hump, and a large abdomen.

D. Hypocortisolism causes severe hypotension and darkened skin pigmentation.

E. Hypoparathyroidism can cause hypocalcemia, tetany, and muscle spasms.

24. C

A radiolucent pear-shaped cyst seen radiographically is a globulomaxillary cyst.

A. A nasopalatine duct cyst is heart-shaped and located at the nasopalatine canal.

B. A dentigerous cyst is a well-defined cyst found in third molar areas.

D. An odontoma is an irregular, calcified mass surrounded by a radiolucent band.

E. A primordial cyst is a solid, well-defined radiolucency in place of a missing tooth.

25. A

Fordyce granules are not abnormalities, but rather, aberrant sebaceous glands.

B. Amalgam tattoo occurs when a particle of amalgam filling embeds in mucosa, leaving a blue-gray tattoo.

B. A nevus is a raised area that is gray–white and resembles a mole.

D. Petechiae are minute, round purplish-red spots on the palate that are the inflamed orifices of mucous glands. They are caused by intradermal or submucous hemorrhage.

Chapter Eleven: **Pharmacology**

Pharmacology is important to the dental hygienist for several reasons. First, patients may need a pharmacological agent before or after dental treatment. Second, pharmacology may be needed to remedy an unhealthy dental ailment. Third, pharmacological agents can have a direct effect on the tissues of the oral cavity.

Pharmacological agents come in many forms and from various sources: animals (e.g., insulin, oxytocin), plants (e.g., foxglove [digitalis]), minerals (e.g., sodium bicarbonate), or synthetics (e.g., lidocaine). Drugs have different actions, properties, and toxic effects.

LAWS AND AGENCIES GOVERNING PHARMACOLOGY

- The **Harrison Narcotics Act** regulates the production, importation, distribution, and use of opiates.

- The **Food and Drug Administration (FDA)** is the federal government agency that regulates food, drugs, cosmetics, medical devices, biologics, and blood products in the United States.

- The **Drug Enforcement Agency** (DEA) enforces the drug laws and controls the availability of drugs with abuse potential (controlled substances).

- The **Controlled Substances Act** (CSA) is the government's fight against the abuse of drugs and other substances. This act regulates substances for their medicinal value.

Controlled Substances Act

Schedule	Abuse potential	Medical use	Prescription	Examples
I	High potential for abuse, lack of accepted safety	None	None	Heroin, hallucinogens, opium derivatives
II	High potential for abuse, may lead to severe psychological or physical dependence	Some medical use with severe restrictions	Requires DEA#, cannot be refilled	Oxycodone, amphetamines, morphine
III	Potential for abuse less than the drugs in schedules I and II, may lead to moderate dependence or high psychological dependence	Accepted for medical use	Requires DEA#, can be refilled	Tylenol #3 (codeine)
IV	Potential for abuse less than the drugs in schedules III, may lead to limited physical dependence or psychological dependence	Accepted for medical use	Requires DEA#, can be refilled	Valium, benzodiazepine
V	Potential for abuse less than the drugs in schedules IV, may lead to limited physical dependence or psychological dependence	Accepted for medical use	Can be refilled	Codeine cough syrup

NOMENCLATURE

- **Agonist** is the drug interaction with a desired receptor cell.

- **Antagonist** is a counteraction or opposition of drugs on a receptor cell, as when **Narcan** counteracts against or releases morphine or opiates that have bound to cells.

- **Brand or trade name** is the manufacturer's name, which can be more than one name. These names may be based on the problem treated and are **capitalized by the first letter** (e.g., Demerol hydrochloride).

- **Chemical name** is the name determined by the chemical structure, e.g., ethyl 1-methyl-4-phenylisonipectorate hydrochloride.

- **Contraindications** are the medical or physical conditions that make the drug harmful to a patient.

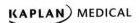

- **Cumulative action** is the increased effect of a drug by its build-up in the bloodstream.

- **Efficacy** is the desired effect that the drug should produce.

- **Generic name** is the shorter version of the chemical name. It is used more often and is **not capitalized by the first letter** (e.g., meperidine hydrochloride).

- **Hypersensitivity** is an exaggerated immune response or an allergic reaction

- **Idiosyncrasy** is a reaction particular to that patient.

- **Loading dose** is an effort to achieve the effective level of drug in blood with initial dose.

- **Official name** is the name used in the U.S. Pharmacopeia; it uses initials USP(e.g., meperidine hydrochloride, USP).

- **Potency** is the ability to achieve a particular effect of a drug.

- **Potentiation** is the enhancement of one drug upon another. Mixing of barbiturates and alcohol, for instance, causes synergistic sedative effects or effects more than desired.

- **Side effects** are undesired effects.

- **Summation** is the exact desired effects of taking two drugs together. (1 + 1 = 2)

- **Synergism** is getting more than desired effects when taking two drugs. (1 + 1 = 3)

- **Therapeutic action** is the desired action.

- **Tolerance** is the decreased effect of a drug over time, with the patient needing larger doses to achieve the same effect.

- **Trademark name** is specific to a manufacturer's product (e.g., Nitrostat™).

- **Toxicology** is the study of harmful or toxic effects.

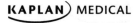

METRIC CONVERSIONS

kilo = 1000 (k)	1 kg = 1000 g
hecto = 100 (h)	1 hg = 100 g
deka = 10 (D)	
gram = 1g	
deci = 0.1(d)	1 dg = 0.1 g
centi = 0.001(c)	1 cg = 0.001 g
milli = 0.0001 (m)	1 mg = 0.0001 g
1 grain = 0.065 g = 65 mg	
2.2 lb = 1 kg	1 in = 2.54 cm

PHARMACOLOGY ABBREVIATIONS

ac	before meals
bid	twice a day
d	day
h	hour
hs	at bedtime
pc	after meals
po	by mouth
prn	as needed
q	every
qd	once a day
qid	4 times a day
s	without
tid	3 times a day

TOXICOLOGIC EVALUATION OF DRUGS

The evaluation of a drug is based initially upon animal experiments. When approved by the FDA, human participants then volunteer in blind studies to evaluate the drug's effectiveness and safety.

Effective dose (ED)50: The dose that produces a specific response in 50% of the participants.

Lethal dose (LD)50: The dose that is lethal in 50% of the participants. In this case, laboratory animals are utilized.

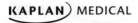

Therapeutic index (TI): Determines the safety of a drug. The larger the therapeutic index, the safer the drug. Divide the LD50 by the ED50 to determine the safety of the drug.

PHARMACOLOGIC ROUTES OF ADMINISTRATION

Enteral indicates medications that are administered by way of the digestive tract.

- **Oral:** safest but slowest
- **Sublingual:** absorbed by capillary network of mucous membranes, e.g., nitroglycerine
- **Rectal:** suppository or enema, e.g., Compazine

Parenteral indicates other routes of administration not including the digestive tract.

- **Inhalation:** pulmonary absorption (nitrous oxide, albuterol)
- **Intradermal:** slow, injected into dermal layer (allergy testing, TB skin test)
- **Intramuscular:** injected into muscle, slower than IV (Benadryl)
- **Intraosseous:** injected into bone, IV route for small children
- **Intravenous:** fastest route (IV solutions, Narcan, 50% dextrose)
- **Subcutaneous:** injected under skin but not into muscle, slow absorption (epinephrine)
- **Topical/Transdermal:** absorbed slowly by capillaries under the skin, lasts a long time through slow absorption (topical anesthesia, nitropatch)

Drug absorption depends on the route of administration, the concentration of the drug, the physical state of the drug, metabolic differences, disease/condition present, and body temperature.

PHARMACODYNAMICS

Pharmacodynamics is concerned with drug effects and how those effects are produced.

Drugs combine **with a receptor cell**, that is, the "lock." The drug is the "key" that unlocks the receptor cell to yield a biochemical reaction. When a drug is bound in a cell, it is called an **agonist**. Drugs that unlock the key of a previously bound receptor cell are called **antagonists**.

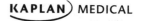

Drugs can also affect the **autonomic nervous system** (ANS) which sends chemical signals between cells. A vast array of drugs can influence the **sympathetic nervous system** and **parasympathetic nervous system** of the autonomic nervous system.

The **sympathetic nervous system (SNS)** utilizes **epinephrine** and **norepinephrine** as its neurotransmitter to mediate responses at **adrenergic receptors**. The SNS is the "fight or flight" system that dilates the bronchi and the pupils, accelerates heart rate and respiration, and increases perspiration and arterial blood pressure while reducing digestive activity.

The adrenergic receptors that respond to **epinephrine** and **norepinephrine** have four subtype receptors: α_1, α_2, β_1, and β_2. In addition, dopamine is a neurotransmitter of the SNS that controls movement, emotional response, and the ability to experience pleasure and pain. **Epinephrine, norepinephrine** and **dopamine** are **catecholamines.**

The **parasympathetic nervous system** (PNS) utilizes **acetylcholine** as its neurotransmitter to mediate responses at **cholinergic** receptors. The PNS is the "feed or breed" system that counteracts the SNS by constricting pupils, decelerating the heart rate and respiration, and decreasing perspiration and arterial blood pressure while increasing digestive activity. The **cholinergic receptors** that respond to **acetylcholine** have three subtype receptors: muscarinic, nicotinic N, and nicotinic M.

Neurotransmitters influence many organ systems, so a drug meant for one organ can have side effects on another organ. Certain drugs can have an effect on receptors that may mimic, diminish, or prevent the effects of the ANS neurotransmitters.

- Sympathomimetics mimic or stimulate the SNS
- Sympatholytics inhibit the SNS
- Parasympathomimetic mimic or stimulate the PNS
- Parasympatholytics inhibit the PNS

DRUGS

Drugs are used therapeutically in the human body to alleviate disease or symptoms. However, in addition to alleviating disease, drugs can cause negative side effects.

Adrenergic & Cholinergic Drugs

Adrenergic drugs stimulate adrenergic receptors to produce the effects that the SNS would produce. These drugs can accelerate heart rate and respiration, increase perspiration and blood pressure, and reduce digestive activity. Adrenergic drugs such as epinephrine are used in local anesthetics as vasoconstrictors.

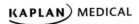

Adrenergic Drug Examples

Generic	Brand name	Action	Indications
epinephrine	Primatine, Adrenaline	Vasoconstricts	Asthma, anaphylaxis
clonidine	Catapress	Decrease in peripheral resistance in blood vessels	Antihypertensive
albuterol metaproterenol	Proventil, Ventolin Alupent	Bronchodilates by stimulating receptors on the smooth muscles	Asthma
methylphenidate	Ritalin	Central nervous system stimulant	Attention deficit disorder

Antiadrenergic drugs block adrenergic receptors. α-adrenergic blockers inhibit vasoconstriction by adrenergic drugs, decreasing blood pressure. This particular action is termed **epinephrine reversal** since the blood pressure is lowered. β-adrenergic drugs block β receptors causing bradycardia and bronchoconstriction with the effect on the heart more profound than on the lungs with bronchoconstriction. Generic drugs with the suffix –olol are beta-blockers that slow the heart rate and cause bronchoconstriction.

Adrenergic-Blocking Drug Examples

Generic	Brand name	Action	Indications
propranolol	Inderal	Reduces heart rate	Arrhythmias, angina, hypertension
atenolol	Tenormin	Reduces heart rate	Hypertension, angina, rapid heart rate
metoprolol	Lopressor, Toprol	Reduces abnormally rapid heart rhythms	Hypertension, angina, rapid heart rate

Cholinergic drugs stimulate cholinergic receptors to produce the effects that the PNS would produce. These drugs can decelerate the heart rate and respiration, decrease perspiration and arterial blood pressure, and increase digestive activity. **Pilocarpine is important in dentistry for patients with xerostomia.**

Adverse reaction to an overdose of cholinergic drugs is increased "SLUD."

Salivation
Lacrimation
Urination
Defecation

Cholinergic Drug Examples

Generic	Brand name	Action	Indications
pilocarpine	Salagen	Increase salivation	Xerostomia
pilocarpine	Isopto Carpine	Pupil constriction and fall in intraocular pressure	Glaucoma

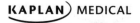

Anticholinergic drugs block the action of the PNS at cholinergic receptors by preventing the action of acetylcholine. These drugs are called antimuscarinics since they do not block the nicotinic receptors. Anticholinergic drugs stimulate the CNS, reduce exocrine gland flow, relax smooth muscle, and increase heart rate. **Sal-Tropine** is a low-dose atropine sulfate that has a duration of about 2 hours. **Drugs such as atropine are important in dentistry for patients with too much saliva-flow.**

Anticholinergic Drug Examples

Generic	Brand name	Action	Indications
atropine sulfate	Sal-Tropine	Reduces exocrine gland function	Excessive saliva

Analgesics

Analgesics treat pain. They can be categorized in two classifications: **non-opioids** and **opioids**. Non-opioids include salicylates, nonsteroidal anti-inflammatory agents (NSAIDs), and acetaminophen.

Patients who place an aspirin by a tooth that hurts can cause a chemical burn to the gingiva.

Salicylates are antipyretic (fever-reducing), anti-inflammatory (inflammation-reducing), and analgesic (pain-relieving). Salicylates also inhibit prostaglandin synthesis for platelet aggregation (adhesiveness). Salicylates are **contraindicated** for patients who are on anticoagulants, who have Reye's syndrome, and who have aspirin-sensitive asthma. **Percodan** is a combination of aspirin and oxycodone.

Antipyretics affect the hypothalamus, which controls fever.

NSAIDs or **NAIDs** are antipyretic, anti-inflammatory, and analgesic. NSAIDs also inhibit prostaglandin synthesis for platelet aggregation (adhesiveness). The NSAIDs of ibuprofen and naproxen work particularly well as anti-inflammatories. NSAIDs should not be taken with Coumadin (will increase bleeding), lithium (increases the effect of lithium), or Lasix (decreases the effect of Lasix).

Acetaminophen is antipyretic and analgesic but it is *not* anti-inflammatory. Acetaminophen is the drug of choice if aspirin is contraindicated. If taken in large doses, however, it can cause damage to the kidneys and liver. **Percoset** is a combination of acetaminophen and oxycodone.

Narcan is an opioid antagonist.

Opium is derived from the poppy plant that has been recorded in history for centuries. Opioids depress the central nervous system (CNS) and are regulated under law by the Harrison Narcotic Act. These drugs suppress pain pathways by attaching to opioid receptors of mu (μ) and kappa (κ). Opioids are used as analgesics, for sedation, and in cough suppressants. **Codeine** in Tylenol #3™ is a **Schedule III** drug that is commonly used in dentistry.

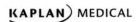

Analgesic Drug Examples

Generic	Brand name	Action	Indications
acetaminophen	Tylenol, Datril	Analgesic	Pain, fever
ibuprofen naproxen ketoprofen	Motrin, Advil, Aleve Naprosyn Orudis	Analgesic, anti-inflammatory	Pain, fever, inflammation
oxycodone hydrocodone propoxyphene meperidine hydromorphone	Percodan, Percoset, Tylox Vicodin Darvon Demerol Dilaudid	Analgesic	Pain

Antianxiety Agents

Antianxiety drugs help to suppress patient fears. Included in this group are benzodiazepines, barbiturates, non-barbiturate sedative-hypnotics, and muscle relaxants.

Benzodiazepines reduce anxiety, induce sleep, act as anticonvulsants (diazepam), and relax muscles. These drugs act on the CNS by mediating γ-aminobutyric acid (GABA) which is a primary inhibitory transmitter of the CNS. Benzodiazepines such as diazepam can be used in dentistry to control anxiety and possible panic attacks. Adverse effects include CNS suppression, decreased blood pressure and pulse rate, respiratory depression, xerostomia, amnesia, and thrombophlebitis.

Barbiturates—derivatives of barbituric acid—enhance and mimic the action of GABA complex. They are used as mild sedatives, hypnotics, as pre-anesthetics, and for general anesthesia. Side effects might be CNS suppression, vasodilation leading to blood pooling, respiratory depression, and depression of kidney and liver function.

Non-barbiturate sedative-hypnotics are not widely used but chloral hydrate is a sedative that has been used for children in dentistry.

Many antianxiety drugs cause xerostomia.

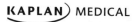

Antianxiety Drug Examples

Generic	Brand name	Action	Indications
alprazolam diazepam clonazepam temazepam lorazepam midazolam	Xanax Valium Klonopin Restoril Ativan Versed	Antianxiety, CNS depression	Acute or chronic anxiety, preoperative sedation, treat insomnia, muscle relaxation, seizures, panic disorders
zolpidem chloral hydrate meprobamate	Ambien Noctec Equanil, Miltown	Sedative hypnotic	Sedation and promotes sleep
buspirone	Buspar	Anti-depressant effect	Generalized anxiety disorder

Barbiturate Examples

Generic	Brand name	Action	Indications
Ultra short acting			
thiopental sodium	Pentothal	Low-dose tranquilizer	Seizure, short-acting general anesthetic
methohexital	Brevital	High-dose hypnotic	Insomnia
Short acting			
phenobarbital	Luminal	Pre-anesthetic, hypnotic	Anesthesia
secobarbital	Seconal	Anti-anxiety, insomnia	Anxiety, insomnia
Immediate acting			
pentobarbital	Nembutal	Anti-seizure, hypnotic	Seizures
amobarbital	Amytal	Treats insomnia, anxiety	Insomnia, anxiety
butabarbital	Butisol	Hypnotic, sleep inducer	Short-term for anxiety, insomnia
Long acting			
phenobarbital	Luminal	Anti-seizure	Seizures
mephobarbital	Mebral, Mebaral	Anti-anxiety	Anxiety

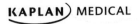

Anti-Infective Agents

Anti-infective agents include many antibiotics (produced by microorganisms) that are used to treat dental infections, such as infection from caries, periodontal disease, and localized infections. Antimicrobials are broad-spectrum medications that treat multiple microorganisms. Antifungals are used for fungal infections such as oral candidiasis. Antivirals treat viruses such as herpes simplex.

Bactericidal agents kill bacteria, while bacteriostatic agents inhibit growth.

Antibiotics are used not only to treat dental infections but also to premedicate those individuals with specific concerns: mitral valve prolapse, hip replacement, kidney dialysis, transplants, or heart valve problems. It is also suggested that premedication be used for those with unstable heart problems, uncontrolled diabetes, spina bifida if with a particular shunt, systemic lupus erythematosis, inflammatory rheumatoid arthritis, or hemophilia.

Penicillin is a bactericidal agent used to treat gram-positive cocci such as *Staphylococcus*, *Streptococcus*, and *Neisseria* infections. Dentistry commonly uses penicillin G, penicillin V, and amoxicillin. Amoxicillin is the drug of choice for premedication in a patient with heart problems, assuming the patient does not have a penicillin allergy.

> Penicillin inhibits cell wall synthesis of bacteria in the multiplication stage. Tetracycline blocks the protein synthesis of bacteria.

The macrolide group of antibiotics includes erythromycin, clarithromycin, and azithromycin. Erythromycin is a bacteriostatic that is effective against some of the same bacteria as the penicillins. Erythromycin used to be the drug of choice for premedication for heart valve problems, but it can cause gastrointestinal cramps and nausea. Clarithromycin and azithromycin are bacteriostatic agents that have similar actions as erythromycin.

The tetracycline groups are bacteriostatic broad-spectrum antibiotics. Tetracycline is the drug of choice for periodontal infection since it has a longer half-life in gingival crevicular fluid. However, it can cause discoloration of unerupted teeth and should not be prescribed for children under 9 years of age, pregnant women in their last half of pregnancy, or nursing mothers.

> Milk or antacids inhibit tetracycline absorption.
>
> Tetracycline has a longer half-life in gingival crevicular fluid.

Clindamycin is a bacteriostatic agent that interferes with bacterial protein synthesis. It is the recommended drug of choice for premedication if a patient is allergic to penicillin. Since one side effect of Clindamycin is pseudomembranous colitis, it is not widely used to treat dental infections.

Cephalosporins are bactericidal agents that inhibit cell-wall synthesis of bacteria. This antibiotic is the premedication of choice for somone who has had a hip or joint replacement.

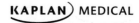

Antibiotic Regimen for Patients Needing to Premedicate

Adult		Child
2 g	Amoxicillin 1 hr prior to appt	Amoxicillin 50 mg/kg orally 1 hr prior to appt.
If penicillin allergic:		
600 mg	Clindamycin 1 hr prior to appt	Clindamycin 20 mg/kg orally 1 hr prior to appt.
2 g	Cephalexin 1 hr prior to appt	
2 g	Cefadroxil 1 hr prior to appt	
500 mg	Azithromycin 1 hr prior to appt	
500 mg	Clarithromycin 1 hr prior to appt	

Patients at highest risk

- Prosthetic heart valves
- Previous history of endocarditis
- Certain congenital heart defects such as
  - Unrepaired cyanotic congenital heart disease, including those with palliative shunts and conduits
  - Completely repaired congenital heart disease with prostetic material or device, whether placed by surgery or catheter intervention, during the first 6 months after the procedure.
  - Repaired congenital heart disease with residual defects at the site of or adjacent to the site of a prosthetic patch or prosthetic device (which inhibit endothelialization)

Metronidazole (Flagyl) is an anti-infective agent that is not only bactericidal, but also amebicidal (effective against amoeba) and trichomonacidal (effective against trichonosis). It is effective in treating periodontal disease and can be used in conjunction with penicillin to treat refractory or juvenile periodontitis. **Alcohol cannot be consumed** when one is on Flagyl, since it will cause an **Antabuse-type reaction of nausea, vomiting, cramps, and headache.**

Antituberculosis agents are used to treat the *Mycobacterium tuberculosis* microbe, which can be a very resistant bacterium. Patients frequently neglect to complete their medications for this disease, so the microbes have mutated and become multi-drug resistant. These agents inhibit DNA-dependent RNA of *M. tuberculosis*.

The RIP drugs used to treat TB are rifampin, isoniazid, and pyrazinamide.

Antifungals are effective against fungal infections including *Candida albicans* intraorally. Fungal infections occur more often in patients who are immunosuppressed. Nystatin is fungicidal and fungistatic, and is used most often to treat candidiasis. **Antiviral** agents are specific in treating viruses. Viruses need a host to live off, making viruses hard to

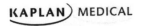

Antiviral agents are specific in treating viruses. Viruses need a host to live off, making viruses hard to treat. **Acyclovir** inhibits DNA replication of viruses and is useful for treating herpes simplex 1 (HSV1), herpes simplex 2 (HSV2), mononucleosis (Epstein-Barr virus), shingles (varicella-zoster), and cytomegalovirus (CMV). **Zidovudine** is an antiviral that treats HIV by blocking viral replication.

Anti-Infective Drug Examples

Generic	Brand name	Action	Indications
Antibiotics			
penicillin G, V	Pentids, V-Cillin K	Bactericidal	Abscess, dental infections, premedication heart
amoxicillin	Amoxil		
ampicillin	Polycillin		Dental or orofacial infections
erythromycin	Erythrocin	Bacteriostatic	
azithromycin	Zitrhomax, Z-pak		
clarithromycin	Biaxin		
tetracycline	Achromycin	Bacteriostatic	Periodontal infections
doxycycline	Vibramycin		
clindamycin	Cleocin	Bacteriostatic	Premedication heart, periodontal infections
			Premedication for joint of hip replacement
cephalexin	Keflex	Bactericidal	
cefaclor	Ceclor		
cefadroxil	Duricef		
Antituberculins			
rifampin	Rifadin	Bactericidal specific to TB	Tuberculosis
isoniazid	INH, Laniazid		
pyrazinamide	PZA		
Antifungals			
nystatin	Mycostatin	Fungicidal	Oral candidiasis
fluconazole	Diflucan		
clotrimazole	Mycelex		
Antivirals			
acyclovir	Zovirax	Blocks viral replication	Herpes simplex
zidovudine	AZT, Retrovir		HIV

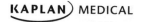

Anticonvulsants

Anticonvulsants treat seizures. Specific types of seizures are discussed in Chapter 20, Medical Emergencies in the Dental Office.

One side effect of phenytoin is gingival hyperplasia.

Phenytoin is commonly used to treat generalized tonic-clonic and partial seizures. It works by blocking the sodium channels of rapidly discharging nerve cells.

Phenobarbital is a barbiturate used to treat epilepsy. It inhibits the neurotransmitter GABA. **Valproic acid**'s mechanism of action is not totally understood, though it is believed that it increases brain levels of GABA. Other drugs include carbamazepine and clonazepam.

Anticonvulsant Drug Examples

Generic	Brand name	Action	Indications
phenytoin	Dilantin	Blocks sodium channels of firing nerve cells	Tonic-clonic, partial seizures
phenobarbital		Inhibits GABA neurotransmitter	Tonic-clonic, partial seizures
valproic acid	Depakote	Not totally understood	Simple and complex partial seizures, absence seizures, generalized tonic-clonic
carbamazepine	Tegretol	Blocks sodium channels of firing nerve cells	Partial simple or complex seizures
clonazepam	Klonopin	Inhibits GABA neurotransmitter	Absence seizures (petit mal) and panic disorders

Antihistamines

Antihistamines block histamines, which are produced by mast cells during allergic reactions. A patient may never have had a problem premedicating with an antibiotic before, yet might develop an allergic reaction with a subsequent dose. Diphenhydramine is the most commonly used antihistamine.

Antihistamine Drug Examples

Generic	Brand name	Action	Indications
diphenhydramine	Benadryl	Blocks the release of histamine	Allergic reaction
loratidine	Claritin	Blocks the release of histamine	Allergies

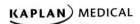

Antineoplastic Agents

Antineoplastic agents treat neoplasms or malignancies but are also used for inflammatory diseases such as rheumatoid arthritis and lupus erythematosus. Their mode of action is to interfere with the metabolism of neoplastic or tumor cells. **Tamoxifen** is an antagonist of estrogen-receptor cancer cells; it works by blocking the estrogen receptors that stimulate breast-cancer cell growth.

Antineoplastic Drug Examples

Generic	Brand name	Action	Indications
tamoxifen	Nolvadex	Blocks estrogen receptors	Breast cancer
methotrexate	MTX	Blocks cell metabolism of abnormal, rapidly growing cells	Cancer, lupus, psoriasis, arthritis

Cardiovascular Agents

According to the CDC, the leading cause of death in the United States is heart disease. Patients with cardiac problems may be on several drugs at once, and it is essential that their health history be updated with each dental visit.

Antianginal drugs relieve the pain of angina pectoris when the heart muscle isn't receiving enough oxygen. Constricted blood vessels keep oxygen from reaching the heart muscle when the workload is demanding more oxygen. **Nitroglycerin** compounds vasodilate the blood vessels to allow a better flow of oxygen to the heart muscle.

Calcium channel blockers inhibit the movement of calcium that muscle needs for contraction. They also vasodilate vessels to relax peripheral resistance. **β-Adrenergic blocking** drugs prevent heart muscle stimulation by β catecholamines.

Antiarrhythmic drugs are used to treat irregular or abnormal heart rhythms produced by the interruptions of the heart's pacemakers. Irregular rhythms include tachycardia (100+ beats per minute [BPM]), bradycardia (< 60 BPM), atrial fibrillation (atria beat at 350+ BPM, causing the ventricles to beat at 80–180 BPM), and heart blocks, where the pathway(s) below the AV node become disabled.

Anticoagulants drugs interfere with the vitamin K production of prothrombin (by the liver) and Factors VII, IX, and X that are needed for clotting. Patients taking these drugs must be monitored for their clotting ability. The test for monitoring is called the **prothrombin time test (PTT).**

Nitroglycerine disintegrates easily. If it comes out of the bottle in a powder form or with a fetid smell, it is no longer usable.

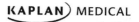

Antihyperlipidemic drugs reduce hyperlipoproteinemias, which are **abnormally high levels of lipids** (cholesterol and triglycerides) transported by lipoproteins in blood. High blood lipoprotein levels are a risk factor for atherosclerosis.

Antihypertensive drugs lower abnormally high blood pressures. **Diuretics** such as HCTZ or Lasix interfere with **sodium reuptake in the loop of Henle in the kidney**. With sodium unable to re-enter the loop, excessive water is excreted from the body. That decreases cardiac output, which means the heart won't have to work as hard. That, in turn, decreases peripheral resistance.

Calcium channel blockers such as nifedipine cause gingival hyperplasia.

β-Adrenergic-blocking drugs decrease cardiac output by blocking catecholamine stimulation of the beta receptors of the heart. **Calcium channel blockers** inhibit the movement of calcium into heart muscle cells, which is necessary for muscle contraction. Calcium channel blockers can cause **gingival hyperplasia**. α_1-Adrenergic blocking drugs block α_1-receptors from being stimulated, causing peripheral vasodilation.

Cardiac glycosides treat congestive heart failure (CHF). CHF occurs when the heart muscle is pumping inadequately. Right- and left-sided heart failure is discussed in Chapter 20. Cardiac glycosides increase the strength of the contraction and improve the electrophysiology properties of the heart. Digoxin increases myocardial contractility in both the failing and the non-failing heart, by allowing more calcium to enter the myocardial cells during depolarization.

Cardiovascular Drug Examples

Loop diuretics such as furosemide (Lasix) work in the loop of Henle—part of the glomerulus of the kidney.

Generic	Brand name	Action	Indications
nitroglycerine	NTG, Nitrostat	Vasodilate, antianginal	Angina pain
nifedipine	Procardia	Vasodilate, antianginal	Angina pain
verapamil	Calan, Isoptin	Inhibit calcium movement, calcium channel blocker	Arrhythmias
propranolol	Inderal	Vasodilate, antianginal	Angina pain
metoprolol	Lopressor	Inhibit calcium movement, calcium channel blocker	Hypertension Arrhythmias
digoxin	Lanoxin	Increase contractility, cardiac glycoside	CHF
furosemide	Lasix	Loop diuretic, antihypertensive	Hypertension
thiazides	HCTZ, Diuril		

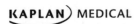

Endocrine Agents

Adrenocorticosteroids have two major classifications: glucocorticoids and mineralcorticoids. **Glucocorticoids** affect the metabolism of carbohydrates, fats, and proteins, but also work as anti-inflammatories and antiallergens. **Mineralcorticoids** affect electrolytes (minerals) and water in the body, by increasing sodium retention and decreasing potassium retention. With adrenal insufficiency, the adrenal glands do not produce enough cortisol, which can place a patient in "crisis." If someone who has been on cortisone for an extended period feels greatly stressed while at the dental office, he could have an adrenal crisis.

Diabetes mellitus is an inability of the pancreas to produce **insulin,** which unlocks cells to allow glucose to enter and sustain cell life. Diabetes has been discussed in depth in Chaper 20. Insulin-dependent diabeties mellitus (IDDM) patients will be on Humulin, Novolin, or Lantus to name a few. These insulin-replacement medications can be short-acting, intermediate-acting, or long-acting. Non-insulin-dependent diabeties mellitus (NIDDM) patients may be able to control the condition with diet, or may be taking one of the medications listed below.

Hypothyroidism is insufficient production of thyroid hormone, and in severe cases, can cause cretinism in children and myxedema in adults. Patients with hypothyroidism need thyroid hormone supplements in order to prevent weakness, lethargy, and a puffy face. **Hyperthyroidism** is the opposite: It produces too much thyroid hormone, and causes Grave's disease. Treatment involves radioactive iodine or partial thyroidectomy.

Endocrine Drug Examples

Generic	Brand name	Action	Indications
methylprednisolone	Solu-Medrol	Anti-inflammatory glucocorticoid	Anti-inflammatory
humulin	Humulin	Insulin replacement	IDDM
insulin glargine	Lantus	Time-released insulin replacement	
glyburide	Diabeta, Micronase	Stimulate the release of insulin	NIDDM
glipizide	Glucotrol		
chlorpropamide	Diabinese		
Levothyroxine	Synthroid, Levoxyl, Levothroid	Thyroid hormone replacement	Thyroid insufficiency

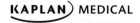

Psychotherapeutic Agents

Antidepressant agents help in the restoration of an individual's mental status, though they can also serve other purposes—migraine alleviation, for one. Antidepressant drugs increase the release, inactivation, or reuptake of norepinephrine. It is believed that depression stems from a deficiency of norepinephrine which controls moods, and that mania arises from an overabundance of norepinephrine. It is also theorized that serotonin levels can manipulate a rise in norepinephrine.

Tricyclics and **monoamine oxidase** (MAO) inhibitors are older-generation antidepressants that use both norepinephrine and serotonin as independent antidepressants. Newer-generation antidepressants (**selective serotonin reuptake inhibitors** [SSRI]) inhibit the firing rate of serotonin neurons. Tricyclics are more effective for severe depression, while the newer-generations drugs are more effective for mild to moderate depression.

A patient who constantly brushes his teeth suffers from obsessive-compulsive disorder.

Antipsychotic agents treat psychosis such as schizophrenia, or neurosis such as obsessive-compulsive disorder. They work by blocking the receptors of dopamine, acetylcholine, norepinephrine, and histamine. Since every patient's metabolism responds differently to each agent, there is a broad range of antipsychotics available.

Bipolar disorder is a manic-depressive illness that causes shifts in a patient's mood, energy, and ability to function. These occur as dramatic mood swings—from very high to sad and hopeless.

Many, many psychotherapeutic agents cause xerostomia.

Psychotherapeutic Agent Examples

Generic	Brand name	Action	Indications
amitriptyline	Elavil	Unknown	Depression, anxiety
fluoxetine	Prozac	Inhibits CNS neural uptake of serotonin	Depression
sertraline	Zoloft	Selective serotonin reuptake inhibitors (SSRIs)	Treat mental depression, obsessive-compulsive disorder
paroxetine	Paxil	Action of SSRIs not totally understood	Major depression and/or obsessive-compulsive disorder
bupropion	Wellbutrin	Not known, weakly blocks serotonin and norepinephrine	Depression
venlafaxine	Effexor	Inhibits the reuptake of serotonin and norepinephrine	Depression
haloperidol	Haldol	Not entirely known but may inhibit the transport mechanism of cerebral monoamines	Acute and chronic psychosis, schizophrenia and manic states
chlorpromazine	Thorazine	Blocks dopamine receptors	Psychosis, schizophrenia, and acute mania
lithium	Lithobid	Mood stabilizer	Manic depression

Other Drugs

Cyclosporines are anti-rejection agents prescribed for patients who have had transplants. Macrophages and T cells mediate inflammation in the transplantation site. Cyclosporines function by inhibiting T cell proliferation, though they can cause **gingival hyperplasia.**

Agents that treat **respiratory diseases** are **sympathomimetic** agents. Beta-adrenergic agonists are the treatment of choice for managing acute asthma, as they relax bronchial smooth muscle. One side effect of **inhalers is xerostomia.** Also, anyone using an inhaler should rinse with water after usage.

Drug Examples

Generic	Brand name	Action	Indications
cyclosporine	Sandimmune	Inhibits T-cell proliferation	Organ transplant, lupus, psoriasis
albuterol terbutaline	Ventolin, Proventil Brethine, Brethaire	Stimulates β2-receptors of bronchial smooth muscles	Asthma

General Anesthetics

General anesthetics provide pain suppression during surgical procedures, and can be administered as inhaled gas or injectable liquid. They are usually administered in combinations since no one agent is able to produce all the desired affects. Some of the mechanisms of action of general anesthetics are not fully understood. General analgesia causes loss of pain sensation. Excitement then causes the patient to become delirious, until surgical anesthesia relaxes the skeletal muscles and surgery is begun.

Halothane (Flurothane) inhibits sympathetic response to painful stimuli but additional muscle relaxation from other drugs is required. **Isoflurane (Forane)** produces profound muscle relaxation and is used in conjunction with nitrous oxide. **Enflurane (Ethrane)** is also used in conjunction with nitrous oxide to provide muscle relaxation and analgesia. **Thiopental (Pentothal)** is an ultra-short-acting barbiturate that has a rapid onset of action.

Succinylcholine is a short-acting muscle relaxant used during endotracheal intubation.

Nitrous oxide is a colorless, non-flammable gas that is also known as **laughing gas.** It is commonly used in dentistry to relax the patient, or used in combination with other drugs such as thiopental to produce surgical anesthesia. The exact mechanism of action is not totally understood but nitrous oxide may mediate the

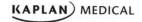
KAPLAN MEDICAL

interaction of opioid receptors in the brain. The use of nitrous oxide in the dental office is discussed in Chapter 17, Anxiety and Pain Management.

Nitrous oxide is **contraindicated** for patients with the following conditions: COPD (pulmonary disease), respiratory obstruction or infection, pregnancy, hepatitis, emotional illness, untreated pneumothorax, or drug abuse.

Chloral hydrate is a rapid-onset, short-duration sedative used to relieve anxiety and induce sleep prior to surgery. In dentistry, it is used with children.

Local Anesthetics

Anesthesia can be defined as the "loss of bodily sensation with or without the loss of consciousness." **Analgesia** is the absence of pain without loss of consciousness.

Two kinds of anesthetics are used in dentistry: esters and amides. **Esters** (with one *i* in their generic name) are metabolized or biotransformed in **blood plasma**. Their usage dropped recently, after many people developed **allergic** reactions. As such, **amides** have become the anesthesia of choice. Amides (with two *i*'s) are biotransformed in the **liver**. Patients with liver complications cannot metabolize amides.

Vasoconstrictors such as epinephrine can prevent local blood vessels from absorbing anesthesia not yet absorbed into the nerve cells. Some anesthetics, such as mepivicaine and prilocaine, are available with or without epinephrine.

Local anesthetics are discussed in greater length in Chapter 17.

DRUG ELIMINATION AND ACID–BASE BALANCE

The **liver** is the primary site for **drug metabolism**. Enzymes in the liver and throughout the body function to eliminate drugs by oxidation, reduction, or hydrolysis. Phase I of drug metabolism occurs with the enzyme cytochrome P-450 with the most common phase II reaction of glucuronidation. Drugs metabolized by the liver are largely excreted in bile.

Drug excretion occurs primarily at the **renal level of the glomerulus** but other sites for smaller excretion include the intestines, saliva, sweat, breast milk, and lungs. Elderly patients, patients with liver disease, and newborns with underdeveloped livers may have suppressed function to metabolize drugs.

Oxygen is stored in a green tank. Nitrous oxide is stored in a blue tank.

The **glomerulus** filtrate and blood plasma have the same pH, but changes in the pH affect the rate of drug excretion. Some drugs are more acidic, while others are more alkaline. Alkalinizing urine increases the rate of elimination while acidic urine decreases that same rate.

DRUGS CAUSING GINGIVAL HYPERPLASIA

Certain drugs can cause gingival hyperplasia, which has a direct effect on the oral cavity and its health. Working with a patient on these drugs can help to reduce the severity of disease in the oral cavity.

- diltiazem (Cardizem, Dilacor)
- felodipine (Plendil)
- nifedpine (Adalat, Procardia)
- phenytoin (Dilantin)
- verapamil (Calan, Isoptin, Verelan)

DRUGS FOR ORAL INFECTIONS

Achromycin (tetracycline): localized JVP, refractory aphthous stomatitis

Amoxil (amoxicillin): NUG, pericoronitis, periapical abscess

Diflucan (flucanzole): oral candidiasis

Mycelex (clotrimazole): oral candidiasis

Mycostatin (nystatin): oral candidiasis

Nizoral (ketoconazole): oral candidiasis

Penicillin VK: NUG, pericoronitis, periapical <u>and</u> periodontal abscess

Vibramycin (doxycycline): localized JVP, periodontal abscess

Zovirax (acyclovir): primary herpes

DRUGS CAUSING XEROSTOMIA

Many drugs cause xerostomia (dry mouth). Xerostomia can seriously affect a patient's quality of life.

ANOREXIANT

Adipex-P, Fastin, Ionamin, Zantryl	phentermine
Anorex SR, Adipost, Bontril PDM	phendimetrazine
Mazanor, Sanorex	mazindol
Pondimin, Fen-Phen	fenfluramine
Tenuate, Tepanil, Ten-Tab	diethylpropion

ANTICHOLINERGIC / ANTISPASMODIC

Anaspaz	hyoscyamine
Atropisol, Sal-Tropine	atropine
Banthine	methantheline
Bellergal	belladonna alkaloids
Bentyl	dicyclomine
Daricon	oxyphencyclimine
Ditropan	oxybutynin
Donnatal, Kinesed	hyoscyamine with atropine, phenobarbital, scopolamine
Librax	chlordiazepoxide with clidinium
Pamine	methscopolamine
Pro-Banthine	propantheline
Transderm-Scop	scopolamine

ANTIDIARRHETIC

Imodium AD	loperamide
Lomotil	diphenoxylate with atropine
Motofen	difenoxin with atropine

ANTIHISTAMINE

Actifed	triprolidine with pseudoephedrine
Benadryl	diphenhydramine
Chlor-Trimeton	chlorpheniramine
Claritin	loratadine
Dimetane	brompheniramine
Dimetapp	brompheniramine with phenylpropanolamine
Hismanal	astemizole
Phenergan	promethazine
Pyribenzamine (PBZ)	tripelennamine
Seldane	terfenadine

ANTI-INFLAMMATORY ANALGESIC

Dolobid	diflunisal
Feldene	piroxicam
Motrin, Advil	ibuprofen
Nalfon	fenoprofen
Naprosyn	naproxen

ANTI-PSYCHOTIC

Clozaril	clozapine
Compazine	prochlorperazine
Eskalith	lithium
Haldol	haloperidol
Mellaril	thioridazine
Navane	thiothixene
Orap	pimozide
Sparine	promazine
Stelazine	trifluoperazine
Thorazine	chlorpromazine

DIURETIC

Diuril	chlorothiazide
Dyazide, Maxzide	triamterine and hydrochlorothiazide
HydroDIURIL, Esidrix	hydrochlorothiazide
Hygroton	chlorthalidone
Lasix	furosemide
Midamor	amiloride

NARCOTIC ANALGESIC

Demerol	meperidine
MS Contin	morphine

ANTIACNE

Accutane . . . . isotretinoin

ANTIANXIETY

Atarax, Vistaril . . . . hydroxyzine
Ativan. . . . . lorazepam
Centrax. . . . . .prazepam
Equanil, Miltown. . . . . .meprobamate
Librium . . . . chlordiazepoxide
Paxipam . . . . halazepam
Serax . . . . .oxazepam
Valium . . . . diazepam
Xanax. . . . . alprazolam

ANTICONVULSANT

Felbatol. . . . . .felbamate
Lamictal . . . . .lamotrigine
Neurontin . . . . .gabapentin
Tegretol . . . . .carbamazepine

ANTIDEPRESSANT

Anafranil. . . . . clomipramine
Asendin . . . . amoxapine
Elavil. . . . . amitryptaline
Luvox . . . . fluvoxamine
Norpramin . . . . desipramine
Prozac. . . . . .fluoxetine
Sinequan . . . . doxepin
Tofrani . . . . .imipramine
Wellbutrin. . . . . bupropion

ANTIHYPERTENSIVE

Capoten . . . . .captopril
Catapres. . . . . clonidine
Coreg. . . . . carvedilol
Ismelin . . . . guanethidine
Minipress . . . . prazosin
Serpasil. . . . . reserpine
Wytensin . . . . guanabenz

ANTINAUSEANT/ANTIEMETIC

Antivert . . . . meclizine
Dramamine. . . . . .dyphenhydramine
Marezine . . . . cyclizine

ANTIPARKINSONIAN

Akineton. . . . . biperiden
Artane . . . . .trihexyphenidyl
Cogentin . . . . benztropine mesylate
Larodopa . . . . levodopa
Sinemet . . . . carbidopa with levodopa

BRONCHODILATOR

Atrovent. . . . . ipratropium
Isuprel. . . . . isoproterenol
Proventil, Ventolin. . . . . .albuterol

DECONGESTANT

Ornade . . phenylpropanolamine with chlorpheniramine
Sudafed . . . . pseudoephedrine

MUSCLE RELAXANT

Flexeril . . . . cyclobenzaprine
Lioresal. . . . . .baclofen
Norflex, Disipal . . . . orphenadrine

SEDATIVE

Dalmane. . . . . .flurazepam
Halcion. . . . . triazolam
Restoril. . . . . temazepam

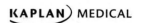

REVIEW QUESTIONS

1. Antibiotics can be bacteriostatic or bactericidal. When does penicillin have an effect on bacterial growth?

   A. During ATP production
   B. During DNA replication
   C. During septum formation
   D. During cell wall synthesis at the multiplication stage
   E. When the centrioles divide

2. Which of the following local anesthetics is an ester that is metabolized in plasma?

   A. Articaine
   B. Lidocaine
   C. Procaine
   D. Mepivacaine
   E. Bupivacaine

3. A functional heart murmur results in damage to the heart. This type of murmur requires prophylactic antibiotic premedication before dental treatment.

   A. Both statements are true.
   B. The first statement is false because the function murmur does not cause damage to the heart valve. The second statement is true.
   C. The first statement is true. The second statement is false because functional murmurs do not require medication.
   D. Both statements are false. A functional murmur does not cause damage to the heart valve, nor does it require medication.

4. A patient taking warfarin might experience which of the following side effects?

   A. Gingival hyperplasia
   B. Bleeding gingiva
   C. Excessive urination
   D. Xerostomia
   E. Hyperkeratosis

5. The drug used to treat copious amounts of saliva is

   A. Salagen
   B. Isopto Carpine
   C. Urecholine
   D. Sal-Tropine

6. The following agents used in dentistry may also be used in emergency cardiac care except one. Which one is this EXCEPTION?

   A. Propoxycaine
   B. Atropine
   C. Lidocaine
   D. Epinephrine
   E. All of the above

7. Lichen planus can be asymptomatic or can cause extreme pain. The drug of choice to treat lichen planus is

   A. Dexamethasone
   B. Metronidazole
   C. Penicillin VK
   D. Doxycycline
   E. Acyclovir

8. If a patient is allergic to sulfa drugs, you would not anesthetize him with

   A. Procaine
   B. Articaine
   C. Mepivacaine
   D. Prilocaine

9. Every medication taken into the body has different routes of elimination. Unlike esters, amides are metabolized or biotransformed in the

   A. Kidneys
   B. Blood
   C. Pancreas
   D. Thyroid
   E. Liver

10. A new patient explains that she had a bad experience with novocaine at her previous dentist; she had passed out after experiencing light-headedness and palpitations. This patient mostly likely

    A. Has a dental phobia.
    B. Is allergic to novocaine.
    C. Needs a referral to an allergist.
    D. Is frightened about dental procedures.
    E. Will have a worse reaction with the next injection of novocaine.

11. A patient has developed a tolerance for a drug. One can assume that he

    A. Has experienced more side effects than desired.
    B. Has reached the desired, correct effects of the drug.
    C. Has reached the maximum response to the drug.
    D. Needs the dosage increased in order to get the desired effect.
    E. Has had an exaggerated immune response to the drug.

12. Some medications have oral side effects. Which of the following medications does NOT cause gingival hyperplasia?

    A. Cyclosporin
    B. Verapamil
    C. Phenytoin
    D. Nifedipine
    E. Cyclophosphamide

13. The most serious side effect of nitrous oxide usage is

    A. Pulmonary embolism
    B. Oxygen deprivation
    C. Electronic throbbing in the ear
    D. Nausea

14. Warfarin acts on the body by

    A. Increasing vitamin K for the production of prothrombin.
    B. Decreasing vitamin K production of thrombin.
    C. Increasing intrinsic factor-absorption of vitamin B12 in the stomach.
    D. Decreasing the protein needed to become hemoglobin.

15. Of the following terms, which one indicates that a drug is safe for use by the public?

    A. Effective dose (ED)$_{50}$
    B. Therapeutic index (TI)
    C. Lethal dose (LD)$_{50}$
    D. Margin of safety

16. What is the drug of choice for the immediate allieviation of a severe anaphylactic reaction?

    A. Diphenhydramine
    B. Diazepam
    C. Epinephrine
    D. 50% dextrose
    E. Lidocaine

17. Which of the following medications might a practitioner prescribe for someone mildly anxious about dental appointments?

    A. Versed
    B. Diazepam
    C. Phenobarbital
    D. Scopolamine

18. What route should be used to administer 50 mg of diphenhydramine to an adult for anaphylaxis?

    A. Intravenous
    B. Intraosseus
    C. Intramuscular
    D. Oral
    E. Rectal

19. While reviewing your patient's health history, you learn that she takes Accutane once a day. How is "once a day" abbreviated?

    A. qid
    B. bid
    C. hs
    D. qd

20. Aspirin is sometimes used in conjunction with another drug to generate a more profound effect. When oxycodone is combined with aspirin, the resulting drug is

    A. Percoset
    B. Percodan
    C. Tylox
    D. Hydromorphone

21. In response to the IV sedation at the oral surgeon's office, a patient develops a sudden anaphylactic reaction. Which of the following medications would help relax the pharynx so that he can be intubated?

    A. Succinylcholine
    B. Propoxyphene
    C. Sufentanil
    D. Propoxycaine
    E. Propulsid

22. A patient presents with a toothache and inflammation around Tooth #28, which has been getting worse over the past week. You deliver the maximum number of cartridges to achieve numbness but the patient still finds it painful when you touch the area. Why might not the anesthetic be working?

    A. Because of the vasoconstriction of vessels in the inflamed area, the anesthetic cannot block the sodium channels.
    B. Because of the proliferation of blood vessels in the inflamed area, the anesthetic is absorbed into the bloodstream quickly.
    C. Because of the alkaline pH in the area (8.5) the inflammation decreases the anesthetic affect.
    D. Edema in the inflamed area concentrates the anesthetic.

Scenario for Questions 23–25

John Thomas is a 16-year-old insulin-dependent diabetic who also has mild asthma. As you review his health history, you discover that his physician has just placed him on an inhaled corticosteroid to manage his mild asthma.

23. Which of the following is NOT true of corticosteroids?

   A. Corticosteroid can elevate the blood-sugar levels of a diabetic.

   B. Corticosteroids have little to no effect on diabetes and blood sugar levels.

   C. Corticosteroids cause or uncover diabetes in many people who don't yet know they have it.

   D. Corticosteroids can counteract insulin.

   E. If corticosteroid use is stopped on a corticosteroid-induced diabetes, the diabetes can reverse itself.

24. Inhaler use can cause all of the following except one. Which one is this EXCEPTION?

   A. Impaired growth in children

   B. Glaucoma or cataracts

   C. Unexpected narrowing of the airways

   D. Tremors

   E. Increased potassium levels in the blood

25. Which of the following statements is true of Humulin?

   A. The most serious side effect of any insulin is hypoglycemia.

   B. Humulin may cause warning symptoms of hypoglycemia more than any other insulin.

   C. Medications such as birth control pills tend to lower blood-sugar levels of those on Humulin.

   D. Beta-blockers including eye drops that contain beta-blockers can reveal some of the signs of low blood sugar.

ANSWER EXPLANATIONS

1. D

Penicillin affects bacterial growth during cell wall synthesis at the multiplication stage. This is when bacteria are susceptible to destruction by penicillin.

A. ATP production of the Kreb's cycle occurs during cell metabolism of glucose during the lag phase.

B. DNA replication occurs during interphase.

C. Septum formation occurs as the cell elongates before it divides.

E. Centrioles divide in the prophase, moving to opposite poles of the cell.

2. C

Procaine is an ester that is metabolized in plasma. It has only one *i*. Articaine, lidocaine, mepivacaine, and Bupivacaine are amides (have two *i*'s).

3. D

Both statements are false. A functional murmur does not cause damage to the heart valve, nor does it require medication.

4. B

Bleeding gingiva can result from warfarin usage.

5. D

Sal-Tropine can help patients who have copious amounts of saliva. It is a low-dose atropine sulfate.

A. Salagen produces saliva.

B. Isopto Carpine produces saliva.

C. Urecholine is therapeutic for urinary retention.

6. A

Propoxycaine is a cardiac agent that is not used in dentistry.

B. Atropine is used in dentistry to dry saliva and in emergency cardiac care to increase cardiac rate.

C. Lidocaine is used as a local anesthetic in dentistry and to treat disrhythmias in emergency cardiac care.

D. Epinephrine is used in dental anesthetics to constrict blood vessels so that local anesthesia can be maintained longer; in emergency cardiac care, it is used to stimulate heart contraction.

7. A

The drug of choice for lichen planus is dexamethasone.

B. Metronidazole is used for periodontal infections.

C. Penicillin VK is used to treat NUG or pericoronitis.

D. Doxycycline is used for localized JVP or periodontal abscess.

E. Acyclovir is for treating herpes simplex.

8. B

For someone allergic to sulfa drugs, you would not anesthetize with articaine, because it has a sulfa preservative.

9. E

Amides differ from esters in that they are metabolized in the liver.

A. Kidneys filter materials but do not metabolize.

B. Blood plasma metabolizes esters.

C. Pancreas aids in digestions with enzymes and produces insulin.

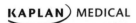

10. D

A patient who passed out after feeling light-headedness and palpitations during her last dental procedure is likely frightened about dental procedures.

B. The symptoms described are not true allergic reactions of novocaine.

E. She would have a worse reaction with novocaine next time only if she were allergic to it, and that has not been determined.

11. D

If a patient has a tolerance for a drug, he needs to increase the dosage to get the desired effect.

B. If the patient has reached the desired effects of the drug, that is efficacy.

C. If the patient has reached the maximum response to the drug, that is potency.

12. E

Cyclophosphamide does not cause gingival hyperplasia.

13. B

Oxygen deprivation would be the most severe complication from nitrous oxide usage.

A. Pulmonary embolism occurs when a thrombus breaks loose and travels to the lungs.

C. Electronic throbbing in the ear is a side effect but not a danger.

14. B

Warfarin works by decreasing vitamin K production of thrombin.

A. Prothrombin becomes thrombin for clotting in the liver with the synthesis of vitamin K. Note that answers A and B are *complete opposites*. Take note with such answers.

15. B

Therapeutic index (TI) indicates that a drug is safe for the public to use. The safety of the drug is determined by dividing the LD_{50} by the ED_{50}. The larger the therapeutic index, the safer the drug.

A. Effective dose $(ED)_{50}$ is the dose that produces a specific response in 50% of the participants.

C. Lethal dose $(LD)_{50}$ is the dose that would be lethal in 50% of participants.

D. Margin of safety is the ratio of the dose within the lethal range (LD_{01}) to the dose that is in the 99% effective range.

16. C

Epinephrine should be used right away for a severe anaphylactic reaction, since it will bronchodilate.

A. Diphenhydramine is an antihistamine that is administered IM after epinephrine has been administered.

B. Diazepam is a drug used with convulsions.

D. 50% dextrose is used when a patient has low blood sugar.

E. Lidocaine is used to treat cardiac disrhythmias.

17. B

Diazepam might help a patient who is mildly anxious about a dental appointment.

A. Versed treats convulsions and is a pre-anesthetic for conscious sedation.

C. Phenobarbital is an anticonvulsant.

D. Scopolamine is used for nausea, vomiting, and dizziness associated with motion sickness and recovery from anesthesia and surgery.

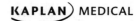

18. C

An intramuscular route should be used to administer 50 mg of diphenhydramine for anaphylaxis, AFTER a subcutaneous injection of 0.4 mg of epinephrine.

A. Intravenous route would be too fast for this medication.

B. Intraosseus would be used for a small child.

D. Oral would be too slow, since epinephrine is short-acting.

19. D

Once a day is abbreviated as qd.

A. qid indicates 4 times a day.

B. bid indicates 2 times a day.

C. hs signifies "at bedtime."

20. B

Oxycodone plus aspirin results in Percodan.

A. Percoset is a combination of oxycodone and acetaminophen.

C. Tylox is a combination of oxycodone and acetaminophen.

D. Hydromorphone or Dilaudid is an opioid that manages pain.

21. A

Succinylcholine would help to relax the pharynx for an emergency intubation.

B. Propoxyphene is an opioid analgesic.

C. Sufentanil is a narcotic analgesic used for surgeryand obstetrics.

D. Propoxycaine is a local anesthetic.

E. Propulsid is a GI tract medication.

22. B

The area is probably still painful because of the proliferation of blood vessels in the inflamed area. The anesthetic is absorbed into the bloodstream much more quickly.

A. The vessels are vasodilated in the areas of inflammation.

C. Inflammation is acidic (ph 5.5), not alkaline.

D. Edema dilutes the anesthesia.

23. B

That corticosteroids have little to no effect on diabetes and blood sugar levels is absolutely not true.

24. E

Inhaler use does not cause increased potassium levels in the blood. It decreases K levels.

A. Corticosteroids can cause impaired growth in children.

B. When taken for long periods of time, inhalers can cause glaucoma or cataracts.

C. Unexpected narrowing of the airways can occur with inhaler usage.

D. Inhaler use can cause tremors.

25. A

The most serious side effect of Humulin or any other insulin is hypoglycemia.

B. Humulin may be less, not more, likely to cause warning symptoms of hypoglycemia than other insulin.

C. Medications such as birth control pills tend to *raise* rather than lower blood sugar levels of patients on Humulin.

D. Beta-blockers including eye drops containing beta-blockers can *mask* rather than reveal the signs of low blood sugar.

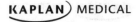

Chapter Twelve:
Nutrition and Biochemistry

Proper nutrition is important for maintaining good dental health. An unbalanced diet can have a direct effect on the body and, indirectly, on the tissues within the oral cavity. In addition, frequent and high intake of carbohydrates promotes tooth decay.

CARBOHYDRATES

Carbohydrates, which are sugar and starch molecules, are necessary for life since cells use glucose for energy. Glucose and fructose supply the energy that the body needs for all cells. Carbohydrates are found in fruit, vegetables, and grains, to name a few, as simple carbohydrates or complex carbohydrates.

Simple Carbohydrates

Simple carbohydrates can be broken down into **monosaccharides** and **disaccharides**. **Monosaccharides** are the simplest type of carbohydrate; they produce **hexoses** of glucose, galactose, and fructose. Glucose and galactose can be readily absorbed into the bloodstream for immediate use. **Glucose**, also known as **dextrose**, is also **absorbed** in the **small intestine** by the hepatic portal system, and is then transported to the **liver** to be **stored as glycogen**. Glycogen that is stored in the liver is used when blood glucose levels fall. The brain absolutely needs glucose in order to function. If blood sugar gets too low in the brain, the body goes after the stores of fat for fuel, breaking fat down into ketones. The brain cannot utilize ketones to function. **Galactose** is the byproduct of the breakdown of **lactose**. **Fructose** is the sweetest sugar derived from fruits and honey.

Disaccharides are more complex. They are made up of **two monosaccharides** or **two hexoses**, and are metabolized into monosaccharides in the digestive tract where absorption takes place. The members of this group include sucrose, lactose, and maltose.

Sucrose, derived from maple syrup, cane sugar, and beet sugar, is hydrolyzed into **glucose** and **fructose**. **Lactose** is derived from milk, and is hydrolyzed into **glucose** and **galactose**. **Maltose** is derived from sweet potatoes, fruits, and vegetables, and is hydrolyzed into two glucose molecules.

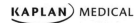

Complex Carbohydrates

Complex carbohydrates include homopolysaccharides and heteropolysaccharides. Since their molecules form **long chains** of **simple carbohydrates**, they are more complex and take longer to hydrolyze. Homopolysaccharides consist of starch, glycogen, and cellulose. **Starchy** foods include pasta, rice, cereals, bread, and legumes.

Glycogen is also known as "animal starch," and is stored in the liver for use if blood-glucose levels fall. **Cellulose** contains not only complex carbohydrates, but also dietary fiber that the body cannot digest. Fiber increases the **peristalsis** of food along the digestive tract for elimination in a softer stool.

Sugar Alcohols

Sugar alcohols should never be recommended for patients on antabuse or flagyl; the alcohol will make them very ill.

Dietary sweeteners include synthetic sweeteners (**saccharine, aspartame**) and sugar alcohols (**mannitol, xylitol, sorbitol**). Synthetic sweeteners break down in cooking. All of these sweeteners are noncariogenic, although large amounts of the sugar alcohols can cause diarrhea.

Starch digestion begins in the mouthby salivary amylase.

Carbohydrate Enzymes and Actions

Location	Enzyme	Acts on	Becomes
Mouth	Amylase	Starch	Maltose
Stomach	None	—	—
Small intestine—bile	None	—	—
Small intestine—pancreas	Pancreatic amylase	Starch	Maltose becomes 2 glucose molecules

Lipoproteins

Lipoproteins contain both proteins and lipids. Lipoproteins which are manufactured in the liver are how cholesterol is transported in the blood stream. They are contained in enzymes, antigens, toxins, structural proteins and membrane transporters.

High denisty lipoproteins (HDL) rid the body of cholesterol, while low density lipoproteins (LDL) attracts cholesterol and clogs arteries.

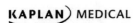

FATS

Fats are **not soluble in water**, and as a result, congeal into masses. **Bile** emulsifies fat so that it is more easily digestible by pancreatic lipases as a fat globule. **Simple lipids** are true fats that are in the form of saturated fats and unsaturated fats. **Saturated fats** are derived from **animal origins** and are **solid** at room temperature. **Unsaturated fats** are derived from **plant origins** and are **liquid** at room temperature.

Essential fatty acids (EFA)—"good fats"—cannot be synthesized by the body and are a very necessary part of our diet since the body cannot make essential fatty acids. They produce **prostaglandins** which boost the immune system, and they regulate blood circulation and blood pressure.

Two important essential fats are alpha-linolenic acid and linoleic acid. Alpha-linolenic acid is an omega-3 fatty acid (EFA) that aids in the formation of cell walls, reduces the risk of thrombosis or stroke, lowers blood pressure, and decreases triglycerides. If the body is deficient in omega-3 fatty acids, mental health symptoms such as depression can occur. Other deficiencies include brittle nails, dry hair, flaking skin, and joint pain. It is found in flaxseed, walnuts, pumpkin seeds, Brazil nuts, and some green leafy vegetables.

Linoleic acid is an omega-6 fatty acid (EFA) that aids in improving rheumatoid arthritis, PMS, and dermatologic disorders. It also promotes blood clotting, but if deficient can cause dry skin and other skin related problems. However, too much omega-6 fatty acids is strongly correlated with a high incidence of cardiovascular disease and can contribute to cancer growth. It is found in flaxseeds, grapeseed oil, pumpkin seeds, pine nuts, pistachio nuts, olive oil, chestnut oil, and chicken.

Synthetic fats, such as the derived lipids of steroids and sterols, help reduce serum cholesterol by interfering with cholesterol absorption. This category also includes the artificial fats **Olestra**, which has large molecules that aren't absorbed in the intestinal tract, and **Simplesse**, which is derived from the whey in milk and has the texture of fat.

Fat Enzymes and Actions

Location	Enzyme	Acts on	Becomes
Mouth	None	—	—
Stomach	Gastric lipase	Fats	Fatty acids & glycerol
Small intestine—bile	Cholecystokinin (hormone)	Emulsifies fats	Fat globules easier to be digested by lipases
Small intestine—pancreas	Pancreatic lipase	Triglycerides	2 monoglycerides & fatty acids

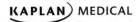

PROTEINS

Proteins are complex substances made up of thousands of amino acids. They are found in food. A daily intake of **protein** is important since it is something **the body cannot store.**

Proteins contain both **essential** and **nonessential amino acids.** The **essential amino acids** are tryptophan; lysine; methionine; phenylalanine; threonine; valine; and leucine. **Complete proteins**—found in meat, fish, poultry, eggs, and dairy—contain all essential amino acids. **Incomplete proteins**—found in legumes, grains, and leafy greens—contain only some amino acids.

Protein Enzymes and Actions

Location	Enzyme	Acts on	Converts to
Mouth	None	—	—
Stomach	Pepsin	Proteins	Peptides
Small intestine—bile	None	—	—
Small intestine—pancreas	Trypsin	Proteins	Peptides & small peptides
	Chymotrypsinogen	Proteins	Peptides & small peptides
	Carboxypeptidase	Proteins	Removes amino acid from peptides

> Excess protein can cause liver or kidney damage, increase the excretion of calcium, and/or become dehydrated. Too much protein can make it harder to loose weight.

MINERALS

Minerals are important to help balance the organ systems in the body. Among other things, they help to maintain acid–base balance and fluid levels, as well as to aid in nerve conduction and muscle contraction.

> Lack of protein can cause muscle atrophy, oedema, and anemia

Calcium is essential for muscle **contraction. Calcium, fluoride,** and **phosphorus** are essential for the formation of **bones** and **teeth. Deficiencies** in these elements could make an individual **susceptible to caries** and have poor bone formation (**osteoporosis**). **Vitamin D** is needed for the absorption of **calcium** and **phosphorus.**

Sodium and **potassium** are essential for both **acid–base balance** and for the proper function of the **sodium–potassium pump** of the heart. Both are also essential for proper nerve conduction. A deficiency in sodium and potassium minerals could cause **cardiac arrhythmias.**

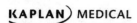

Essential Minerals

Mineral	Essential for	Deficiency	Foods
Calcium	Bones & teeth mineralization, muscle contraction	Osteoporosis (adults), rickets (children), decay susceptible, & periodontal disease	Dairy products, beans, oysters, broccoli
Chlorine	Fluid and acid/base balance, forms gastric juices (HCl)	Hypotension, hair loss	Table salt, ripe olives, rye flour
Fluorine	Bones & teeth mineralization	Decay susceptible	Fluoridated water, seafood
Iodine	Thyroid function & hormones	Enlarged thyroid (goiter), hypothyroidism	Iodized salt, seafood
Iron	Combines with protein to form hemoglobin	Anemia, fatigue, glossitis, angular cheilosis, xerostomia	Meat, poultry, fish liver, nuts, beans
Magnesium	Bone mineralization, neurotransmission, heart muscle contraction, enzymes	Disorientation, muscle tremors (tetany), gingival hypertrophy, arrhythmias	Green vegetables, soybeans, milk, seafood
Manganese	Activates enzymes to synthesize fat & cholesterol, regulate glucose	Inability to remove sugar, uncoordinated muscles, convulsions	Egg yolks, nuts, legumes, whole-grain cereals
Phosphorus	Bone & teeth mineralization, ATP energy to replicate DNA & RNA, muscle contraction	Decay susceptible, stunted growth from poor bone quality	Milk, meats, eggs, beans, cheese, poultry, fish
Potassium	Acid/base balance, sodium potassium pump of the heart, nerve conduction	Arrhythmias, loss of muscle tone, lethargy, impaired CNS	Bananas, sweet potatoes, meat, fruits, vegetables
Selenium	Antioxidant protection, thyroid hormone, tissue elasticity, immune function	Tissue constriction, cardiomyopathy, inability to fight off viruses	Meats, dairy products, fish, grains, broccoli
Sodium	Acid/base balance, sodium potassium pump of the heart, nerve conduction	Arrhythmias, hypotension	Table salt, ripe olives, soy sauce, seafood, meat

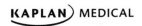

VITAMINS

Vitamins also help the body to maintain homeostasis. They are organic molecules that cannot be produced by the body, and as a result, need to be ingested daily. Since the body does not have to break down the vitamin molecules, they can be utilized by cells immediately. When taken daily—either in food or as a supplement—these micronutrients aid in growth, immunity, digestion, and mental alertness. The body is able to store some vitamins, such as vitamin A.

Water-Soluble Vitamins

Water-soluble vitamins are soluble in water and are excreted by the body when they are not needed. A deficiency in **vitamin B1 (thiamin)** can cause **beri beri**, the degeneration of the nervous system, digestive system, and heart. **Vitamin B3 (niacin)** can be synthesized from **tryptophan**; a deficiency in this can cause **pellagra**.

Vitamin B12 is **absorbed** in the stomach because of **intrinsic factor**. Intrinsic factor is a protein, produced by glands in the stomach lining, that is needed for absorption of vitamin B12. Alcoholics lack intrinsic factor to absorb B12 and are prone to pernicious anemia.

Vitamin C prevents **scurvy** but also aids in healing connective tissue by helping to produce collagen. **Folic acid** is important for women before and during **pregnancy**, in the prevention of **neural tube defects**.

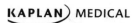

Water-Soluble Vitamins

Vitamin	Essential for	Deficiency	Foods
B1 (thiamin)	Neurotransmission of acetylcholine, heart function, digestion	Beriberi, myocardial failure, loss of appetite, disorientation, burning of oral mucosa	Pork, nuts, legumes, grains, fish, brown rice
B2 (riboflavin)	Metabolism of carbohydrates, fats & protein, red blood cell formation	Oral inflammations, glossitis, cheilosis, cornea problems, anemia	Dairy products, green vegetables, nuts, grains, lean meats
B3 niacin (nicotinic acid)	Metabolism of carbohydrates, fats & protein, neural function, healthy skin	Angular cheilosis, glossitis, neuritis, dermatitis, dementia, loss of appetite, diarrhea, pellagra	Legumes, dairy products, meats, green leafy vegetables, yeast
B5 (pantothenic acid)	Metabolism of carbohydrates, fats & protein, growth, reproduction	Impairs all body systems, depression, weakened immune system, cardiac instability	Organs meats legumes, fish, dairy products, avocado
B6 (pyridoxine)	Enzymes cofactor for 120 enzymes, metabolism of amino acids	Dermatitis, glossitis, cheilosis, anemia, mental impairment	White meats, legumes, bananas, grains, cabbage
B12 (cobalamin)	Nucleic acid synthesis, blood cell formation	Pernicious anemia, weakness, neuritis	Meats, dairy products, eggs, fish
Biotin (vitamin H)	Enzyme function to catalyze fats and glucose	Impaired fat metabolism, dermatitis, gingivitis, cheilosis	Eggs, dairy products, legumes
Folic acid B9 (folate)	Amino acid metabolism, red blood cell formation, cell division	Prebirth neural tube defects, megaloblastic anemia, tongue depapillation	Citrus fruits, green leafy vegetables, grains, legumes
C (ascorbic acid)	Controls infection, aids connective tissue healing, healthy gingiva	Scurvy, swollen gingiva, hemorrhages, delayed healing	Citrus fruits, tomato, green pepper, melon, strawberries

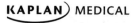

Fat-Soluble Vitamins

Fat-soluble vitamins are soluble in fats and can be stored in the body. **Vitamin A** is necessary for good vision. **Vitamin D** absorbs and retains **calcium** and **phosphorus** to aid in the formation of healthy bones and teeth. Too much **vitamin E** interferes with the absorption of **vitamin K**, which is essential for **blood clotting**. Vitamin K is absorbed in the large intestine and goes to the liver to produce prothrombin for clotting.

Fat-Soluble Vitamins

Vitamin	Essential for	Deficiency	Foods
A (beta carotene) Chemical name: Retinol	Eyesight, white blood cells, bone formation, healthy skin, cell growth & repair	Night blindness, poor bone formation, weakened immune system, xerostomia	Carrots, colored fruits and vegetables, dairy
D (calciferol) called the sunshine vitamin	Bone & teeth mineralization, calcium absorption, blood clotting	Caries prone, rickets (children), osteomalacia (adults), myopia, tetany	Dairy, fatty fish, cereals, egg yolks, tuna, margarine
E (tocopherol)	Prevention of blood clots & heart disease, antioxidant properties, potency	Sterility, hemolytic anemia, weakened immune system	Vegetable oil, seed oils, dark green leafy vegetables, wheat germ
K (phylloquinone)	Blood clotting, normal liver function	Prolonged bleeding	Dark green leafy vegetables, kiwi, cauliflower, cabbage

WATER

Water is the primary medium for determining how cells interact at the intracellular and the extracellular levels. Needless to say, it is an essential nutrient. Its functions are many. Water:

- Keeps in check the acid–base balance and the sodium–potassium pump in the heart
- Aids in the transport of blood, nerve conduction, osmotic pressure, and nutrients
- Eliminates waste and toxins
- Repairs and builds cells
- Lubricates
- Regulates body temperature
- Aids in cellular respiration and in organ-system function

Normally, the body cannot survive without water for more than three days.

ANTIOXIDANTS

Free-radicals are unstable atoms that need an electron to complete their shell. An unstable atom will attack another atom to steal its electron, making the newly attacked cell a free-radical. That free-radical goes on to look for another atom to steal away its electron.

When the free-radical production become excessive, the free-radicals join together in groups of molecules. At that stage, they form into a chain and do damage to cell membranes or DNA. Cells will perform poorly or die.

Antioxidants interfere with the free-radical chains before they can damage cells. Antioxidants include vitamins E, C, and beta carotene.

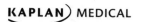

NUTRITIONAL DISORDERS

Nutritional disorders have a direct effect on the body systems and their ability to function properly, whether they involve insufficient nutritional intake or cause an inability to absorb nutrients.

Anorexia Nervosa

Anorexia nervosa means literally, "starving to death." It is commonly seen in over-achievers or perfectionists. The patient is typically a female who has an intense fear of gaining weight, and denies that her weight is too low. She stops eating, and multiple-organ system failure can lead to death.

Many individuals with anorexia are withdrawn and irritable, and suffer from depression.

Signs & symptoms: Weigh 85% or less of ideal body weight, **lanugo** (downy hair growth), low blood pressure and pulse, low body temperature, body system failure

Bulimia Nervosa

With **bulimia nervosa**, a patient eats but also purges afterward in private, with the feeling that her eating is out of control. Usually, these individuals are at normal or near-normal weight, though this could also be the result of the use of laxatives or diuretics.

Many individuals with bulimia suffer from self-doubt, deep anger, and depression.

Signs & symptoms: Calloused knuckles from purging, swelling of the parotid glands, erosion of the maxillary anterior teeth from stomach acid when purging, inflamed esophagus

Kwashiorkor

Kwashiorkor is a nutrition disorder that is seen in children living in impoverished areas. It is caused by a **lack of protein**. A child with this disorder may not reach his full growth potential, and in severe cases, may have permanent disabilities.

Signs & symptoms: Large abdomen due to liver enlargement, low weight, dermatitis

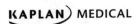

Marasmus

Marasmus is a protein-energy deficiency seen in children from impoverished areas. It results after chronic **inadequate protein** consumption during the first year of life. It causes growth retardation and the wasting away of fat and muscle.

Signs & symptoms: Low weight, loss of fat stores, weakness

Phenylketonuria

Phenylketonuria (PKU) is a genetic disorder caused by a deficiency in the enzyme phenylalanine hydroxylase. Loss of this enzyme could result in mental retardation and organ damage once phenylalanine builds up in the blood. If put on a proper diet, children born with this disorder can live a normal life.

Celiac Disease

People with Celiac disease cannot absorb glutens such as wheat, rye or barley. Glutens absorbed in the villi actually destroy the villi of the small intestine causing malnourishment. A dental visit may be the first time a dentist may send a patient to a gastroenterologist to be diagnosed with this disease. Defects in the enamel such as white, yellow, or brown spots may be an indication of celiac disease as well as pitting, banding, poor enamel formation, mottled or translucent teeth. It may be genetic, can occur during pregnancy, postpartum, with stress or after a viral infection.

Treatment is a gluten free diet and cosmetic dentistry.

Signs & Symptoms: White, yellow, or brown spots on enamel, pitting, banding, poor enamel formation, mottled or translucent teeth

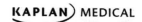

REVIEW QUESTIONS

1. Carbohydrates are stored in the liver as

   A. Glucose
   B. Glucagon
   C. Glycoside
   D. Glycoprotein
   E. Glycogen

2. Which of the following vitamins is found in broccoli, strawberries, green peppers, tomatoes, and melons?

   A. Ascorbic acid
   B. Biotin
   C. Vitamin B1
   D. Vitamin B5
   E. Vitamin E

3. Which of the following conditions causes knuckles to be calloused and parotid glands to swell?

   A. Marasmus
   B. Anorexia nervosa
   C. Bulimia nervosa
   D. Kwashiorkor

4. Omega-3 fatty acids help to improve all of the following conditions EXCEPT

   A. High blood pressure
   B. Rheumatoid arthritis
   C. Triglycerides
   D. Increases blood clotting
   E. Depression

5. Which of the following is NOT a fat-soluble vitamin?

   A. A
   B. C
   C. D
   D. K
   E. E

6. A high intake of which of the following vitamins interferes with synthesis of vitamin K, necessary for blood clotting?

   A. D
   B. E
   C. Biotin
   D. Folic acid
   E. C

7. The body can synthesize triglycerides from

   A. Animal products
   B. Saturated fats
   C. Alcohol
   D. All of the above

8. Simple and complex carbohydrates break down into different simpler sugars that are absorbed by cells. The breakdown of maltose results in

   A. Galactose
   B. Fructose
   C. Sucrose
   D. Lactose
   E. Two glucose molecules

9. Bile is produced by the liver and stored in the gallbladder. Which of the following hormones stimulates bile release?

    A. Cholecystokinin
    B. Chymotrypsinogen
    C. Amylase
    D. Prostaglandins

10. Which of the following vitamins aids in the absorption of calcium and phosphorus?

    A. Vitamin C
    B. Vitamin D
    C. Vitamin E
    D. Vitamin K
    E. Vitamin B12

11. Trace minerals help to keep our bodies in balance. The minerals essential for water balance in the body are

    A. Sodium and iodine
    B. Potassium and phosphorus
    C. Chlorine and iron
    D. Sodium and potassium
    E. Calcium and magnesium

12. Phenylketonuria (PKU) is a genetic disorder that can cause mental retardation. It is caused by a deficiency in which of the following enzymes?

    A. Tyrosine hydroxylase
    B. Tryptophan hydroxylase
    C. Phenylalanine hydroxylase
    D. Phenyl
    E. Phenytoin

13. Carboxypeptidase is an enzyme needed for

    A. Removing amino acids from peptides.
    B. Converting carbohydrates into maltose.
    C. Converting triglycerides into monoglycerides.
    D. Converting fats into glycerol.

14. All the following statements are true about free-radicals EXCEPT

    A. They do damage to DNA and cell membranes.
    B. They are unstable atoms looking to steal an electron from another cell.
    C. Vitamin D interferes with them.
    D. They form together in chains.
    E. Cell performance becomes poor.

15. Which of the following hormones aids in increasing blood-glucose levels?

    A. Oxytocin
    B. ACTH
    C. Insulin
    D. Thyroxine
    E. Thymosin

16. All of the following are symptoms of anorexia nervosa EXCEPT

    A. Lanugo
    B. Brittle nails
    C. Weight less than 50% of normal weight for height
    D. Low blood pressure
    E. Low body temperature

17. A patient on blood thinner would have to be cautious about eating too many green leafy vegetables that contain

    A. Vitamin E
    B. Vitamin K
    C. Vitamin A
    D. Folic acid
    E. Ascorbic acid

18. Beri beri causes cardiac and neuromuscular problems and is still common in southeast Asia. A deficiency in which of the following vitamins causes beri beri?

    A. Vitamin A
    B. Vitamin C
    C. Vitamin E
    D. Vitamin B1

19. Years ago, sailors who were out at sea for long periods acquired scurvy, a breakdown of connective tissue in bones, dentin, and capillaries that ultimately causes bleeding. Scurvy is caused by a deficiency in

    A. Vitamin B1
    B. Vitamin D
    C. Vitamin B2
    D. Vitamin C

20. Water is essential for all life forms. It helps human beings with all of the following EXCEPT

    A. The regulation of body temperature
    B. Waste elimination
    C. Lubrication
    D. Cellular respiration
    E. Muscle contraction

21. To prevent neural tube defects in infants, which of the following vitamins must a mother take before and during pregnancy?

    A. Niacin
    B. Biotin
    C. Folic acid
    D. Ascorbic acid

22. When the body is deficient in vitamins, it tries to correct those deficiencies by synthesizing from other substances. What vitamin can be synthesized from tryptophan?

    A. Vitamin B1 (thiamin)
    B. Vitamin B2 (riboflavin)
    C. Vitamin B3 (niacin)
    D. Vitamin B6 (pyridoxine)
    E. Vitamin B12 (cobalamin)

23. Oral manifestations can occur as a result of nutritional deficiencies. A deficiency in which the following vitamins can cause oral inflammation, glossitis, and cheilosis?

    A. Vitamin A
    B. Vitamin B2
    C. Vitamin B5
    D. Vitamin C

24. Cheilosis is caused by a deficiency in all of the following EXCEPT

    A. Vitamin B2
    B. Vitamin B3
    C. Vitamin B6
    D. Vitamin B9

25. Which of the following dietary habits would put a patient at greatest risk for a high caries rate?

    A. Sipping soda during the day
    B. Eating a candy bar for a quick snack
    C. Having cake for dessert
    D. Drinking unsweetened tea

ANSWER EXPLANATIONS

1. E

Glycogen is carbohydrate that is stored in the liver.

A. Glucose is used by cells to maintain life.

B. Glucagon is produced in the pancreas by the alpha cells. Glugagon utilizes the stores of glycogen in the liver when blood glucose gets too low.

C. Glycoside is a sugar derivative that, after bonding with a non-sugar molecule, hydrolyzes it into a sugar.

D. Glycoprotein is a protein that bonded to a glucose molecule.

2. A

Ascorbic acid—vitamin C—is found in broccoli, strawberries, green peppers, tomatoes, and melons.

B. Biotin, or vitamin H, is found in eggs, dairy, and legumes.

C. B1 is thiamine found in pork, nuts, legumes, and fish.

D. B5 is pantothenic acid found in organ meats, fish, and dairy.

E. Vitamin E is found in vegetable oil, seed oils, dark green leafy vegetables, and wheat germ.

3. C

Symptoms for bulimia nervosa include calloused knuckles, swelling of the parotid glands, and erosion of the maxillary anterior teeth due to significant stomach acid.

A. Marasmus is a protein deficiency that can lead to low growth potential and permanent disabilities.

B. Anorexia nervosa is starving to death due to no caloric intake.

D. Kwashiorkor is a protein deficiency that can lead to the wasting away of fat and muscle tissue.

4. D

Omega-6 fatty acids help to promote blood clotting. Omega-3 reduces one's chances for thrombosis with blood clotting.

5. B

Vitamin C is not fat-soluble. A, D, E, and K are fat-soluble.

6. B

Vitamin E interferes with synthesis of vitamin K.

7. D

Triglycerides can be synthesized from animal products, saturated fats, and alcohol. Triglycerides are stored in fat tissue, and have been linked with heart disease and high cholesterol.

8. E

The breakdown of maltose results in the formation of two glucose molecules.

A. Galactose is the byproduct of lactose breakdown.

B. Fructose is the breakdown of fruits and honey.

C. Sucrose breaks down into glucose and fructose.

D. Lactose breaks down into glucose and galactose.

9. A

Cholecystokinin, a hormone, stimulates bile release.

B. Chymotrypsinogen is a pancreatic enzyme that breaks down proteins into peptides.

C. Amylase is a starch enzyme that breaks down carbohydrates.

D. Prostaglandins are fats, not enzymes, that help to regulate blood pressure and circulation.

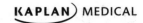

10. B

Vitamin D aids in the absorption of calcium and phosphorus.

11. D

Sodium and potassium are essential for water balance in the body.

A. Sodium is necessary in acid–base balance, but iodine is needed for thyroid function and hormones.

B. Potassium is necessary but phosphorus is necessary for bone and teeth mineralization.

C. Chlorine is necessary but iron is needed for hemoglobin to transport oxygen.

E. Calcium is necessary for muscle contraction and magnesium activates protein enzymes.

12. C

Phenylketonuria (PKU) is a genetic disorder. Lack of the hormone phenylalanine hydroxylase causes a build-up of phenylalanine in the blood. That, in turn, can cause mental retardation.

A. If deficient, tyrosine hydroxylase results in rigid arms and legs.

B. Tryptophan hydroxylase can be synthesized by the body from niacin.

D. Phenyl is a benzene derivative.

E. Phenytoin is a seizure medication.

13. A

Carboxypeptidase is an enzyme necessary for removing amino acids from peptides.

B. Amylase converts carbohydrates into maltose.

C. Pancreatic lipase converts triglycerides into monoglycerides.

D. Gastric lipase converts fats into glycerol.

14. C

Vitamin D does not interfere with free-radicals. Vitamins E and C do, as does beta carotene.

15. D

Thyroxine helps to increase blood glucose levels.

A. Oxytocin produced in the hypothalamus contracts the uterus before and after birth, to reduce it to its normal size.

B. ACTH is produced by the anterior pituitary gland to influence the adrenal glands to release cortisol.

C. Insulin is the hormone produced by the pancreas that allows glucose to enter into cells, thereby decreasing blood glucose levels.

E. Thymosin is produced in the thymus to stimulate immunity.

16. C

A patient suffering from anorexia nervosa weighs less than 85% of the ideal weight for her height.

17. B

A patient on blood thinners would not want to ingest a lot of vitamin K (needed for blood clotting), something found in green leafy vegetables. An excessive amount of vitamin K will reverse the effects of the blood thinner.

A. Vitamin E interferes with the absorption of vitamin K.

C. Vitamin A aids in white blood-cell formation.

D. Folic acid aids in red blood-cell formation.

E. Ascorbic acid is vitamin C necessary for healthy connective tissue.

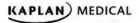

18. D

Beri beri is a deficiency in vitamin B1.

A. Vitamin A deficiency causes night blindness, poor bone formation, and xerostomia.

B. Vitamin C deficiency causes scurvy.

C. Vitamin E deficiency causes hemolytic anemia and a weakened immune system.

19. D

Vitamin C deficiency results in scurvy.

A. Vitamin B1 deficiency causes beri beri, myocardial failure, disorientation, and burning mucosal tissues.

B. Vitamin D deficiency causes poor bone and tooth formation.

C. Vitamin B2 deficiency causes oral inflammations and glossitis.

20. E

Muscles contain water and do have cellular respiration, but it is calcium that actually makes muscles contract.

21. C

To prevent neural tube defects, folic acid is essential before and during pregnancy.

22. C

Vitamin B3 (niacin) can be synthesized from tryptophan.

23. B

Oral inflammations, glossitis, and cheilosis can be caused by a deficiency of vitamin B2.

A. Vitamin A deficiency can cause night blindness, poor bone formation, and xerostomia.

C. B5 deficiency can impair the immune system and cause cardiac instability.

D. Vitamin C deficiency can cause scurvy, hemorrhages, and delayed healing.

24. D

A deficiency in B9 (folic acid) does not cause cheilosis.

25. A

Drinking soda all day would put a patient at greatest risk for a high caries rate. Drinking so much soda bathes the teeth in sugar all day.

Chapter Thirteen: **Dental Materials**

When a patient has restorative needs, he is bound to have related questions. There are many options available to those needing to replace diseased or missing teeth. Having knowledge about the different materials available will enable the dental hygienist to help the patient make an informed decision.

STRUCTURES AND PROPERTIES

Dental materials can be classified into four categories: ceramics, composites, metals, and polymers. Each category has its own properties: biological, chemical, electrical, mechanical, physical, and thermal.

Mechanical Properties

The mechanical properties needed to withstand the dynamic forces of mastication include stress and strain. The biting force of human beings is about 125–150 pounds at the molar areas, with less force moving anteriorly. People with dentures or partials have a lower biting force of about 25–30 pounds.

Stress is a measure of how much force is applied to a material and also how the material resists that force. Strain measures how a portion or length of a material deforms when a force is applied.

A stress-strain curve measures different types of forces applied to a material, such as elasticity, resilience, hardness, strength, and compression.

The elastic modulus measures how stiff a material is—a material's ability to resist deformity. Resilience is its ability to absorb energy and not become deformed when force is applied.

Hardness is the ability of a material to resist indentation. The most widely used test for hardness is Knoops hardness, which uses a diamond indenter. Other tests include Brinell, which uses a steel ball; Vickers, which uses a square-based diamond point; and Rockwell, which measures the difference in depth caused by two different forces. Mohs scale measures rigidity and resistance to pressure and being scratched.

Stress Forces

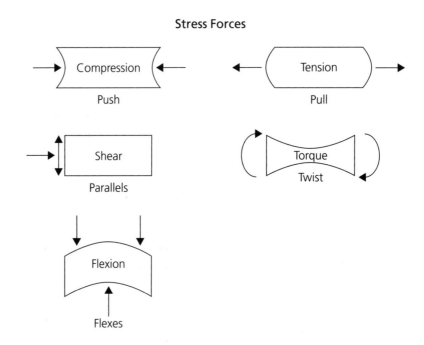

Materials need to have strength to withstand the forces of mastication. Ultimate strength is the point at which you can apply the most force to a material just before it breaks or fails. If a material fails due to a compressive stress, then it withstood a compressive strength. If it fails due to a shear stress, then it withstood a shear strength. A failure under tension is a tensile strength.

Physical Properties

The physical properties of a material—its composition—always remain constant. These properties include weight, volume, density, mass, boiling point, melting point, and vapor pressure.

Percent of elongation is the extent to which a material can be stretched before it ruptures or breaks. Compression measures how ductile or malleable a material is. Both ductility and malleability go hand-in-hand with deformation. If deformation occurs <5% of fracture, then a material is considered brittle. If deformation occurs >5% of fracture, it is considered ductile.

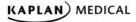

Thermal Properties

Restorative materials need to withstand the properties of thermal changes, with metal having a higher conductivity rate than polymers or ceramics. Restorative materials do not have the same thermal expansion rates as do the different tooth structures. A coefficient of thermal expansion measures a material's change in length per degree of temperature change. In the illustration below, a change in temperature (heating) caused a fractional expansion of length of the material.

Linear Thermal Expansion:
Material Change (Δ) in Length from Heat

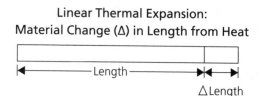

Since amalgam and composites restorations have 2–5 times the expansion and contraction rates as tooth structures, they have a direct effect on fluids penetrating the junction of restoration and tooth structure. The penetration or movement of fluids in and out of this juncture is called **percolation**. Microleakage goes hand-in-hand with percolation, causing recurrent decay. Creep is the permanent breakdown of a restoration's margin where percolation and microleakage have occurred.

> With percolation, microleakage occurs down the side of a restoration.

Thermal conductivity is the amount of heat transferred. Some dental materials have greater thermal conductivity than others. Think of a metal pan on a stove, for instance, that has a metal handle. The pan itself is over the heat and becomes hot, but heat is also transferred to the metal handle. Amalgam fillings have a higher thermal conductivity than other dental restorations such as composites.

Wettability

Wettability is the ability of a dental material to flow and contact all the surfaces it needs to touch. For instance, a cement liner is wettable in that it needs to flow and make contact with all surfaces of the cavity preparation. Flow also depends on the viscosity or thickness of a material. How much wetting occurs also depends on the surface energy that the material is being applied to.

Sorption

Sorption or sorb is a material's ability to pick up and retain fluids by absorption or adsorption. Some dental materials exposed to saliva are more soluble in the mouth. An example of sorption would be the loss of an onlay due to the dissolution of the cement that was retaining it.

Imbibition is a material's ability to take up fluids, such as mixing water with an alginate impression material. Syneresis is the loss of fluid, as in a dried alginate impression that was not poured right away. The distorted dried impression would not be a representation of the model it needed to be.

Chemical Bonds

Chemical bonding occurs with the juncture of two or more atoms. A **primary bond** is a strong bond between the atoms of a dental material. Primary bonds include ionic, covalent, and metallic bonds. An **ionic bond** occurs when one or more electrons from an atom are displaced and attach to another atom. The end result is positive and negative ions that attract each other. A **covalent bond** occurs when one or more pairs of electrons are shared by two atoms. A **hydrogen bond** is a common bond where hydrogen is attracted to highly electronegative elements like oxygen and fluorine. This makes a weaker bond. A **metallic bond** shares outer electrons by all of the atoms in an electron cloud. Since the electrons are free to move about, this allows for good electrical and thermal conductivity.

A **secondary bond**—a weak bond—provides a fragile link that can deform or fracture easily. In van der Waals forces, the moving electrons tend to shift to one side of the atom, causing that side to be slightly more negative. The negative side tends to attract a positive atom.

Electrical Properties

Some dental materials such as metal have the ability to conduct electrons. This can occur with galvanization or corrosion. Galvanization occurs when two dissimilar metals touch and produce an electrical current, and cause a sharp pain. Corrosion occurs when two dissimilar adjacent metals produce galvanic corrosion, or oxidation of the metal. Corrosion may also occur from substances in different foods, causing tarnish on the surface of the amalgam.

Biological Properties

Biological properties are the effects that dental materials can have on tissues or cells. Patients can have a sensitivity to certain dental materials, such as an allergy to nickel. In response to the sensitivity, tissues become fibrous or inflamed, requiring replacement with a less reactive material.

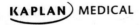

FILLING MATERIALS

Amalgams

One of the oldest filling materials is dental amalgam filling, a mixture of metal powders triturated with mercury. Dental amalgam is a cost-effective material that has a prolonged longevity. When mixed or triturated, the putty-like metal is condensed easily into the cavity preparation, flowing into proximal contacts. After the cavity preparation is filled to excess, it is carved easily to the proper tooth anatomy.

The particles of amalgam can have an irregular or spherical shape, or they can be a bit of both (called admixed alloy). The metal powders are made up of silver, copper, tin, and zinc. Silver and copper give the filling strength, while the tin reduces expansion. Tin, however, has a strong affinity for the mercury, and it attracts it away from the copper, thus weakening the restoration. Zinc, if present, minimizes oxidation of the metal.

Mercury is a metal that is liquid at room temperature. Mercury dissolves the metals but is also absorbed into the particles of the powder. Before the invention of precapsulated amalgams, mercury was mixed with the powder by mortar and pestle. Excess mercury was squeezed out with a cheesecloth, exposing dental personnel to mercury through both the handling of the substance and the inhalation of its vapors. Today, precapsulation of the compressed powder with mercury provides the proper mixing ratio.

There has been much controversy over mercury toxicity for individuals with amalgam fillings. Research has shown that a minute amount of mercury vapor (1–2 μg per day) is indeed given off, though this miniscule amount has not been proven to have adverse health effects (except, perhaps, for someone who is allergic to mercury).

Years ago, the metals had a lower content of copper, but over time, that changed. More copper, it was discovered, produces a stronger, less-corrosive amalgam with greater longevity. The higher copper content allows more of the copper to react with the tin, thus eliminating a tin–mercury reaction. The specific amount of copper contained depends on the gamma (γ) reaction that occurs.

Gamma Reaction of Amalgam Fillings

Phase	Strength	Copper content	Metal reaction	Corrosiveness	Amalgamation reaction
Gamma (γ)	Strongest	High	Ag alloy	Resistant	Contraction
Gamma 1 (γ_1)		Low or high	Ag-Hg		Expansion
Gamma 2 (γ_2)	Weakest	Low	Sn-Hg	Prone	
εια (η)			Cu-Sn		Expansion

Low copper = Gamma 2 (γ_2) reaction yields a weak restoration

High copper = Elimination of the gamma 2 (γ_2) reaction

Proper manipulation during trituration and condensation yields a successfully placed restoration.

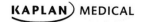

If an amalgam filling is undertriturated (mixed), it will appear to have a dull, crumbly surface. Undertrituration produces voids, which make the filling less strong due to insufficient $\gamma 1$ and η particles cohering. Overtriturated restorations are soupy and have less strength. They are more prone to corrosion because they have excessive $\gamma 1$ and η particles.

If the restoration is not properly condensed, it produces gaps, making it prone to leakage. The cavity preparation is packed in excess of what is needed and then carved to the desirable tooth anatomy. If moisture contamination occurs during condensation and setting, the integrity of the restoration is disturbed.

Creep occurs when the margin of an amalgam restoration loses its integrity. Creep allows microleakage to occur, causing recurrent decay, though this occurs more often with low copper restorations than with high copper ones.

Tarnish of the amalgam restoration can occur from acidic food substances reacting with the surface of the amalgam. Corrosion, however, is a deeper penetration of an acidic or chemical reaction into the amalgam restoration, and it compromises the integrity of the restoration.

> Tin oxide is used to polish amalgam fillings.

Once the restoration has been placed, polishing can be performed after 24 hours. For polishing, a green stone or finishing bur may be used, followed by fine pumice, silex, or tin oxide.

Composites and Resins

Composites are made up of a matrix and filler. The filler contributes mechanical properties to the composite, while the matrix forms the structural skeleton network. Composites contain poly-ceramic materials that mix with resin matrixes, such as dimethacrylate (Bis-GMA) or urethane dimethacrylate (UDMA) oligomers.

The thermal conductivity of composite material nearly matches the thermal conductivity of the tooth structure, providing exceptional thermal insulation. Though thermal expansion rates of composites are higher than tooth structure, more filler and less resin minimizes shrinkage during polymerization. This, in turn, decreases the rate of thermal expansion of composites.

Composites are typically used for Class III, IV, and V restorations, but are also useful for low-stress Class I and II restorations. Composites have fillers. First-generation composites contained macrofilled quartz materials that were rough to the eye and tactile sense, and are not typically used today except for orthodontic brackets.

Some newer generation composites have microfine fillers or particles composed of lithium aluminum silicate or quartz. Others include barium, strontium, ytterbium, or zinc glass.

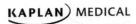

Microhybrid composites contain both fine and microfine fillers. Microfilled composites contain only microfine particles. The surfaces of the fillers are treated with silane-coupling agents that ensure that the fillers chemically bond to the resin matrix. The silanated particles are then mixed with pigments, initiators, accelerants, and monomers.

Common resin matrixes such as dimethacrylate monomer are 2,2-bis[4-(2-hydroxy-3-methacryloyloxypropoxy)phenyl]propane (Bis-GMA) or urethane dimethacrylate (UDMA) oligomers. These viscous liquids combine with the fillers or particles to become the composite polymer.

Initiators commence the polymerization (setting up) of the composite by exposing it to an intense blue light. Light-cured composites have nearly an unlimited amount of time to work with the material, and are set or polymerized in 20–40 seconds. With self -curing composites, the initiator is organic peroxide, which is mixed with an organic amine accelerator. When mixed, self-curing composites have 1–2 minutes of working time.

Since most people have various shades of teeth, pigments from yellow to gray are added.

To condition the tooth, the tooth surface is etched before the composite is placed. A gel or solution of 37% phosphoric acid for 30 seconds is recommended for fourth- and fifth-generation composites. The tooth is rinsed thoroughly for 5–10 seconds, then dried for another 5–10 seconds.

Single-use compules of composites can be flowed via a syringe directly into the preparation. 20–30-second light exposure is required for polymerization.

When self-cured composites are properly mixed, they can be placed in a preparation with a plastic instrument within 1–2 minutes of mixing. Self-cured composites set 4–5 minutes from the onset of mixing.

Finishing composites may be accomplished with carbide bur, diamonds, or stones for gross reduction. For a finer finish, special diamonds, finishing disks, or a rubber prophy cup with polishing pastes can be used.

Glass Ionomers

Glass ionomers are an ideal restoration for anyone with a high caries index or for class V restorations. Research has shown that glass ionomers have a better retention rate in class V areas than do composites.

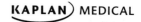

Glass ionomers contain an aluminosilicate glass that includes ground fluoride and is mixed with a liquid solution of polyacrylic acid (copolymer). When the components are mixed, an acid-base chemical reaction occurs as aluminum and calcium ions react with the acid groups in the polymers. Half the powder is incorporated into the polymer until a creamy texture is achieved, at which point the second half is incorporated. With that, a viscous restoration is produced. Mixing time is 30–40 seconds with a set time of about 4 minutes.

Glass ionomers are ideal for Class V restorations. | The fluoride seeps out of the restoration for about 2 years after placement, and is absorbed into neighboring tooth structures. Research has show that significantly fewer *S. mutans* reside on the tooth surface in the area of the glass ionomers.

Compomers

Compomers are a new type of material that combine the advantages of composites ("comp") with the benefits of glass ionomer ("omer"). This polyacid-modified composite resin contains a filler that incorporates a fluoride ion-leachable glass, similar to the one in glass iomoners. This resin releases a low level of fluoride that is reported to discharge into surrounding tooth structures for about 300 days.

One disadvantage of compomers is that they do not bond to hard tooth structure, so they must be placed in low-stress bearing areas. Compomers have a low compressive and flexural strength.

Bonding Agents

Many improvements have been made in bonding materials and techniques over the years. Dentistry is now using what are termed 6th- and 7th-generation materials. These materials adhere to surfaces by micromechanical bonding, which adheres to both dentin and enamel.

After a tooth is prepared for a restoration, a smear layer (a thin layer of dentinal debris) remains in the dentin tubules. The smear layer weakly adheres to the preparation surface, and is ultimately eliminated by etching the tooth surface with 37% phosphoric acid. The acid also decalcifies dentin into microspaces for micromechanical adhesion of the bonding material.

After etching the tooth, the surface needs to be primed with a hydrophilic resin. This resin flows into and penetrates surface irregularities that occur from etching. Next, an adhesive material or bond is applied to the surface with viscous resin, which penetrates any exposed collagen. This provides retention to dentin.

Newer generations of bonding materials contain acidic primers/adhesives that eliminate the etching step. Once the bonding is completed, the restoration material adheres to the bonding layer.

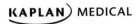

Liners and Cements

Cements are poor thermal conductors that provide superb thermal insulation for deep carious lesions. When the lesion is deep, a smaller amount of remaining dentin does not provide ample thermal insulation. Cement's primary role is to aid in the retention of restorations. In lower strengths, it may also be used for pulp capping.

Cement is also used for the cementation of crowns, bridges, inlays, onlays, veneers, and orthodontic appliances. A thicker application may be used as a temporary filling.

Used in conjunction with a varnish, cement can provide an electrical insulating barrier. Varnishes decrease the amount of percolation that contributes to thermal expansion thus preventing corrosive amalgam products from entering the tooth surface. Varnishes include copal resin (Copalite). The varnish solvent evaporates after application, yielding a permeable resinous coating. Composites or resins interfere with the varnish coating and so are contraindicated with its use.

Glass ionomer cement contains fluoride-releasing powder in aluminosilicate glass, which mixes with polyacrylic acid. This combination makes for the strongest, least-permeable cement that provides a superior high-strength base. Its ability to leach fluoride makes it an ideal cement for someone with a high caries rate. Plus, its nonirritating qualities allow for a superior compatibility with many alloys—including stainless steel crowns. All and all, it is a popular luting or bonding material.

Hybrid ionomer cement is permanent water-based cement that is ideal for crowns, bridges, orthodontic appliances, core build-ups, and posts. It contains fluoroaluminosilicate glass that mixes with aqueous polyacrylic acid, making it a high-strength base. This type of cement is known for its compressive and tensile strength, minimal sensitivity, and release or leach of fluoride.

Resin cement is used with ceramic crowns, inlays, onlays, veneers, and bridges such as Maryland bridges. It is composed of microhybrid or microfilled glass dimethacrylate resin, with the latter resin being the stronger of the two. The tooth and ceramic restoration are etched prior to placement or sandblasting with alumina. Silane is also applied before placement, to provide for a good bond.

Compomer cement is used for gold inlays and onlays, cast alloy crowns, bridges, and porcelain fused to metal crowns and bridges. This polyacid modified composite resin contains strontium aluminum fluorosilicate glass with sodium fluoride, and is noted for its high retention and bond strength.

Zinc phosphate cement is used for luting (bonding) crowns, bridges, inlays, and orthodontic appliances and bands. It is a water-based cement that contains zinc oxide powder and phosphoric acid in water. The acidity of this porous mixture is

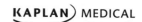

a pulp irritant, so a base, liner, or varnish is needed to protect the pulp. Powder should be added in small increments to liquid and done on a cool glass slab, since an exothermic chemical reaction occurs. When the mixture is thin, it can be used as a luting (bonding) agent; if thicker, it can be used as a base.

Zinc polycarboxylate cement is an aqueous permanent cement used as an intermediate base for crowns and bridges. It lacks the compressive strength of glass ionomers, and has moderate solubility. It is a powder of zinc oxide and a viscous polyacrylic acid in water, mixed on a pad or cool glass slab. Ninety percent of the powder should be mixed into aqueous acid, and then added in small increments.

Zinc oxide and eugenol (ZOE) is widely used in dentistry as an impression material, temporary cement, temporary filling, bonding agent, periodontal dressing, and base. ZOE cement is a low-strength base that is an oil-based obtundant when used for its sedative effects. It is a temporary cement because of its solubility. When mixed to a thin consistency, it can be used as a luting (bonding) material. With a putty-like consistency, it can be used as a base or temporary restoration. ZOE may also be used for root canal sealing, surgical dressings, or periodontal dressings. A large amount of powder should be mixed into the liquid on a paper or glass slab, and then added in small increments. It is also available in two-paste systems that mix equal lengths of paste.

Calcium hydroxide cement is a low-strength base that provides good thermal and electrical insulation. It can be used as a based for composite restorations or with direct or indirect pulp-capping to stimulate reparative dentin. Since newer bonding materials with higher strengths have been developed, it is not widely used today. It is a two-paste system of a base paste and catalyst paste, placed in equal lengths on a paper pad for mixing. The base paste contains calcium phosphate, calcium tungsten, and zinc oxide in glycol salicylate. The catalyst paste contains calcium hydroxide, zinc oxide filler, and zinc stearate radiopacifier in ethyl toluene sulfonamide dispersant.

DENTAL IMPLANTS

Chapter 7 discusses the implant itself, as used in periodontal procedures. Here, we will discuss the materials used for the implants, in addition to the prostheses required.

The most commonly used implant materials are "pure" titanium and titanium alloy. Both materials promote osseointegration (the border of bone develops within 100 angstroms of the implant surface) into bone. "Pure" titanium is not 100% titanium, but contains varying percentages of oxygen less than 0.5% by weight. The amount of oxygen it contains depends on the grade of the alloy. Pure titanium also

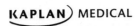

contains trace amounts of carbon, hydrogen, iron, and nitrogen. Titanium alloy contains 6% by weight aluminum, and 4% by weight vanadium, to increase twice over its tensile strength.

**Pure Titanium Trace Minerals
by Percentage of Weight**

Pure Titanium	Oxygen
Grade 1	0.18%
Grade 2	0.25%
Grade 3	0.35%
Grade 4	0.4%

Prior to implantation, the surface is coated with oxygen and titanium oxide. Research has revealed that coating the surface with ceramic contributes to a strong biointegration (fusion with no gaps) into bone.

Ceramic implants had more success than earlier polymer implants and were used prior to titanium implants. Their biological reactions and brittleness, however, make them less desirable. On the other hand, the material is nontoxic and noncorrosive, making it an ideal coating for biointegrating titanium into bone.

Fixed or removable appliances or restorations can be used with the implant. Removable over-dentures may be retained with a snappable ball and O-ring attachment or a bar implant with clips in the dentures.

A denture may also be placed permanently with screw retention. A small screw is placed into the implant or cemented permanently onto the implant. The screwed-on type of prosthesis can be removed by a dental clinician when necessary. Fixed restorations can be a single crown or multiple-unit bridges constructed of acrylic resin, porcelain, or metal.

DENTAL CERAMICS

Dental ceramics have varied uses. They can be used as ceramic teeth in dentures, porcelain fused to metal (PFM) crowns and bridges, all porcelain or ceramic crowns, veneers, inlays, and onlays. Ceramic materials consist primarily of feldspar, silica, and alumina. Porcelain also contains quartz. While ceramic can be brittle, it is known for its compressive and tensile strength, coefficient of thermal expansion, and ability to match the color of other teeth.

Resin-bonded all ceramic crowns are translucent and aesthetically pleasing, not to mention stronger than earlier ceramic crowns. Porcelain fused to metal (PFM) crowns bond layers of porcelain to a metal foundation (high gold, nickel-chromium,

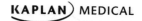

or palladium silver alloys), giving it more strength. The ceramic material that chemically bonds to the metal foundation is crucial for the prevention of fracturing of the porcelain from the metal.

An inlay is an intracoronal restoration that incorporates the occlusal and proximal surfaces and lies within the cusp tips. An onlay is a restoration that incorporates the occlusal and proximal surfaces, along with one or more of the cusps. These ceramic restorations are produced in the dental laboratory on a die, or engineered by computer on a CAD/CAM system. In addition to lab systems, there are chair-side and in-office systems.

Veneers are generally anterior extracoronal restorations that conceal stains, fractures, and defects. They are wafer-thin shells of porcelain laminate that are bonded to facial and incisal surfaces.

CASTING ALLOYS AND SOLDERS

Casting alloys are made of the noble metals of gold (Au), silver (Ag), platinum (Pt), and palladium (Pd) that are used for inlays, onlays, crowns, and bridges. Other metals include nickel, copper, titanium, zinc, and others. Gold combats corrosion, and along with silver, makes these alloys more aesthetically pleasing by hindering a coppery color. Platinum and palladium contribute to their hardness, and help to increase the melting point should solder need to be added. Copper, too, helps to strengthen them in the same way it strengthens amalgam fillings.

ADA Classification of Casting Alloys

Type	Noble metals by weight	Uses	Strength
High noble alloys	Noble metal ≥ 60%(Au, Pt, Pd) & ≥ 40% gold	Inlays, onlays	Least strong
Titanium and titanium alloys	Titanium ≥ 85%	Implants, prostheses	Strong
Noble alloys	Noble metal content ≥ 25% (gold, platinum, palladium)	Bridges, crowns	Stronger
Predominantly base alloys	Noble metal content < 25% (gold, platinum, palladium)	Bridges, crowns, partial denture fame	Strongest

[as of March 2003]

Solders join metals together, as in the case of a bracket to an orthodontic band, for instance. Flux cleanses the surface of oxides in preparation for soldering or brazing. Different fluxes are used for different metals. Silver flux is used for base metal alloys while gold flux is used for high content gold alloys.

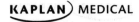

CARE OF RESTORATIONS AND POLISHING AGENTS

Polishing a restoration removes any surface irregularities that could retain plaque, which in turn could cause gingivitis or corrosion of material. Initially, a bur or coarse abrasive should be used to shape the restoration to follow the contour of the tooth. Gradual use of finer abrasives will reduce any scratches created by the higher grit abrasives.

Amalgam fillings are carved and burnished after placement and need 24 hours to set. Marginal irregularities can first be reduced with a stone or polishing disks and strips. Then, polishing takes place with slurries of pumice and tin oxide with a rubber cup or polishing cup. Care should be taken not to overheat the tooth, since amalgams have a high thermal conductivity.

Excess from composites and compomers can be finished or removed with a carbide bur, finishing bur, or diamond stone. Contouring of the tooth surface to its original shape is next, with polishing disks or white stones. Diamond polishing pastes create a high glass surface. Hybrid ionomers are finished in a similar fashion, but an unfilled resin glaze is smoothed onto the surface.

Gold restorations and other precious metals are polished in the laboratory with rouge, a red powder of iron oxide, before placement in the oral cavity.

> Rouge is used in a laboratory for polishing.

PIT AND FISSURE SEALANTS

Pit and fissure sealants have proven to be extremely beneficial as a preventive measure in the reduction of carious lesions in grooves and pits. The materials consist of filled or unfilled resins, similar to composite materials. Filled resins contain glass and quartz materials; these flowable materials can be light- or self-cured. Sealant application is discussed in Chapter 15.

> Topical fluoride is least effective in pits and fissures, and most effective on smooth surfaces.

Sealants are composed of a dimethacrylate monomer such as Bis-GMA (bisphenol A-glycidyl methacrylate) or UDMA (urethane dimethacrylte) with TEGDMA (tri-[ethylene glycol] dimethacrylte). Light exposure initiates the setting (polymerization) of an organic amine accelerator with diketone.

Sealants may be clear, white, or tinted, with some tinted materials changing to white when light-cured. The colored sealant allows the clinician to monitor placement and to remove any excessive areas prior to setting.

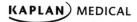

If a sealant fails, it is usually due to operator error.

Sealants mechanically bond to teeth after being etched by 37% phosphoric acid, which is applied for 15–60 seconds as per the manufacturer's recommendations. The acid should be rinsed thoroughly before the sealant is applied, since acid interferes with the bonding process.

Sealants should be placed as soon as possible after molar eruption at around age 6–12. Sealants also protect patients who have xerostomia or are in orthodontic treatment.

DESENSITIZERS

Hypersensitivity is a brief, though sharp, pain caused by painful stimuli such as extreme temperature change, chemicals, or mechanical force. The most widely accepted theory about why this occurs is the hydrodynamic theory, where fluid passes in and out of the dentinal tubules and stimulates nerve-endings (A-delta fibers).

While the application of desensitizing agents to teeth is crucial, controlling plaque is equally important. That's because an accumulation of bacterial plaque releases toxins that break down tooth structure. Carious lesions expose dentin where the tubules are open to transmit pain.

Treatment may include the application of a desensitizing agent, varnish, or bonding material. Since individual tooth structures and sensitivity levels differ, there is no single material that can be universally applied. It may be necessary to try different agents if the patient's sensitivity does not abate.

Fluoride gels, pastes, and rinses include neutral sodium and/or stannous fluoride. If they are applied at bedtime, uptake of the fluoride ion occurs overnight. Iontophoresis utilizes an electrical current to impregnate fluoride ions into the tooth surface.

FLUORIDE AND FLUORIDE VARNISHES

Whether taken orally in water, by prescription, or applied topically with toothpaste, gels, rinses, or varnishes, fluoride can significantly reduce an individual's carious lesions. See more on fluoride in Chapter 15, Oral Health Promotion.

Varnish contains 5% sodium fluoride; when applied topically, it impregnates the tooth with fluoride ions for 3–4 hours.

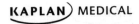

Acidulated phosphate fluoride is an ideal fluoride of 2% sodium fluoride with 0.34% hydrogen fluoride and 0.98% phosphoric acid, available in gels and foam. Application should be every 6 months. Since its acidity causes a layer of enamel to demineralize, it should not be used on those with crowns, bridges, veneers, or composite restorations.

Neutral sodium fluoride is available in 2% foam or gel. It should be applied 4 times at one-week intervals.

Stannous fluoride is an unstable fluoride with two parts that need to be mixed prior to application. It is also available as a 0.4% gel or 0.63% solution that is used as an antimicrobial to reduce gingival inflammation. Stannous fluoride can stain; it also has a harsh taste that irritates tissues.

> Neutral sodium fluoride is safe to use with crowns, veneers, bridges, and composites, though stannous and acidulated fluorides are not safe.

WAXES

Wax is used for bite registrations and impressions, and to fabricate restorations such as inlays. In the early years of dentistry, beeswax was used for this purpose.

Pattern waxes produce a reproduction of a desired restoration. Processing waxes are used to create models or aid with impressions.

Waxes Used in Dentistry

	Type	Use	Material
Inlay	Pattern	Inlays, onlays, crowns, bridges	Paraffin, ceresin, carnauba, beeswax
Casting	Pattern	Metal framework partial denture	Paraffin, ceresin, carnauba, beeswax
Baseplate	Pattern	Baseplate of denture, holds teeth	Ceresin, carnauba, beeswax
Sticky	Processing		Beeswax, rosin
Boxing	Processing	Establish base for poured impression	Paraffin, beeswax
Utility	Processing	Outline periphery of impression tray	Paraffin, beeswax
Bite registration	Processing	Model articulation	Paraffin, ceresin, beeswax
Corrective impression	Processing	Register soft tissue in an impression	Paraffin, ceresin

FLEXIBLE IMPRESSION MATERIALS

Impression materials create a duplicate of a person's teeth and surrounding tissues. The model is the positive, and the impression is the negative. Colloids are particles of polysaccharides derived from seaweed that are suspended in a liquid. Hydrocolloid means that these particles are suspended in water.

Some impression materials are considered irreversible; when set, they cannot be unset or reversed after the chemical reaction occurs. With reversible impression materials, no chemical reaction occurs, so they can exist as a sol (liquid) or a gel by raising or lowering the temperature.

All impressions should be rinsed and then properly disinfected according to the manufacturer's directions prior to pouring up the models.

Alginate Hydrocolloid

Alginate hydrocolloid impression material is one of the most popular flexible impression materials. It is an **irreversible hydrocolloid** that is frequently used for study models and bleaching or fluoride trays since it lacks the accuracy of reversible hydrocolloids. It is composed of either sodium alginate or potassium alginate powder that is mixed with water.

The water temperature controls the **set (gel) time**. For patients with a strong gag reflex, warmer water shortens the set time. Spatulation incorporates a measured amount of powder into a measured amount of water in a rubber mixing bowl until a creamy consistency is obtained.

An alginate impression is removed with a quick motion.

After placing the mixed alginate into the impression tray, **setting** or **gelation** occurs in 2–5 minutes depending on water temperature. The impression is **removed with a quick motion** to not distort the impression.

After disinfection, the alginate impression material needs to be **poured up** as soon as possible in plaster or stone to prevent **syneresis** (shrinkage from air exposure). If soaked in water, the impression takes on more water through **imbibition** causing expansion of the impression material.

Agar Hydrocolloid (Agar Agar)

The **agar** hydrocolloid impression material is a very **accurate elastic** impression material that is reversible and flexible. This particular material can be **used in undercut areas**. Agar hydrocolloid is composed of 12–15% agar, borax, potassium sulfate, benzoates, and 85% water.

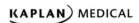

There are two "bodies." The light body (12–15% agar) is placed in the impression tray, while the heavy body (6–8% agar) is flowed by a syringe around the prepared tooth (teeth).

Agar agar may be supplied in tubes as a gel or as hardened cylindrical rolls. A roll of the agar agar is placed in a water bath at 100° C for 10-15 minutes until it becomes a sol. It is then placed in a second water bath at 60-66° C until ready for usage in an impression tray. It is squeezed into the tray and placed in a third water bath at 43-46° C, for cooling to near normal body temperature so the patient is not burned. The heavy body is flowed by syringe around the preparation prior to placement of the light body in the impression tray. When set, it is **removed with a quick snap** to prevent distortion.

Agar agar is removed with a quick snap.

Agar materials are not as widely used as the newer impression materials. Also, the expense of the three-chamber bath equipment necessary to heat the materials can be high.

Polysulfides

Polysulfide impression material is a flexible elastomer consisting of a base paste and a catalyst paste. The **base** contains low molecular-weight **mercaptan polymer** that **vulcanizes** into **polysulfide rubber** when mixed with the **catalyst** of **lead dioxide** or **copper hydroxide**. This chemical reaction yields a sulfur odor from the **mercaptan**.

The base paste and catalyst paste are placed with equal lengths onto a paper-mixing pad. The accelerator is mixed into the base for about 45 seconds until the color is homogeneous and is then placed into the tray. When set, the impression is removed with a constant force.

Silicones

There are two types of elastomer silicones; each polymerize differently. The two will be discussed separately. The silicones are supplied in different viscosities according to their molecular weight.

Composition silicones are composed of a base paste of dimethysiloxane (silicone liquid) and catalyst of ortho-ethyl silicate. The putty is scooped out and onto a mixing pad, and an indentation is made for the liquid or paste catalyst to be placed. It is mixed for 30 seconds until homogenous and placed into a perforated tray.

An initial impression is taken prior to tooth preparation by rocking the impression into place. Rocking allows for an open space around the tooth and for a wash material to be applied with the final impression. The impression is allowed to gel (set). After the tooth is prepared, a wash (thin) material is added by syringe to the initial impression. The impression is retaken until the wash is set. The impression is removed with a direct pull.

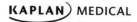

Addition silicones, known as polyvinylsiloxanes, are composed of two-putty or two-paste systems, which are used widely for crowns and bridges. A vinyl-terminated silicone monomer along with chloroplatinic acid combines with silicone hydrogen groups and fillers.

Addition silicones are supplied in 2 putties of a catalyst and base or in a gun with mixing cartridges. The putties are mixed with bare hands or with vinyl gloves until homogenous and placed into the impression tray. The gun triggers the plunger to expel the uniformly mixed base and catalyst as it spirals out the end into the impression tray. This material has a low tear strength so it should be cautiously removed.

One advantage of this impression material is that it may be disinfected and sent to the lab without pouring it up.

Polyether

Polyether is dispensed in a base of polyether with ethylene imine paste and catalyst of aromatic sulfonic acid ester. It is supplied in a two-paste system, or in a gun with mixing cartridges, or in an automatic mechanical mixer.

For mixing the pastes, equal strips are placed on a paper mixing pad and mixed until homogenous in about 45 seconds and then placed in the impression tray. The gun and automated mechanical mixer expel the uniformly mixed base and catalyst as it spirals out the end into the impression tray.

This impression is removed by gently breaking the seal and then snapping out along the long axis of the tooth.

RIGID IMPRESSION MATERIALS

Rigid impression materials have no flexibility and cannot be used on under cuts. They are best used for edentulous patients with no undercut and bite registration. Since the inception of newer materials, rigid impression materials are not widely used.

Zinc Oxide and Eugenol

Zinc oxide and eugenol is supplied in a tube of zinc oxide and oils, along with a tube of eugenol, oils, and resins. Equal strips are placed on an oil-resistant mixing pad or glass slab, mixed until homogenous and then placed in an impression tray. Set time is 3–5 minutes.

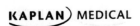

Impression Compound

Impression compounds are used for the following purposes: inspection of a cavity preparation when there is a possibility of an undercut; for preliminary impressions for a denture; and to add to the periphery of an impression or custom tray. They are supplied in cakes and sticks that are heated over a flame or by placing in hot water until softened. For the cavity preparation, the compound is gently pressed into place, cooled with a water spray, and removed. For denture patients, it is pressed over the tissues.

Impression Plaster

Impression plaster is no longer used as an impression material but is useful for mounting casts on an articulator. It is very accurate and has a short set-time.

PLASTER AND STONE

Impressions are the negative while models are the positive. Models are poured up in gypsum materials such as plaster, dental stone, or die stone, which all contain calcium sulfate hemihydrate. These products were fabricated from mineral gypsum which is a calcium sulfate dihydrate. These compounds differ in strength due to the structure and size of the hemihydrate, and the amount of excess water still held within the material when set.

When water is mixed with any of these gypsum products, the calcium sulfate hemihydrate is transformed back into a dihydrate. The water-powder ratio varies with each compound due to particle shape and size. Excess water locked into a set material reduces its strength by creating spaces.

As models set, an exothermic reaction occurs. Typically, set time is 45–60 minutes.

Plaster

Plaster is generally used for study models, bleaching trays, and fluoride trays. It is a beta (β) hemihydrate made up of small, irregular crystals. Irregular crystals need a fair amount of water, which decreases the strength of the material. Plaster has the lowest compressive strength.

Stone

Stone is used for making casts. It is an alpha (α) hemihydrate made up of large regular particles that require less water than plaster, yielding a strong material. Stone has a larger tensile strength than plaster.

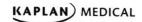

Die Stone

Die stone is used to make casts and dies. Die stone is alpha (α) hemihydrate made up of larger, dense cuboidal particles that require even less water than stone, creating an even stronger material. Die stone has 4 times the compressive strength, along with a higher tensile strength, than plaster.

ACRYLICS

Acrylic plastics are used in dentistry for full and partial dentures, resin teeth, temporary crowns and bridges, custom trays, orthodontic appliances, and mouth guards. Monomers are single organic molecules that polymerize (manufacturing of small molecule monomers into large molecules of polymer) into polymers.

Polymer = Powder
Monomer = Liquid

A frequently used dental acrylic is produced from the powder poly-methyl methacrylate resin, added to the monomer liquid of methyl methacrylate. Hydroquinone is used as an inhibitor to prevent polymerization during storage. Titianium oxide influences the amount of translucency the finished product may have. Pigments may also be added for any specific application of the material. An organic amine is used as an accelerator for cold-cured resins.

Cold- or chemical-cured acrylic resin is created when the monomer liquid of methyl methacrylate is gradually added to the poly-methyl methacrylate resin. As more powder dissolves in the liquid and the material goes from runny to a pie-dough consistency, more polymerization (linking monomers together in chains) takes place. The reaction generates heat as it becomes thicker and more rigid, as polymerization transpires.

Heat-cured acrylic resins lack the organic amine accelerator. The mixing process is the same as for the cold-cured. In this case, after the material is shaped into its desired purpose, the fabrication is placed into a heated water bath.

MOUTH PROTECTORS

Mouth protectors are advocated for all athletes playing contact sports. Custom-made mouth protectors have the best fit, are the most resilient and comfortable, and produce less gagging and speech impediment. The material used most often is polyvinyl acetate-polyethylene, created over a model of the patient's mouth.

Mouth-formed protectors are made from thermoplastic copolymer or polyurethane. The protector is lined with acrylic or rubber. The material is boiled in water for 10–45 seconds, then cooled in cold water, and then placed in the patient's mouth (with the patient biting into the material until it sets).

Stock mouth protectors are the least desirable type and are made of thermoplastic polyvinyl acetate-polyethylene copolymer in limited sizes. Fit adjustment is limited and the bulkiness impedes speech. Since the mouth must be closed to hold the protector in, breathing may be inhibited.

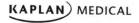

REVIEW QUESTIONS

1. With time, dental materials wear. Amalgam fillings can lose their marginal integrity to allow the penetration of fluid between the restoration and tooth surface. This phenomenon is called

   A. Imbibition
   B. Syneresis
   C. Percolation
   D. Wetting
   E. Creep

2. Your patient has a strong gag reflex but study models are needed for a treatment plan. Which of the following procedures might help better control the gag reflex?

   A. Decreasing the water temperature.
   B. Increasing the water temperature.
   C. Slowly adding mixed impression material to the tray.
   D. Not placing the impression material at the posterior segment of the tray.

3. With respect to dental properties, strain measures resilience. Another property is stress, which measure expansion.

   A. Both statements are true
   B. The first statement is true. The second statement is false because stress measures conductivity.
   C. The first statement is false because strain measures strength. The second statement is true.
   D. Both statements are false. Strain measures deformation per unit length while stress measures force per unit area.

4. Of the metals in an amalgam filling, which attracts tin away from mercury?

   A. Zinc
   B. Silver
   C. Copper
   D. Gold
   E. Lead

5. An example of an impression material that sets by a physical reaction is agar agar. An example of an impression material that sets by a chemical reaction is zinc oxide and eugenol.

   A. Both statements are true
   B. The first statement is false because agar agar is a chemical reaction. The second statement is true.
   C. The first statement is true. The second statement is false because zinc oxide and eugenol is a physical reaction.
   D. Both statements are false. The reactions in the statements are reversed.

6. Undertrituration affects the set of an amalgam filling. Which of the following is NOT a result of undertrituration?

   A. Amalgam can fracture.
   B. Amalgam appears dull.
   C. Amalgam hardens too quickly.
   D. Amalgam appears crumbly.
   E. Amalgam appears like a mirror.

7. The dental metal alloy element that causes the greatest amount of allergic reaction is

   A. Mercury
   B. Tin
   C. Silver
   D. Copper
   E. Nickel

8. Dental materials are gauged by their different properties. Knoop's test measures

   A. Resilience
   B. Hardness
   C. Malleability
   D. Dynamic modulus
   E. Flexibility

9. A patient should return to the dental office 24 hours to 7 days after the placement of an amalgam filling. Which of the following polishing agents is used to polish dental amalgam filling?

   A. Pumice
   B. Rouge
   C. Tin oxide
   D. Strips of alumina

10. Dental hygienists can assist in the prevention of disease with the placement of sealants. Which of the following reasons accounts for the greatest number of sealant failures?

    A. Water contamination
    B. Improper set time
    C. Acid not properly rinsed
    D. Tooth not properly etched
    E. Clinician inaccuracy

11. Some impression materials are rigid while others are flexible. All the following are flexible impression materials except one. Which one is this EXCEPTION?

    A. Polysulfide
    B. Silicone
    C. Polyether
    D. Polyvinyl siloxane
    E. Zinc oxide and eugenol

12. Water temperature can affect the set-time of an alginate impression. This process of setting up of an alginate impression is called

    A. Imbibition
    B. Syneresis
    C. Gelation
    D. Polymerization
    E. Sintering

13. Permanent molars should be sealed as soon as possible after they erupt before the grooves and pits are affected. The most appropriate time to perform this service is

    A. First and third grades
    B. Kindergarten and sixth grades
    C. First and sixth grades
    D. Second and seventh grades

14. A patient's tongue has just contaminated the occlusal surface that you had just etched for a sealant. What should be the next step?

    A. Rinse the tooth thoroughly to get rid of saliva contamination, then dry thoroughly and apply sealant.

    B. Saliva is not a contaminant so proceed with the next step of drying and then applying the sealant.

    C. Begin over again by re-etching the tooth for the same amount of time, thoroughly dry the tooth, and apply sealant.

    D. Re-etch the tooth for a shorter amount of time, thoroughly dry the tooth, and apply sealant.

    E. Dismiss the patient and reappoint for another day.

15. Some types of impression materials are more accurate than others. Which of the following impression materials is the most accurate?

    A. Alginate

    B. Plaster

    C. Silicone

    D. Agar agar

16. When there is amalgamation of a low-copper-content silver alloy with mercury, the result is an elimination of the gamma-2 reaction which is weak. When there is amalgamation of a high-copper-content silver alloy with mercury, the result is an elimination of the gamma-2 reaction, which is a stronger alloy.

    A. Both statements are true

    B. Statement 1 is true. Statement 2 is false because high copper produces a weak gamma-2 reaction.

    C. Statement 1 is false because low copper content of a silver alloy produces a weak gamma-2 reaction. Statement 2 is true.

    D. Statement 1 is false because low copper content of a silver alloy produces a weak gamma-2 reaction. Statement 2 is false because high copper produces a gamma-1 reaction with silver.

17. Grit is used in the dental operatory as well as in the dental lab and toothpastes. The word grit refers to

    A. Shape

    B. Hardness

    C. Size

    D. Firmness

    E. Strength

18. Before applying sealant, a clinician will use an acid etch, which provides a surface that allows for a _____ bond.

    A. Chemical

    B. Physical

    C. Micromechanical

    D. Macromechanical

    E. Thermal

19. A restoration varnish or liner performs all of the following functions except one. Which one is this EXCEPTION?

    A. Protects against thermal conduction
    B. Reinforces the floor of the preparation
    C. Increases the ingress of fluids
    D. Seal dentinal tubules

20. An impression material that sets by both a chemical and physical reaction is

    A. Agar agar
    B. Alginate
    C. Poly sulfide
    D. Polyether
    E. Plaster compound

21. During a long procedure, zinc oxide and eugenol were not immediately removed from the spatula. Which of the following would best remove the set material?

    A. Wax solvent
    B. Benzalkonium chloride
    C. Soap and water
    D. Orange solvent

22. Iontophoresis uses an electrical current to impregnate desensitizing agents into a tooth surface. When fluoride is used with this electrical device, what action takes place with the tooth surface?

    A. Fluoride–ion penetration incorporates 2–6 times more fluoride into dentinal tubules.
    B. Ameloblastic activity is stimulated
    C. Fluoride applied with an electrical current provides short-term relief.
    D. Fluoride applied in this manner stimulates secondary dentin formation to insulate the tooth.

23. If an impression is not poured up within 60 minutes, _____ can occur.

    A. Imbibition
    B. Creep
    C. Cohesion
    D. Retardation
    E. Syneresis

24. A disinfectant not acceptable for use as an laboratory disinfectant is

    A. Iodophors
    B. Glutaraldehydes
    C. Quarternary ammonium compounds
    D. Chlorine compounds

25. If a fork should touch an amalgam and a sudden pain is produced in the tooth, which of the following occurs?

    A. Corrosion
    B. Adhesion
    C. Burnishing
    D. Galvanization

ANSWER EXPLANATIONS

1. C

Percolation occurs when amalgam fillings lose their marginal integrity to allow fluid to penetrate between the restoration and tooth surface.

A. Imbibition is the taking on of extra fluid.

B. Syneresis is the loss of fluid.

D. Wetting is the spreading a liquid over a solid mixing surface.

E. Creep is the slow-dimensional change of a dental material that occurs from stress.

2. B

Increasing the water temperature will speed up the set time. This might help the patient better control the gag reflex.

C. Adding impression material to the tray might cause it to set before it is placed in the mouth.

D. Not placing the impression material at the posterior segment of the tray would yield inaccurate study models.

3. D

Both statements are false. Strain measures deformation per unit length while stress measures force per unit area.

4. C

Copper attracts tin away from mercury in an amalgam-filling reaction.

A. Zinc minimizes oxidation.

B. Silver increases strength.

D. Gold is not in an amalgam.

E. Lead is not in an amalgam.

5. A

Both statements are true. Agar agar is an impression material that sets by a physical reaction, while zinc oxide and eugenol sets by a chemical reaction.

6. E

Undertrituration does not cause an amalgam to appear like a mirror, which is an ideal amalgam. Undertriturating or undermixing can cause an amalgam to fracture, appear dull, harden too quickly, and appear crumbly.

7. E

Nickel causes the greatest amount of allergic reaction.

8. B

Knoop's test measures the hardness of dental materials.

A. Resilience measures the amount of energy needed to cause permanent deformation.

C. Malleability measures the resistance to fracture when the material is rolled out into a sheet.

D. Dynamic modulus measures the ratio of stress to strain when applying dynamic load.

E. Flexibility measures the degree that a material can stretch until it fractures.

9. C

Tin oxide should be used to polish a dental amalgam filling after it is placed.

A. Pumice is used intraorally and in the lab.

B. Rouge is used in the lab but not intraorally.

D. Strips of alumina are used for composite fillings.

10. E

Sealant failures are primarily due to clinician error or inaccuracy. It is the clinician who leaves water on the surface, does not allow for proper set time, does not rinse the acid off, or does not allow the acid to etch properly.

11. E

Zinc oxide and eugenol is a rigid impression material.

12. C

The setting-up of an alginate impression is called gelation.

A. Imbibition takes on extra water.

B. Syneresis is a liquid that forms on the surface of a hydrocolloid due to loss of water within the hydrocolloid.

D. Polymerization produces large polymer molecules from small molecules.

E. Sintering is the fabrication of ceramic restorations from ceramic particles through heat fusion.

13. C

The most appropriate time to place sealants is in the first and sixth grades, ages 6 and 12.

14. D

When a patient's tongue contaminates the surface just etched for a sealant, you would re-etch the tooth for a shorter amount of time, thoroughly dry the tooth, and apply sealant.

15. D

The most accurate impression material is agar agar.

A. Alginate is not accurate so it is used for study models or bleaching trays.

B. Plaster is used to mount casts on an articulator.

C. Silicone impressions have a moderate amount of shrinkage upon setting.

16. C

Statement 1 is false because low-copper content of a silver alloy produces a weak gamma-2 reaction. Statement 2 is true.

17. C

Grit refers to size of the grit.

18. C

Etching a tooth prior to sealing allows for micro-mechanical retention of the sealant.

19. C

A restoration varnish or liner does not increase the ingress of fluids. It prevents fluids from entering at the margin.

20. E

Plaster compound sets by chemical and also physical reaction.

A. Agar agar is a physical reaction.

B. Alginate is a chemical reaction.

C. Poly sulfide is a chemical reaction.

D. Polyether is a chemical reaction.

21. D

Removing hardened ZOE from a spatula is accomplished with orange solvent, an essential-oil-disintegrating solvent. It is especially effective for zinc oxide and eugenol sealer.

A. Wax solvent cleans waxes.

B. Benzalkonium chloride can be used as a surge evacuation system cleaner.

C. Soap and water are not strong enough.

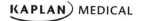

22. A

Iontophoresis utilizes an electrical current to impregnate fluoride ion into a surface causing penetration that incorporates 2–6 times more fluoride into dentinal tubules.

B. Ameloblasts are not stimulated because the enamel is already formed.

C. Fluoride applied with an electrical current does not provide short-term relief.

23. E

If an impression is not poured up within an hour, syneresis occurs. The loss of water causes the impression to shrink.

A. Imbibition absorbs more water.

B. Creep occurs with amalgam fillings.

C. Cohesion occurs when a gold foil is bonded to a tooth.

D. Retardation slows a reaction.

24. C

Quarternary ammonium compounds would not be acceptable for disinfecting a laboratory.

25. D

Galvanization occurs when a fork produces pain in an amalgam filling.

A. Corrosion may occur with fillings but a shock is not felt.

B. Adhesion is a tenacious bond between 2 compounds.

C. Burnishing smoothes an amalgam filling.

Chapter Fourteen:
Dental Hygiene Process of Care

The dental hygienist's first step in building a treatment plan for a patient should be to complete an overall evaluation or assessment. Collection of data should include medical history, vital signs, current symptoms, diagnostic radiographs if available, and an initial screening with extraoral and intraoral clinical findings. All of this information provides baseline data on which to identify patient needs.

MEDICAL HISTORY

A patient's medical history determines the general health of the patient. This information is necessary to determine any **health condition** that may manifest itself in the oral cavity or that may affect the patient's response to dental treatment. By identifying risk factors, the dental hygienist can determine if there is a need to postpone dental treatment. Active infection, for example, might be potentially infectious to dental personnel. Elevated blood pressure might put the patient at risk if treatment were to take place. In addition, knowledge of risk factors helps in identifying potential medical emergencies.

Medications that patients take for pre-existing conditions such as calcium channel blockers for hypertension can cause gingival hyperplasia. Another side effect intraorally can be excessive bleeding for patients on anticoagulants. Therefore, it is important to have the exact list of medications for a patient.

It is also essential that the dental hygienist know what medication **allergies** a patient has, should something need to be prescribed. Certain drugs become less effective when taken with other drugs. Birth control pills, for instance, become less effective when a woman takes antibiotics. Latex allergies, especially, are vital to know, since latex gloves are a big part of infection control.

The medical history should be updated at every visit—without fail—since patients often forget to advise you of changes. The original medical history and each update needs to be signed in ink.

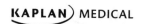

VITAL SIGNS

Vitals signs include **pulse rate**, **respiratory rate**, and **blood pressure**. Taking vital signs provides a screening for a patient who may not be aware of a condition such as hypertension. Vital signs also provide a baseline for a patient should a medical emergency occur.

Normal Vital Signs

	Heart Rate	Respiratory Rate	Blood Pressure	Plan for Hypertension
Infant	120–160	25–40	60–90 / 30–35	
Toddler	80–130	20–35	70–110 / 40–65	
School-age	70–110	15–25	90–110 / 50–70	
Adult	60–100	12–20	<120 / <80	Normal treatment
			<140 / <90	Normal treatment, annual check
			140–160 / 90–100	Recheck next 3 subsequent visits
			160–180 / 100–110	Recheck in 5 min., if unchanged, no dental treatment, medical consult
			>180 / >110	No treatment, immediate medical consultation

A blood pressure cuff is called sphygmomanometer.

The National Institutes of Health describes Stage I hypertension as 140–159/90–99, and Stage II hypertension as ≥160 / ≥100.

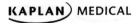

ASA CLASSIFICATION OF PHYSICAL STATUS

The **American Society of Anesthesiology** (ASA) has created a classification system in order to categorize a patient's medical health and if a risk factor exists for a potential medical emergency. These categories can help in the determination of whether a specific dental treatment should be performed.

ASA Classification of Physical Status

Classification	Color	Risk	Types of Ailments
Category I	Green Able to receive treatment	Normal, healthy; Can climb a flight of stairs and not get tired.	None
Category II	Yellow Treatment still advisable but it may need to be slightly altered	Mild systemic condition; can climb a flight of stairs but stops to rest or rests en route though completes task	Allergies, pregnancy, anxiety, well controlled non-insulin dependent diabetes, epilepsy, asthma, thyroid ailments, controlled hypertension
Category III	Yellow Elective treatment still advisable but it may need to be altered if patient's condition changes	Severe condition but not incapacitating. Cannot complete climbing a flight of stairs	Insulin controlled diabetic, stable angina pectoris, history of myocardial infarction or cerebrovascular accident greater than 6 mo. ago, COPD, congestive heart failure, exercise-induced asthma, thyroid problems accompanied by symptoms
Category IV	Red Medical consultation with physician prior to dental treatment. Utilize caution with non-invasive dental emergencies	Continual life-threatening, severe systemic condition	Unable to climb a flight of stairs, end-stage renal failure, uncontrolled diabetic, unstable angina, myocardial infarction or cerebrovascular accident less than 6 months ago, uncontrolled hypertension, respiratory distress from CHF or COPD, uncontrolled hypertension
Category V	Red Palliative treatment only	Patient has less than 24 hours to survive	Terminal illness

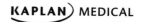

ENDOCARDITIS PROPHYLAXIS INFORMATION

For patients with heart conditions, the American Heart Association (AHA) recommends premedicating with antibiotics before certain types of dental treatment.

AHA Guidelines for Cardiovascular Disease

Patients at highest risk

- Prosthetic hear valves

- Previous history of endocarditis

- Certain congenital heart defects such as

  - Unrepaired cyanotic congenital heart disease, including those with palliative shunts and conduits

  - Completely repaired congenital heart disease with prostetic material or device, whether placed by surgery or catheter intervention, during the first 6 months after the procedure.

  - Repaired congenital hear disease with residual defects at the site of or adjacent to the site of a prosthetic patch or prosthetic device (which inhibit endothelialization)

Dental procedures for which endocarditis prophylaxis is recommended[1]

- Dental extractions
- Periodontal procedures including surgery, scaling, and root planing, probing, and recall maintenance
- Endodontic (root canal) instrumentation or surgery only beyond the apex
- Subgingival placement of antibiotic fibers or strips
- Initial placement of orthodontic bands but not brackets
- Intraligamentary local anesthetic injections
- Prophylactic cleaning of teeth or implants where bleeding is anticipated

[1]Prophylaxis is recommended for patients with high- and moderate-risk cardiac conditions

PROPHYLACTIC REGIMENS FOR DENTAL, ORAL, RESPIRATORY TRACT, OR ESOPHAGEAL PROCEDURES

(Follow-up dose is no longer recommended.) Total children's dose should not exceed adult dose.

Standard

Amoxicillin: Adults, 2.0 g (children, 50 mg/kg) given orally 1 hour before procedure.

If Unable to Take Oral Medications

Ampicillin: Adults, 2.0 g (children 50 mg/kg) given IM or IV within 30 minutes before procedure.

If Allergic to Amoxicillin/Ampicillin/Penicillin

Clindamycin: Adults, 600 mg (children 20 mg/kg) given orally 1 hour before procedure

OR:

Cephalexin* or Cefadroxil*: Adults, 2.0 g (children 50 mg/kg) orally 1 hour before procedure

OR:

Azithromycin or Clarithromycin: Adults, 500 mg (children 15 mg/kg) orally 1 hour before procedure.

Amoxicillin/ampicillin/penicillin allergic patients unable to take oral medications

Clindamycin: Adults, 600 mg (children 20 mg/kg) IV within 30 minutes before procedure.

OR:

Cefazolin*: Adults, 1.0 g (children 25 mg/kg) IM or IV within 30 minutes before procedure.

* Cephalosporins should not be used in patients with immediate-type hypersensitivity reaction to penicillin.

OTHER CONDITIONS REQUIRING PREMEDICATION

There is some disagreement about whether antibiotics should be required before dental treatment for patients with certain other conditions.

Joint and hip replacement: The **American Academy of Orthopedic Surgeons** suggests that individuals who have had a total joint or hip replacement premedicate with the same dosages listed above for the AHA:

- Joint replacement less than 2 years ago
- Previous infections in an artificial joint
- Inflammatory type of arthritis such as rheumatoid arthritis
- Systemic lupus erythematosis
- Weakened-immune system from disease, drugs, or radiation
- Insulin-dependent (Type I) diabetes
- Undernourished or malnourished
- Hemophilia

—Recommended by the AAOS, 2002

End-stage renal failure: A patient who has had end-stage renal failure is classified by the American Society of Anesthesiology as ASA IV. It is recommended that a patient in this category receive **dental treatment** the **day after dialysis**. The patient's physician should be consulted about premedication with an antibiotic. Care should be taken not to prescribe an antibiotic that is eliminated in the kidney.

Spinal bifida: Patients with spinal bifida often have latex allergies, so care should be taken not to use latex products. Premedication with an antibiotic for spinal bifida patients before dental treatment is dependent on what type of shunt the patient has, so the patient's physician should be consulted.

DENTAL HISTORY

With every office visit, a complete dental history should be taken. It should include past orthodontic, endodontic, or periodontic treatments. Additionally, a patient's "chief complaint" for that visit should be written in quotes. Frequency of previous dental visits gives insight into the patient's motivation for maintaining a healthy oral cavity.

Extraoral Examination

- Inspect the head, face, and nose for symmetry and equal function. Observe for unusual skin pigmentations and lesions as well as texture. Inspect the pupils of the eyes for equal reactivity, dilation, or constriction.

- Inspect the function of the temporomandibular by palpating the joint when the patient open and closes. Check for deviations, joint sounds, crepitus, and tenderness.

- Palpate the occipital, preauricular, postauricular, parotid, superficial cervical, deep cervical, submental and submandibular lymph nodes for lymphadenopathy (chronic abnormal swelling) or adenopathy (enlargement).

- Bilaterally inspect the masseter and temporalis muscle with circular palpation to determine if there are any nodules, swelling, tenderness, or tension.

- Observe the patient swallowing to determine if there are any difficulties or abnormalities.

- Inspect the lips for cracks, dryness, pigmentations, lesions, and irritations.

Intraoral Examination

Inspect the labial and buccal mucosa as well as the vestibule for abnormalities such as lesions, ulcerations, nodules, injuries, amalgam tattoos, scars, and Fordyce granules which are normal sebaceous glands. Observe Stenson's duct.

Inspect the tongue's dorsal and ventral surfaces by gently holding with gauze. Look for fissuring, migratory glossitis, coatings, hairy leukoplakia, black hairy tongue, beefy tongue, or tenderness. Observe and palpate the floor of the mouth for nodules, ranula, lesions, varicosities, and ankyloglossia. Observe duct openings and the possibility of mandibular tori.

Inspect the hard and soft palates for palatal tori, lesions, injuries, nodules, clefts, inflammations, and petechiae. Observe the oropharynx for inflammation, lesions, and injuries as well as inspect the tonsils for enlargement, inflammation, and signs of infection.

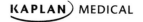

Gingival Assessment

The gingiva should also be inspected for lesions, tattoos, injuries, nodules, fibromas, and inflammation. The gingiva will be **pink** and **stippled** if healthy. Redness and loss of stippling indicates disease. **Pigmentation** can be inherited in certain races.

Contour is dependent on the relationship of the gingiva to the teeth. In **healthy** dentitions, the margins will be **knife-edged**. In the presence of **disease** they may be **blunted**, **cratered**, **rolled**, or **bulbous**. If there is **disease** present, the tissues may be **soft** and **spongy**.

PERIODONTAL EXAM

There are many types of periodontal charts on which to record the pocket depths of patients. This charting is used to evaluate the patient's periodontal health. Six measurements are taken per tooth, with three measurements on the facial surfaces and three on the lingual surfaces. Bleeding upon probing is also annotated, along with recession, furcation involvement, and mobility.

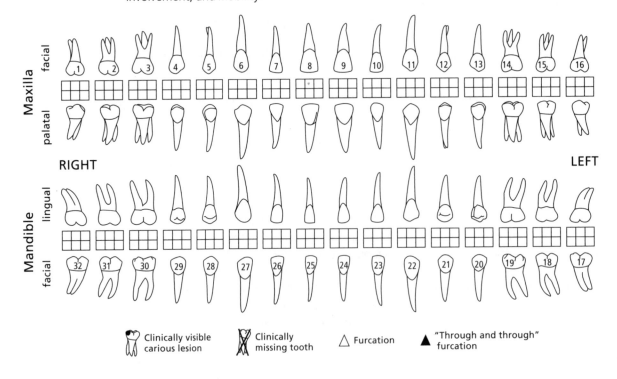

Periodontal Screening and Reporting

A periodontal screening and report is a quick, proficient way to check patients for the presence of periodontal disease. A **color-coded probe** with a ball on the end is calibrated at 0.5 mm (allows for the ball), 3.5 mm to 5.5 mm (colored section), and 8.5 mm to 11.5 mm. The **worst score** for each sextant is recorded in its respective box.

PSR Scores

Score	Depth	Deposits	Bleeding
0	Depths inserted to first clear band		No bleeding
1	Depths inserted to first clear band	Plaque, no calculus	Bleed upon probing
2	Depths inserted to first clear band	Calculus present	Bleed upon probing
3	Depths inserted to color section	Supra- and/or sub-gingival calculus	Mild to moderate bleeding
4	Depths inserted past color section	Subgingival calculus	Moderate to severe bleeding
*	Denotes furcation involvement, mobility, recession		

Periodontal screening and report probe

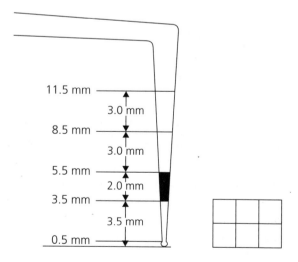

The worst score for the sextant is placed in the box.

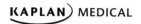

In the presence of disease, the dental hygienist will need to **assess the gingiva** for **inflammation** and **bleeding**, and also note change in contour and consistency. Furcation involvement and mobility should be noted as well. See Chapter 8 for more on Periodontics.

Furcation Involvement

Class	Involvement	Bone level
I	Notch felt	No interradicular bone loss
II	Into furcation but not completely through	Some loss between roots
III	Through and through but gingiva covers opening	Complete loss between roots
IV	Through and through	Complete loss between roots

Mobility

Class	Degree of movement
I	Slightly more than normal
II	> 1 mm
III	Severe, tooth depressible

Fremitus is a sensation or vibration that occurs when teeth contact each other in normal occlusion. This vibration can lead to tooth mobility. Fremitus can be experienced by sitting the patient in an upright position, then having him "tap his teeth" together, while putting a finger on the cervical third of each maxillary tooth. Note each tooth that the vibration was felt on.

Fremitus Scores

Fremitus Class	Degree	Sensation/Visual
N	Normal, no vibration	None
+	1° Slight vibration	Felt but not visual
++	2° Movement clearly felt	Felt and visual
+++	3° Movement obviously felt	Seen and felt with certainty

Fremitus may cause occlusal trauma or insult to a tooth and its periodontium. If a tooth is receiving heavy occlusal forces but the **periodontium is intact** this force is termed **primary occlusal trauma**. If the tooth is involved with heavy occlusal trauma and the **periodontium becomes involved** resulting in mobility and/or sensitivity, it is termed **secondary occlusal trauma**.

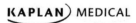

Dentition Assessment

A dentition assessment is needed for treatment formulation. Documentation should include **missing teeth** and the reason for their loss; any **restorative work**; **caries** as indicated with Black's classifications; **overhangs**; **anomalies** that have affected any teeth; and **evidence of occlusal forces** by charting wear-patterns on the dentition.

Root caries are *not* classified with Black's classification.

Black's Classification of Caries

Class	Location	Examples	Region	Detection
I	Pits and fissures	O, F	Posterior teeth	Explorer, visual
II	Proximal molars, premolars	MO, DO, MOD	Posterior teeth	Radiograph, change in tooth color, explorer
III	Proximal incisors, canines **not including** incisal edge	ML, DL, MF, DF, MFL, DFL	Anterior teeth	Radiograph, explorer, color change, transillumination, visual
IV	Proximal incisors, canines **including** incisal edge	MI, DI, MIL, DIL, MIF, DIF, MIFL, DIFL	Anterior teeth	Radiograph, explorer, color change, transillumination, visual
V	Cervical $\frac{1}{3}$ facial or lingual	F, L	All teeth	Visual, radiographs
VI	Incisal edge, cusp tip	O, I	All teeth	Visual

Root caries are also called **cemental** or **cervical** caries. They can result from **xerostomia, radiation therapy, poor oral hygiene, recession,** or **a high-sugar diet.**

Nursing-bottle decay is seen in a small percentage of young people. The **maxillary anterior teeth** are affected first, since that is where the milk tends to pool in the mouth. The **maxillary deciduous molars** are affected next, followed by the **mandibular deciduous molars.** Mandibular anterior teeth are not usually affected since the tongue covers them and the milk is not as likely to pool there.

Overhang Classifications

	Region	Detection	Correction
Type I	$< \frac{1}{3}$ of interproximal space	Radiograph	Margination procedure and repolish
Type II	$\frac{1}{3} - \frac{1}{2}$ of interproximal space	Radiograph and clinical palpation	Margination procedure
Type III	$> \frac{1}{2}$ of interproximal space	Radiograph and clinical palpation	Replace restoration

Everything should be recorded on a dentition chart numbered with the **universal coding system** from **1–32** for the **permanent,** and from **a–t** for the **primary dentition.**

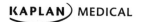

Occlusion

Patient occlusion should also be noted as to Angle's Classification of Occlusion, as noted in Chapter 5. **Overbite** and **overjet** evaluations are also necessary. Along with the molar and canine relationship-wear patterns should be noted the **attrition** (tooth-to-tooth wear), **abrasion (**tooth wear with another force besides teeth), and **erosion** (chemical wear).

Abfraction is the flexation and fatigue of a tooth at the point of load or juncture. When you bend a stick too many times, it breaks. In the same way, when you flex a tooth, stress occurs at the cementoenamel junction. Microscopic fractures of the enamel occur at the CEJ.

Universal Chart Numbers

			a	b	c	d	e	f	g	h	i	j					
Maxillary Right	1	2	3	4	5	6	7	8	9	10	11	12	13	14	15	16	Maxillary Left
Mandibular Right	32	31	30	29	28	27	26	25	24	23	22	21	20	19	18	17	Mandibular Left
			t	s	r	q	p	o	n	m	l	k					

Radiographs

Radiographic surveys should be taken for any new patients on an **as-needed basis**. The survey will show any work that needs to be done, look for subgingival calculus, check bone levels, evaluate all hard structures, and look for abnormalities. For more on radiology, see Chapter 9.

Oral Hygiene Assessment

All patients have different oral hygiene habits, and of course some are more motivated than others. It is the dental hygienist's responsibility to help motivate each patient to reach a higher standard of homecare.

The **plaque index** (PI) assesses the amount of plaque present on each tooth. **Four scores** are taken for each surface (facial, mesial, lingual, distal) of a tooth. The scores for each tooth are added up and divided by 4. These scores are then added up and divided by the number of teeth scored.

Plaque Scores[†]

Score	Plaque Amount
0	No plaque
1	Plaque film at gingival margin
2	Moderate soft debris within the gingival margin
3	Gross soft debris within gingival pockets and/or margins

[†] Adapted from Silness and Löe Plaque Index

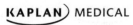

Plaque Index [†]

Score	Rating
0	Excellent
0.1–0.9	Good
1.0–1.9	Fair
2.0–3.0	Poor

[†]   Adapted from Silness and Löe Plaque Index

The **calculus index** (CI-S) measures calculus on surfaces. Along with plaque index, pocket depths, and gingival health, the amount of calculus a patient has determines what type of care she will receive. CI-S is used along with the **debris index** (DI-S) to create the **simplified oral hygiene index** (OHI-S).

Calculus Rating [‡]

	Calculus amount
0	None
1	Supragingival calculus covering not more than $\frac{1}{3}$ of exposed tooth
2	Supragingival calculus covering more than $\frac{1}{3}$ but less than $\frac{2}{3}$ of exposed tooth or subgingival flecks of calculus at CEJ
3	Supragingival calculus covering more than $\frac{2}{3}$ of exposed tooth

[‡] Adapted from Greene, Vermillion, and
WHO Oral Health Country/Area Profile Programme

Calculus Index Rating [‡]

	Hygiene Rating
0.0–0.6	Good
0.7–1.8	Fair
1.9–3.0	Poor

[‡] Adapted from Greene, Vermillion, and
WHO Oral Health Country/Area Profile Programme

NEEDS ASSESSMENT

General assessment is determined by the following: intraoral and extraoral exams, periodontal status, dentition assessment, occlusal assessment, radiographs, oral hygiene assessment, and dental and medical history. Systemic diseases and the medications possible taken for them may have a direct impact in the mouth. They can also affect the healing process.

Periodontal assessment is determined by pocket depth probing, assessing the gingiva for color, texture, and contour, loss of gingival attachment, recession, bone loss radiographically, furcation involvement, and tooth mobility.

Dentition assessment provides the information necessary to create a treatment plan for the patient's **restorative needs.** Previous restorative work also needs to be assessed on its present condition and quality.

All dental findings should be precise and documented in ink. From all of this information, a treatment plan can be formulated for the patient but it can also be used to educate the patient as to his needs. Education provides a direct way to get the patient to become involved with home care, fluoride therapy, and effective plaque removal with adjuncts if necessary.

TREATMENT PLAN

A treatment plan can be formulated to restore the dentition and its supporting structures to full health. Prioritization of the each individual's dental hygiene needs should be a part of the treatment plan. Sound supporting structures (periodontium) will support any restorative needs.

The dental hygienist can provide the patient with the dental hygiene treatment plan, ensuring that the periodontium be in sound condition. The plan should include the amount of appointments and time necessary to complete treatment.

The treatment plan should list not only risk factors that would go along with the benefits of receiving care, but also risk factors that could occur if the patient fails to receive care. The plan should list alternatives; for example, replacing a missing tooth with a partial denture, fixed bridge, or dental implant. It should also list any referrals to specialists such as oral surgeons, orthodontists, endodontists, or periodontists.

Providing the information to the patient as a verbal or written agreement is termed **informed consent**. A **written document** of **informed consent** should be signed by both the dentist or dental hygienist and the patient and becomes a permanent part of the record. If the patient decides not to proceed with the treatment plan provided, it is termed **informed refusal**. This also should be carefully documented with the patient signing a written form of the treatment plan stating he does not wish to proceed with part or all of the treatment.

REVIEW QUESTIONS

1. A new patient has arrived for a thorough examination. Upon reviewing her health history, you find that she has checked off heart murmur, though she states that she had it only as a child. Your next step is to

   A. Go on with the exam since it was only as a child that she had the murmur.

   B. Take any necessary radiographs today and go on with the exam.

   C. Take radiographs only today and reappoint the patient until she checks again with her doctor about the murmur.

   D. Explain that, since she has not had medical clearance for the murmur, you are unable to continue today. Have the patient seek a medical consultation with her physician.

2. Your new patient seems to have a very weak pulse that is thready and hard to detect. The next best place to take a pulse is the

   A. Popliteal artery

   B. Femoral artery

   C. Jugular artery

   D. Palmer artery

   E. Brachial artery

3. Your patient has presented for a 6-month recare visit. He did not feel well this morning and even hesitated about coming for the appointment. You take his temperature and find it slightly elevated. What is a normal temperature range?

   A. 93.5–96.7° F

   B. 95.8–97.7° F

   C. 97.0–99.5° F

   D. 99.6–101.9° F

4. A patient arrives today who has not been in for 2 years. Typically, this patient has had moderate to heavy calculus. Today. he presents with a heavy bridge of calculus on the mandibular anterior teeth. After you remove it with an ultrasonic, you decide to reinspect for any remaining calculus. What is the best way to check for remaining calculus?

   A. Direct vision

   B. Indirect vision

   C. Cavitron tip exploration

   D. Overhead light inspection

   E. Transillumination

Scenario for Questions 5–10

Mrs. Jones who has been a type 1 brittle diabetic has returned for a 6-month visit. She states that her physician has been monitoring her blood sugar and put her on humulin twice daily since her diabetes was out of control. Prior to her appointment today, her blood sugar test results showed her level at 135 mg/dL. Her pulse reading is 72 BPM, respiratory rate of 16, and blood pressure reading of 140/86 mm Hg. Mrs. Jones states that the gingiva around the crowns on #6, #7, #8, #9, and #10 feels very tender lately, and bleeds easily with her home care. Upon inspection, you find generalized mild redness with moderate redness around all of the anterior crowns. There is light generalized gingival plaque and some interproximal plaque on the anterior crowns that she has not been flossing due to the tenderness. Calculus is light on the mandibular anterior teeth and not detectable in other areas with the PSR.

Pocket depth comparison from her last appointment has gone from generalized 3-4 mm readings to 4-5 mm. Radiographs reveal insipient carious lesions on # 4M, #5D, and #19D with a deeper carious lesion under a large filling on # 15 MO that she says has been very sensitive lately.

5. With respect to the patient's statements about her diabetes, what would be your course of action?

    A. Advise a medical consultation with her doctor since she said her diabetes had been out of control.

    B. Do nothing and reappoint when her diabetes is under control.

    C. Address her problem with Tooth #15 and address her gingival problems.

    D. Give her flossing instructions.

    E. Tell her she is going to need premedication with an antibiotic since her diabetes had been out of control.

6. Mrs. Jones's condition today could be classified as

    A. ASA I

    B. ASA II

    C. ASA III

    D. ASA IV

7. Mrs. Jones's inflamed tissues are exacerbated by her poor plaque-control and health condition. What would be the most important step in today's treatment?

    A. Instruct her with an electric toothbrush

    B. Explain that even though the gingiva is tender she needs to floss daily to eliminate the breeding ground of microbes.

    C. Perform an oral prophylaxis and give flossing instructions.

    D. Ask her to buy a Waterpik to aid in getting the tissues under control.

    E. Perform a root debridement and reappoint for evaluation in 6 weeks.

8. What would be the most appropriate recare interval for the patient in this scenario?

    A. 1 month

    B. 3 months

    C. 4 months

    D. 6 months

9. Even though the patient is reluctant to floss, she states she will do so. Which of the following statements would help to motivate her with better homecare?

    A. Flossing will help to reduce the redness and microbes

    B. An electric toothbrush will aid in better plaque removal

    C. Research shows that gingival disease can contribute to systemic diseases such as diabetes

    D. Use a rubber stimulator

10. This patient's periodontal status would be classified as

    A. Aggressive periodontal disease

    B. Chronic periodontitis

    C. Chronic plaque-induced periodontitis

    D. Systemic and plaque-induced aggressive periodontal disease

    E. Systemic and plaque-induced chronic periodontitis

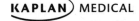

11. A new patient who is a veterinary assistant has arrived at the dental office with a toothache. Upon reviewing her medical history, you find that she has not only environmental allergies, but also food allergies to banana, shellfish, melons, kiwi, and pineapple. What other conditions might this patient be at risk for?

    A. Chronic bronchitis

    B. Asthma

    C. Hemophilia

    D. Diabetes

    E. Latex allergies

12. Upon radiographic evaluation and oral inspection, you find the patient in question #11 has a periodontal abscess on Tooth #31. The periodontal probe reveals a 4 mm pocket and class II furcation involvement. A class II furcation can best be described as

    A. Early bone loss

    B. Bone loss into the furcation with the presence of disease

    C. Moderate bone loss into the furcation

    D. Moderate bone loss with the presence of disease

    E. Severe bone loss into the furcation

13. A new patient has not received dental treatment in 4 years. Upon discussing his pocket depths and periodontal disease, he becomes reluctant to return to the office for the necessary procedures and asks for just a cleaning today. What would be the best course of action for this patient?

    A. Just do the cleaning as he has asked

    B. Suggest more frequent recall appointments

    C. Perform oral hygiene instructions

    D. Discuss his right to refuse treatment

    E. Have him sign an informed refusal form

14. All of the following conditions can put a patient at high risk for endocarditis except one. Which one is this EXCEPTION?

    A. Previous history of bacterial endocarditis

    B. Mitral valve prolapse

    C. Complex cyanotic congenital heart disease

    D. Surgically constructed shunts or conduits

    E. Artificial heart valves

15. The floor of the mouth is inspected by pressing a finger from one hand in the floor while pressing a finger from the other hand externally under the chin. This type is tissue inspection is termed:

    A. Digital

    B. Bidigital

    C. Bimanual

    D. Bilateral

    E. Circular

16. When recording a periodontal screening, one sextant has a score of 2. This determines that the pocket depths are:

    A. Within the first clear band

    B. Within the first clear band with bleeding

    C. Within the first clear band with bleeding and calculus

    D. Within the first clear band with no bleeding and calculus

    E. Within the black mark on the probe

17. Which of the following nodes is NOT palpated upon examination of the patient?

    A. Anterior and posterior auricular

    B. Superficial cervical

    C. Submandibular

    D. Submental

    E. Tonsillar

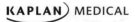

18. Which of the following is NOT an important part of the dental history?

    A. Past dental treatment

    B. Insurance carrier

    C. Chief complaint

    D. Water fluoridation

    E. Injuries to the face and teeth

19. When speaking with your patient about her periodontal condition, you state that periodontal disease has been found to contribute to many systemic diseases. Periodontal disease, however, does NOT contribute to which of the following?

    A. Heart attack

    B. Stroke

    C. Diabetes

    D. Pre-term low birth weight in babies

    E. Obesity

20. When assessing the gingiva, which of the following lesions is considered to be a blisterform?

    A. Papule

    B. Plaque

    C. Nodule

    D. Bulla

    E. Tumor

21. All of the following except one are descriptive terms used to assess a lesion. Which one is this EXCEPTION?

    A. Exophytic

    B. Indurated

    C. Sessile

    D. Punctate

    E. Inebriate

22. Which of the following food snacks would you suggest for a patient with a history of asthma?

    A. Cheese

    B. Apples

    C. Peanuts

    D. Raisins

    E. Carrots

23. To perform an inspection of the TMJ, you would use

    A. Percussion

    B. Bilateral palpation

    C. Bimanual palpation

    D. Transillumination

24. The term that measures vibration is which of the following?

    A. Buccal space

    B. Fremitus

    C. Creep

    D. Percussion

25. Blood pressure is taken with a(n)

    A. Sphygmotonometer

    B. Sphygmomanometer

    C. Otoscopes

    D. Sphygmo-oscillometer

ANSWER EXPLANATIONS

1. D

Explain to the patient since she has not had medical clearance for the murmur, you should not proceed. She must first present clearance from her doctor that as per an echocardiogram, there is no longer a murmur.

2. E

The next best place to take a pulse is the brachial artery.

A. The popliteal artery is behind the knee joint.

B. The femoral artery is in the groin area.

C. There is no jugular artery. There is a jugular vein; the carotid is the artery used in CPR.

D. The palmer artery is too deep in the palm to feel.

3. C

Normal temperature range is 97.0–99.5° F.

4. E

Transillumination will help to detect subgingival and interproximal calculus.

A. Direct vision will not help subgingivally & interproximally.

B. Indirect vision will not be sufficiently thorough.

C. With Cavitron-tip exploration, the Cavitron tip is not sensitive enough for tactile inspection.

D. Overhead light inspection would help to detect supragingival calculus.

5. C

With respect to the diabetes, her readings are 135 mg/dL today which is near the normal 80–120 mg/DL. You would address the problem with Tooth #15 and address her gingival problems.

A. A medical consult is unnecessary since it seems to be under control today. All of her vitals and blood-sugar levels are normal.

6. C

Mrs. Jones's status is ASA III; her diabetes is typically not well-controlled though her readings are good today and she can be treated.

A. ASA I is healthy with no medical history.

B. ASA II has some mild form of a medical history and would include a diet-controlled or oral hypoglycemic medicated diabetic.

D. ASA IV would be her classification if she were out of control today.

7. C

The most important step today would be to perform an oral prophylaxis and give flossing instruction.

E. Performing a root debridement and reappointing for evaluation is not appropriate since she had only light calculus on the mandibular anterior teeth.

8. B

Recare should be in 3 months, since the patient has systemic risk factors and inflammation.

A. 1 month would be for someone with advanced disease and multiple systemic factors.

C. 4 months would be for someone who has had good findings for 1 year or more as per NSPT.

D. 6 months would be for someone who has had good findings for 1 year or more as per NSPT, maintained healthy tissues, and has low risk factors.

9. C

The most powerful piece of information is that gingival disease can contribute to systemic diseases such as diabetes.

A. Flossing will help but the patient has systemic factors that contribute to the disease.

B. An electric toothbrush would help in plaque removal only if she were brushing correctly.

D. A rubber stimulator would be of limited help.

10. E

The patient's periodontal status would be classified as systemic and plaque-induced chronic periodontitis.

11. E

The patient might be at risk for latex allergies. Research has found that foods such as kiwi, banana, shellfish, pineapple, avocado, tomato, and melons are most likely to trigger latex sensitivity. This patient is also a veterinary assistant who wears latex gloves.

A. Chronic bronchitis is not a risk factor for food allergies.

B. Asthma could be induced from the animal environment and latex usage as a veterinary assistant but this is not the best answer.

12. D

A Class II furcation is moderate bone loss with the presence of disease, visible radiographically with the periodontal probe just entering into the furcation.

A. Early bone loss is not detected radiographically, probe enters flute of furcation.

B. Bone loss into the furcation with the presence of disease would be just into the notch without a 4 mm pocket reading.

C. Moderate bone loss into the furcation occurs when the probe just enters into the furcation but does into pass through.

E. Severe bone loss into the furcation radiographically and probing would be a clear through and through opening into the furcation.

13. E

The best thing to do would be to have the patient sign an informed refusal form.

A. To just do the cleaning as he has asked will not truly help him.

B. To suggest more frequent recalls is a part of the formal case presentation after root debridement.

C. To instruct in oral hygiene is part of the formal case presentation.

D. Discussing his right to refuse treatment is a part of the formal case presentation.

14. B

Having mitral valve prolapse would put a patient at moderate risk—not high risk—for endocarditis.

15. C

Bimanual tissue inspection uses the fingers of two hands.

A. Digital uses one finger only.

B. Bidigital uses two fingers on the same hand.

D. Bilateral uses two hands.

E. Circular uses fingers of one hand for rotation on an area.

16. C

When one sextant has a score of 2, the pocket depths are within the first clear band with bleeding and calculus.

A. Within the first clear band would be a score of 0.

B. Within the first clear band with bleeding would be a 1.

D. Within the first clear band with no bleeding and calculus is not a classification.

E. Within the black mark on the probe would be a 3.

17. E

Tonsillar nodes are internal and so are not palpated upon examination.

18. B

An individual's insurance carrier has nothing to do with dental history.

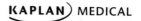

19. E

Periodontal disease does not contribute to obesity, though it does contribute to heart attack, stroke, diabetes, and pre-term low birth weight in babies.

20. D

Bulla is a blisterform. It is a fluid-filled sac of more than 1 cm.

A. Papule is a small, solid lesion of nonblisterform.

B. Plaque-like lesions ae nonblisterform raised lesions with a flat top.

C. Nodule is a large papule 5 mm to 1 cm in size. It is a nonblisterform.

21. E

Inebriated means drunk, and would never be used to describe a lesion.

A. Exophytic means growing outward.

B. Indurated means hardened.

C. Sessile means it has a broad, flat base.

D. Punctate indicates differentiated points or dots.

22. D

Raisins have the fewest food allergies, so they would advisable for someone with asthma.

Cheese, apples, peanuts, and carrots are more likely to be allergens.

23. B

To inspect the TMJ, you would use bilateral palpation, which uses two hands.

A. Percussion would not be used for this joint, as it can cause damage.

C. Bimanual palpation uses a finger of each hand.

D. Transillumination will not help with this joint.

24. B

Fremitus measures vibration.

A. Buccal space is the fascial area between the buccinator and masseter muscles.

C. Creep is the change in a dental material under stress.

D. Percussion is used to test for hollowness.

25. B

A sphygmomanometer measures blood pressure.

A. A sphygmotonometer measures the elasticity of the arterial walls.

C. An otoscope inspects the middle ear.

D. A sphygmo-oscillometer is a form of sphygmo-manometer that measures the disappearance and reappearance of the pulse, as indicated by an oscillating needle.

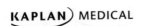

Chapter Fifteen: **Oral Health Promotion**

With a goal of prevention, oral health promotion strives to expand the awareness of the origins of oral disease. By educating patients about the importance of reducing plaque, for instance, attitudes can be changed; the reduction of plaque-levels typically reduces carious lesions—and the inflammation and bleeding gingiva of periodontal disease.

We now have evidence that periodontal disease can have a direct effect on the body. It contributes to coronary heart disease, diabetes, arthritis, and low birthweight in newborns. Therefore, keeping the oral cavity in good health has a clear effect on our general health.

ORAL ENVIRONMENT

The oral cavity contains a normal flora of microorganisms that contribute to a healthy mouth. Though only about 200 species have been identified, over 500 species are present—some of which can become pathogenic. Different microorganisms produce different dental diseases, such as carious lesions, gingivitis, and periodontitis.

Microorganisms

The first microorganisms to become organized on the tooth surface are aerobic gram-positive rods and cocci. As plaque accumulates and matures, more facultative bacteria such as *Streptococcus sanguis,* *Streptococcus mutans,* *Streptococcus mitis,* and *Actinomyces viscosus* enter into the picture.

S. sanguis and *S. mutans* compete with each other, though *S. sanguis* exists in higher numbers in a low-sugar diet, and *S. mutans* is more prevalent—and cariogenic—in high sugar diets.

The fimbriae (hair-like projections) of the bacteria attach to the dental pellicle, firmly adhering to the tooth surface. Then, the bacteria begin to replicate.

The next microorganisms that enter into the picture are the gram-negative groups of *Prevotella intermedia,* *Fusobacterium nucleatum,* and *Capnocytophaga* spirochetes. This set has a very strong affinity for the gram-positive bacteria previously attached to the tooth surface.

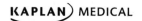

As plaque matures and migrates apically, more of the **gram-negative** bacteria associated with periodontal disease join in. This includes *Treponema* spirochetes, *Actinobacillus actinomycetemcomitans*, *Eikenella corrodens*, *Campylobacter rectus*, *Porphyromonas gingivalis*, and vibrios.

Biofilm Maturation

Days	Gram +	Gram –	Appearance
1–2	Cocci, *S. mutans*, *S. sanguis*, *S. mitis*		Invisible
2–4	Cocci, filamentous bacteria, *S. sanguis*, *Actinomyces viscosus*		Biofilm
4–7	Rods, cocci, filamentous bacteria	*Fusobacterium nucleatum*, *Capnocytophaga* species, *Prevotella intermedia*, spirochetes	Thickens
7–14		*Porphyromonas gingivalis*, *Campylobacter rectus*, *Eikenella corrodens*, *Actinobacillus actinomycetemcomitans*, *Treponema* spirochetes, vibrios	"Corn cob"
14–21		Motile rods, streptococcus, *Porphyromonas gingivalis*, *Treponema* spirochetes, vibrios	Denser biofilm

Acquired Pellicle

The **acquired pellicle** is a very tenacious, acellular coating on the tooth surface to which plaque adheres. It is composed primarily of **salivary glycoproteins** that adhere directly to the hydroxyapatite crystal of the tooth. When it is removed from the tooth surface, it takes only minutes to begin reforming again on the newly cleaned surface.

Bacterial Biofilm

Plaque is a **nonmineralized biofilm** comprising of the colonizing **microorganisms** and **food debris** that adhere to the **acquired pellicle**. According to the American Society of Microbiology, with over 500 microorganisms in the mouth, plaque biofilm contains not only bacteria but also protozoa, mycoplasmas, and yeasts.

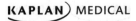

Supragingival biofilm is a heterogeneous, mostly gram-positive, bacterial soft deposit on the clinical crown of a tooth. **Subgingival biofilm** is supragingival biofilm that migrated apically with more gram-negative microorganisms, producing inflammatory alterations in the sulcus of the gingiva.

Subgingival biofilm—also called **tooth-associated subgingival biofilm**—may be attached to the tooth surface or loosely adherent. It is affiliated with the formation of subgingival calculus and root caries. **Loosely adherent subgingival biofilm** is also called epithelial-associated subgingival biofilm, and it proliferates from the apical gingival margin to the base of the pocket at the junctional epithelium. As the microorganisms produce toxins, pathogens begin to invade connective tissue.

A **matrix** protects and surrounds unevenly distributed **microcolonies** of bacteria as they replicate in biofilm. These bacteria convey chemical signals to each other via fluid channels, while microcolonies form destructive enzymes or toxins that produce periodontal disease. Eventually, the microcolonies become confluent as they merge together.

Gingivitis occurs about 2–3 weeks after the collecting plaque accumulates.

Biofilm adheres to the tooth surface as a result of the breakdown of dietary sucrose into glucans, fructans, and polysaccharides. **Dextrans** are high molecular weight macromolecules produced from polysaccharides by bacteria in the mouth.

Biofilm is a soft deposit that can be removed by mechanical means. Cariogenic biofilm initiates carious lesions in diets that contain a high sugar intake. Calculogenic biofilm mineralizes the soft deposits into calculus, though not all biofilm mineralizes.

Calculus

Calculus formation or mineralization of the biofilm dental plaque can occur within 48 hours of accumulation of plaque. Calculus is a haven for the collection of bacteria.

Coronal to the gingival margin is **supragingival calculus**, which obtains its minerals from saliva. **Apical** to the gingival margin is **subgingival calculus**, which obtains its minerals from crevicular fluid.

Like biofilm, calculus begins with the formation of the pellicle and then the formation of biofilm, which mineralizes into calculus. Calculus is an irregular, tenacious deposit composed of biofilm, inorganic salts, microorganisms, and epithelial cells. The biofilm mineralizes as hydroxyapatite crystals organize in the intracellular matrix. The color may be white, yellow, gray, or brown, from tobacco or food pig-

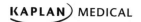

ments, though subgingival calculus may be black from blood pigments. It may be localized or generalized with the heaviest on the proximal surfaces.

Calculus adheres to the tooth surface in different ways: by direct attachment to the acquired pellicle, by "locking" into tooth irregularities, or by latching into the hydroxyapatite crystals of the tooth as the dental biofilm mineralizes.

Supragingival calculus can be detected with a mirror and air syringe, while subgingival calculus can be detected through exploration with a light lateral pressure.

Carious Lesions

Carious lesions occur from the demineralization of the tooth surface by cariogenic bacteria. The **normal pH** of the mouth is **6.75–7.25**, but with **carious enamel lesions**, the **pH is 4.5–5.5** for dissolution to the crown portion. **Root caries** occur when the pH is **6.0–6.7**, since cementum is less calcified than enamel. Root surface caries are common in older adults with recession.

As mentioned earlier, *S. sanguis* and S. *mutans* compete with each other intraorally. *S. sanguis* exist in higher numbers in a low-sugar diet, while *S. mutans* is more cariogenic and prevalent in a high-sugar diet. **Lactobacilli** are present in **deep carious lesions** and break down sucrose to form acid, which demineralizes the tooth surface.

Frequency of carbohydrate intake has a direct effect on the pH of the oral cavity. A continual intake of sucrose produces more acid by the bacteria. So someone who sips on soda all day might have a higher caries experience than someone who eats high carbohydrate desserts on occasion after a meal.

Saliva acts as a **buffer** to slow caries formation. A high flow rate of saliva increases the pH of the oral cavity to make it less acidic.

Radiographically, carious lesions can be detected at 200 microns.

A **carious lesion** starts off as a **demineralized** area that enters in the porous micro-channels of tooth structure. Later, a **white spot** appears on the enamel, with the surface area appearing undisturbed. This area can acquire stain, remineralize, or be arrested before cavitation occurs. **Cavitation** occurs when considerable tooth structure disintegrates from the demineralization. **Arrested caries** are lesions that began, but remineralized before further destruction occurred into cavitation.

Caries are seen frequently in **pits and fissures**, on **smooth surfaces**, and on **root surfaces**, especially in patients with recession. Chapter 14 discusses Black's classifications of carious lesions.

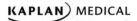

Oral Stains

Oral stains can appear in the oral cavity from different things:

- **Intrinsic stain** has become embedded into external tooth structure.

- **Extrinsic stain** exists on the surface of external tooth structure.

- **Endogenous stain** occurred within the tooth structure as the tooth developed.

- **Exogenous stain** developed from external sources. Exogenous stain can be extrinsic or it can become intrinsic.

Nasmyth's membrane is a membrane that covers newly erupted teeth. It can stain green and is not discussed in the table of stains.

Stain Removal

The polishing of stain is mainly for aesthetic reasons. Though it has no impact on oral health, stain should be removed as much as possible during scaling procedures. After scaling, the patient should be evaluated for **selective polishing**.

Polishing is beneficial for removing stains that have not been removed with toothbrushing or scaling. It is also beneficial for occlusal surfaces with plain pumice, before sealant placement.

One problem that polishing creates is an aerosol by rotary and air-polishing technique. This aerosol can stay airborne for hours, and is a contamination source for the clinician and other dental personnel.

Polishing can also induce **bacteremias** in a patient, by passing a rubber cup along the gingiva. Abrasive polishing paste may be driven into the gingival sulcus and may cause an inflammatory response and delayed healing of traumatized tissue.

In addition, polishing can remove tooth structure (**4 μm** with **30 seconds** of polishing), and can also scratch the tooth surface with coarse abrasives. It can remove the abundant outer fluoride layer of enamel.

Patients with **communicable diseases** and who are **susceptible to infection** are contraindicated for polishing. Dental contraindications would include **tooth hypersensitivity, implants, inflamed bleeding gingiva,** and **demineralized areas**.

Types of polishing include the rubber cup with abrasive paste and air-polishing. With the rubber cup, the most widely used polishing agent is a powered pumice with **varying coarseness**: fine (**F**), finer (**FF**), and finest (**FFF**).

> Stain does not contribute to caries formation or periodontal disease.

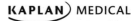
KAPLAN MEDICAL

Types of Stains

Type	Intrinsic Endogenous	Extrinsic Exogenous	Intrinsic Exogenous	Characteristics	Occurrence	Etiology
Brown from tobacco		X	X	Light to very dark brown	Mainly cervical third lingual surfaces	Tobacco
Brown from other sources		X		Dispersed in acquired pellicle, interproximal surfaces, or exposed roots	Varied, may be veneered or adherent to calculus	Coffee, tea, soy, betel leaf, stannous fluoride, mouth rinses
Black line		X		Thin line at gingival third, gingiva healthy	Cervical third of surface, mainly maxillary lingual posterior teeth	Unknown, clean mouths
Green		X	X	Yellow-green, embedded plaque biofilm, tooth may demineralize	Facial surface at gingival margin	Chromogenic bacteria
Orange		X		Orange to red	Cervical third anterior teeth	Chromogenic bacteria
Yellow		X		Yellow plaque biofilm	Biofilm at gingival margin	Food pigments
Tetracycline	X			Yellow to gray-brown	Generalized or confined to limited areas during tooth development	Tetracycline ingestion during tooth development
Amelogenesis imperfecta	X			Yellow-brown, gray-brown	Generalized	Genetic
Dentogenesis imperfecta	X			Opalescent gray-blue to brown	Generalized	Genetic
Enamel hypoplasia	X			White to brown in color	Systemic or localized	Ameloblast disturbance
Dental fluorosis	X			White to brown	White flecks to general pitting	Ingestion of excess fluoride
Non-vital tooth	X			Gray to brown-black in color	Reflected throughout	Pulp necrosis
Industrial metallic salts			X	Copper – green Brass – green Bismuth – brown Lead – black Cadmium – yellow	Mainly anterior cervical thirds	Oral inhalation of dust at industrial plants
Pharmacological stains			X	Iron – black Antidiarrhetic – brown	Biofilm, calculus	Drug ingestion

The **low-speed prophylaxis angle** can be a contra-angle or right-angle with a rubber cup or a bristle. The rubber cup should be passed over the tooth surface at a low r.p.m., with light pressure so that the tooth isn't heated and the gingival tissue isn't damaged. The brush allows the bristles to remove stains and debris from grooves and pits.

Air polishers utilize **air**, **water** and **powder** to remove stain from teeth. The most widely used powder is **sodium bicarbonate**, though it *should not* be used on patients with **high blood pressure** or with **restricted sodium diets**. New, safer powders for these patients have been developed, such as **aluminum trihydroxide**. Newer instruments have also been developed that function with air pressure between 40–100 psi and water pressure between 20–60 psi.

One way to greatly reduce a dental hygienist's aerosol contamination risk is to have the patient rinse with an **antibacterial mouth rinse** before using the air polisher. Another way is to use high-speed suction during the procedure. A consistent circular motion should be used at a **60-degree** angle to the facial and lingual surfaces of the **anterior teeth**; an **80-degree angle** for the **posterior teeth**; and a **90-degree** angle for the **occlusal surfaces**.

Polishing may be performed interproximally with dental floss or tape after a polishing agent is applied to the tooth surface. Finishing strips made of linen or plastic have an abrasive on one side, and may be used for interproximal stain removal.

> Air-polishing is contraindicated for those with respiratory diseases, communicable diseases, end-stage renal disease, Addison's disease, Cushing's syndrome, or metabolic alkalosis.

TOOTH BRUSHING

Toothbrushes provide mechanical action to break up plaque on the tooth surface. There are many manual and electric toothbrushes to choose from.

Bristle stiffness is determined by the **diameter** of each bristle. The smaller the diameter, the softer the brush. **Soft brushes** are recommended to prevent tissue injury. Microfine bristles have a diameter of 0.005 inches, with most soft bristles having a diameter of 0.007–0.009 inches. Each bristle tip should be rounded.

Quite recently, a new generation of power toothbrushes has been developed, designed specifically for those who lack dexterity, have orthodontic appliances, have dental implants, or are physically or mentally challenged. Two of these toothbrushes are the sonic and ultrasonic head. The **sonic head** operates at a low frequency of 200 Hz, and a vibration of 31,000 brush strokes per minute. The **ultrasonic head** operates on 1.6 MHz, and utilizes Piezo-electric emitters for its vibration. The cavitation of the heads of both brush types penetrates further than the area that the bristles touch. Other types of new-generation power toothbrushes are the rotary head and oscillating brushes, which also pulsate.

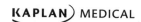

Tooth-Brushing Techniques

Method	Bristle Direction	Movement	Advantage
Bass	45° apically into sulcus	Short back and forth vibration	Efficient plaque removal
Modified Bass	45° apically into sulcus	Combines Bass movement with roll technique	Cleanses lingual and facial supragingival surfaces
Charters	45° to occlusal surface	Short back and forth vibration	Useful for orthodontic appliances and after periodontal surgery
Stillman	45° to long axis of tooth at gingival margin	Gentle rotary vibration of stationary bristles	Gingival stimulation
Modified Stillman	45° to long axis of tooth at gingival margin	Combines Stillman movement with roll technique	Cleanses lingual and facial supragingival surfaces
Fones	90° to long axis of tooth	Wide circular motion	Easy for children or patients with disabilities
Roll	Bristles directed apically	At gingival margin roll brush toward occlusal or incisal	Cleanses lingual and facial supragingival surfaces
Scrub	90° to long axis of tooth	Back and forth vertical and horizontal scrubbing	Easy for children or patients with disabilities
Leonard	90° to long axis of tooth	Up and down vertical motion from maxillary to mandibular teeth	Not recommended
Collis	45° apically into sulcus with curved filaments over crowns	Short back and forth vibration	Good for care givers of disabled patients

DENTIFRICES

Dentifrices are accepted by the ADA because of their effectiveness in preventing caries and gingivitis, and in reducing calculus formation, sensitivity, and bacterial plaque. They are available in paste, gel, or powder.

Pyrophosphate in anti-tartar toothpaste is not the reason a toothpaste is accepted by the ADA. The ADA approves toothpastes for their fluoride content, which prevents caries.

Detergents lower surface tension to loosen bacterial plaque and debris with foaming action. **Cleaning** and **polishing agents** use abrasives to remove stain, plaque, and debris. **Binders** prevent the separation of the components, while **humectants** maintain the moisture and prevent drying. **Sweetening** and **flavoring agents** deliver an enjoyable taste. **Preservatives** prolong shelf-life by deterring bacterial growth. **Coloring agents** are added to make the dentifrice more appealing for use.

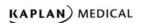

DISCLOSING AGENTS

Disclosing agents are available in pill and liquid form, and can be used as an educational tool to identify supragingival bacterial plaque. Plaque is invisible unless stained by foods or tobacco. Making plaque visible with disclosing solution allows the dental hygienist to gear her instruction to the needs of the patient.

Erythrosin is one of the most widely used disclosing agents. **Two-tone disclosing solutions** stain new plaque red and mature plaque blue, allowing the hygienist to educate the patient with home care. **Fluorescein dye** utilizes yellow sodium fluorescein and an ultraviolet light. Iodine solutions are not widely used today because of their severe allergic potential, nor are merbromin, Mercurochrome, or Bismarck Brown.

MOUTHWASH

Mouthwash is a supragingival procedure that may have cosmetic or therapeutic effects. The ADA recommends mouthwashes with therapeutic effects, such as over-the-counter fluoride rinses, chlorhexidine gluconate, and phenol-related essential oil compounds.

Chlorhexidine gluconate 0.12% (Peridex, PerioGard) is an effective bactericidal agent that has the ability to be retained in the oral cavity after rinsing and is slowly released into saliva, prolonging its therapeutic effect. It is an effective preprocedural mouth rinse to reduce aerosol spray contamination. Some side effects include tooth staining, temporary taste sensation loss, or burning sensation.

Phenol-related essential oils such as Listerine are over-the-counter mouth rinses that inhibit bacterial plaque growth and gingivitis. Listerine also reduces *S. mutans*, and is an effective preprocedural rinse to reduce aerosol spray contamination.

Over-the-counter fluoride rinses help to reduce carious lesions and to minimize tooth sensitivity.

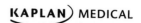

INTERDENTAL CARE

Since dental floss is pulled taut to remove plaque and debris, it will not remove plaque from a surface concavity on a tooth such as the mesial surface of the maxillary first premolar.

Flossing is the most effective way to remove interdental debris and plaque. Floss is now available in various types: waxed, unwaxed, tape, ribbon, tufted, variable diameter with a tufted segment and built-in threader, polytetrafluoroethylene, and braided nylon.

Floss should be inserted gently past the contact area into the embrasure and wrapped around the interproximal surface of one tooth in the **form of a "C."** It should slide gently beneath the gingival margin. Then, an up-and-down motion should be used to cleanse the tooth's interproximal surface. Finally, that motion should be repeated on the interproximal surface of the other tooth that shares that embrasure.

Floss aids include a **floss holder**, for those patients who lack dexterity; a **floss threader** for bridges and orthodontic appliances; **knitting yarn** for open embrasures, diastemas, and dental implants; and **pipe cleaners**, to remove bacterial plaque in furcation-involved areas (though care must be taken not to injure the tissues).

An **interdental brush** can help in open interproximal areas, furcations, concavities, orthodontic appliances, fixed prostheses, and space maintainers. It can also be used to apply chemotherapeutic agents such as chlorhexidine or fluoride. Size and shape selection depends on the size of the embrasure. The brush itself is a **soft filament** fiber, **twisted onto a steel wire**. It can be **cylindrical** or **tapered**. For anyone with an implant, the wire should be coated with plastic, so that the implant will not be scratched.

A **rubber tip** can be helpful for gingival margins, interproximal surfaces, and furcation areas. By tracing along the gingival margin, it can remove plaque. By placing the side of the tip onto the gingiva and massaging with a firm rotary motion, it can recontour gingiva.

Wooden devices include interdental wedges and toothpicks. An **interdental wedge** is triangular shaped so that it fits into embrasures. It is pressed in and out interdentally with a moderated amount of pressure. A **wooden toothpick** can be used alone or in a **periodontal aid** (plastic holder) to trace at a 45° angle into the sulcus or pocket.

SUBGINGIVAL IRRIGATION

Oral subgingival irrigation interrupts microbial colonization. Pulsating jet irrigators should be used with **low pressure**, perpendicular, or at a **90° angle** to the tooth surface. A soft rubber tip irrigator can be inserted 2 mm below the gingival margin. Oral irrigators may also be used to deliver antimicrobial agents such as chlorhexidine, stannous fluoride, phenolic mouth rinses, or sanguinaria.

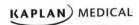

Oral irrigation is useful for patients with malpositioned teeth, open embrasures and furcations, orthodontic appliances, prostheses, and implant maintenance.

Care must be taken to instruct the patient to use a subgingival irrigator correctly since it can have adverse effects such as transient bacteremias. Moreover, it should not be used if the patient has any active lesions, such as a periodontal abscess.

PROSTHESIS CARE

Removable prostheses includes such things as partial dentures, dentures, night guards, and orthodontic appliances. These prostheses accumulate plaque, stain, and calculus and need to have the same cleaning that the rest of the oral cavity receives. If not properly cleansed, chronic *Candida albicans* can occur, especially in older adults whose immune systems are not able to fight off infection as well.

Removable appliances should be removed after eating and brushed with a denture brush, clasp bush if appropriate, and dentifrice. Appliances should be removed at night as instructed by the dentist. The removable appliance may also be immersed in detergent solution for the appropriate time suggested.

Fixed appliances may include space maintainers, bridges, crowns, orthodontic bands and wires, and implants. Implants will be discussed separately.

Care for orthodontic appliances includes both sulcular and Charter's method of tooth brushing. Orthodontic appliances and other fixed appliances may be cleaned with floss threaders and floss, or interdental brushes, and special orthodontic brushes.

IMPLANT CARE

Dental implants are placed within bone to replace missing teeth or to help place fixed or removable prosthesis. Great care needs to be taken during dental visits not to scratch the implant since those areas will harbor bacteria.

Plastic, graphite, or **nylon** instruments may be used for calculus removal from the prosthesis or superstructure with a light lateral pressure. These instruments may be scaler- or curet-shaped, or even hoe-shaped, crescent blade, or wrench-shaped. Scratching the implant will cause further accumulation of deposits.

Pocket depth probing is somewhat controversial but is performed with a plastic probe and a light pressure. Bleeding upon probing should be noted, along with tissue color and consistency. Care should be taken not to breach the fragile biological seal.

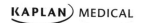

Ultrasonic cleaning causes **severe scratching** and is not recommended, but **air polishers** on a **light setting** with a low pressure may be used for stain removal.

Oral irrigation with an antimicrobial such as **0.12% chlorhexidine** is approved for subgingival irrigation with peri-implantitis. Acidulated fluorides are not recommended, since the acid will etch the implant surface. **Neutral sodium** is **recommended.**

Yarn, floss threaders, and tufted floss are excellent ways for the patient to maintain the implant prosthesis along with brushing twice daily with the Bass method. For patients who lack dexterity, a rotary toothbrush is beneficial. Interdental brushes coated with plastic may be used in open embrasure areas.

> The best way to check for implant failure is with radiographs.

Mobility may not be a loose implant but rather a loose prosthesis. Biannual radiographs are recommended to observe bone levels or radiolucencies around the implant.

FLUORIDE

Fluoride is an effective way to prevent caries. Fluoride was discovered in the early 1900's, when Dr. Frederick McKay noted that residents of an area of Colorado were less prone to carious lesions though they had discolored teeth. Dr. McKay invited a dental researcher by the name of Dr. G. V. Black to help investigate this mystery of discolored teeth. He thought it was because of the local water, but Dr. Black was dubious.

Research in the early 1930's by Dr. H. Trendley Dean, an epidemiologist with the National Institutes of Health, proved that Dr. McKay was correct in connecting dental fluorosis and mottled teeth with a low caries rate.

Dental Fluorosis Classification by H.T. Dean, 1942*

> Fluoride is absorbed in the stomach and small intestine, but is stored in teeth and long bones.

Classification	Criteria–Description of Enamel
Normal	Smooth, glossy, pale creamy-white translucent surface
Questionable	A few white flecks or white spots
Very Mild	Small opaque, paper-white areas covering less than 25% of the tooth surface
Mild	Opaque white areas covering less than 50% of the tooth surface
Moderate	All tooth surfaces affected; marked wear on biting surfaces; brown stain may be present
Severe	All tooth surfaces affected; discrete or confluent pitting; brown stain present

* Table from the American Dental Association site at www.ADA.org/

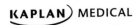

Fluoride can effectively be delivered through **community water** or **prescription**; with **topical treatments** in the office; and in **mouthwashes** and **toothpastes** at home.

The optimal level of fluoride in community water supplies is **1 part per million (ppm)**. **Less fluoride** is required in **warmer environments**, with **0.6 ppm** ideal, since people in those populations tend to drink more water. In **cooler climates** where the population **drinks less water**, the amount can be **1.2 ppm**. Recommended for community water supplies are **sodium fluoride, sodium silicofluoride,** or **hydrofluorosilicic** solution.

If a community water supply is not fluoridated, fluoride may be delivered in institutional water such as a school at 5 ppm. This is a higher concentration, but the students are present only 5 days a week. For children who live in an area that is not fluoridated, the recommend dosage is as follows:

Age	Dosage	
	<0.3	between 0.3-0.6
6 months – 3 years	0.25 mg	0 mg
3 years – 6 years	0.5 mg	0.25 mg
6 years to 16 years	1.0 mg	0.5 mg

Fluoride combines with the calcium **hydroxyapatite crystal** of the tooth to form **fluorapatite**, rendering the surface less soluble to the acid that the bacteria produce. Fluoride also has the ability to remineralize areas that have become demineralized by bacteria. Calcium hydroxyapatite redeposits into the demineralized area, with resurgence of the fluorhydroxyapatite crystals.

Fluoride is least effective in pits and fissures.

In-office fluorides that can be topically applied are neutral sodium fluoride (NaF), stannous fluoride (SnF_2), and acidulated phosphate fluoride (APF).

Neutral sodium fluoride is the **safest fluoride** to use on those with **porcelain veneers, crowns, bridges,** or **composite restorations**. It is also ideal for those on chemotherapy, or suffering from xerostomia or bulimia. It comes in **2%** solution, foam, or gel, and even a 5% varnish. The foam can be applied with a tray, while the solution is painted on. The gel may be painted on or placed in a tray. Fluoride varnish is applied with an applicator to dry teeth. The varnish sets quickly on its own, in the midst of saliva. Fluoride varnish has proved to desensitize sensitive teeth.

Neutral sodium can be applied 4 times at once-a-week intervals that correspond with the eruption of the primary and permanent molars. After that, it can be applied at 6-month intervals.

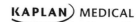

Stannous fluoride (SnF$_2$) **8%** is an unstable fluoride that must be mixed prior to usage. It is available as a gel or a two-part rinse. It can be used in 6-month intervals, with recare appointments. Patients often complain about the taste of stannous fluoride, and there may be some sloughing of gingiva after usage. It can also stain restorations, demineralized areas, and the acquired pellicle.

Stannous fluoride is *not recommended* for those with porcelain veneers, crowns, bridges, or composite restorations. Nor is it ideal for those suffering from xerostomia, bulimia, or undergoing chemotherapy.

Acidulated phosphate fluoride (APF) is the Rolls Royce of fluoride treatments. It comes in **1.23%** solution, gel, or foam. It is applied in the same manner as neutral sodium fluoride at 6-month intervals. Due to its acidity (3.0–3.5 pH), though, it has greater uptake in demineralized areas. Acidulated phosphate fluoride does not irritate tissues and is widely used in the dental office. It does need to be stored in plastic containers to maintain stability.

Due to its pH, APF is *not recommended* for those with porcelain veneers, crowns, bridges, or composite restorations. Nor is it ideal for those suffering from xerostomia, bulimia, or undergoing chemotherapy.

Fluoride Toxicity

Ingesting an excess amount of fluoride can cause fluoride toxicity. If it is ingested **rapidly**, then **acute fluoride toxicity** occurs. If it is ingested over a **longer period**, then chronic **fluoride toxicity** occurs.

A **lethal dose** of fluoride is **5–10 g** when taken all at once. This calculates out to about **32–64 milligrams per kilogram** of body weight. For children who weigh much less, the lethal dose per their body weight would be **0.5–1.0 g**.

A **toxic dose** is considerably less at **8 mg/kg per kilogram** of body weight for adults, and **5 mg/kg for children**. Consider this with a child receiving fluoride application in the office: A fluoride tray should not contain any more than 2 ml of gel per arch, or 4 ml total.

When administering an acidulated phosphate fluoride treatment to an 18-kilogram child with a small F tray holding 4 ml of APF, this would be delivering 50 mg of APF, that is more than half the toxic dose.

18 kg child weight × 5 mg/kg toxic dose = **90 mg of toxic dose**

1.23% of APF = 0.0123 g/ml = 12.3 mg/ml

4 ml of APF × 12.3 mg/ml = **50 mg, which is more than half the toxic dose**

Fluoride Facts:

- Fluoride does not cause cancer or birth defects.
- Topical fluoride does NOT cause fluorosis.
- Bone fluorosis is called osteosclerosis.
- Fluoride toxicity can cause respiratory or cardiac arrest.

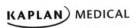

Signs and symptoms of acute fluoride toxicity include **thirst, increased salivation, nausea, vomiting, diarrhea, diaphoresis, tachycardia,** and **irreversible shock from respiratory suppression leading to cardiac suppression.** The gastrointestinal tract shows symptoms because **fluoride is absorbed in the stomach and small intestine.**

Emergency treatment for acute toxicity would include **induced vomiting,** with digital (mechanical) stimulation or syrup of ipecac, followed by ingestion of **milk or limewater** if the vomiting is still not stimulated. Vomiting **should not** be induced with **acidulated phosphate fluoride.** Further treatment may include the administration of calcium gluconate for muscle tremors, monitoring of vital signs for arrhythmias, gastric lavage, endotracheal intubation, and monitoring of blood electrolytes and pH.

DENTINAL HYPERSENSITIVITY

Dentin hypersensitivity is an abnormal response to extreme temperature change, chemicals, or mechanical stimuli. It can be aggravated by the existence of acid-producing bacterial plaque that demineralizes the tooth surface. It typically occurs on root-exposure areas, where recession may have occurred—whether from aggressive toothbrushing, periodontal disease, orthodontic movement, frenum pulling force, or occlusal forces. Hypersensitivity may also be caused by tooth bleaching.

Research seems to point to the **movement of fluids** in and out of the dentinal tubules as the cause of hypersensitivity. The hydrodynamic theory suggests that a stimulus such as a blast of cold air from an air–water syringe causes rapid transport of fluid in the dentinal tubules. This causes the odontoblasts to move, which then **stimulates A-delta nerve** fibers that line the pulp. A-delta nerve fibers are myelinated fibers that can conduct stimuli rapidly, while C-delta nerve fibers are unmyelinated fibers that conduct stimuli more slowly.

Chemicals such as sugar solutions in a fruit drink produce a hypersensitivity in a linear manner, depending on their osmotic strength. Chemicals with stronger osmotic pressure produce a greater proportion of hypersensitivity than do low-pressure chemicals.

Teeth can be desensitized in a number of ways. Adequate plaque removal prevents acid-producing bacteria from demineralizing the tooth surface, which can increase hypersensitivity.

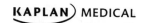

At-home applications include brush-on fluoride gels, fluoride rinses, and desensitizing toothpastes. Active ingredients in desensitizing toothpastes include **potassium nitrate, calcium hydroxide, strontium chloride, sodium citrate, potassium oxalate**, or **ferric oxalate**. Since there is no one desensitizing agent for every patient, you may suggest that your patient try another desensitizing toothpaste if he has not yet had relief.

In-office remedies include **fluoride varnishes, fluoride rinses**, or **gels** of either stannous or neutral sodium, **tooth-bonding materials**, or an **iontophoresis** electrical permeation of fluoride. The iontophoresis electrical current allows for better impregnation of the fluoride ion into the tooth surface.

SEALANTS

Pit and fissure sealants seal the pits and grooves of occlusal surfaces, areas that fluoride cannot protect. Bacteria can thrive in these microscopic areas, producing acid that demineralizes the tooth surface.

Sealants can be **self-cured** (autopolymerize) or **light-cured** (photopolymerize). They can be **filled** with particles of glass or quartz, or **unfilled** containing no particles. Sealant material is discussed further in Chapter 13. Proper administration of a sealant is as follows:

1. Before application, clean the tooth surface of all matter and debris, either with plain pumice and water and a prophy brush or with air abrasive alumina particles. Do not use prophy pastes with fluoride for this purpose. A sharp explorer can help to remove any matter that remains in the grooves.

2. Next, isolate the tooth with a rubber dam or cotton rolls and triangular bibulous pads. Dry it thoroughly and apply the acid-etch material. Phosphoric acid of 15–50% generates micropores to which the sealant can adhere. **Solutions** should be applied with a **gentle dabbing** by a cotton pellet or applicator. **Gels** should be applied with a syringe or brush.

Etching gels are applied and left undistrubed until the rinse. Etching solutions are gently dabbed on.

3. As per the manufacturer's recommendations, leave the acid-etch on the surface for 15–60 seconds.

4. Thoroughly rinse the tooth surface of all etchant and dry for 15–20 seconds or until the surface looks chalky white. Change the cotton rolls and triangular bibulous pads. Take care to prevent saliva contamination of the tooth surface. (If for any reason the surface was contaminated, re-etch for less time.)

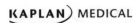

5. After the tooth has been thoroughly dried, apply the sealant material to all pits, fissures, buccal groves, and lingual grooves. If light-cured, place curing light over the surface for 20–30 seconds as per manufacturer recommendations while utilizing eye protection. Self-cured sealants set in 1–3 minutes. Do not disturb self-cured sealants while curing.

6. Examine the sealants for voids, overextensions, and under-curing. Evaluate the patient's occlusion with articulating paper for high spots that may need adjusting with a finishing bur.

TOOTH WHITENING

Tooth whitening occurs as a result of bleaching procedures. Vital teeth may be bleached with no damage to tooth structure, though some patients do experience temperature or gingival sensitivity afterward.

Teeth acquire extrinsic and intrinsic stains. Some extrinsic stains can become intrinsic. Over-the-counter materials may remove the stain but removal by dental professional with a dental prophylaxis may be the only way to remove tenacious stain.

Over-the-counter methods include bleaching strips impregnated with 6.5–14% hydrogen peroxide. Paint-on solutions contain 19% sodium percarbonate that adheres to the tooth surface by a viscous gel called Carbopol. Toothpastes have a chemical or polishing agent that aids in stain removal.

At-home bleaching kits include mouth guards with carbamide peroxide 10, 15, or 22%. In-office bleaching kits use 30–35% hydrogen peroxide, activated with a light or heat.

Non-vital teeth may contain necrotic pulps that require endodontic treatment, which may then turn dark in color. Bleach may be inserted into an unfilled pulp chamber until the correct tooth shade is attained. A composite or glass ionomer-filling is placed afterward.

PIERCINGS

Body piercing has become very popular. Tongue piercing, in particular, can have serious dental consequences, such as fractured teeth, gingival injury, infection leading to **Ludwig angina** (infection of the floor of the mouth), prolonged bleeding, or numbness or loss of taste from nerve damage.

"Mouth jewelry" should be removed before the taking of dental radiographs. The patient should be educated on maintaining a clean site.

TOBACCO USAGE

Tobacco has serious negative consequences on oral health, and the dental hygienist should do what he can to change a smoker's behavior. Habit-forming nicotine is absorbed in the lungs, where it then enters into the bloodstream. Smokeless tobacco (chewing tobacco or snuff) has direct contact with oral membranes. It is absorbed through gingival tissues and also enters into the bloodstream. Smokeless tobacco is sweetened with sugar or molasses, which makes the patient susceptible to caries.

Oral manifestations from tobacco use include exacerbation of periodontal disease, nicotine stomatitis, black hairy tongue, hyperkeratosis, leukoplakia, erythroplakia, xerostomia, basilar melanosis, and oral cancer. An intraoral and extraoral cancer screening should be performed at each routine recare appointment.

CANCER RISK FACTORS

Risk factors for cancer include the use of tobacco, alcohol, sun exposure, a diet high in fat and low in fruit and vegetables, and asbestos or radiation exposure.

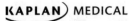

REVIEW QUESTIONS

1. Which of the following disclosing solutions cannot be used on a patient who is on Antabuse?

   A. Skinner's solution

   B. Fluorescein

   C. Erythrosin

   D. Two-tone dyes

2. Which of the following stain colors is produced by chromogenic bacteria?

   A. Brown stain

   B. Black line stain

   C. Orange stain

   D. Yellow stain

   E. Gray stain

3. In the intraoral cavity, which area tends to collect a greater amount of biofilm?

   A. The lingual of the mandibular incisors

   B. The facial of the mandibular anterior teeth

   C. The facial of the maxillary anterior teeth

   D. The lingual of the mandibular molars

   E. The facial of the maxillary third molars

4. What is the most important advice that a dental hygienist can give a patient with respect to oral home health care?

   A. Toothbrushing instruction

   B. Flossing instruction

   C. Guidance on using chlorhexadine rinses

   D. Guidance on using a Perio-Aid for plaque removal

   E. Instruction geared to the patient's current level of learning

5. Dental biofilm accumulates on the tooth surface

   A. Immediately

   B. In 1–2 days

   C. In 2–4 days

   D. In 7–14 days

6. Plaque becomes organized in stages. The micro-organism responsible for early plaque formation is

   A. *A. naeslundii* and *S. oralis*

   B. *Prevotella intermedia* and *Porphyromonas gingivalis*

   C. *Treponema* spirochetes and *Veillonella*

   D. *Streptococcus sanguis* and *Streptococcus mutans*

   E. *A. israelii* and *Bacteroides*

7. Nursing-bottle decay occurs when fluids rich in sugar pool around tooth structures. Nursing-bottle caries can occur on all of the following teeth EXCEPT

   A. Mandibular incisors

   B. Maxillary incisors

   C. Maxillary molars

   D. Mandibular molars

8. Recurrent decay is caused by

   A. Imbibition

   B. Syneresis

   C. Percolation

   D. Flow

9. The normal pH in the oral cavity is 6.75–7.25. The cementum of a tooth starts to demineralize at a pH of ___, while the enamel starts to demineralize at a pH of ___.

    A. 4.5–5.0 cementum and 3.0–3.5 enamel
    B. 5.0–5.5 cementum and 3.5–4.0 enamel
    C. 5.7–6.2 cementum and 4.0–4.5 enamel
    D. 6.0–6.7 cementum and 4.5–5.0 enamel
    E. 6.0–6.7 cementum and 5.0–5.5 enamel

10. The hardness or softness of a toothbrush is determined by

    A. Bristle length
    B. Bristle shape
    C. Amount of bristles in each tuft
    D. Bristle diameter
    E. Bristle color

11. To prevent bacteremias, an oral irrigator should be used at what angle to the long access of the tooth?

    A. 45°
    B. 60°
    C. 75°
    D. 90°

12. The most helpful adjunct for a patient who has difficulty with plaque removal in a Class II furcation would be

    A. Interproximal brush
    B. Floss
    C. Stimudents
    D. Cannula irrigator
    E. PerioAide

13. Although not widely used anymore, someone who is allergic to _____ should not be disclosed with Skinner's solution.

    A. Shellfish
    B. Tomatoes
    C. Chocolate
    D. Peanuts
    E. Milk

14. A patient who has lived for 20 years in a naturally fluoridated community at 10–15 PPM can suffer from

    A. Osteoporosis
    B. Osteopenia
    C. Osteomalacia
    D. Osteosclerosis

15. After the dental hygienist has done a complete root debridement, how long does it take for the acquired pellicle to return?

    A. Within minutes
    B. 1 hour
    C. 2 hours
    D. 24 hours
    E. 1 or 2 days

16. The mode of communication for microorganisms that are distributed unevenly in microcolonies is

    A. Sodium channels
    B. Chemical signals
    C. Via oxygen transport
    D. Through dormant cells

17. Which of the following stains green on newly erupted teeth?

    A. Hertwig's sheath
    B. Nasmyth's membrane
    C. Acquired pellicle
    D. Cementum
    E. Demineralized areas

18. Workers in which of the following industrial plants may accumulate blue-gray stained teeth from breathing in the industrial dust?

    A. Cadmium
    B. Bismuth
    C. Copper
    D. Silver
    E. Lead

19. Dental floss cannot efficiently remove plaque from the _____, because of that tooth's concavity.

    A. Mesial of the mandibular canine
    B. Distal of the maxillary canine
    C. Mesial of the maxillary first premolar
    D. Mesial of the maxillary second premolar
    E. Mesial of the mandibular first premolar

20. Efficient plaque removal around implants prevents peri-implantitis. The most helpful adjunct for cleaning around an implant is

    A. Yarn
    B. Pipe cleaner
    C. Interdental brush
    D. Interdental wedge

21. Air polishers can now be used on patients with high blood pressure. The powder of choice is sodium bicarbonate.

    A. Both statements are true
    B. The first statement is true. The second statement is false because the powder is aluminum trihydroxide.
    C. The first statement is false because patients with high blood pressure should not have an air polisher used on them. The second statement is true of air polishers.
    D. Both statements are false since there are new polishing agents for the air polisher.

22. All the following instruments may be used on dental implants EXCEPT

    A. Plastic
    B. Graphite
    C. Nylon
    D. Gracey curet
    E. Oral irrigator

23. A 6-year-old boy and his family have just moved into an optimally fluoridated water community. The mother asks the new dentist to write a prescription for fluoride tablets. How much fluoride should this child be taking?

    A. 0.25 mg
    B. 0.5 mg
    C. 1.0 mg
    D. None of the above

24. Which of the following fluorides would you suggest for a patient who has had veneers placed on #6, #7, #8, #9, #10, and #11, along with a bridge from #29 – #31?

    A. Fluoride varnish
    B. Neutral sodium fluoride
    C. Stannous fluoride
    D. Acidulated phosphate fluoride
    E. None of the above

25. Lifestyles can promote good health or contribute to bad health. All of the following are risk factors for cancer EXCEPT

    A. A diet low in fat
    B. Tobacco usage
    C. Sun exposure
    D. Asbestos exposure
    E. Alcohol

ANSWER EXPLANATIONS

1. C

Erythrosin cannot be used since it contains 95% alcohol. Someone taking Antabuse for alcoholism would become very ill if any alcohol were absorbed or ingested.

2. C

Chromogenic bacteria produce orange and green stains.

A. Brown stain is produced by coffee, tea and tobacco.

B. Black line stain occurs in clean mouths on the lingual surfaces.

D. Yellow stain occurs from poor oral hygiene and food pigments.

E. Gray stain can occur from smoking marijuana.

3. E

The facial surfaces of the maxillary third molars tend to collect a lot of plaque and biofilm. They are quite difficult to reach with a toothbrush during plaque removal.

4. E

Building a rapport with your patient is important so that instruction can be geared to his current level of learning and so that he will be open to hearing about his oral health needs.

Toothbrushing instructions, flossing instructions, chlorhexadine rinses and the use of a Perio-Aid for plaque removal will all help but getting on the patient's level to motivate them is the most important.

5. B

Dental biofilm or plaque is made up of bacterial polysaccharides that adhere to the tooth surface 1–2 days over the acquired pellicle. The acquired pellicle comes back within minutes of removal.

6. D

Plaque formation organizes in stages, with *Streptococcus sanguis* and *Streptococcus mutans* most prominent early on. The other microorganisms listed develop after that.

7. A

In nursing-bottle decay, the mandibular incisors are not as likely to have caries. That is because when the baby sucks on the bottle, those teeth are generally covered by the tongue and protected from the fluids.

8. C

Recurrent decay is caused by percolation, which allows for fluids containing polysaccharides to move in and out of the area between the tooth and filling. This occurs from breakdown of the filling margins.

A. Imbibition means to absorb more water.

B. Syneresis means to dry out.

D. Flow is concerned with dental materials contacting all surfaces when applied.

9. D

Cementum starts to demineralize at a pH of 6.0–6.7, since it is softer than the enamel (65% inorganic). Enamel starts to demineralize at a lower acidic pH of 4.5–5.0, since it is much harder (95% inorganic).

10. D

The hardness or softness of a toothbrush is determined by bristle diameter. The smaller the diameter (0.007-0.009 inches), the softer the bush. A hard brush ranges from 0.007-0.015 inches.

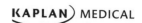

11. D

Oral irrigation should perfomed at a 90° angle to the long access of the tooth on a low-pressure setting. This will prevent transient bacterias.

12. E

For a Class II furcation, the most helpful adjunct for plaque removal is Perio-Aid. This would trace along the gingiva and into the concave furca.

A. Interproximal brush would not be able to penetrate into a Class II and is an interproximal adjunct.

B. Floss will not enter a Class II involvement.

C. Stimudents are used in embrasure areas.

D. Cannula irrigator is not proper for this function.

13. A

A patient with an allergy to shellfish should not use iodine-disclosing solutions. Skinner's solution contains iodine, as does shellfish.

14. D

A patient who has lived for years in a naturally fluoridated community at 10–15 PPM could well suffer from osteosclerosis, bone that is abnormally hardened.

A. Osteoporosis is bone loss through loss of calcium.

B. Osteopenia is the thinning of bones before osteoporosis occurs.

C. Osteomalacia is a reduction of mineral content of bone leading to softening.

15. A

The acquired pellicle takes only minutes to start reforming, as a result of glycoproteins contained in saliva, something constantly flowing in the mouth.

16. B

Microcolonies of microorganisms exchange chemical signals via fluid channels, as they direct colonization to transition into a pathogenic entity.

A. Sodium channels are needed for nerve conduction.

C. Oxygen transport is necessary for some of the bacteria, but not for anaerobic bacteria which cannot survive in an oxygen environment.

D. Some bacteria can become dormant or inactive but can be activated by new bacteria.

17. B

Nasmyth's membrane can stain newly erupted teeth green. It is cuticle—which is a membrane—covering a newly erupted tooth.

A. Hertwig's sheath is on the root and not on the crown of an erupting tooth.

C. Acquired pellicle can be unstained or stained brown or black.

D. Cementum is on the root and not the crown of an erupting tooth.

E. Demineralized areas should not occur on most newly erupted teeth.

18. D

A plant worker who inhales silver will acquire a blue–gray stain.

A. Cadmium stains the teeth yellow when inhaled.

B. Bismuth stains the teeth dark brown when inhaled.

C. Copper stains the teeth green when inhaled.

E. Lead stains gray–black.

19. C

The mesial of the maxillary first premolar has a concavity that is hard to scale or rootplane. In fact, it may be mistaken for a cavity and cannot be penetrated with floss.

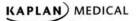

20. **A**

The most helpful adjunct for cleaning around an implant is yarn, because it is soft and will not scratch.

B. A pipe cleaner has metal in the middle and can scratch the implant.

C. An interdental brush would be acceptable only if the metal wire were coated in plastic.

D. An interdental wedge would be of little benefit.

21. **B**

The first statement is true. The second statement is false because the powder of choice is aluminum trihydroxide. Sodium bicarbonate is not recommended for those with hypertension because of its sodium content.

22. **D**

A Gracey curet should not be used on a dental implant. It is metal and would cause scratches.

23. **D**

The child should be taking no fluoride tablets. The water is already optimally fluoridated. More fluoride would cause dental flurosis.

24. **B**

The safest fluoride to use with veneers and bridges is neutral sodium fluoride, since it will not stain or etch these surfaces.

A. Fluoride varnish is colored brown and is not recommended.

C. Stannous fluoride would stain these surfaces.

D. Acidulated phosphate fluoride will etch crowns, bridges, and veneers.

25. **A**

A diet low in fat is not a risk factor for cancer. In fact, that diet is ideal for optimal health.

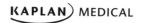

Chapter Sixteen: Instrumentation for Client Assessment and Care

There are three major parts to any dental instrument: the **handle,** the **shank,** and the **working end.** The handle is the part that is grasped during instrument activation; it may be single or double ended, and is available in various diameters, weights, and shapes. The shank connects the handle to the working end of the instrument. It may be straight (simple) or curved/angled (complex), and flexible or rigid. The straight shank allows for access to anterior teeth, while the curved/angled shank allows for access to posterior teeth. The type, amount, and location of deposit will determine which instrument to use for deposit removal. The heavier the deposit, the more rigid the shank should be. For lighter deposits, a flexible shank is sufficient.

The working end of every dental instrument is unique, depending on its function. Sharp instruments such as curets or scalers have a **cutting edge** and **lateral surface.** The cutting edge is where two surfaces meet to form a line, such as the face of the instrument and the lateral surface. The lateral surface is the continuous back of the instrument that meets the cutting edge. Non-sharp instruments, such as a probe, have a dull blade or nib.

INSTRUMENT GRASP AND ACTIVATION

There are two basic grasps used during dental hygiene instrumentation and patient care. The first—the **Modified Pen Grasp**—is used in the activation of most scalers, curets, probes, and explorers. This is a **three-fingered grasp,** where the index, thumb, and middle fingers grasp the instrument. The middle finger plays a pivotal role, serving primarily to prevent instrument slippage during adaptation and activation against the tooth surface. The ring finger acts as the fulcrum during instrument adaptation and activation, and is therefore not considered a finger in this grasp. The fulcrum is always on a tooth adjacent to the tooth being treated, so that deposit removal can be performed properly.

The second most popular grasp is the **Palm Grasp,** which is used to activate the air/water syringe, porte polisher, and the rubber-dam clamp holder. With this grasp, the handle of the instrument lies in the palm of the hand, and the thumb serves as the fulcrum.

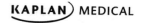

Adaptation refers to the relationship between the instrument and the tooth or the gingival tissue. The instrument is rolled at the line angles of the teeth so it adapts to the tooth surface and prevents laceration of gingival tissue.

Angulation refers to the relationship between the working end of the instrument and the tooth surfaces. **Lateral pressure** refers to the pressure of the instrument against the tooth during instrument activation. This varies with each task. During an exploratory stroke for deposit detection, lateral pressure is light. For **deposit removal, lateral pressure** is **heavier**, to ensure adequate deposit removal. For **root debridement, lateral pressure starts out heavy** and then **becomes lighter** as deposits are removed; this helps to prevent excess tooth tissue removal.

PROBES AND EXPLORERS

Periodontal probes measure the presence or absence of periodontal disease through evaluation of the periodontal pocket, root surface exposure, and bone loss. Their functions are many. Probes can:

- Assess periodontal status for a dental hygiene care plan
- Evaluate the mucogingival junction
- Survey the sulcus and pocket depths
- Evaluate gingival bleeding upon probing or suppuration
- Measure gingival recession
- Appraise the consistency of gingival tissue
- Establish parameters for gingival characteristics
- Evaluate the success of completed treatment
- Measure oral lesions and pathologies

The Nabor's probe is used to evaluate furcation involvement.

Each probe has a straight blade which can be round or flat, tapered, color-coded, or narrow in diameter. The PSR (Periodontal Screening and Recording Probe) has a ball at one tip, and the Nabor's Probe is curved (unlike any other probe) and is used to evaluate furcations.

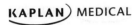

TYPES OF PERIODONTAL ASSESSMENTS

The first type of periodontal evaluation is for **probing periodontal pockets**. During this procedure, the clinician initially considers recession, furcation involvement, mobility, and bleeding. In an **evaluation for pocket depths**, a **walking stroke** is used to evaluate the 6 areas on each tooth: mesiofacial/mesiobuccal, facial/buccal, distofacial/distobuccal, mesiolingual, lingual, and distolingual. Each pocket depth is recorded from the base of the pocket to the height of the gingival margin.

Several things can affect pocket depth evaluation: the severity and extent of periodontal disease, the calibration of the clinician, placement problems due to calculus deposits, tooth contours, restorations, furcation, anatomical anomalies, and the amount of pressure used during the probing process. The amount of pressure needed for adequate periodontal probing of the gingival sulcus is 10–20 grams of pressure.

The second type of periodontal assessment is **clinical attachment Level** (CAL). This is determined by first measuring the distance from the CEJ to the base of the pocket. If recession is present, then a second measurement is taken from the gingival margin to the CEJ. The two numbers are added to determine the CAL. So if there were a 3 mm pocket on the buccal aspect of Tooth #14 along with 2 mm of gingival recession, the CAL would be 5. See illustration in Chapter 8.

Third, the **attached gingiva (AG)** is assessed by first measuring the CEJ to the mucogingival junction, and then measuring the CEJ to the base of the pocket. The second number is subtracted from the first number to determine the attached gingiva. So if the CEJ to the mucogingival junction were 7 mm and the CEJ to the base of the pocket were 3 mm, then there would be a 4 mm zone of attached gingiva.

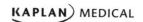

Most Common Periodontal Probes

Types of Probe	Probe Markings	Purpose
Williams	1	Evaluates periodontium
	2	Measures attached epithelium
	3	Measures oral lesions/pathologies
	5	
	7	
	8	
	9	
	10	
Michigan	3	Evaluates periodontium
	6	Measures attached epithelium
	8	Measures oral lesions/pathologies
Color Coded PSR	3.5–5.5	Provides a cursory screening of each sextant in the oral cavity. May be used for individuals or large groups.
	5.5–8.5	
	8.5–11.5	
Nabor	Non-calibrated	Evaluates the degree and severity of furcation involvement

Classification of Furcations

Class I	Feel indentation of furcation with probe. Early involvement
Class II	Probe enters furcation but does not pass through. Bone loss is evident.
Class III	Probe enters furcation and passes through it. Furcation is not visible.
Class IV	Probe enters furcation and passes through it. Gingival recession is present and furcation is visible to the naked eye.

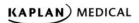

Explorers evaluate several things: tooth surface irregularities; the presence or absence of decay; calculus deposits (both subgingivally and supragingivally); and the effectiveness of existing restorations. When looking at the presence of calculus deposits, one should use a light grasp with small overlapping strokes. (Light lateral pressure = exploratory stroke.) A pull stroke will activate the explorer from the base of the sulcus/periodontal pocket toward the incisal or occlusal surface. For **proper adaptation** to the given tooth, the **explorer is then rolled between the fingers;** this ensures that the toe 1/3 of the explorer is adapted to the tooth and that the gingival tissues will not be damaged. The "point" at the end of the explorer is never used for calculus detection.

> Rolling the explorer allows for better adaption to the tooth surface.

Most Commonly Used Explorers

Types	Shape	Use
Subgingival	Angulated shank Short tip	Subgingival root exam
Sickle or Shepherd's Hook	Wide hook	Examine pit and fissures, supragingival smooth surfaces, and margins of restorations
Pigtail or Cowhorn	Paired curved tips	Proximal surfaces for calculus, margins of restorations, and dental caries

MOUTH MIRROR

The mouth mirror has several surfaces: **plane (flat), concave,** and **frontal.** The diameter of the mirror head can range from $\frac{5}{8}$ of an inch to 2 inches. A disposable mirror is one piece of plastic with a front surface mirror, often used for screenings and patient education. The dental mirror is used for **indirect vision, illumination, transillumination,** and **retraction.** In order to maintain a clear field of vision with a mirror, one can do the following:

1. Warm the mirror with warm water.
2. Rub along buccal mucosa to coat the mirror with film of saliva.
3. Ask the patient to breathe through the nose.
4. Use the mirror dips such as a defogger
5. Discard scratched mirrors.

The hygienist should hold the mouth mirror in her **non-dominant hand.** The fulcrum rests on the incisal or occlusal surface (though it can also rest on the occlusofacial or occlusolingual line angle of a stable tooth), and is set on the same arch as the tooth being instrumented. The fulcrum allows the hand and instrument to move as one unit. Intraoral or extraoral fulcrums are both acceptable.

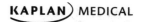

INSTRUMENTS FOR DEPOSIT REMOVAL

Scalers are used to remove heavy supragingival **calculus** and **spicules just below the gingival margin.** Both anterior sickle scalers and posterior sickle scalers are adapted to the tooth surface by placing the tip 1/3 of the cutting edge at a 70–80° angle. A pull stroke will activate the instrument.

A scaler should not be used subgingivally because it is so large: It could cause trauma to the gingival tissues; its pointed tip might not easily adapt to the curved root surface; and tactile sensitivity will drop as a result of the rigid shanks.

The universal curet has 2 cutting edges per end for a total of 4 cutting edges. Area-specific curets have one cutting edge per end, for a total of 2 cutting edges.

Curets are universal (adaptable to any tooth surface) or area-specific. A **universal curet** has two cutting edges per end—called inner and outer cutting edges. Both edges are used for deposit removal. The toe 1/3 of any universal curet may be adapted to any tooth surface in the oral cavity. The face of the universal curet is at a 90° angle from the terminal shank.

For scaling the **distal** aspect of a mesial root, use a **posterior distal curet.** For scaling the **mesial** aspect of a distal root, use a **posterior mesial curet.** Pay attention to the surface—not the root—being curetted.

Area-specific curets have one cutting edge per end that can remove deposits from specific tooth surfaces. Only the lower cutting edge is used for deposit removal procedures. The toe 1/3 of any area-specific curet is adapted to the area of the tooth being instrumented, and the face set at a 70° angle to the terminal shank. The Micro Mini-Five-bladed Gracey curets have a blade which is half the length of a Gracey curet. They also have a 3mm longer shank which yields better access to calculus in intraradicular furcations and developmental depressions. After-Five curets have a longer shank with a standard diameter blade of a Gracey curet. Rigid After-Five curets have a longer terminal shank but have an increased diameter blade. Micro Mini-Five curets have an extended, rigid shank length with a blade that is 50% shorter and 20% thinner to better adapt into furcations for the removal of residual calculus. The most commonly used Gracey curets are listed below:

Gracey Area-Specific Instruments

Anterior	1/2	3/4
Anterior and premolar	5/6	
Posterior: facial and lingual	7/8	9/10
Posterior: mesial	11/12	15/16
Posterior: distal	13/14	17/18

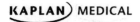

OTHER INSTRUMENTS

Files can crush and break calculus on enamel surfaces, and also be used for smoothing rough amalgams. They are applied to the outer surface of the deposit. Files have multiple cutting edges that line up as a series of miniature hoes. The blades are at a 90 or 105° angle with the shank. The stroke used is a pull-stroke only.

Hoes cannot be adapted to a curved tooth surface. They are used primarily to remove heavy supragingival calculus. They have a straight, single cutting edge with the blade at a 99–100° angle to the shank. The cutting edge is beveled at a 45° angle to the end of the blade. A pull stroke is used to activate the hoe in the direction of the incisal or occlusal surface.

Chisels are used to remove heavy supragingival calculus deposits from the interproximal surfaces of anterior teeth. They have a straight, single cutting edge that is beveled at a 45° angle. The stroke is horizontal only from facial to lingual on the proximal surfaces of anterior teeth.

SHARPENING OF INSTRUMENTS

A sharp cutting edge on a dental instrument will make it easier to remove deposit; easier to improve stroke control and reduce the number of strokes needed; allow for improved patient comfort; and reduce the clinician's fatigue. Dental instruments should be sharpened after each use and at the first sign of dullness. Due to aerosol generation during sharpening, the clinician should wear protective eyewear, a mask, and gloves.

> Instrument sharpening should produce a sharp cutting edge and maintain the integrity of the instrument.

Once it has been determined that an instrument need to be sharpened, the appropriate sharpening stone should be selected and lubricated. The internal angle of all curets and scalers is 70–80°. **The face of the instrument should be placed at a 110° angle in relation to the flat sharpening stone.**

> Honing removes the "wire edge" produced during the sharpening process.
>
> Sterile stone should be in every instrument setup.

For universal instruments, both cutting edges should be sharpened. For an area-specific instrument, only the lower cutting edge of the face is sharpened. Movement of the stone or the instrument should include sharpening of the heel 1/3 of the working end, then the middle 1/3, and finally the toe or tip 1/3. The toe of a curet should be rounded to maintain the integrity of its shape. Honing the face of the instrument allows for removal of the wire edge that was produced during the sharpening procedure. Finally, the instrument should be tested for sharpness; a test stick will determine whether it has been sufficiently sharpened.

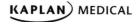

Acoustic microstraining with ultrasonics is the agitation of fluids which remove calculus and exotoxins.

Intense turbulence at the ultrasonic tip interrupts bacterial colonization.

Frequency = Speed of tip

Amplitude = Power

Contraindications: Unshielded pacemaker, implant, demineralized areas, amelogenesis imperfecta, immune compromised, respiratory infections, sensitivity, recession.

Types of Sharpening Stones

Stone	Consistency	Lubrication	Function
Ceramic	Fine Synthetic stone	Water or dry	Routine instrument sharpening
Arkansas	Fine Natural	Mineral oil	Routine instrument sharpening
India	Medium Synthetic	Water or oil	Sharpen very dull cutting edges
Composition	Coarse	Water	Reshape improperly sharpened instruments, exceedingly dull cutting edges, and damaged cutting edges

ULTRASONIC AND SONIC INSTRUMENTS

Ultrasonic and sonic scalers can be used to debride surfaces, making it easier for a dental hygienist to perform her duties. These electrically powered instruments use high-frequency energy in a rapid vibration at the tip of the scaler. Water is used to lavage the area being debrided and also to prevent overheating of the ultrasonic scaler. Minute bubbles are released in a process called **cavitation**. Cavitation aids in destroying microbes and their endotoxins while removing calculus.

Ultrasonic versus Sonic Scalers

Types of of Ultrasonic	Tip Movement	Active Surfaces of Tip	Cycles Per Second (CPS)/Frequency	Method of Activation
Sonic	Elliptical or orbital	All surfaces	2000–8000 cps	Air-pressure to create mechanical vibrations
Magnetostrictive	Elliptical	Face, back, lateral edges	29,000–40,000 cps	Conversion of electrical current into a magnetic field causing the tip to vibrate
Piezoelectric	Linear	Lateral edges	25,000–50,000 cps	Expansion and contraction of the crystals in the housing unit causing the tip to vibrate

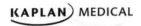

REVIEW QUESTIONS

1. How many cutting edges does a Gracey 11/12 have?

   A. 1

   B. 2

   C. 3

   D. 4

2. In relation to the long axis of the tooth, what position is the terminal shank of a Columbia 13/14 to allow for proper instrument activation to take place?

   A. Horizontal

   B. Perpendicular

   C. Parallel

   D. Oblique

3. When scaling subgingivally on the distal aspect of the mesial root on tooth #30, which instrument should be used for adequate deposit removal?

   A. Gracey 1/2

   B. Gracey 13/14

   C. 204SD

   D. Gracey 11/12

4. During power driven instrumentation, the magnetostrictive scaler moves in what type of pattern?

   A. Vertical

   B. Linear

   C. Elliptical

   D. Horizontal

5. All of the following are sharpening stones used in dentistry EXCEPT one. Which of the following stones is the EXCEPTION?

   A. Arkansas stone

   B. Indian stone

   C. Ceramic stone

   D. Alabama stone

6. What is the angle of the face of a Gracey 13/14 to its shank?

   A. 60–70°

   B. 70–80°

   C. 80–90°

   D. 100–110°

7. When probing the mesial aspect of tooth #3, the gingival margin rests at 3.5 mm. The recording on the periodontal chart should show the reading as

   A. 3 mm

   B. 3.5 mm

   C. 4 mm

   D. 3-4 mm

8. A patient returns for a follow-up appointment 5 weeks after initial root debridement. The root debridement has been successful, as the gingival tissue is pink, firm, and does not bleed upon probing. However upon examination, you see that several root surfaces have brown debris. This is because the patient

   A. Has poor oral hygiene

   B. Is a heavy coffee/tea drinker

   C. Has residual deposits from initial therapy

   D. Accumulates deposits quickly

9. With regard to question #8, what would be the best course of action to take with this patient?

    A. Review oral hygiene habits.
    B. Advise him to reduce the amount of coffee/tea he drinks.
    C. Remove the deposits.
    D. Advise him to use an electric toothbrush.

10. When using an explorer to detect subgingival deposits, what type of stroke should be used?

    A. Grasp the instrument lightly and apply light pressure.
    B. Grasp the instrument lightly and apply heavy pressure.
    C. Grasp the instrument firmly and apply light pressure.
    D. Grasp the instrument firmly and apply heavy pressure.

11. While performing root debridement, the angulation of the instrument against the tissue should be

    A. Less than 45°
    B. 45–90°
    C. 90–100°
    D. Greater than 100°

12. The ultrasonic principle is based on the use of

    A. Pressure
    B. A jet stream of water
    C. Rapid electrical impulses
    D. High-frequency sound waves
    E. None of the above

13. The primary purpose of removal of deposit during root debridement is that it

    A. Acts as a mechanical irritant against the gingiva.
    B. Alters the cementum.
    C. Harbors plaque organisms.
    D. Pushes against the junctional epithelium.
    E. All of the above

14. The most important criterion for determining a patient's recare interval for oral prophylaxis is the

    A. Patient's desire
    B. Amount of calculus deposits present
    C. Previous caries experience
    D. Maintenance of good oral health

15. Definitive exploration is used for all of the following conditions except one. Which of following is the EXCEPTION?

    A. Detection of calculus
    B. Overhanging restoration
    C. An irregular cementoenamel junction
    D. Cemental resorption
    E. Root fenestration

16. During scaling, which of the following could be mistaken for calculus deposits?

    A. Developmental depression
    B. Enamel pearl
    C. Concavity
    D. Convexity

17. All of the following conditions except one are contraindicated for use of the ultrasonic scaler. Which of the following is the EXCEPTION?

    A. Pacemaker
    B. Pregnancy
    C. Diabetes
    D. Tuberculosis
    E. HBV

18. What is the angle of the face of a Gracey 13/14 in regard to the shank?

    A. 60–70°
    B. 70–80°
    C. 80–90°
    D. 95–105°

19. Ultrasonic scalers differ from sonic scalers by

    A. Heat production
    B. Ultrasonics use lower frequency than sonic
    C. Ultrasonics use a higher frequency than sonic
    D. Linear movement

20. Your patient presents with a lingual ledge of calculus on her mandibular anterior linguals. To remove this deposit, the best instrument would be a

    A. Gracey 1/2
    B. Universal curet
    C. Curved sickle scaler
    D. Hoe
    E. 204SD

21. All of the following are difficult areas to scale EXCEPT one. Which of the following is the EXCEPTION?

    A. Convexity
    B. CEJ
    C. Concavity
    D. Developmental depression

22. A periodontal file would not be used to

    A. Perform soft tissue curettage
    B. Crush calculus deposits
    C. Remove calculus from areas of limited access
    D. Complete root debridement procedures

23. All of the following except one would describe the exploratory stroke. Which of the following is the EXCEPTION?

    A. The stroke is vertical to oblique.
    B. The stroke is short and overlapping.
    C. Light pressure is applied to the tooth surface.
    D. The handle of the instrument is grasped firmly.

24. Which of the following strokes would be used during root debridement?

    A. Horizontal
    B. Vertical
    C. Diagonal
    D. All of the above

25. The primary goal of sharpening curets and scalers is to

    A. Reduce the number of strokes
    B. Prevent slippage and trauma to tissue
    C. Reduce clinician fatigue
    D. Allow more lateral pressure to be used
    E. Maintain the integrity of the instrument

26. Using an angulation of less than 30° during instrumentation with a Gracey 13/14 will result in all of the following EXCEPT one. Which of the following is the EXCEPTION?

    A. Improved root debridement
    B. Burnished calculus
    C. Laceration of gingival tissue
    D. Incomplete removal of calculus

27. Which of the following causes fracturing of calculus deposits during ultrasonic scaler use?

    A. Pressure of the water
    B. High frequency sound
    C. Blunt, shearing action of the tip
    D. Vibratory action of the tip

28. When performing root debridement, a dull instrument may cause all of the following conditions EXCEPT one. Which of the following is the EXCEPTION?

    A. Clinician fatigue
    B. Gouged tooth structure
    C. Injury to soft tissue
    D. Increased tactile sensitivity
    E. Burnished calculus

29. Hand sharpening curets on a flat stone is most effective when the face of the Columbia 13/14 curet meets the stone at

    A. 70°
    B. 90°
    C. 110°
    D. 130°
    E. 150°

30. For efficient deposit removal, the blade of a scaler should be adapted to the tooth surface at what angle?

    A. Approximately 15°
    B. Slightly less than 45°
    C. Slightly less than 90°
    D. Slightly more than 90°
    E. At least 100°

ANSWER EXPLANATIONS

1. B

The Gracey 11/12 curet has a cutting edge at each end, so that's 2 edges total. The universal curet has 2 cutting edges per end for a total of 4 cutting edges.

2. C

All terminal shanks should be parallel to the long axis of the tooth so that proper instrumentation can take place. Perpendicular, oblique and horizontal are not desirable positions for the terminal shank during instrumentation.

3. B

The Gracey 13/14 is an area-specific curet designed to remove deposits on the distal aspects of posterior teeth.

A. The Gracey 1/2 is used on anterior teeth.

C. The 204SD is a posterior scaler that removes supragingival deposits.

D. The Gracey 11/12 removes subgingival deposits from the mesial aspects of teeth.

4. C

The magnetostrictive scaler moves in an elliptical movement, as does the sonic scaler. Power driven scalers do not move vertically or horizontally

B. The piezoelectric unit moves in a linear pattern.

5. D

The Alabama stone does not exist.

6. A

The face of all area-specific instruments is 60–70° in relation to the shank.

D. The face of all instruments is 100–110° to the *sharpening stone*, not the shank.

7. C

The recording should be 4 mm, since the gingival margin has extended beyond the 3 mm marking on the probe. A 3 mm reading would be inaccurate, and a 3–4 mm reading would not be acceptable.

8. C

Residual deposits are common when inflammation of the gingival tissue is present during initial therapy. Once the deposits have been removed, the gingival tissue will shrink and reveal deposits that were unable to be removed during the initial therapy.

A. Plaque is soft and white to yellow.

B. Tea and coffee stains do not migrate subgingivally where shrinkage may have occurred.

D. Some deposits may recur but not this quickly.

9. C

The residual deposits must be removed from the tooth surfaces. Oral hygiene instruction, decreasing the consumption of tea/coffee, and utilization of an electric toothbrush will have no effect on the deposits.

10. A

In order to allow for deposit detection, a light grasp and light pressure should be used. A firm grasp and/or firm pressure would be used during deposit removal.

11. B

With root debridement, the angulation of the instrument against the tissue should be 70–80° to the tooth surface.

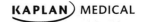

12. D

The ultrasonic principle is based upon the use of high-frequency sound waves.

A. Pressure is not a consideration with the ultrasonic principle.

B. A jet stream of water is used with oral irrigators at a 90° angle to the tooth surface.

C. Transmission of electrical impulses would not benefit patient comfort.

13. C

Deposits are removed during root debridement because they harbor plaque organisms. The calculus acts as a nidus for plaque and will retain the organisms found in plaque.

A. Deposits acting as a mechanical irritant against the gingiva is an old theory.

B. The cementum is not altered by deposits but rather with excessive debridement.

D. Deposits do not push against the junctional epithelium.

14. D

A patient's ability to maintain oral health is the most important factor in determining her recare interval.

A. The patient's desire has nothing to do with determining recare interval.

B. The amount of calculus deposits present depends on the patient's motivation for removal and her particular build-up of deposits. Every patient is different.

C. Previous caries experience has nothing to do with recare intervals.

15. E

Definitive exploration is not used for root fenestration, which is an opening in the bone that looks like a window. The cementum is exposed in the oral cavity. Explorers are used to detect calculus, carious lesions, defects, or irregularities in the margin surfaces of restorations and root surfaces, diseased or altered cementum, and overhanging restorations.

16. B

Enamel pearls are usually found at furcation on multi-rooted teeth. Due to their location, they are often mistaken for calculus deposits.

A. Developmental depressions are true depressions, and cannot be mistaken for deposits that are on the surface as convex deposits.

C. Concavities are concave depressions that occur on certain teeth such as the maxillary first premolars, and are not mistaken as deposits that are convex in nature.

D. Convex natural surfaces are rare but may occur as enamel pearls or cementicles. This answer choice would be the second best answer.

17. C

Diabetes is not contraindicated for the use of the ultrasonic scaler.

18. A

The face of the Gracey 13/14—and all Gracey curets—is 60–70° in relation to the shank.

19. C

Ultrasonic scalers user a higher frequency; they have a frequency of 25,000–50,000 cps, while sonic scalers have 3,000–8,000 cps.

A. Heat production is reduced by water flow with ultrasonics.

B. Ultrasonics use lower frequency than sonic is incorrect.

D. Elliptical rather than linear movements is a true movement of ultrasonic scalers.

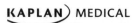

20. D

A hoe is designed to remove ledges of deposit on the anterior teeth.

A. The Gracey 1/2 removes light deposits from the anterior teeth.

B. The Universal Curet is used to remove light to moderate subgingival calculus throughout the oral cavity.

C. The curved sickle scaler removes moderate supra-gingival deposits from the anterior.

E. The 204SD is used to remove moderate supra-gingival deposits from the posterior.

21. A

A convexity is easier to scale than CEJ, concavity, or a developmental depression.

22. A

The periodontal file would not be used to perform soft tissue curettage. It is used, instead, for crushing calculus, removing deposits in areas of limited access, and completing root debridement procedures.

23. D

During an exploratory stroke, the handle is not grasped firmly; light pressure is applied to the tooth.

24. D

All of the strokes listed would be used during root debridement.

25. E

The sharpening of curets and scalers maintains the integrity of the instruments. All of the other answer choices are subsets of this answer choice.

26. A

An angulation less than 30° would not improve root debridement. Ideal angulation for deposit removal is more than 70° but less than 90°.

27. D

During ultrasonic scaler use, the vibratory action of the tip causes the calculus deposits to fracture. The water pressure, high frequency sound, and shearing action have no bearing on the deposit.

28. D

A dull instrument would not cause increased tactile sensitivity. That would occur with a sharp instrument. Dull instruments result in clinician fatigue, burnished calculus, gouged tooth structure, or injury to gingival tissues.

29. C

During hand sharpening, the face of any curet or scaler should be at a 110° angle in relation to the stone.

30. C

To ensure adequate deposit removal, the face of the blade of the scaler should be at an angle greater than 70° but less than 90° to the tooth.

Chapter Seventeen:
Anxiety and Pain Management

Anxiety and pain management are of crucial importance for every patient. Since every person has a different threshold for pain, the level at which a patient is comfortable directly affects the hygienist's clinical performance. Needless to say, it is important to keep the patient as pain-free and anxiety-free as possible.

Definitive familiarity of head, neck, and nerve anatomy is essential in order to properly deliver anesthesia. This chapter entails anatomical landmarks to be considered for that purpose.

Most states today allow dental hygienists to deliver local anesthesia, though there are a few that do not. Some states even allow hygienists to administer nitrous oxide for patient comfort as well.

States Allowing DH Anesthesia

Alaska	New Jersey
Arkansas	New Mexico
Arizona	New York
California	New Jersey
Colorado	North Dakota
District of Columbia	Ohio
Hawaii	Oklahoma
Idaho	Oregon
Illinois	Pennsylvania
Iowa	Rhode Island
Kansas	South Carolina
Kentucky	South Dakota
Louisiana	Tennessee
Maine	Utah
Massachusetts	Vermont
Michigan	Virginia
Minnesota	Washington
Missouri	Washington, DC
Montana	West Virginia
Nebraska	Wisconsin
Nevada	Wyoming
New Hampshire	

States NOT Allowing DH Anesthesia

Alabama	Indiana
Connecticut	Maryland
Delaware	Mississippi
Florida	North Carolina
Georgia	Texas

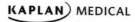

PAIN PHYSIOLOGY

Pain is a basic bodily response to uncomfortable stimuli that are received by **sensory nociceptors**, the peripheral receptors of the central nervous system. Nociceptors are so named after *noci*, a derivative of *noxious*, which means something harmful like pain. Every patient has a different threshold to pain.

Injury releases chemicals, causing nociceptors to become more sensitive. Pain is then detected by these sensory neurons through gateways that allow (or not) transmission to other nearby cells. The stimuli can be either suppressed or passed on to the central nervous system by neurons.

Nerve cells termed **neurons** contain a nucleus and dendrite that conveys nerve impulses between other neuron cells. **Dendrites** within the neuron have branching fibers that extend out from the cell body to receive incoming impulses. **Axons** are a single longer, thicker fiber than dendrites that carry the impulse away from the cell body to other neurons.

All cells have a **resting potential** whether or not they are excitable cells. During the resting potential, three sodium ions are kicked out of the neuron and two potassium ions easily pass back in. This leaves a negative charge in the cell, with more sodium ions "gated" outside of the cell. Calcium and chloride are also present in higher levels outside of the cell. At rest, the inside of the neuron has less voltage than the outside.

Resting Potential in Neurons

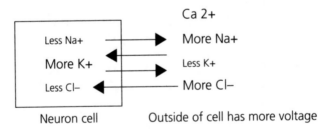

When the neuron receives a stimulus, the charge changes; more **sodium** is **pumped back into** the cell. At the same time, more **potassium** is **pumped out** during **depolarization** of the cell. As the sodium gates open, voltage within the cell changes.

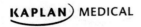

Action potential occurs when depolarization sweeps along the cell, sending information away from the cell body down an axon as a nerve impulse. As sodium ions flood the neuron that was negatively charged, the neuron becomes positively charged.

Depolarization of Neurons

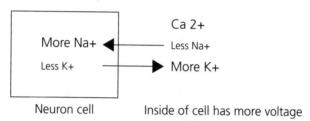

Repolarization occurs when potassium ions are pumped back into the cell by facilitated diffusion. At this time the cell is impermiable to sodium. When the neuron is at rest, sodium ions are actively transported back out of the cell.

Local anesthesia prevents the sodium gates from opening, so that sodium cannot enter back into the neuron. Cell permeability is thus decreased. If the sodium cannot enter the nerve cell, it cannot transmit nerve impulses downstream. And if sodium cannot get in, potassium cannot get out, and that inhibits depolarization of the nerve.

The branches of the **trigeminal nerve (V)** transmit pain stimuli from the teeth and surrounding structures.

PAIN CONTROL MANAGEMENT

Pain can be controlled in different ways. First, relaxation can help. If a patient can relax, his anxiety about being in the dental office will drop and his perception of pain might also decrease. Patients often recall "bad experiences" they had at the dentist in the past, anticipating that something unpleasant will happen again.

Second, anesthesia can help control pain. Local anesthesia can block the potential for pain to a specific area, while general anesthesia blocks the central nervous system from painful stimuli. Third, nitrous oxide or IV sedation can reduce a patient's anxiety and potential reaction to pain.

NITROUS OXIDE

Nitrous oxide is used for **conscious sedation**. It allows the patient to remain awake while it reduces pain. This is especially important if the patient needs to interact with the dentist during a treatment.

Nitrous oxide is delivered by inhalation in a closed system of a **facemask**, **gas hose**, and **regulator**. This system reduces the pressure from the gas cylinder with a **flow meter** that regulates the amount of oxygen and nitrous that the patient receives. A **reservoir bag** contains excess gas should the patient require a deeper breath. A **face-mask scavenger system** allows for the nitrous that is exhaled by the patient to be taken up in the outer portion of the mask where it is then transferred back to a high-speed evacuation system. The high-speed evacuation system protects dental personnel from inhaling expired nitrous oxide by venting it to outside of the building.

> Nitrous gas is stored in a blue tank, while oxygen is stored in a green tank.

Nitrous oxide is stored in a **blue tank**, while **oxygen** is stored in a **green tank**. Nitrous conscious sedation depresses the central nervous system, and thus reduces the amount of anxiety the patient is feeling.

Nitrous oxide is initially delivered to the patient **as 100% oxygen** for 2–3 minutes. The nitrous is then **increased** gradually—in **5–10% increments**—until the desired response is achieved. Onset of desired effect usually occurs within 3–5 minutes. Depending on the patient's metabolism, etc., the desired effects may occur in the **10–50% range**, with the **average** being about **35%** nitrous oxide.

A patient must be closely monitored during this procedure. When the procedure is complete, the patient should be **flushed with 100% oxygen for 3–5 minutes** or until no more nitrous effects are present. This is so that the patient does not become hypoxic, leaving too much nitrous oxide in his system. Hypoxia from nitrous oxide does not allow for the alveoli to exchange oxygen and carbon dioxide properly.

Contraindications and Indications for Nitrous Oxide Usage

Indications for N_2O_2	Contraindications for N_2O_2
Anxious patient	Someone who cannot speak well
Intolerant to long appointments	Respiratory tract infections
Stress induced asthma	COPD (emphysema, chronic bronchitis)
Strong gag reflex	Nasal obstructions
Cardiovascular disease	Claustrophobia
Hypertension	Pregnancy
Mental retardation	Emotional instability/losing control
Cerebral palsy	Epilepsy
	Multiple sclerosis

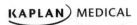

Advantages and Disadvantages of Nitrous Oxide

Advantages	Disadvantages
Rapid onset	Nausea, vomiting
Easy to control	Nose mask interferes with instrumentation
Rapid recovery	
Patient able to respond	
Acceptable for children	
Oxygen enrichment for cardiovascular patients	
No accompaniment needed	

Guedel's Stages of Anesthetics

	Induction	Condition
Stage I	Analgesia	Conscious Reduced pain
Stage II	Delirium/excitement	Loss of consciousness Irregular respirations Tachycardia
Stage III	Surgical anesthesia	Unconscious Regular respirations Normal pulse rate
Stage IV	Respiratory paralysis	Respiratory arrest Cardiac arrest

TOPICAL ANESTHESIA

Topical anesthesia comes in **ointment, spray, gel, liquid,** or **patch** forms, to desensitize tissue prior to injection. Topical anesthesia is higher in concentration than injectable local anesthesia, to better penetrate mucous membranes.

Topical anesthesia can be used for discomfort during probing and scalings, to prevent gag reflex with dental impressions, and during radiography exposure. It also can be used to ease discomfort of any prior lesions during a dental visit.

The **transoral patch** provides an intense level of anesthesia to soft tissues. It is a **lidocaine-impregnated strip.** To apply, dry the tissue for 30 seconds and press firmly into place. It is effective for 35–45 minutes. **Lidocaine** is an **amide** that can also be found as an ointment, spray, liquid, or gel.

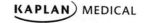

Amides have 2 *i*'s in their generic name and are metabolized or biotransformed in the **liver**.

Esters have 1 *i* in their generic name and are metabolized or biotransformed in **blood plasma**.

With the exception of lidocaine (Xylocaine), all other topical anesthetics are esters. One of the most popular topical anesthesias is **benzocaine** (ester), which comes in spray, liquid, or gel. It is effective for 30 minutes and offers minimal toxicity. Topical anesthesia should be applied with the **least amount possible to a small area**.

LOCAL ANESTHESIA ARMAMENTARIUM

Armamentarium is defined as the equipment and methods used in medicine. The armamentarium necessary for delivering local anesthesia include the syringe, anesthetic cartridge, and the needle.

Syringe and Needle

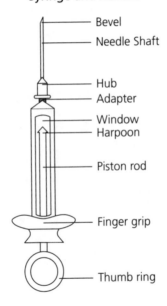

The **beveled needle** contains a **hollow shaft** with a **lumen** or opening for the anesthesia. The larger the gauge of the needle, the smaller the lumen opening. The **hub** connects the needle to the **adapter** of the syringe.

The **syringe** has an **adapter** to screw on the hub of the needle, a **barrel** with a **window** to hold the cartridge, a **piston** with a **harpoon** attached to it to embed into the stopper of the cartridge, a **finger grip** to grasp the syringe with the middle and index fingers, and a **thumb ring** that is attached to the piston that advances the rubber stopper into the cartridge to aspirate or express fluid into the tissue.

Cartridge

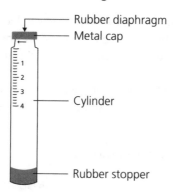

Rubber diaphragm
Metal cap

Cylinder

Rubber stopper

A **rubber diaphragm** seals the cartridge at one end. It is this area, surrounded and protected by a **metal cap**, that the needle penetrates to deliver the anesthesia. The **cylinder** contains the **anesthetic** and the information about its content, which is called **inscription**. The **rubber stopper** seals the other end of the cartridge, acting as the plunger to deliver anesthesia to the tissue.

LOCAL ANESTHETICS

Local anesthetics block pain, thus allowing the clinician to better perform the dental procedure. As mentioned earlier, local anesthesia works by closing the gates to the sodium which wants to enter the nerve cell. It is sodium that transmits nerve impulses to other cells. At the same time, it also keeps the potassium in the cell, preventing it from depolarizing.

There are two kinds of anesthetics used in dentistry: esters and amides. **Esters** have not been used for the past few years because they were **allergenic** to so many patients. **Amides** have become the anesthesia of choice. (They are **biotransformed in the liver** so people with liver complications cannot metabolize amides.) **Esters** are metabolized or biotransformed in **blood plasma**.

Anesthetic pH

Normal body pH is 7.35–7.4. **Anesthetics are processed as weak bases**, and then combined with an acid to form a salt that is more soluble in solution. Anesthetics need to cross the lipid cell membrane to enter into the cell, as a free base (uncharged) form. The positively charged ion combines with the uncharged anesthesia radical. With a normal pH, the anesthetic can enter the cell at a faster rate.

If there is inflammation, the tissue pH is lowered to the acidic range of 5–6. This shift does not allow for as many uncharged anesthesia radicals to diffuse into the cell.

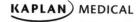

Vasoconstrictors

Vasoconstrictors such as **epinephrine** are used widely to prevent local blood vessels from absorbing anesthesia that is not yet absorbed into the nerve cells. They reduce the flow of blood and plasma into the injection site area, slowing vascular absorption of the anesthetic.

Some anesthetics—mepivicaine and prilocaine, for instance—come with or without epinephrine. Without the epinephrine, they become short-acting anesthetics and should be considered for brief appointments.

Maximum Safe Dose of Vasoconstrictors

Generic	Brand	Concentration	mg per ml	mg per Cartridge	MSD Healthy Adult # of Cartridges	MSD Cardiac Patient # of Cartridges
Epinephrine	Adrenaline	1:50,000	0.02	0.036	5	1
Epinephrine	Adrenaline	1:100,000	0.01	0.018	11	2
Norepinephrine	Levophed	1:30,000	0.033	0.059	5	2
Levonordefrin	Neo-Cobefrin	1:20,000	0.05	0.09	11	2
Phenylephrine	Neo-Synephrine	1:2,500	0.4	0.72	5	2

Local Anesthetics

Generic	Brand	Type	Epinephrine	Conc.	MSD by mg/kg	MSD mg	Action
Procaine	Novacaine	Ester	1:200,000	2%	6.6 mg/kg	500	Inter.
Tetracaine*	Pontocaine	Ester		0.15%	1 mg/kg	20	
Lidocaine	Xylocaine Octocaine	Amide	Plain 1:50,000 1:100,000	2%	4.4 mg/kg 4.4 mg/kg 4.4 mg/kg	300 300	Short Inter. Inter.
Bupivacaine	Marcaine	Amide	1:200,000	0.5%	2 mg/kg	90	Long
Mepivacaine	Carbocaine Isocaine Polocaine	Amide	None	3%	5.7 mg/kg 5.7 mg/kg	300 300	Inter. Inter.
Mepivacaine w/levonordefrin		Amide	1:20,000		4.4 mg/kg	300	Inter.
Prilocaine no epi	Citanest Plain	Amide	none	2%	6 mg/kg	400	Inter.
Prilocaine	Citanest Forte	Amide	1:200,000	4%	6 mg/kg	400	Inter.
Articaine	Septocaine	Amide	1:200,000	4%	7 mg/kg	500	Inter.
Etidocaine	Duranest	Amide	1:200,000	1.5%	8 mg/kg	400	Long

*Tetracaine is very toxic and is generally used topically in a 2% concentration.

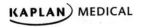

Adverse Reactions

An allergic response can be immediate or delayed. Symptoms can be delayed (a mild rash) or immediate (anaphylactic symptoms of difficulty in breathing, urticaria, tachycardia, hypertension, and altered level of consciousness). Local side effects may include hematoma, trismus, parasthesia, burning sensation, and tissue sloughing.

Adverse Reactions to Vasoconstrictors

Health Condition	Clinical Implications
Uncontrolled hypertension	Elevates blood pressure
Patients on ß blockers	Elevates blood pressure
Unstable angina	Elevates blood pressure
Severe arrhythmias	Worsens arrhythmia
Hyperthyroidism	Increases thyroid hormone
Patient on tricyclic antidepressant	Elevates blood pressure and heart rate
Patient on anti-psychotic	Leads to hypotension
Patient on anti-depressant	Hypertensive crisis
Monoamineoxidase (MAO) inhibitors	Elevates blood pressure, cannot metabolize vasoconstrictor
Cocaine abuse	Hypertensive crisis, arrhythmia, MI, CVA

Delivery of Anesthesia

Local infiltration blocks nerve conduction to a specific area such as an area **surrounding 1 or 2 teeth**. The injection occurs near the **apices** of the teeth to be anesthetized and the surrounding tissue.

Nerve blocks affect a broader area when the anesthesia is infiltrated the area near the nerve trunk.

NERVE LOCATIONS AND INJECTION SITE

As studied in dental anatomy, as well as head and neck anatomy, nerves travel to different locations to supply sensation to those locations. Knowing the proper injection site and delivery of anesthesia to that site is essential for patient comfort.

Maxillary Branch of Trigeminal Nerve (V$_2$)

- **Nerve:** The **infraorbital nerve** (IO) that enters into the oral cavity by way of the infraorbital foramen, where it passes posteriorly to the infraorbital canal. There, it **joins** the ascending branches of the **anterior superior alveolar nerve** (ASA) and **middle superior alveolar nerve** (MSA) as part of the dental plexus. It is the choice nerve for anesthesia if both the maxillary anterior teeth and maxillary premolars are indicated for treatment.

  Teeth Anesthetized: Maxillary incisors, canines, and bicuspids, as well as the mesiobuccal root of the first molar

  Soft Tissue: Facial gingival tissue of the maxillary incisors, canines, and bicuspids as well as the upper lip, cheek, and side of the nose

  Penetration Site: Mucobuccal fold close to the apex of the maxillary premolar where the ASA and MSA ascend to join the IO nerve

  Needle: Long

- **Nerve:** The **anterior superior alveolar nerve** (ASA) eventually joins the infraorbital (IO) nerve at the infraorbital canal.

  Teeth Anesthetized: Maxillary central incisors, lateral incisors, and canines

  Soft Tissue: Facial gingival tissue of the maxillary incisors and canines

  Penetration Site: Mucobuccal fold just mesial to the canine eminence

  Needle: Short

- **Nerve:** The **middle superior alveolar nerve** also ascends to the infraorbital canal to join the infraorbital nerve (IO).

  Teeth Anesthetized: Maxillary first and second premolars and the mesiobuccal root of the first molar

  Soft Tissue: Facial gingival tissue of the maxillary first and second premolars and the gingival tissue near the mesiobuccal root of the first molar.

  Penetration Site: Mucobuccal fold close to the apex of the maxillary second premolar

  Needle: Short

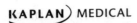

- **Nerve:** The **posterior superior alveolar nerve** (PSA) ascends along the maxillary tuberosity. It exits through various posterior superior foramen, then travels to the pterygopalatine fossa where it rejoins the maxillary nerve.

  Teeth Anesthetized: The distal-buccal and lingual roots of the maxillary first molar, as well as all the roots of the maxillary second and third molars

  Soft Tissue: Facial gingival tissue of the maxillary first molar distal-buccal root and the facial tissues of the second and third molars

  Penetration Site: Mucobuccal fold just distal to the maxillary second molar

  Needle: Short

- **Nerve:** The **greater palatine** (GP) nerve conveys afferent sensation for the posterior hard palate and lingual tissues of the posterior teeth as it enters the greater palatine foramen in the vicinity of the maxillary second and third molars.

  Teeth Anesthetized: None, but does anesthetize the posterior portion of the hard palate

  Soft Tissue: Palatal tissue distal to the maxillary canine, includes the premolars and molars

  Penetration Site: Blanch tissue with pressure anesthesia prior to injection. Inject anterior to the greater palatine foramen and just distal to the maxillary second molar.

  Needle: Short

- **Nerve:** The **nasopalatine** (NP) nerve arises at the lingual mucosa of the maxillary anterior teeth as it passes through the **incisive foramen**. It also corresponds with the greater palatine nerve.

  Teeth Anesthetized: None, but does anesthetize the anterior hard palate

  Soft Tissue: Palatal tissue of the maxillary anterior teeth

  Penetration Site: Blanch tissue with pressure anesthesia prior to injection. Inject the base of the incisive papillae.

  Needle: Short

Mandibular Branch of Trigeminal Nerve (V3)

- **Nerve:** The **mandibular block** includes the **inferior alveolar** (IA) and **lingual nerves.** The **inferior alveolar nerve** (IA) is formed by the merger of the **mental nerve** and **incisive nerve.** It also connects with the pulpal nerve branches of the posterior teeth to form the dental plexus. The **lingual nerve** carries afferent sensation for the floor of the mouth, lingual mandibular gingival surfaces, and two-thirds of the anterior surface of the tongue. The lingual nerve also provides taste sensation for the same two-thirds of the tongue.

  Teeth Anesthetized by the inferior alveolar block: Molars, premolars, canines, and incisors to the midline line of the mandible on the side anesthetized

  Soft Tissue by the inferior alveolar block: Facial gingival tissue of the molars, premolars, canines, and incisors to the midline of the mandible on the side anesthetized

  Teeth Anesthetized by the lingual block: None

  Soft Tissue by lingual block: Lingual tissue from the posterior molars to the midline of the mouth as well as anterior two-thirds of the tongue

  Penetration Site: Pterygomandibular triangle at the medial border of the coronoid notch

  Needle: Long

- **Nerve:** The **buccal nerve** descends from the trigeminal nerve as it branches out over the surface of the buccinator muscle to supply sensation to the skin and mucous membranes.

  Teeth Anesthetized: None

  Soft Tissue: Facial gingival tissue and periodontium of the mandibular molars

  Penetration Site: Mucobuccal fold distal to the last mandibular molar parallel to the retromolar pad of the anterior ramus

  Needle: Long

- **Nerve:** The **mental nerve** joins with the incisive nerve at the mental foramen to form the inferior alveolar nerve (IA) nerve.

  Teeth Anesthetized: None

  Soft Tissue: Facial periodontium of the mandibular premolars and molars, as well as the lower lip and chin on the side anesthetized

  Penetration Site: Vertical injection near the depression of mental foramen between the mandibular first and second premolars

  Needle: Short

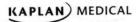

- **Nerve:** The **incisive nerve** connects with the mental nerve at the mental foramen near the roots of the mandibular premolars to become the IA nerve.

  Teeth Anesthetized: Mandibular anterior teeth and first premolar on the side anesthetized.

  Soft Tissue: Facial gingival tissue of the mandibular anterior teeth and first premolar on the side anesthetized.

  Penetration Site: Applied with **pressure** near or slightly anterior to the depression of mental foramen between the mandibular first and second premolars. Pressure or massaging the site propels more solution into the mental foramen for better anesthesia.

  Needle: Short

- **Infiltration** blocks nerve conduction to a specific area of one or two teeth without having to block a large area.

  Tissues anesthetized: Tooth pulp, facial periosteum, and facial gingival tissue of the teeth chosen to be anesthetized.

  Penetration site: Mucobuccal fold above the apex of the tooth for maxillary teeth and below the apex for mandibular teeth.

  Needle: Short

ADVERSE EFFECTS OF ANESTHESIA

Anesthesia can cause anything from a **drug reaction** to an **iatrogenic** problem. A drug reaction could be anaphylaxis due to an allergic response, overdose from too much anesthesia, or heart palpitations from anesthesia absorption into the bloodstream. An iatrogenic problem could be a hematoma resulting from the penetration of a blood vessel with the injection, parathesia from piercing the myelin sheath, or burning during the injection.

In addition, if a patient has kidney or liver disease, he may have a problem eliminating the anesthesia.

DRUG CALCULATIONS

If you have a cartridge of an anesthetic with 1:100,000 epinephrine, how many milligrams of epinephrine are in that cartridge?

1:100,000 = 1 gram per 100,000 mL of epinephrine

1 g = 1000 mg of epinephrine

$$\frac{1,000 \text{ mg}}{100,000 \text{ mL}} = 0.01 \text{ mg/mL}$$

Each cartridge holds 1.8 mL, so: 0.01 mg/mL × 1.8 mL = 0.018 mg per cartridge.

What is the maximum safe number of cartridges of 2% lidocaine with 1:100,000 epinephrine that a healthy adult can receive?

$$\frac{2\% \text{ lidocaine}}{100\%} = 0.02 \text{ g} \qquad 0.02 \text{ g} \times \frac{1,000 \text{ mg}}{1 \text{ g}} = 20 \text{ mg per 1 cc (or mL)}$$

Each cartridge has 1.8 cc or mL   1.8 cc (or mL) × 20 mg = 36 mg per cartridge

The maximum safe dose (MSD) of lidocaine is 300 mg

$$300 \text{ mg MSD} \times \frac{1 \text{ cartridge}}{36 \text{ mg}} = 8.333333 \text{ cartridges} \text{ or round to 8 cartridges}$$

REVIEW QUESTIONS

1. During the resting potential of a cell,

   A. Three sodium ions are pumped out of the neuron, while two potassium ions are let back in.

   B. Three potassium ions are pumped out of the neuron, while two sodium ions are let back in.

   C. Sodium ions flood the negatively charged neuron so that it becomes positively charged.

   D. Depolarization sweeps along the cell, sending information away from the cell body and down an axon as a nerve impulse.

2. Most cartridges hold a set amount of local anesthesia. That set amount is

   A. 0.18 mL

   B. 0.36 cc

   C. 1.8 cc

   D. 3.6 mL

   E. 18.0 mL

3. Topical anesthesia is effective for controlling sensations arising from

   A. Sensory receptors in the oral mucosa

   B. Meissner's corpuscles

   C. Pacini's corpuscles

   D. Nodes of Ranvier

4. A dentist has just learned that he was allergic to procaine when he developed a rash. Which of the following anesthetics would he not want to use?

   A. Lidocaine

   B. Articaine

   C. Mepivacaine

   D. Propoxycaine

   E. Prilocaine

5. To make sure that a blood vessel has not been penetrated, you would perform _____ before injecting the anesthesia.

   A. Deposition

   B. Aspiration

   C. Positive pressure

   D. Lumen

6. Epinephrine causes vasoconstriction. How much vasoconstrictor is in one milliliter if the epinephrine is 1:100,000?

   A. 10.0 mg

   B. 1.0 mg

   C. 0.1 mg

   D. 0.01 mg

   E. 0.001 mg

7. When administering nitrous oxide, in what increments would you would increase the anesthetic to until you get the desired effect?

   A. 2–5 %

   B. 4–8 %

   C. 5–10 %

   D. 10–15 %

8. Your patient has no posterior maxillary teeth, but you need to perform a root debridement on #6, #7, #8, and #9. What nerves would you anesthetize to get profound gingival anesthesia?

   A. ASA and NP

   B. MSA and NP

   C. MSA and GP

   D. ASA and GP

9. Numbness on the lower half of the lip, tongue, and mandible on one side a month after an extraction might be caused by all of the following except one. Which of the following is the EXCEPTION?

   A. Piercing of the myelin sheath

   B. Anesthetic solution was contaminated

   C. Hemorrhage

   D. Concentration of the anesthesia was too high

   E. Burning feeling

10. A patient with an emergency toothache just walked in the door. Tooth #14 has a deep carious lesion and periapical lesion on the radiograph. Which nerves would need to be anesthetized for an extraction?

    A. MSA, ASA, GP

    B. MSA, PSA, NP

    C. IO, PSA, NP

    D. IO, PSA, GP

    E. MSA, PSA, GP

11. A cartridge holds 1.8 mL of 4% prilocaine solution. How many mg of lidocaine are in that cartridge?

    A. 0.072 mg

    B. 0.72 mg

    C. 7.20 mg

    D. 72.0 mg

    E. 720.0 mg

12. When injecting 3% mepivacaine for anesthesia, the maximum number of cartridges that can be injected into a healthy adult is

    A. 3.5 cartridges

    B. 5.6 cartridges

    C. 6.6 cartridges

    D. 7.5 cartridges

    E. 8.5 cartridges

13. Tanks that carry gases are color-coded. A nitrous oxide tank is color-coded in which of the following colors?

    A. Blue

    B. Green

    C. Gray

    D. Red

    E. Yellow

14. The body has the ability to rid itself of toxins including anesthesia. Which of the following anesthetics is metabolized or biotransformed in the liver?

    A. Procaine

    B. Tetracaine

    C. Choloroprocaine

    D. Prilocaine

15. When receiving local anesthesia, it is impossible to be allergic to

    A. Latex allergy

    B. Sodium bisulfite

    C. Epinephrine

    D. Topical anesthesia

16. According to Guedel's stages of anesthesia, which stage creates delirium?

    A. Stage I
    B. Stage II
    C. Stage III
    D. Stage IV
    E. Stage V

17. Nitrous oxide has all of the following effects except one. Which of the following is the EXCEPTION?

    A. Depresses the CNS
    B. Makes the patient feel warm
    C. Reduces anxiety
    D. Reduces gag reflex
    E. Blocks pain reception

18. All of the following except one are signs of minimal sedation by nitrous oxide. Which of the following is the EXCEPTION?

    A. Slower eye movement
    B. Tingling in the fingers and toes
    C. Heavy feeling in the legs
    D. Feeling cold
    E. Nasal-sounding voice

19. Your patient has anxiety over the treatment she is about to receive. To relax her, you explain that the anesthesia will be delivered slowly. How much time should it take to deliver 1.8 mL of a local anesthetic at the slow-flow rate?

    A. 1 minute
    B. 2 minutes
    C. 3 minutes
    D. 4 minutes

20. Your patient was previously seen for one quadrant of root debridement, during which he received local anesthesia. Today, he is in for the second quadrant, though he refuses anesthesia. He recently quit smoking and is experiencing heavy bleeding with flossing. After discussing the problem with the dentist, it is decided that local anesthesia is indeed necessary to control the bleeding. What compound in anesthesia helps to control the bleeding?

    A. Saline solution
    B. Local anesthetic salt
    C. Epinephrine
    D. Sodium bisulfite
    E. Sterile water

21. What might have caused the patient in Question #20 to bleed more today?

    A. Not being able to use the anesthetic at the early onset of the appointment
    B. His lack of home care
    C. The fact that he quit smoking
    D. None of the above

22. Which of the following actions in anesthesia administration helps create a faster onset of action?

    A. Decrease the anesthetic pH
    B. Increase the anesthetic pH
    C. Inject it into an area that is not inflamed
    D. Increase the salts in the anesthetic

23. Which of the following minerals is prevented from going back into the nerve cells when local anesthetics take effect?

    A. Potassium
    B. Calcium
    C. Sodium
    D. Chlorine
    E. Phosphorus

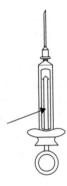

24. In the picture above, the arrow is pointing to the

    A. Spool finger grip
    B. Shaft
    C. Barrel
    D. Piston rod
    E. Harpoon

25. Which of the following is true of a needle?

    A. The larger the number of the gauge, the smaller the diameter of the lumen.
    B. The smaller the number of the gauge, the larger the diameter of the lumen.
    C. A short needle is 1.25 inches.
    D. A long needle is 1.75 inches.
    E. Presterilized needles still need to be sterilized.

ANSWER EXPLANATIONS

1. A

During the resting potential of a cell, three sodium ions are pumped out of the neuron while two potassium ions are let back in.

B. This answer choice has the ions reversed.

C. When sodium ions flood the negatively charged neuron that so it becomes positively charged, that is action potential.

D. When depolarization sweeps along the cell, sending information away from the cell body down an axon as a nerve impulse, that, too, is action potential.

2. C

The set amount of local anesthesia is most cartridges is 1.8 cc.

3. A

Topical anesthesia is effective for controlling sensations arising from sensory receptors in the oral mucosa.

B. Meissner's corpuscles are found in the papillae of the skin, especially in the fingers and toes

C. Pacini's corpuscles are pressure sensors found in the fingers, mesentery, and tendons.

D. Nodes of Ranvier are gaps between the Schwann cells.

4. D

If the dentist were allergic to an ester such as procaine, he would not want to use another ester such as Propoxycaine.

5. B

Aspiration would help ensure that a blood vessel will not be penetrated. It requires pulling back on the plunger with the thumb, and checking for blood in the cartridge.

A. Deposition is the application of anesthesia into the tissue.

C. Positive pressure is the pressure application of the thumb to the plunger, allowing for injection of the anesthetic.

D. Lumen is the opening at the end of the needle.

6. D

If the epinephrine is 1:100,000, there would be 0.01 mg of vasoconstrictor in one milliliter.

1,000 mg = 1 g

1:100,000 mL = 1 g epinephrine per 100,000 mL

1,000 mg ÷ 100,000 mL = 0.01 mg/mL

7. C

When administering nitrous oxide, you would increase the anesthetic by 5–10% until the desired amount was reached.

8. A

In this situation, the nerves that need to be anesthetized are ASA, which provides pupal and facial gingival anesthesia to the anterior teeth, and NP, which provides lingual tissue anesthesia to the maxillary anterior teeth.

9. E

A burning feeling upon injection would not produce a lasting effect. It occurs as a result of the pH of the solution.

10. E

Tooth #14 requires anesthesia for the MSA, which provides anesthesia to the MB root of #14, PSA which provides anesthesia for the DB and lingual root of #14, and GP, for lingual anesthesia for #14.

11. D

If a cartridge has 1.8 mL of 4% prilocaine solution, it contains 72.0 mg of lidocaine.

$$\frac{4\% \text{ prilocaine}}{100\%} = 0.04 \text{ g} = 40 \text{ mg/mL in the cartridge}$$

1.8 mL × 40 mg/mL = 72 mg in the cartridge

12. C

No more than 6.6 cartridges should be injected into an adult. The maximum safe dose for 3% mepivacaine is 360 mg. Each cartridge holds 0.03 g = 30 mg/mL.

Each cartridge also holds 1.8 mL of solution.

1.8 mL × 30 mg/mL equals 54 mg per cartridge. 360 mg (maximum safe dose) is divided by 54 mg per cartridge, so the result is 6.66 cartridges.

13. A

A nitrous oxide tank is blue.

B. An oxygen tank is green.

14. D

Prilocaine is an amide metabolized in the liver.

15. C

Contrary to what many people believe, people cannot be allergic to epinephrine. That's because it occurs naturally in our bodies.

A. Latex allergy can occur at anytime once an allergen has been introduced to the body but latex does not have to do with an anesthetic allergy.

B. Sodium bisulfite is sprayed onto fruit to keep it fresh-looking, but it also is contained in local anesthetics and can become an allergen.

D. Topical anesthesia is mostly esters, for which patients can develop an allergy.

16. B

Stage II of anesthesia produces delirium.

A. Stage I causes the patient to focus less on the pain.

C. Stage III provides surgical anesthesia.

D. Stage IV is given in a hospital setting; it provides respiratory paralysis.

E. Stage V does not exist.

17. E

Nitrous oxide does not block pain reception.

18. D

Minimal nitrous oxide sedation will not cause patients to feel cold. In fact, patients will feel warm as the drug vasodilates.

19. B

2 minutes is the slow rate.

A. 1 minute is the fast flow rate.

20. **C**

Epinephrine is a vasoconstrictor.

A. Saline solution dilutes the salt to an isotonic solution.

B. Local anesthetic salt is the anesthetic.

D. Sodium bisulfite is a preservative.

E. Sterile water is used as an inert ingredient.

21. **C**

The patient quit smoking. Smoking constricts the vessels and so by quitting, his clotting factors changed with the vessels being more dilated.

22. **B**

A faster onset of action of local anesthetics relies on an increase of the anesthetic pH for delivery.

A. A decrease in the anesthetic pH reduces the local anesthetic to a pH of 3.3–5.5.

C. Inflamed tissues carry off the anesthetic faster.

D. An increase in the salts of the anesthetic can make it less potent.

23. **C**

Sodium cannot go back into the nerve cells when a local anesthetic takes effect.

24. **D**

The arrow is pointing to the piston rod.

A. The spool finger grip is where the index and middle fingers rest.

B. The shaft is on the needle.

C. The barrel is the main area that holds the anesthetic.

E. The harpoon is at the end of the piston rod.

25. **A**

The larger the number of the gauge in a needle, the smaller the diameter of the lumen.

C. A short needle is not 1.25 inches; it is 1 inch.

D. A long needle is not 1.75 inches; it is $1\frac{5}{8}$ inches.

E. Presterilized needles do not need to be sterilized.

Chapter Eighteen:
Community Health Education

For the dental hygienist, effective community health education can provide individuals and groups with information on larger issues of health and wellness; that is, lifestyle, values, behavioral patterns, and environment.

HEALTH AND WELLNESS

The concept of health and wellness cannot simply be defined as "free of disease or disability." That would not be a true picture of health. The WHO has defined health as "a state of complete physical, mental, and social well-being and not merely the absence of disease or infirmity." The Human Needs Theory certainly plays a role in defining the concept of health.

The paradigms and models of healthcare can be described as the following:

Disease Treatment

The Disease Treatment Model is based purely on the health definition of "being free from disease." This is obviously the most costly model of healthcare since it treats disease only once it is present. At that point, the disease must be eradicated.

Disease Prevention

The Disease Prevention model places emphasis on identifying the causative agents of disease and disability, and avoiding exposure to these agents.

Health Promotion

The Health Promotion model of treatment is structured on communities taking control of their current and future health. All aspects of the community take on the role of improving the overall health of that community.

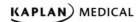

PRINCIPLES OF LEARNING AND PATIENT MOTIVATION

For learning to occur, several factors must be in place. First, an individual must be physiologically and psychologically ready to learn. Since not all individuals learn at the same rate or in the same way, individual learning styles must be taken into account. Second, the individual must be motivated to learn. And third, the individual must recognize and understand the material to be learned.

The most effective learning is when an individual obtains a sense of satisfaction. In order to determine if learning has taken place, evaluation is necessary.

Steps in a learning ladder

Unawareness = Ugly
Awareness = Apes
Self-Interest = Sit
Involvement = In
Action = A
Habit = Hut

Steps in the Learning Ladder

Unawareness
Awareness
Self-Interest
Involvement
Action
Habit

Let's look at the learning ladder from the standpoint of patient motivation. The benefits of regular flossing have been well-documented. But let's say your patient flosses only when she has food caught in her teeth. How can you motivate her to begin a healthy habit of regular flossing every day? Obviously, she is **unaware** of the health benefits that regular flossing would bring.

By following the steps in the Learning Ladder, one can initiate change with a patient or community. Habits are extremely difficult to change since they require a person to alter his value system.

THE HUMAN NEEDS THEORY AND THE HIERARCHY OF NEEDS

The Hierarchy of Needs is a prioritized human-needs categorization that was created by Abraham Maslow. In it, he identifies that some human needs are more basic than others.

The first need we all have is **physiological need**. This includes the need for food, water, and shelter. Once these needs have been met, humans have a need for **safety and security**. One must feel secure in his environment. Following this comes the **love and belonging or social** need; that is, the need to have loving relationships and feel part of a community. **Self-esteem or ego** comes last—only after the three earlier needs have been met—since a person will acquire self-esteem after those things are in place. Finally, **self-actualization** helps people to reach their full potential as human beings.

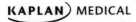

Maslow's Hierarchy of Needs

Self-Actualization
↑
Self-Esteem
↑
Social Needs
↑
Safety and Security
↑
Physiological Needs

COMMUNITY PROGRAM PLANNING

Community health planning is similar to patient planning, though with a few differences:

Community Planning	Patient Treatment
Assessment	Examination
Analysis of need	Diagnosis
Program planning	Treatment Planning
Implementation	Treatment Implementation
Financing	Payment
Evaluation	Evaluation

In community planning, the needs of the community must first be assessed. Once the needs have been determined, the appropriate program plan can be formulated. Depending on the type of community, financing of the program will be determined by the scope and level of intervention. After implementation and then completion of the program, evaluation will determine the level of effectiveness.

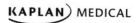

EPIDEMIOLOGY

Epidemiology is the study of the distribution and determinants of disease in a population. There are two major types of studies that are performed in epidemiology: descriptive studies and analytical studies. **Descriptive studies** focus on an epidemic with respect to a person, place, or time. **Analytical studies** focus on testing a theory or hypothesis. We will be comparing the various types of epidemiological studies.

Epidemiological Studies

Case control

Convenience

Cross section

Double blind

Longitudinal

Non-randomized

Randomized

Endemic =
Expected disease prevalence
(flu season)

Epidemic =
Higher than normal prevalence
(high measles outbreak)

Pandemic =
Spread worldwide (SARS)

In a **case control study**, a comparison is made between the **control** and **experimental groups**. The individuals in a control group do not receive the treatment being tested. Instead, they are given a placebo or no treatment at all. The experimental group receives the treatment or drug being tested. By using the appropriate index on both groups prior to treatment and after it has commenced, one can measure a change for drug or treatment effectiveness. **Stratified sampling** allows for randomized selection of the subjects into the control and experimental groups.

Convenience studies allow participation of individuals who are conveniently located to the examiner. Dental hygiene students, for instance, may conduct a study comparing the effectiveness of patient education on patients being treated at their school's dental hygiene clinic. A Patient Hygiene Performance index would be used to measure their plaque levels. Keep in mind that this type of study is not considered the most reliable, since it does not include the general population. It includes only those people convenient to the examiner.

A **cross-sectional study** is considered to be a true reflection of an entire population.

A **double-blind study** is the most valid of all studies. Neither the examiner nor the participant knows which is the control or experimental group. This minimizes the bias in the data collection and prevents the study from being skewed.

Longitudinal studies are performed over a long period of time. One may study the survival rate of women who have undergone treatment for breast cancer. The study may last 10 years, so that the success of treatment can be tracked. One could compare the effectiveness of different treatments, such as mastectomy, chemotherapy and radiation.

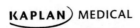

Non-randomized studies are the least valid since the groups that participate are not randomized. This, of course, jeopardizes the validity of the study; the participants are not randomly assigned and so the results are skewed.

In **randomized studies**, the participants are randomly assigned to their groups. The cross-section result improves the validity and decreases the examiner's bias.

Once the data has been collected, the **rate** (a numerical ratio) is calculated with the following formula:

$$\text{Rate} = \frac{\text{\# of people with disease}}{\text{\# of people in the community}}$$

The incidence of something is the rate that measures the number of new cases for a specific amount of time. So the incidence rate of heart disease in New York City from 1/1/04–12/31/04 might look like this:

$$\text{Incidence Rate} = \frac{\text{\# of new cases of heart disease in 2004 in New York City}}{\text{Population of New York City}}$$

A prevalence rate measures the *percentage* of the population that is affected. The prevalence rate here would be calculated as follows:

$$\text{Prevalence Rate} = \frac{\text{Total \# of cases of heart disease in 2004 in New York City}}{\text{Population of New York City}}$$

Once the data has been collected, analyzed, and interpreted, the **statistical data** is produced. The statistical data is a summary of the numerical data. The data is then tested for **correlation,** which measures the linear relationship of 2 or more variables. The coefficient ranges from −1.0 to +1.0. Correlation may be positive or negative. **Positive correlation** occurs when an increase in one variable will increase the second variable. The perfect positive correlation is +1.0. A **negative correlation** occurs in an inverse relationship of the 2 variables. The perfect negative correlation is −1.0. The closer the variables are to 1—whether they are positive or negative—the stronger the correlation.

A +0.95 or −0.95 would be a strong correlation.

Data is also evaluated for its mean, median, and mode. The **mean** is merely an average or statistical ratio. All of the numerical data are added together and then divided by the number of values that were added together. So if 10 subjects participated in a Patient Hygiene Performance Index and the final score was 50, the average PHP score would be 5. The calculation is as follows:

$$\text{Mean} = \frac{\text{Total PHP score (50)}}{\text{Total \# of Participants (10)}} = 5$$

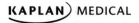

The **median** is the middle score: half of the values fall below, and half fall above. Sometimes the mean and the median are the same number, but often they are not. The median of the values 1,2,3,4,5 would be 3. The mean here would be 3.

The **mode** in an array of values is the most frequently occurring value. There can be more than one mode. So for the following values, which would be the mode?

1,1,1,2,2,2,2,3,3,4,5,5,5

The mode would be 2, since it is the most frequently occurring value. The number 1 appears 3 times, the number 2 appears 4 times, the number 3 appears 2 times, the number 4 appears only 1 time and the number 5 appears 3 times.

There can be more than one mode in a question as follows.

1,1,3,1,5,6,2,5,2,6,1,8,6,5,7,6

Mean = Average

Median = Middle number(s)

Mode = How often the same number appears

In this example, 1 appears four times, and 6 appears four times. So 1 and 6 are both the mode.

Parametric tests measure variables that follow the normal distribution. These types of tests assume that the variables being tested or compared are distributed in a particular way.

Non-parametric tests measure variables in which the distribution is not standard. Fewer assumptions are made with a non-parametric test when it looks at the statistics of a parametric test. The **ratio** is measured by the presence of an absolute zero.

The **p-value** is a numerical value calculated by using a statistical test of a hypothesis. The p-value helps to measure things that occurred by chance during an experiment.

If the p-value is <0.05, then there was a significant statistical result.

If the p-value is >0.05, then the statistical result was insignificant.

If the p-value is 0.05, then the difference occurred by chance.

The *t*-test—also known as the Student's *t* test, named for the developer of the test—is used to compare the relationship of two test results in different studies. It can be independent or dependent. The **Chi square test (x2)** provides a comparison of actual results versus independent results. It measures the significance of observed and expected frequency.

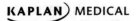

The **significance level** of a study will determine if the results were noteworthy. Did the results have statistical significance without being clinically significant? **Standard deviation** measures variation around the mean. All scores will fall around the standard deviation. The **variance would be the deviation of the mean.**

So, if you have a mean of 8 with a standard deviation of 1, the score would represent which number?

    a.   5-9

    b.   6-10

    c.   7-9

The answer is C, since the standard deviation is 1. One is the variance.

DENTAL INDICES

Many questions about dental indices appear on the National Board Exam. They relate to whether a certain index should be used to determine measurement of disease in a community.

Just what is an index? An index is a numerical measurement of the presence or absence of disease, whether in an individual or community. There are several criteria used to determine if an index is a good one.

1.   The index should have **validity.** It must measure what it is intended to measure.

2.   The index should have **reliability**. It measures consistently at different times. In other words, by following the same criteria, different examiners would gather the same data and the outcome would be the same.

3.   The index should be **clear, simple, and objective.**

4.   The index should be **quantifiable.**

5.   The index should be **acceptable.** It is safe for the subjects involved in the study.

<u>**Criteria for a Good Index**</u>

Valid
Reliable
Clear
Simple
Objective
Quantifiable
Acceptable

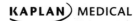

Indices assess both reversible and irreversible disease. A **reversible index** measures conditions that can be reversed, such as gingivitis. Gingivitis is a reversible disease because no bone loss occurs. An **irreversible index** measures conditions that cannot be reversed, such as decay. Once decay is present, it cannot be reversed. It must be treated with a restoration since tooth tissue has been destroyed.

Which index you select depends on the condition being studied, the age of the community being studied, and the purpose of research being conducted. Regardless, examiners must be calibrated to the index that will be used when surveying the presence or absence of disease. **Intrarater** and **intraexaminer reliability** is when each examiner is scoring consistently with each measurement taken. This has been described as "the extent to which the same investigator remains consistent in scoring techniques when using a data collection instrument"(Drury).

Interrater and **interexaminer reliability**, on the other hand, is when there is consistency between examiners. If different examiners were to measure the same population, the data that is collected would be the same. **Calibration** among examiners ensures that each will measure the data in the exact same manner.

Indices are used in **epidemiological studies**, to measure both dependent and independent variables. The **dependent variable** is when a change occurs because of an absence, presence, or control of the variable. The **independent variable** is when the investigator manipulates or controls the experimental condition.

Know if an index is reversible or irreversible, what it measures, and how it is scored.

Suppose you gave one group of people diet soda and another group regular soda, so that you could measure enamel decalcification. The dependent variable is the enamel decalcification, and the independent variable is the presence or absence of sugar in the soda.

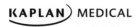

Most Common Dental Indices

Dental Caries Indices

DMFT: Decayed, Missing, Filled Teeth

▷ Used to measure past and present caries experience of a population

▷ Is an **irreversible index**

▷ Performed on individuals age 12 and older

▷ Evaluates 28 teeth
(Hint: BIG LETTERS = BIG TEETH)

▷ Excludes the following:

- Primary retained teeth
- Congenitally missing teeth
- Teeth extracted for orthodontic purposes
- 3rd molars
- Unerupted teeth

▷ The percentage of decayed teeth would be calculated in the following manner:

$$\frac{D}{\text{Total DMFT}} = \% \text{ of decayed teeth}$$

▷ The percentage of missing teeth would be calculated in the following manner:

$$\frac{M}{\text{Total DMFT}} = \% \text{ of missing teeth}$$

▷ The percentage of filled teeth would be calculated in the following manner:

$$\frac{F}{\text{Total DMFT}} = \% \text{ of filled teeth}$$

$$\frac{D + F}{\text{Total DMFT}} = \% \text{ of total caries experience}$$

deft: decayed, exfoliated, filled teeth

▷ Used to **measure past and present caries** experience of a population

▷ Is an **irreversible index**

▷ Performed on individuals age 11 and younger

▷ Evaluates 20 teeth
(Hint: small letters = small teeth)

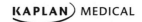

▷ Excludes the following:

- Missing teeth that are unerupted or congenitally missing
- Supernumerary teeth
- Teeth that have been restored for reasons other than dental decay

▷ $\dfrac{d}{\text{Total deft}}$ = % of decayed teeth

▷ The percentage of exfoliated (missing) teeth would be calculated in the following manner:

$\dfrac{e}{\text{Total deft}}$ = % of exfoliated teeth

▷ The percentage of filled teeth would be calculated in the following manner:

$\dfrac{f}{\text{Total deft}}$ = % of filled teeth

RCI: Root Caries Index

▷ Used to **measure the extent of root caries** experience and identifies those at risk for developing root caries

▷ Is an **irreversible index**

▷ Evaluates four surfaces of the root: mesial, distal, facial and lingual. If multiple surfaces are affected, then the surface most severely affected is the one that is recorded.

▷ $\dfrac{(R\text{–}D) + (R\text{–}F)}{(R\text{–}D) + (R\text{–}F) + (R\text{–}N)}$ = X 100 = RCI

- R–D = Root surface with decay
- R–F = Root surface that is filled
- R–N = Root surface that is not filled

Gingivitis Indices

GI: Gingival Index

▷ Used to **determine prevalence and severity of gingivitis**

▷ Is a **reversible index**

▷ Assigns a score of 0–3 to four gingival areas: mesial, distal, facial, and lingual. This score is calculated by totaling all surfaces and then dividing by 4.

▷ Scoring criteria are as follows:

- 0 = Normal gingival
- 1 = Mild inflammation, slight color change, slight edema, no bleeding on probing
- 2 = Moderate inflammation, redness, edema and bleeding upon probing
- 3 = Severe inflammation, marked redness, edema, ulceration, and spontaneous bleeding

SBI: Sulcular Bleeding Index

▷ Used to detect **early symptoms of gingivitis**

▷ Is a **reversible index**

▷ Assigns a score of 0–5 to four gingival areas: mesial, distal, lingual, and facial. This score is calculated by totaling all surfaces and dividing by 4.

$$SBI = \frac{Total\ Surfaces\ Scored}{4}$$

▷ Scoring criteria are as follows:

- 0 = Healthy appearance of the gingiva, no bleeding upon sulcus probing
- 1 = Healthy appearance of gingiva, no change in color, no swelling or bleeding from sulcus on probing
- 2 = Bleeding on probing, change of color caused by inflammation, but no swelling or macroscopic edema
- 3 = Bleeding on probing, change in color, slight edematous swelling
- 4 = Bleeding on probing, change in color, obvious swelling
- 5 = Bleeding on probing, spontaneous bleeding change in color, marked swelling with or without ulceration

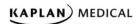

Periodontal Indices

PDI: Periodontal Disease Index

▷ Used **to measure** the presence and severity of **periodontal disease**

▷ Is an **irreversible index** since bone loss is permanent

▷ Assigns a score of 0–8, calculated by totaling all of the scores for each tooth and dividing by the number of teeth present and examined.

$$PDI = \frac{\text{Total Score of Teeth Examined}}{\text{Number of Teeth Examined}}$$

▷ Scoring criteria are as follows:

- 0 = Negative. No inflammation present or loss of function caused by destruction of supporting tissue

- 1 = Mild Gingivitis. Overt area of inflammation in the free gingiva that does not circumscribe the tooth

- 2 = Gingivitis. Inflammation completely circumscribes the tooth without affecting the epithelial attachment

- 6 = Gingivitis with Pocket Formation. Breakdown of the epithelial attachment with pocket formation. There is no change in masticatory function and the tooth is firm in its socket.

- 8 = Advanced Destruction with Loss of Masticatory Function. Tooth may be loose, drifted, and depressible in its socket.

CPITN: Community Periodontal Index of Treatment Needs

▷ Used to **measure** group **periodontal needs**

▷ Is an **irreversible index** (if periodontal disease is recorded)

▷ Developed by the World Health Organization (WHO)

▷ Assigns a score for two groups: children and adolescents, and then adults age 20 and over

▷ The CPITN and the Periodontal Screening and Recording (PSR) by the American Academy of Periodontology and the ADA are both performed using the exact same scoring criteria and scoring box.

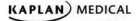

Scoring parameters for children and adolescents ages 7–19

▷ The dentition is divided into sextants.

▷ Evaluation of one tooth per sextant. Teeth #'s 3, 9, 12, 19, 25, 28. (Ramfjord teeth). Some schools use teeth# 3, 8, 12, 19, 24, 28.

▷ When a designated tooth is missing, the sextant is recorded as missing and an X is recorded for that sextant.

Scoring parameters for adults age 20 and older

▷ The dentition is divided into sextants and all teeth are evaluated

▷ A sextant must have two or more functional teeth. In order for a tooth to be considered functional, it must not be treatment planned for an extraction. In the event there is only one tooth present, it is to be evaluated with the adjacent sextant. If only one tooth is present, or if a sextant is edentulous, then an X will be recorded for that sextant.

▷ Third molars are included in a sextant's evaluation only if the second molars are missing and the third molars function in place of the second molars.

▷ Scoring criteria are as follows for CPITN and PSR:

- Code 0 = Healthy periodontal tissues
- Code 1 = Bleeding after gentle probing
- Code 2 = Supragingival or subgingival calculus or defective margin of a restoration or crown
- Code 3 = 4–5 mm pocket
- Code 4 = 6 mm or deeper pathologic pocket

CPITN and PSR recording scores

▷ Use a simple box chart to recordings

▷ An X is placed in any box that has a missing sextant

▷ The highest score in each sextant is the only one recorded

▷ Once a code 4 is reached in a sextant, there is no need to examine the remaining teeth in that sextant

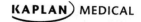

Periodontal Treatment Needs Scale

Once the scores have been recorded, the patient's or community's needs are classified according to the highest coded score during the screening.

▷ O = No need for treatment

▷ I = Oral hygiene instruction needed

▷ II = Oral hygiene instruction with root debridement, elimination of plaque, retentive margins on restorations and crowns

▷ III = Oral hygiene instruction with root debridement, elimination of plaque retentive margins on restorations and crowns, periodontal therapy that may include surgical intervention and/or root debridement with local anesthesia

PSR: Periodontal Screening and Recording

▷ Used to **measure** an individual's **periodontal needs**

▷ Is an **irreversible index** (if periodontal disease is recorded)

▷ Developed by the World Health Organization (WHO)

▷ Assigns a score for two groups: children and adolescents, and then adults age 20 and over

▷ Criteria and Scoring: Same as CPTIN above. See previous page.

PI: Periodontal Index

▷ Used to **measure the periodontal disease status of a community** in epidemiologic studies

▷ Is an **irreversible index**

▷ Assigns each tooth a score according to the tissues that surround it. Each tooth is assigned a score from 0 (no disease)–8 (severe disease with loss of function). For an individual's score, the scores of each tooth are totaled and divided by the number of teeth present and examined. For a group's score, all individual scores are totaled and divided by the number of individuals examined. The average will range from 0–8.

$$PI = \frac{\text{Total Score of Teeth Examined}}{\text{Number of Teeth Examined}}$$

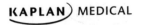

▷ Scoring criteria are as follows:

- 0 = Negative. No inflammation present, no loss of function caused by destruction of supporting tissue

- 1 = Mild Gingivitis. Inflammation is present in the free gingival but does not circumscribe the tooth.

- 2 = Gingivitis Inflammation completely circumscribes the tooth but there is no loss in the epithelial attachment.

- 6 = Gingivitis with Pocket Formation. There is a loss in the epithelial attachment, the tooth is firm in its socket, there is no loss of masticatory function.

- 8 = Advanced Destruction with Loss of Masticatory Function. The tooth may be loose, may have drifted, may sound dull upon percussion, and may be depressible in its socket.

Scoring Ranges

▷ 0.0–0.2 Clinically normal supportive tissues

▷ 0.3–0.9 Simple gingivitis

▷ 0.7–1.9 Early phase of periodontal disease

▷ 1.6–5.0 Moderate phase of periodontal disease

▷ 3.8–8.0 Advanced phase of periodontal disease

Oral Hygiene Indices

OHI-S: Simplified Oral Hygiene Index

▷ Used to **measure oral cleanliness** by examining the tooth surface covered with debris and/or calculus

▷ Is a **reversible index**

▷ Evaluates 6 specific teeth, one in each sextant (the first fully-erupted teeth distal to each 2nd premolar, #8 facial, #24 facial). Each surface is assigned a score of 0 (no debris)–6 (debris present). All surfaces are totaled and divided by the number of teeth assessed

$$\text{OHI-S} = \frac{\text{Total Score of Teeth Examined}}{\text{Number of Teeth Examined}}$$

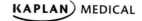

Scoring Ranges

▷ 0.0–1.2   Good oral hygiene

▷ 1.3–3.0   Fair oral hygiene

▷ 3.1–6.0   Poor oral hygiene

▷ OHI-S Score $= \dfrac{\text{Total number of tooth surfaces scored}}{\text{Number of teeth that have been scored}}$

PI: Plaque Index

▷ Used to **measure** the amount of **debris** present on the tooth surface

▷ Is a reversible index

▷ Assigns four plaque scores per tooth: M, D, B, L. The score is calculated by totaling the scores of all the teeth involved and dividing by 4

▷ Evaluates the entire dentition or selected teeth

PI for a Tooth

▷ PI $= \dfrac{\text{Total of all areas of a tooth}}{4}$

PI for Groups of Teeth

▷ PI $= \dfrac{\text{Total of scores for group of teeth}}{\text{Number of teeth scored}}$

Score Criteria

▷ 0 = No plaque

▷ 1 = Film adheres to attached gingiva

▷ 2 = Moderate soft debris within the gingival margin

▷ 3 = Gross soft debris within gingival pockets and/or margins

Scoring Ranges

▷ 0   Excellent

▷ 0.1–0.9   Good

▷ 1.0–1.9   Fair

▷ 2.0–3.0   Poor

PHP: Patient Hygiene Performance

▷ Used to **measure** the effectiveness of a patient's **oral hygiene** regimen

▷ Is a **reversible index**

▷ Evaluates #3–Buccal, #8–Facial, #14–Buccal, #19–Lingual, #24–Labial, #30–Lingual in five areas: Vertically (3 divisions)—mesial, middle, and distal. Horizontally (middle 1/3)—subdivided into gingival, middle, and occlusal or incisal thirds

▷ Disclosing solution is applied to the teeth. Each subdivision of the tooth is scored 1 if debris is present. Scores for all of the teeth are totaled and divided by 6 or the number of teeth used in the index. If one of the teeth used in the index scoring is missing, the examiner will substitute it with the tooth that is adjacent to it in the same class. So if #3 is missing, #2 would be used in the scoring—not tooth #4.

$$PHP = \frac{\text{Total Debris Score}}{\text{\# of Teeth Scored}}$$

Score Criteria

▷ 0 = No debris present

▷ 1 = Debris is present

▷ M = All three molars or both incisors are missing

▷ S = A substitute tooth is used

Scoring Ranges

- ▷ 0–0.9   Excellent
- ▷ 0.1–1.7   Good
- ▷ 1.8–3.4   Fair
- ▷ 3.5–5.0   Poor

Fluorosis Indices

Dean's Classification of Fluorosis

- ▷ Used to **measure severity and degree of fluorosis**
- ▷ Is an **irreversible index**
- ▷ Evaluates all teeth
- ▷ Assigns a score based on the severity or absence of fluorosis

Score Criteria

- ▷ 1 = Very mild. Small opaque, paper white areas, with less than 25% of tooth affected
- ▷ 2 = Mild. White opaque areas, 25–50% of tooth surfaces affected
- ▷ 3 = Moderate. All teeth affected, brown stains, surface is subject to attrition
- ▷ 4 = Severe. All surfaces are affected with hypoplasia. Brown stains and the tooth appears to be corroded

PUBLIC FINANCING OF DENTAL CARE

Title XVIII Medicare Insurance provides insurance for individuals over the age of 65 to cover medical needs though it offers little dental coverage. It was one of the federal government's first amendments to the Social Security Act of 1935, which helped remove barriers to healthcare for the elderly.

Title XIX Medicaid provides assistance to individuals from low-income and needy backgrounds. The federal and state governments formed a coalition to help provide both medical and dental care. Dental care is not mandatory except for individuals under the age of 21.

Title XXI, amended in 1997, created the state Children's Health Insurance Program. The program—both state and federally funded—was designed for those whose income exceeds the limitations for Medicaid assistance but at the same time, does not have an ability to pay for private medical insurance.

The U.S. Department of Veterans Affairs provides medical and some dental care through its network of hospitals to many veterans. Public Health Service provides healthcare services to individuals who are institutionalized (prison) and to the general public. Indian Health Services (IHS) provides medical and dental care to the Native American and Alaskan American Indian tribes.

REVIEW QUESTIONS

<u>Questions 1-4 are based on the scenario below.</u>

Members of the Franklin County School District
are concerned about the high decay rate in students
who attend the public elementary schools. They have
appealed to the Public Health Department to help rec-
tify the situation. Franklin County is a rural county with
85% of residents living outside of the city limits. Those
individuals have well water, which is not fluoridated.

1. Which of the following indices would be used to
    measure the decay rate of the elementary-school
    children?

    A. DMFT
    B. DEFT
    C. deft
    D. dmft
    E. PHP

2. Based upon the needs of this population, what step
    is next in program planning with the statistics used
    in this index?

    A. Treatment planning
    B. Diagnosis
    C. Evaluation
    D. Examination
    E. Assessment

3. Since the Franklin County School District water is
    not fluoridated, which of the following would be
    the most cost-effective way to address the decay
    issue?

    A. Start a school sealant program
    B. Fluoridate the school's water supply
    C. Start a school fluoride rinse program
    D. Professionally applied fluoride treatments

4. Treatment of the active decay would be considered
    _____ preventive treatment.

    A. Secondary
    B. Primary
    C. Endemic
    D. Tertiary
    E. Quarternary

5. When other individuals in a community suffer
    from a similar condition at the same time, it is
    known as

    A. Incidence
    B. Epidemiology
    C. Epidemic
    D. Prevalence
    E. Mortality

6. When various examiners measure in the same
    manner while using the same measurement tool, it
    is called

    A. Mean
    B. Interrater reliability
    C. Intrarater reliability
    D. Validity

7. Which of the following correlation coefficients
    demonstrates the strongest relationship?

    A. −0.05
    B. +0.75
    C. −0.35
    D. +3.0
    E. −0.95

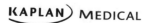

<u>Questions 8-10 are based on the scenario below.</u>

The first-year dental-hygiene clinic coordinator at Jones Community College needs to calculate the final scores for students at the end of the semester. Listed below are the grades of the 15 dental hygiene students.

80	90	85	75	82
67	87	83	82	85
85	86	90	89	88

8. What is the mode of the values listed above?

    A. 67
    B. 90
    C. 87
    D. 82
    E. 85

9. How many modes are found in the values listed above?

    A. 1
    B. 2
    C. 3
    D. 4

10. What is the mean score for the values listed above?

    A. 82
    B. 83.6
    C. 84
    D. 86.3
    E. 85.5

11. For an epidemiology study, which of the following indices would be used to measure the degree of oral debris remaining on a tooth surface?

    A. GI
    B. CPTIN
    C. OHI-S
    D. DMFT
    E. PHP

12. In the context of comparing private dental care to public health care, the first step in private dental care is examination. In public health care, the first step is

    A. Analysis
    B. Diagnosis
    C. Survey
    D. Treatment
    E. Evaluation

13. In the study of epidemiology, the term *morbidity* refers to which of the following?

    A. Disease and disability
    B. Occurrence of disease within a population at a given point in time
    C. Number of new cases within a population in time
    D. Death

14. The expected level of disease found within a population is called

    A. Pandemic
    B. Epidemic
    C. Epidemiology
    D. Endemic

15. Community X has an optimally fluoridated water supply. What would be the dosage of supplemental fluoride for a 3-year-old living in this community?

    A. None
    B. 0.25 mg
    C. 0.50 mg
    D. 1.0 mg
    E. 2.0 mg

16. The percentage of individuals within a given area suffering from a particular condition at the same time is known as

    A. Need for care
    B. Frequency
    C. Prevalence
    D. Incidence

Questions 17–22 are based on the scenario below.

The freshman class at Wakefield High School has 60 girls and 40 boys, aged 14–16. Two public-health hygienists decide to conduct a study on the decay rate of this group of teenagers by using the DMFT to assess their oral health status. In order to calibrate the hygienist as examiners, 20 sophomore students are used to prepare the examination technique of the hygienists. Once calibrated, the hygienists decide to examine and determine the DMFT on the freshman class. The total DMFT for this class is 175.

17. The following formula was used in a study involving 60 girls and 40 boys: DMFT ÷ 100. What does this formula determine?

    A. DMFT per teenager
    B. DMFT per teenage boys in the group
    C. DMFT per teenage girls in the group
    D. DMFT of the entire school
    E. DMFT of the entire group

18. The DMFT index refers to

    A. The adult patient
    B. The child patient
    C. The geriatric patient
    D. None of the above

19. During calibration, what type of reliability was demonstrated by the hygienists in the evaluation of the DMFT?

    A. Intrarater
    B. Interrater
    C. Independent
    D. Dependent

20. If D = 35, M = 25, and F = 115, what percentage of teeth has untreated decay?

    A. 20%
    B. 25%
    C. 30%
    D. 35%
    E. 40%

21. The relatively high F value (115) for filled teeth would indicate that this group of students

    A. has no access to care.
    B. has a high incidence of tooth extraction.
    C. is in need of periodontal treatment.
    D. has access to restorative dental care.

22. The public health hygienists decide to conduct annual DMFTs on these 100 students for 10 years. This type of study is called

    A. Retrospective
    B. Cross-sectional
    C. Longitudinal
    D. Cohort
    E. Double-blind

23. Which of the following indices would be most helpful for public dental hygienists in assessing the periodontal treatment needs of a population?

    A. CPTIN
    B. GI
    C. OHI-S
    D. PHP

24. Which federal agency provides for dental treatment of children who live at or below poverty level?

    A. Headstart
    B. Medicaid
    C. Medicare
    D. CHAMPUS

25. In planning a presentation about oral healthcare to a state prison population, which of the following is important?

    A. Distribution of free samples
    B. Use of multimedia presentations
    C. Use of a combination of teaching strategies
    D. Focus on personal well-being
    E. Both C and D

ANSWER EXPLANATIONS

1. C

The index that would be used to measure the decay rate of the elementary school children is the deft for children who still have primary teeth.

A. The DMFT is used on individuals age 12 and older.

B. The DEFT is not a true index.

D. The dmft is not a true index

E. The Patient Hygiene Performance measures plaque and oral debris and the effects of patient motivation on improvement of oral hygiene.

2. E

The next step in program planning is assessment— the gathering of information.

A. Treatment planning is used in private dental care settings, not in those of public health.

B. Diagnosis is also used in the private dental care setting.

C. Evaluation is the appraisal for program effectiveness.

D. Examination gathered the information for the statistics in Question #1.

3. B

The most cost-effective way to address the decay issue would be to fluoridate only the school's water supply. All other methods would be more expensive to implement.

4. A

Secondary preventive treatment includes placement of dental restorations.

B. Primary preventive treatment is placement of sealants, prophylaxis, and professionally applied fluoride treatments.

C. Endemic refers to the level of expected disease.

D. Tertiary treatment refers to treatment that will restore normal function, such as crown and bridge or removable dentures.

E. Quarternary is not a dental option here.

5. D

Prevalence is when other individuals in a community suffer from a similar condition at the same time.

A. Incidence refers to the number of new cases of a condition that occur in a given period.

B. Epidemiology is the study of the determinants and distribution of disease.

C. Epidemic refers to the higher than normal occurrence of a disease or condition.

6. B

Interrater reliability is when different examiners measure in the same way with the same measurement tool.

C. Intrarater reliability is when an individual examiner measures all subjects in the same manner.

7. E

The strongest correlation relationship is -0.95 since it is closest to -1.0.

8. E

Mode is the most frequently occurring value. Here, that would be 85, since it appears 3 times.

9. A

There is only one mode. No other value is equal in occurrence to 85.

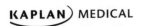

10. B

The mean is the average of all the values (scores). Add all of the values here to get 1,254. Next, divide 1,254 by 15 (the number of values). The result is 83.6.

11. C

The Oral Hygiene Index Simplified measures the amount of oral debris remaining on a tooth surface.

A. The Gingival Index measures the presence and severity of gingival disease.

B. CPTIN measures group periodontal needs.

D. DMFT measures decayed, missing, and filled teeth.

E. PHP measures patient hygiene performance.

12. C

When developing a public health community program, the first step is to survey the needs.

A. Analysis or evaluation is the final step for measuring program effectiveness.

B. Diagnosis is the second step in private care settings.

D. Treatment is a dental term, not a community planning term.

13. A

Morbidity refers to disease or disability.

B. Prevalence is the occurrence of disease within a population at a point in time.

C. Incidence is the number of new cases within a population in time.

D. Mortality refers to death.

14. D

The expected level of disease found within a population is called endemic.

A. Pandemic refers to a disease or condition that is widespread throughout a country or even the world.

B. Epidemic refers to a higher than normal prevalence of disease.

C. Epidemiology is the study of new cases in the community.

15. A

The water is optimally fluoridated, so no supplement is needed.

16. C

Prevalence is when people of a certain area suffer from a particular condition at the same time.

D. Incidence is the number of new cases of a condition that occurred in a given period of time.

17. E

The entire group is being measured for DMFT.

18. A

The DMFT is for the adult patient.

B. The deft would be used on the child patient.

19. B

Interrater reliability was used, since both hygienists used the same instrument of measurement in the same manner.

20. A

The number of teeth with decay (35) is divided by the total number of surfaces affected by decayed, missing, and filled teeth. So 35 ÷ 175 = 0.2, or 20%.

21. D

The relatively high F value (115) for filled teeth suggests that these students have access to care.

22. C

A longitudinal study is conducted over a long period of time.

A. A retrospective occurs after an event has occurred.

B. A cross-sectional study looks at a wide sample of a population.

D. A cohort study looks at a population with a similar characteristic or condition.

E. A double-blind study occurs when neither the examiner nor the participant knows which is the control or experimental group.

23. A

The CPTIN would help public dental hygienists to assess the periodontal treatment needs of a population.

D. The PHP measures the oral hygiene status of an individual or group.

24. B

Medicaid is the federal agency that provides dental treatment of children living at or below poverty level.

A. Headstart involves infants and toddlers in school programs by addressing family literacy needs.

C. Medicare is a federally funded medical insurance for adults over the age of 65.

D. CHAMPUS (Civilian Health and Medical Program of Uniform Services) provides healthcare for military personnel and their dependents.

25. E

A presentation to a prison population should incorporate various teaching strategies (to enhance learning) and emphasize personal well-being.

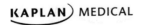

Chapter Nineteen:
Patients with Special Needs

As per the Americans with Disabilities Act, individuals with disabilities are guaranteed equal access to any public facility—including a dental office. Treatment, as well, needs to be the same for those with disabilities as those without.

ADRENAL PROBLEMS

More than 50 steroids are produced within the adrenal cortex of the adrenal glands, with cortisol and aldosterone the most abundant and physiologically active. These steroids have many functions. They:

- Balance the effects of insulin to maintain sugar levels in the blood
- Activate amino and fatty acids
- Increase RBC and platelet levels in blood serum
- Take part in the inflammatory response
- Produce estrogens that affect sexual development and reproduction

Adrenal Crisis/Hypocortisolism

An adrenal crisis can occur when there is an insufficiency of cortisol, which is produced by the adrenal glands. It can be exacerbated by stress.

- **Addison's disease** is a hormonal disorder that damages the adrenal glands. Someone with this disease produces insufficient adrenal hormones needed for normal daily functions. This occurs due to the gradual destruction of the adrenal cortex (outer layer of the adrenal glands) by the body's own immune system. Risk factors are stress, trauma, surgery, or infection. The disease is characterized by weight loss, low blood pressure, weakness, fatigue, and **dark skin pigmentation** (melanoderma).

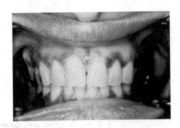

Addison's Disease

Contributed by Dr. Michael Finkelstein,
DDS College of Dentistry, University of Iowa

- **Etiology**: Hypocortisol secretion by the adrenal glands

- **Symptoms**: Skin pigmentations, weakness and fatigue, headache, nausea and/or vomiting, low threshold for stress, abnormally low blood pressure, altered level of consciousness, susceptibility to infections, rapid heart and respiratory rates

- **Oral manifestations**: None

- **Oral care**: Maintain a nonstressful atmosphere in the dental setting. Keep in mind that a patient with Addison's can give himself an emergency injection of hydrocortisone in times of stress.

- **Hypercortisolism (Cushing's syndrome)** is an **overproduction** of cortisol by the adrenal glands. It is an endocrine disorder caused by excessive levels of cortisol.

  - **Etiology**: Hypersecretion of cortisol by the adrenal glands

  - **Symptoms**: Weight gain, fatty tissue deposits in the face creating a **"moon" face**, **buffalo hump**, large abdomen, excess sweating, thin and easily bruised skin, and purple pigmentation on the trunk and legs

  - **Oral manifestations**: None

  - **Oral care**: Provide oral hygiene instruction for the maintenance of healthy tissues.

ATTENTION DEFICIT HYPERACTIVITY DISORDER (ADHD)

ADHD is characterized by improper behavior and/or failure to pay attention, with deficits in learning. It is estimated that 3–5% of the population has this disorder. Patients lack concentration and direction, and are easily distracted.

- **Etiology**: Possibly smoking or alcohol-use during pregnancy. Other causes include high levels of lead exposure, brain injury, refined sugar, food additives, or genetics.

- **Symptoms**: Inattentiveness, hyperactivity, impulsiveness, and possible learning disability

- **Oral manifestations**: None. Drugs such as Ritalin or Concerta (time-released formula) have no oral side effects.

- **Oral care**: Gear home-care instruction to the caregiver. Consider not leaving this patient in your room unattended.

ALCOHOL-RELATED PROBLEMS

Alcohol-related problems affect people of all ages. Researchers estimate that 1 in every 13 adults abuse alcohol to some degree. Alcoholics can develop **pernicious anemia** as a result of **insufficient intrinsic factor** in the stomach. Plus, they are at high risk for cancer.

- **Etiology**: Possibly genetics, though not every child of an alcoholic parent becomes an alcoholic. Stress plays a significant role.

- **Symptoms**: Craving for alcohol. And in cases where an alcoholic suddenly stops drinking, nausea, shakiness, and anxiety.

- **Oral manifestations**: Xerostomia, glossitis, periodontal disease, and possible poor oral hygiene

- **Oral care**: You may need to perform root scaling and debridement for periodontal problems to return the tissues to health. Diet consulting is needed to help the patient realize he is at risk for pernicious anemia. Place the patient on a frequent recall basis. Recommend nonalcoholic mouthwashes.

> Patients on Antabuse should use a non-alcoholic mouthwash, since alcohol absorption can cause a severe reaction.

ALZHEIMER'S DISEASE

Alzheimer's disease is a severe disorder that brings about the gradual loss of brain cells. Over time, the patient's memory and ability to learn are wiped out.

- **Etiology**: Unknown

- **Symptoms**: For early stage: Inability to recall recent events, make judgments, manage routine chores. For moderate stage: Difficulty getting dressed, bathing and using the bathroom. For severe stage: Inability to say more than a few words, walk, smile, or hold up the head.

- **Oral manifestations**: Xerostomia, angular cheillitis, glossitis, loss of taste, root caries, or periodontal disease

- **Oral care**: Advise the care giver about oral hygiene for the patient. The patient may need an adapted handle on a manual brush or a power-assisted toothbrush. Nightly fluoride rinses or pastes may help to control root caries. Xerostomia may be relieved with saliva substitutes such as Biotine.

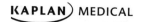

ARTHRITIS

Osteoarthritis is the most common type of arthritis in the United States. It starts with the **breakdown of the cartilage in joints, causing pain and stiffness. Rheumatoid arthritis** is an inflammation of the lining of the joints. Arthritis is more common in women than in men.

- **Etiology**: For osteoarthritis, likely due to mechanical stress to joints, and might also be due to genetics, age, joint overuse, and obesity. For rheumatoid arthritis, likely due to an autoimmune disease when the body attacks healthy joint tissue, and might also be due to genetics and environmental factors.

- **Symptoms**: For osteoarthritis: Initial joint tenderness when exercising or performing tasks. With disease progression, swelling, stiffness, and pain occur in the joints with possible crepitus. For rheumatoid arthritis: Stiffness and joint swelling, warmth, and tenderness.

- **Oral manifestations**: None, though patients may experience xerostomia caused by many arthritis medications.

- **Oral care**: Patient may require an adapted handle on a manual brush or a power-assisted toothbrush. A floss holder may help the patient with flossing.

AUTISM

Autism is a neurological disorder that results in developmental disabilities. It occurs within the first 3 years of life, and is far more prevalent in boys than in girls. Patients have trouble with verbal and non-verbal communication, social interactions, and play activities. **Asperger syndrome** is a high-functioning autism, where the patient seems of normal intelligence and communicates well, but has autistic characteristics.

- **Etiology**: Theories point to genetics or medical problems such as fragile-X syndrome, untreated phenylketonuria (PKU), or congenital rubella syndrome.

- **Symptoms**: Range from mild to severe: repetitive routines, speech difficulties, preference for being alone, lack of eye contact, abnormal attachment to things, learning disabilities, spinning of objects, no fear of danger

- **Oral manifestations**: None

- **Oral care**: Instruct the caregiver in oral hygiene, keeping in mind that the patient may be uncooperative. Nutritional counseling may reveal that the child has a diet high in sugar set up as a reward system for good behavior. During the dental appointment, provide repetitive encounters in a quiet atmosphere.

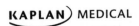

BELL'S PALSY

Bell's palsy is an idiopathic, unilateral facial muscle paralysis affecting the facial or 7th cranial nerve. Most patients recover in 3 weeks or up to 6 months, though some experience permanent paralysis.

- **Etiology**: Possibly a viral infection, where a latent virus travels along the sensory nerves, though more recent research suspects the herpes simplex virus. Possibly after a tooth extraction or parotid gland surgery.

- **Symptoms**: Unilateral facial paralysis, drooling, loss of turgor, and inability to close the eye on the side affected

- **Oral manifestations**: Inadequate oral care on the affected side, causing tissue inflammation and/or carious lesions

- **Oral care**: Focus on home care techniques and adjuncts for better plaque removal.

BLOOD DISORDERS

Anemias

Anemia indicates a drop in oxygen-carrying hemoglobin in red blood cells. There are several types of anemia.

- **Etiology**: **Iron-deficiency anemia** is due to insufficient iron. The body needs iron to make hemoglobin, a substance in red blood cells that enables them to carry oxygen. **Pernicious anemia** is caused by insufficient B12 vitamin, usually the result of an intrinsic factor shortage in the stomach. **Aplastic anemia** is the failure of the bone marrow to produce enough red and white blood cells, and platelets.

- **Symptoms**: For iron-deficiency anemia: Weakness, paleness, shortness of breath, sore tongue, brittle nails, and headache. For pernicious anemia: Add to that tachycardia, tingling/numbness in feet and hands, unsteady gait, beefy red tongue, angular cheilosis, and impaired smell. For aplastic anemia: Low blood counts, shortness of breath, tachycardia, and rash.

- **Oral manifestations**: For iron-deficiency anemia: Pale gingiva and mucosa, angular cheilitis, and painful glossitis. For pernicious anemia: Burning glossitis and bleeding gingiva. For aplastic anemia: None.

- **Oral care**: Focus on good oral hygiene, since any gingival disease may cause an abnormal amount of bleeding.

Hemophilia

Hemophilia is a genetic disorder that affects men with hemophilia A and B, that is carried by females in their X chromosome. **Hemophilia A** lacks **factor VIII** clotting factor, while **hemophilia B** (Christmas disease) lacks **factor IX**.

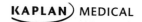

- **Etiology**: Inherited. For hemophilia A and B, the female carries the X-linked recessive gene.

- **Symptoms**: Bruising with ease, blood in the urine (hematuria), bleeding intojoint with swelling, intracranial bleeding without injury, backache or paralysis due to bleeding into the spinal column, and frequent nosebleeds.

- **Oral manifestations**: Ecchymosis, hematoma, or prolonged bleeding with dental procedures.

- **Oral care**: Screen for clotting factors. Home care should include oral hygiene instruction to maintain healthy soft tissues so that bleeding gingiva is prevented. Include instruction on antimicrobial mouth rinses, soft-bristle tooth brushing, and flossing. Routine prophylaxis and examination, routine restorative work or local infiltration anesthesia may be performed without administering any factors. Deep scaling, root debridement and planing, extractions, or nerve block anesthesia require **a slow IV infusion of pure preparation factor VIII** (hemophilia A) **or factor IX** (hemophilia B) **concentrate**.

Leukemia

There are four major types of leukemia that affect white blood cells.

Acute myelogenous leukemia occurs from genetic damage to the DNA of developing cells in the bone marrow. This form of the disease is caused by excessive growth of abnormal cells ("leukemic blasts") and the obstruction of bone marrow production of normal red blood cells, platelets, and normal white blood cells.

Chronic myelogenous leukemia is caused by an injury to the DNA of a stem cell in the marrow. The DNA is then altered, causing an overproduction—and ultimately, a massive proliferation—of white blood cells (WBC). Unlike acute myelogenous leukemia, chronic myelogenous leukemia does allow for the production of normal white blood cells.

Acute lymphocytic leukemia is the most common type of leukemia in children under age 19. It is caused by a genetic injury to the DNA in a single cell in bone marrow. Normal leukemic cells of normal bone marrow are exchanged with abnormal lymphoblastic-producing cells. These new cells do not perform as do regular white blood cells, and they block the production of normal red blood cells, platelets, and normal white blood cells.

Chronic lymphocytic leukemia is caused by an acquired injury to the DNA in a single cell of bone marrow. The DNA change results in abnormal, malignant cells that proliferate excessively. The leukemic cells do not inhibit normal blood cell production as greatly as in acute lymphocytic leukemia.

A subtype of chronic lymphocytic leukemia is **hairy cell leukemia**, a slow-growing malignant disorder that affects lymphocytes. It earned its name because the lymphocytes exhibit short, thin projections on the cell membranes, resembling hairs when inspected microscopically. Hairy cell leukemia is difficult to diagnose since its symptoms are indistinguishable from other illnesses.

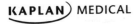

- **Etiology**: Genetic or via acquired injury to the DNA of white blood cells.

- **Symptoms**: Shortness of breath, fatigue, unexplained bruising, mild fever, swollen gums, frequent minor infections, slow healing of cuts, enlarged lymph nodes, and paleness. Chronic myelogenous leukemia may also include enlarged spleen, sweating, and weight loss.

- **Oral manifestations**: Gingivitis with bleeding, petechiae and ecchymoses of the hard and soft palate, chemotherapy-induced mucositis, xerostomia, herpes simplex ulcers, and oral candidiasis

- **Oral care**: If neutrophil count is less than 500/mm^3, preprocedural prophylactic antibiotic should be administered. Avoid elective procedures in acute stages. Oral hygiene instructions will help to maintain healthy oral tissues to prevent bleeding, palliative treatment of any lesions, fluoride treatments, antimicrobial rinses, and saliva substitutes for xerostomia.

Polycythemia

Polycythemia is a stem-cell disorder that causes an overproduction of red blood cells. It is more common in men than in women.

- **Etiology**: Unknown

- **Symptoms**: Sludging blood flow and thromboses, causing headache, dizziness, vertigo, tinnitus, visual disturbances, dyspnea, and angina pectoris. Also, enlarged spleen, GI bleeds, epistaxis, and ecchymoses. Pruritus often occurs after a hot bath.

- **Oral manifestations**: Bleeding gingiva, deep red–purple oral tissues

- **Oral care**: Focus on oral hygiene instruction so that bleeding can be kept to a minimum, palliative treatment for any lesions, and antimicrobial rinses.

Sickle-Cell Disease

Sickle-cell disease is an inherited hemolytic anemia affecting African-Americans. It is distinguished by chronic anemia and periodic episodes of pain.

Normal red blood cells are donut-shaped. With sickle-cell anemia, they are crescent or sickle-shaped. With this disorder, hemoglobin molecules are defective within the red blood cell; when they relinquish oxygen to cells, the hemoglobin molecules within the red blood cell stack up together in a rod-like configuration. Round red blood cells can move easily through small vessels but the crescent-shaped sickle cells cannot. Instead, they stack up and act as a dam, stopping red blood cells from going through. This starves organs of oxygen and causes pain.

- **Etiology**: Inherited as an autosomal recessive genetic disorder.

- **Symptoms**: Shortness of breath, pallor, osteoporosis, fatigue, and general weakness.

- **Oral manifestations**: Pallor of oral tissues, with liver involvement, jaundice, delayed tooth eruption, and tooth hypoplasia

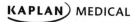

- **Oral care**: Focus on oral hygiene instruction so that bleeding can be kept to a minimum, and on antimicrobial rinses. Consider prophylactic antibiotics prior to treatment. For dental treatment, use local anesthesia without epinephrine.

Thalassemia

Thalassemia is an inherited disorder that affects children of Mediterranean origin younger than age 2. It is the impaired creation of either the alpha or beta hemoglobin chain, producing reduced or erroneous hemoglobin.

The hemoglobin of each parent contributes 2 alpha globin sub-unit genes and 1 beta globin sub-unit gene, for a total of 4 alpha globin sub-unit genes and 2 beta globin sub-unit genes. Thalassemia occurs if one or more of the genes are missing producing a shortage of sub-unit protein. If an alpha sub-unit is missing, the individual has alpha thalassemia. Likewise if an individual lacks a beta sub-unit, they have beta thalassemia. Since the combination of missing sub-unit genes can vary, there are many types of thalassemia.

- **Etiology**: Inherited.
- **Symptoms**: Jaundice, fatigue, shortness of breath, spleen and liver enlargement, skull deformity with Mongoloid features, and heart enlargement.
- **Oral manifestations**: Bleeding gingiva, malocclusions
- **Oral care**: Focus on oral hygiene instruction so that bleeding can be kept to a minimum, and antimicrobial rinses.

Von Willebrand's Disease

Von Willebrand factor is a protein in blood that **mediates platelet cohesiveness** when endothelium is injured and also **maintains factor VIII levels** in blood.

Von Willebrand's disease is a hereditary bleeding disorder that can affect both **men and women**. Von Willebrand factor is a **protein released by the lining of blood vessels** that allows for platelets to adhere to each other. This same factor also transports the protein factor VIII for clotting. With von Willebrand's disease, the factor is either deficient or defective and occurs in about 1% of the population. The disease is usually so mild that is can go undiagnosed.

There are 3 types of von Willebrand's disease. Type 1 has low levels of factor VIII.

Type 2 is a defect in the function of the von Willebrand factor. Type 2A is a less efficient factor of holding platelets together. Type 2B occurs when platelets adhere together in the bloodstream rather than at the injury site. Type 2N is a rare form that is sometimes mistaken for hemophilia A. In this case, 2N von Willebrand factor does not bind to factor VIII creating a low level of factor VIII which mimics hemophilia A.

Type 3 is a very rare type when the von Willebrand factor is totally absent or extremely low.

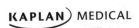

- **Etiology**: Hereditary

- **Symptoms**: History of bleeding. Bruising, recurrent nosebleeds, prolonged bleeding, bleeding gums, blood in the stool or urine, and heavy menstruation.

- **Oral manifestations**: Prolonged bleeding after dental procedures, petechiae, hematomas.

- **Oral care**: Lab screening test for clotting factors. Home care instructions to maintain healthy tissues to prevent bleeding.

CANCER

In 2002, the CDC stated that "approximately 75% of oral cavity and pharyngeal cancers are attributed to the use of smoked and smokeless tobacco." Alcohol abuse also contributes to oral cancer. Approximately 2–4% of all cancers are diagnosed as oral cancer, with the survival rates among the lowest of all cancers. Over 90% of all oral cancers are squamous cell carcinomas.

Oral cancer lesions can involve the anterior two-thirds of tongue, lips, buccal mucosa, gingiva, floor of the mouth, hard palate, and retromolar area. The lower lip accounts for over 90% of oral cancers. Oropharyngeal cancer lesions may involve the base of tongue (posterior one-third), soft palate, tonsils, tonsillar pillars, and posterior pharyngeal wall.

> Oral cancer lesions appear on the lower lip in over 90% of cases.

Other risk factors for all cancers not only include smoking and alcohol but also secondhand smoke, sun exposure, radiation exposure, viruses, chronic trauma, nutritional deficiencies, high fat intake, and genetics.

Carcinoma in situ is a precancerous condition when dysplasia of epithelial tissue occurs. The cancer is encapsulated in lining epithelial cells and has not metastasized into deeper layers. **Dysplasia** is the abnormal development of adult cells that can alter the cell's genetic make-up, size, and shape.

- **Etiology**: Mostly unknown. Possibly viral but risk factors contribute to cancer.

- **Symptoms**: For oral cancer, a lip or mouth sore that won't heal, unusual bleeding, jaw swelling, voice change, persistent sore throat, or difficulty swallowing.

- **Oral manifestations**: Early oral tissues changes include erythroplakia and leukoplakia. Later symptoms include epithelial lesions that are red, white, or mixed red and white with raised borders. Xerostomia and mucositis from radiation therapy, candidiasis, loss of taste, cervical caries, osteonecrosis, and trismus.

- **Oral care**: Good oral hygiene care with home and in-office fluoride treatments, saline/baking soda, or chlorhexidine mouth rinses. Saliva substitutes and sugarless gum are helpful for xerostomia. All necessary dental treatment should be done prior to radiation therapy if possible.

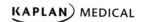

Types of Cancer

Originate	Benign	Malignant	Tissues Affected
Bone	Osteoma	Osteosarcoma	Bone
Cartilage	Chondroma	Chondrosarcoma	Cartilage
Fat	Lipoma	Liposarcoma	Mature fat cells
Fibrous tissue	Fibroma	Fibrosarcoma	Fibrous connective tissues
Nerve	Neurofibroma	Neuroblastoma	Nerve tissue
Epithelium	Papilloma	Squamous or basal cell carcinoma	Skin and mucous membranes
Smooth muscle	Leiomyoma	Leiomyosarcoma	Digestive tract, blood vessels, respiratory system
Striated muscle	Rhabdomyoma	Rhabdomyosarcoma	Skeletal muscle, tongue

CARDIOVASCULAR DISEASE

Coronary artery disease (CAD) is the build-up of plaque in arterial walls that results in narrowing of the arteries. This greatly reduces the amount of blood flow of the coronary arteries that feed oxygen to heart muscle. This can result in angina, myocardial infarction, or sudden death.

Angina pectoris occurs when the heart muscle does not get enough oxygen in relation to the amount of work that it is performing. This condition is relieved with rest, oxygen, or nitroglycerine. A **myocardial infarction** occurs when the heart muscle is not getting enough oxygen and an infarction occurs. That cuts off the oxygen supply to that part of the heart muscle (myocardium). The pain is not relieved by rest or oxygen or nitroglycerine.

Sudden death is the sudden interruption of electrical activity by an arrhythmia such as ventricular fibrillation.

CAD can also damage the heart causing **congestive heart failure**, resulting in the loss of pumping action of the heart muscle. When right-sided failure occurs, fluids from the blood leak back out into the extremities. When left-sided failure occurs, fluids from the blood leak out into the lungs.

Arrhythmias involve abnormal electrical conduction to the heart muscle. Some arrhythmias require a **pacemaker** or an **implanted defibrillator**. **Mitral valve prolapse** with regurgitation and **rheumatic heart disease** with permanent valve damage require premedication of an antibiotic before certain dental procedures.

- **Etiology**: Coronary artery disease for congestive heart failure, angina, myocardial infarction, and sudden death.

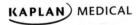

- **Symptoms**: Symptoms for angina, myocardial infarction, and sudden death may include difficulty in breathing (dyspnea), edema, diaphoresis, or chest pain that may radiate into the arms, neck, jaw and/or epigastric area. Symptoms for cardiac failure may include pitting edema, chest pain, and difficulty in breathing.

- **Oral manifestations**: Gingival hyperplasia for patients taking calcium channel blockers.

- **Oral care**: Since research now shows that periodontal disease contributes to coronary artery disease, a dental hygienist can have a direct influence on a patient with this condition. Building a rapport is crucial; and it will help motivate the patient to perform good oral hygiene.

> Calcium channel blockers such as **nifedipine (Procardia)**, verapamil (Calan, Isoptin), and diltiazem (Cardizem) cause gingival hyperplasia.

If a patient suffers from chest pain, dyspnea, or diaphoresis during a dental procedure, terminate the procedure and administer nitroglycerine. Check his vital signs and summon EMS if the pain is not relieved by the nitroglycerin.

Patients with left-sided heart failure have fluid leakage from blood into their lungs, causing them difficulty in breathing. These patients may not be able to lie back for long periods. They are often on diuretics and may need frequent bathroom breaks.

Antibiotic premedication for dental procedures is required for those with certain heart defects, heart valve replacement, mitral valve prolapse with regurgitation, and rheumatic heart disease with valve damage.

Newer **cardiac pacemakers** have shielded leads to protect the pacemaker. There have been no reports in interference with piezoelectric scalers; however, **magnetostrictive ultrasonic scalers should be avoided**. New pacemakers are built with ceramic shields to prevent interference from cellular phones.

CEREBRAL PALSY

Cerebral palsy (CP) is a condition where the brain cannot transmit nerve impulses for coordinated muscle movements. Motor skills and muscle coordination are affected. It is caused by damage (anoxia) to the brain at the fetal, prenatal, with birth or postnatal stage of early infancy.

There are different types of CP: **spasticity** involves muscles that are stiffly and permanently contracted; **athetoid** affects the extremities with uncontrolled, slow, writhing motions; **ataxia** affects balance, depth perception and has an unsteady gait; and **mixed** with a combination of all of these types.

- **Etiology**: Lack of oxygen to the brain in the fetal period, prenatal, natal, or postnatal period.

- **Symptoms**: Depends on where in the brain the damage took place. Uncoordinated movements, involuntary contractions, lack of manual dexterity, tendency to fall, drooling, difficulty swallowing, speech defects, seizures, mental retardation, bladder and bowel control, postural difficulties, and learning disabilities.

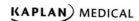

- **Oral manifestations**: Gingival hyperplasia from seizure medications (25–30% of CP patients), malocclusion, **fractured teeth from repeated falling**, periodontal disease or gingivitis, bruxism causing attrition, enamel hypoplasia, and caries due to soft diets.

- **Oral care**: The caregiver should be involved with homecare instructions. An electric toothbrush can be used. Many patients are wheelchair-bound and coordinated transfer to the dental chair is necessary. A pediwrap or papoose board may need to be used to control uncoordinated movements. A bite block should be used to prevent sudden closure.

CEREBROVASCULAR ACCIDENT

Cerbrovascular accidents (CVA) or **strokes** are a form of cardiovascular disease in the brain. A blood vessel in the brain becomes occluded from a cerebral thrombosis or embolism, blocking the flow of oxygen delivery to that part of the brain. Alternatively, a vessel may rupture and bleed into the brain. Bleeding into the brain may be caused by an aneurysm or arteriovenous malformation. That portion of the brain becomes ischemic since oxygen is not reaching brain tissue.

- **Etiology**: Caused primarily by an arterial occlusion to a portion of the brain, though occasionally by a hemorrhage into the brain.

- **Symptoms**: Sudden weakness to half the body, unsteady gait on the side affected, difficulty speaking, severe headache, dizziness, loss of balance, visual impairment, and/or drooling on affected side

- **Oral manifestations**: Hemiplegia may lead to food becoming trapped in the buccal mucosa; xerostomia from medications.

- **Oral care**: Due to impaired dexterity, oral hygiene instruction may be geared to use of an adapted handle for a manual toothbrush or electric toothbrush. Patients tend to be afraid of losing their independence so guidance with home hygiene is essential. Due to loss of dexterity on the affected side (right or left-handed), the caregiver should also receive instruction. Plan dental appointments in the morning and keep them short.

CLEFT LIP/PALATE

Cleft lip can occur at 4-7 week of the embryonic period while cleft palate occurs at 8-12 week time frame of fetal development.

Cleft lips occur from the incomplete merger of one or both maxillary processes with medial nasal process processes. Cleft palates, on the other hand, occur from the incomplete merger of the palatal shelves with the primary palate or each other. Cleft palates are also associated with Pierre Robin syndrome.

- **Etiology**: Genetics, nutritional deficiencies, medication, smoking, alcohol, infections, and rubella virus

- **Symptoms**: See table below.

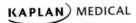

Types of Clefts

Location
Tip of uvula
Bifed uvula
Soft palate
Hard & soft palate
Hard & soft palate with one side of an alveolar ridge
Hard & soft palate with bilateral alveolar ridge with a "floating" premaxilla
Submucosa cleft with incomplete muscle merger of the soft palate. Uvula may be bifed with a groove at the midline.

- **Oral manifestations**: Open palate, speech impediments, missing or hypoplastic teeth, malocclusions, high caries rate, and/or periodontal disease.

- **Oral care**: Cleft lip surgery may take place as early as 10 weeks of age or when the baby weighs 10–12 pounds. Surgery to close the palate may take place at 9–18 months of age.

- If the cleft was not closed surgically, the patient may be wearing an **obturator** (acrylic appliance that resembles a retainer). For the majority of the prophylaxis, it can be left in place. This allows the patient to rinse more comfortably and keeps debris from flowing into the cleft. Oral hygiene instruction and adjuncts should be adapted to individual needs. Fluoride treatments at home with a rinse or brush-on fluoride are recommended, as is nutritional counseling to prevent caries.

CROHN'S DISEASE

Crohn's disease is a chronic disorder of inflammation of the digestive tract. It is related to ulcerative colitis. The immune system of the gastrointestinal tract mistakes food, bacteria, and other substances as foreign or invading substances. White blood cells enter into intestinal linings and generate chronic inflammation, which then produces ulcerations and bowel injury.

- **Etiology**: Unknown

- **Symptoms**: Loss of appetite, weight loss, persistent diarrhea, abdominal discomfort, fever, and occasional rectal bleeding

- **Oral manifestations**: Non-necrotizing granulomas in the submucosa, angular cheilitis with lip enlargement, fissured lips, and "cobblestone" buccal mucosa.

- **Oral care**: Schedule appointments during remission. Oral hygiene instruction to maintain healthy tissues.

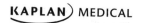

CYSTIC FIBROSIS

Cystic fibrosis is a genetic disease that affects the lungs and endocrine glands. The lungs produce abnormally thick and sticky mucous which blocks the alveoli and can produce infections. Larger areas such as the bronchioles may also become blocked, preventing oxygen from entering the lungs. These patients are prone to lung infections. Other secretions can be thick or solid and can block endocrine glands such as the pancreas from secreting digestive enzymes. This causes digestive problems such as poor absorption of fats and proteins. Most CF patients have an average life expectancy of about 33 years or longer.

- **Etiology**: Many people carry the cystic fibrosis gene without experiencing any symptoms. It is inherited from two defective CF genes—one from each parent.

- **Symptoms**: Mucous accumulation in the lungs with poor air exchange, barrel chest from an inability to exhale properly, persistent cough or wheezing, poor weight gain, excessive sweating, or nasal polyps

- **Oral manifestations**: Xerostomia from mouth-breathing and/or inhalers, enlarged salivary glands, or tetracycline staining.

- **Oral care**: More frequent recalls and nutritional counseling to avoid carbohydrates.

DIABETES

Diabetes is a metabolic disease that affects insulin production of the pancreas. Diabetes is also discussed in depth in Chapter 20, Medical Emergencies.

Patients suffering from diabetes experience polyuria, polydipsia, and polyphagia.

The **alpha** cells of the pancreas produce **glucagon**, which seek out stores of glycogen in the liver if the blood-glucose levels get to low. The **beta** cells produce **insulin** to unlock cells, allowing glucose to enter into cells. Glucose is necessary for cell life.

Type I diabetes (IDDM) mellitus occurs with the body's inability to produce insulin. **Type II** diabetes (NIDDM) mellitus occurs with the body's inability to produce enough insulin, along with the body's inability to use the insulin properly.

Hyperglycemia is too much sugar in the blood. **Hypoglycemia** is not enough sugar in the blood. The brain needs glucose to survive and cannot use ketones, which are broken down from fats in ketoacidosis.

- **Etiology**: Genetics and environmental influences, such as obesity

- **Symptoms**: Extreme hunger, thirst, and urination, weight loss, vision problems, vascular disease, and organ failure

- **Oral manifestations**: Poor wound healing, periodontal disease, xerostomia, and oral candidiasis.

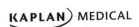

- **Oral care**: Schedule dental appointments after meals, preferably in the morning, since the stress of a dental appointment can quickly use up blood-glucose levels. Uncontrolled diabetics should not be treated until their diabetes is under control, but in an emergency, a medical consultation may result in premedication with an antibiotic. Meticulous oral hygiene will help prevent periodontal disease, which has an effect on blood glucose levels. Plaque reduction improves periodontal tissues as well as reduces carious lesions. Nutritional counseling to keep blood glucose levels at an optimum level may be necessary. Regular fluoride therapy is suggested.

DOWN SYNDROME

Down syndrome is a mental retardation disorder where the person has prominent physical features and limited intelligence potential. The retardation may be from very mild to severe.

- **Etiology**: Genetics: Normal cells have 46 chromosomes. However, the sperm and an egg each have only 23 chromosomes, with 22 of them carrying genetic information and the 23rd determining a baby's sex. During cell division, a sperm or an egg with an extra 21st chromosome joins with a cell with the proper amount of chromosomes. In Down syndrome patients, there is an extra chromosome 21, with the patient having 3 chromosome 21's, which go into every cell replicated in the body. Hence the name **trisomy 21.**

- **Symptoms**: Smallness in stature, high incidence of congenital heart defects, different ranges of mental retardation, microcephaly, slanted eyelids (epicanthic fold at eye corners), depressed nasal bridge, small mouth, poor muscle tone, stubby fingers, and small hands and feet

- **Oral manifestations**: Prone to periodontal disease and caries, prognathic mandible with Class III malocclusion, macroglossia, gingival hyperplasia from medications, open bite due to tongue-thrusting, mouth-breathing due to small nasal passage, delayed exfoliation and tooth development, fissured tongue, cracked lips, microdontia with malformed teeth, and congenitally missing teeth.

- **Oral care**: Advise the caregiver to be involved with oral hygiene, depending on the degree of retardation. If the patient is of small stature, in-office care may require a papoose board or support straps, in addition to a mouth prop or bite block.

EATING DISORDERS

Anorexia nervosa is an eating disorder whereby the patient literally starves herself to death. It occurs most often in adolescent girls who have an intense fear of gaining weight. The patient weighs 85% or less of her normal expected body weight.

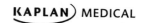

With **bulimia nervosa**, the patient binge eats but purges the food afterward. Laxatives and water pills may also be used.

- **Etiology**: Those who are perfectionists and overachievers tend to be prone to this disorder.

- **Symptoms**: Depression and withdrawal. With **anorexia nervosa**: refusal to eat full meals, excessive exercise, sensitivity to cold, absent or irregular menstruation, and excessive facial/body hair (**lanugo**). With **bulimia nervosa**: preoccupation with food, binging then purging, laxative and diuretic abuse, and compulsive exercise.

- **Oral manifestations**: Nutritional deficiencies may occur from lack of vitamins and minerals such as glossitis, angular cheilosis bleeding gingiva, and hypertrophy of the papillae. With **anorexia**, poor oral hygiene. With **bulimia**, esophageal inflammation, burning tongue, perimylolysis, or **tooth erosion to the lingual surfaces of the maxillary teeth** (anterior teeth, in particular, from the stomach acid), tooth sensitivity, xerostomia, and enlarged parotid gland.

- **Oral care**: Provide oral hygiene instruction. Tell patient to rinse thoroughly after purging to rid the oral cavity of acids, glass ionomer restorations if indicated, home fluoride rinse or dentifrice.

END-STAGE RENAL DISEASE

End-stage renal disease is the bilateral deficiency of renal function. The main filtration system in the kidney—the glomerulus—becomes damaged and cannot properly remove excretions. **Uremia** is the build-up of excretions in the blood, causing a severe and toxic situation. Patients must undergo dialysis and have an arteriovenous fistula as an access line. This fistula is created by joining an artery and a vein under the skin on an arm. Another route for access is through an arteriovenous graft, whereby an artery and vein are joined by a plastic tube. The hemodialysis machine is hooked up to this access line 3–5 hours twice or three times a week. Eventually, this patient will need a transplant.

- **Etiology**: Hypertension, diabetes, glomerulonephritis, congenital diseases, infectious diseases, neoplastic tumors, or sickle cell disease.

- **Symptoms**: Depression, uremia, hypertension, electrolyte imbalances, skin hyperpigmentaion, anemia, and susceptibility to infections.

- **Oral manifestations**: Candidiasis, metallic taste from urea in saliva, mucosal pallor, xerostomia, stomatitis, increased calculus formation, bleeding gingiva, and radiographic bone lucency from renal osteodystrophy. If the patient has a transplant, antirejection drugs can cause gingival hyperplasia.

- **Oral care**: Schedule dental appointments the **day after dialysis**. Prior to any dental procedure, consult with the physician about appropriate antibiotic premedication. During any dental procedure, monitor blood pressure. Provide oral hygiene instruction to maintain optimal health.

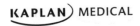

FETAL ALCOHOL SYNDROME

Alcohol-use during pregnancy can significantly affect fetal development, since alcohol can cross the placenta. The fetus can develop abnormal growth patterns and mental retardation, as the brain is very vulnerable during the last trimester. The child will be small in stature with abnormal facial features; the eyes will be abnormally narrow (short palpebral fissure) with epicanthal folds (elongated fold of the upper eyelid on the inner corner), smooth philtrum (lack of a groove from the upper lip that runs to the nares of the nose), upturned nose with a flat face, and micrognathia.

- **Etiology**: Alcohol consumption during pregnancy

- **Symptoms**: Mental, behavioral, and/or learning disabilities (hyperactivity), seizures, sociopathic behavior, facial deformities (craniofacial dysmorphia), growth deficits, poor muscle coordination, and vision and hearing problems. Heart, liver, and kidney defects are common as well.

- **Oral manifestations**: Tooth malformations, malocclusion, and gingivitis

- **Oral care**: Provide oral hygiene instruction to manage gingivitis.

GERIATRICS

Today's aging population has a much longer life expectancy than ever before. "Older" patients, these days, can be over age 55, while "elderly" patients are those age 75 and up. The aging process can diminish the capability of different organ functions. Elderly patients tend to have a variety of illnesses and may be on numerous medications.

Some patients are afraid of losing their independence if they become ill. Depression and loneliness especially from the loss of a spouse can have a profound effect on their well being. Some have economic limitations that limit their personal care.

They can suffer more commonly from osteoporosis, arthritis, Alzheimer's disease, dementia, cardiovascular disease, hypertension, diabetes, pulmonary disorders, gastrointestinal diseases, and renal failure among other illnesses as well.

- **Etiology**: Aging process

- **Symptoms**: Symptoms such as loss of hearing and visual problems will vary with the type of illness

- **Oral manifestations**: Abrasion, attrition, root caries, and tooth sensitivity. Many medications can cause xerostomia. Some people suffer from oral candidiasis from weakened immune systems and lack of proper nutrition.

- **Oral care**: Removing barriers to care is essential for the patient to remain completely mobile. Careful updating of the medical history can reveal something the patient forgot to disclose, and knowing his full list of medications can help you gauge the type of treatment he should receive—if at all (as with a surgical procedure if the patient is on blood thinners, for instance).

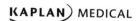

Plaque control is essential for the control of root caries and periodontal disease. Great care should be taken with oral hygiene instruction to allow the patient a feeling =of independence. Some patients have economic limitations while others lack interest in preparing meals.

Recession, along with root exposures, may expedite carious lesions, so home fluoride treatments are recommended. Arthritis may cause patients to lose manual dexterity, needed for good oral hygiene. Work with the patient to find the appropriate adjunct. Also, nutritional counseling can reveal any dietary deficiencies that generate oral conditions, such as angular cheilitis or glossitis.

HYPERTENSION

Hypertension is an abnormally high blood pressure that is commonly the result of hypertensive cardiovascular disease. Contributing factors are arteriosclerosis, atherosclerosis, coronary heart disease, congestive heart failure, and diabetes. See more on hypertension in Chapter 14, Dental Hygiene Process of Care.

Primary hypertension occurs in 90% of hypertensive cases where the etiology is unknown. Risk factors include genetics, obesity, race, climate, age, gender, sodium intake, smoking, and the use of oral contraceptives.

Secondary hypertension accounts for 10% of hypertensive cases where the patient may have an underlying, though correctable, cause: obstructive sleep apnea, renal parenchymal disease, Cushing's syndrome, or endocrine disorders.

According to the American Heart Association, normal blood pressure should be less than 120/80 mm/Hg for an adult. A range of 120–139/80–89 mm/Hg is considered prehypertension, while 140/90 mm/Hg or higher is considered hypertension.

AHA Blood Pressure Classifications for Adults Over Age 18*

Category	Systolic in mm/Hg	Diastolic in mm/Hg
Normal	< 120	< 80
Prehypertensive	120–139	80–89
Hypertension		
Stage 1	140–159	90–99
Stage 2	160–179	100–109
Stage 3	180–209	110–119
Stage 4	> 210	> 120

* If the patient's blood pressure falls into two categories, the higher category should be selected. 160/92, for instance, is Stage 2, while 174/118 is Stage 3.

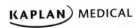

- **Etiology**: 90% of unknown etiology, 10% from an underlying cause

- **Symptoms**: Headaches, dizziness, dyspnea, tingling in extremities

- **Oral manifestations**: Xerostomia and/or gingival hyperplasia from medications, ulcerations, stomatitis.

- **Oral care**: Dental care causes great anxiety and stress for some patients. This stress can, in turn, cause their blood pressure to increase, making them more susceptible to angina, myocardial infarction, or sudden death. If the pressure is **<140/<90,** normal dental **treatment can be received**, but the pressure should be **checked annually**. If the pressure is **140-160/90-100**, the pressure should be rechecked for the **next 3 subsequent visits**. If the pressure is **160-180/100-110**, the pressure should be **rechecked in 5 minutes**, and if the individual has not improved, refer him to a physician. If the pressure is **greater than 180/110, dental care should be delayed and the individual should see a physician.**

IMMUNODEFICIENCY DISEASE (AIDS/HIV)

Immunodeficiency disease occurs when the immune system becomes compromised and cannot identify—or destroy—invading pathogens. Viruses are moochers who need a host cell in order to replicate. As viruses penetrate a cell, they inject their RNA into that cell. These viruses take over during the replication stage of that cell producing hundreds of new virus particles instead. Then the new viruses look for more cells in which to do the same.

HIV or human immunodeficiency virus occurs when the HIV virus invades its favorite T lymphocyte cells, called CD4 helper cells. These cells are important in defending our body from invading pathogens. If the CD4 count becomes too low, the body cannot protect itself against infection. HIV affects the CD4 to CD8 ratio to defend the body. The CD8 suppressor or killer cells go up proportionately with HIV infections as the CD4 goes down. The lower the ratio, the more damage that has been done.

- **Etiology**: HIV virus

- **Symptoms**: Early onset has flu-like symptoms of fever, chills, and rashes. Later lymphadenopathy, fever, lethargy, headache, diarrhea, vaginal yeast infections, night sweats, and weight loss.

- **Oral manifestations**: Oral **candidiasis, Kaposi's sarcoma,** herpes, **hairy leukoplakia, linear gingival erythema, angular cheilitis,** and periodontal disease.

- **Oral care**: Good oral hygiene instructions, scaling and root debridement. Antifungal treatments when indicated.

Kaposi's Sarcoma

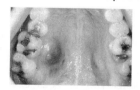 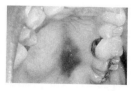

Contributed by Dr. Michael Finkelstein, DDS College of Dentistry, University of Iowa

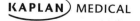

LUPUS ERYTHEMATOSUS

Lupus erythematosus is an autoimmune disease that causes inflammation and damage to the joints, skin, kidneys, heart, lungs, blood vessels, and brain. Brief flare-ups tend to follow long periods of remission. Though there is no cure for lupus, most patients can lead an active life with medication.

Systemic lupus erythematosus can present mild or serious symptoms on many parts of the body. **Discoid lupus erythematosus** is a chronic skin disorder that usually appears on the face or scalp as a thick, scaly, red, raised rash. The rash can last for days or years. **Subacute cutaneous lupus erythematosus,** caused by sun exposure, presents as skin lesions.

The nose can have butterfly shaped lesions of white patches with red and white lines that radiate.

- **Etiology**: A combination of genetic, environmental, and hormonal factors but can also be drug-induced.

- **Symptoms**: Extreme weariness, painful arthritis, unexplained fever, skin rash, unusual hair loss, and kidney problems

- **Oral manifestations:**Drug-induced stomatitis

- **Oral care**: Provide oral hygiene instruction on maintaining healthy tissues

MENTAL DISORDERS

According to the American Psychiatric Association, there are over 200 types of mental disorders. Patients may be extremely apprehensive or anxious about their dental appointments, but they could also suffer from one of the following disorders.

Anxiety disorder occurs when the patient worries excessively about everything.

Bipolar disorder or manic depression is a mood disorder characterized by varying cycles of extreme highs to extreme lows (depression).

Brief psychotic disorder is characterized by delusions, hallucinations, impaired speech, and/or catatonic behavior for at least 24 hours but less than 1 month.

Depression is a deep feeling of sadness that negatively affects how one feels, thinks, and acts.

A patient who constantly brushes his teeth all day is obsessive compulsive.

Obsessive-compulsive disorder is characterized by images, ideas or thoughts that repeat themselves.

Panic attacks are an anxiety disorder that occurs for no apparent reason. The patient has a fear of losing control.

Post-traumatic stress disorder follows a traumatic event. After the initial stressful event there may be intense emotions of horror, fear, or helplessness.

Psychotic disorders are characterized by delusions and hallucinations.

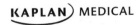

Schizophrenia is a major psychiatric disorder that involves loss of contact with reality, false beliefs, abnormal thinking, and reduced motivation.

- **Etiology**: Chemical imbalance, mental disturbance, stress, and/or genetics

- **Symptoms**: Symptoms vary with each illness.

- **Oral manifestations**: Patients may neglect their oral hygiene, resulting in periodontal disease and/or carious lesions. Some medications can result in xerostomia and/or gingival hyperplasia.

- **Oral care**: Review medical history and medications, have a nice atmosphere and music, explain procedures to be performed, review oral hygiene care, for xerostomia recommend daily home fluoride and saliva substitute.

MULTIPLE SCLEROSIS

Multiple sclerosis (MS) is an autoimmune disease that affects the central nervous system. Most patients experience bouts of symptoms followed by periods of remission. With MS, the protective myelin sheath that surrounds and protects nerves is damaged. It is believed that T cells circulating in the central nervous system injure the protective myelin sheath, secreting toxins that damage nerve fibers. Sclerotic tissue replaces the destroyed sheath, damaging the nerve even further.

"Clusters" or high incidences of MS have been found to occur in certain areas, suggesting environmental factors as a cause. MS is not inherited, though families with more than one MS member might share a gene(s) and a predisposition toward an environmental trigger. Anti-amalgamists claim a link between amalgam and MS, which has not been supported by any medical or dental research.

There are different types of MS: In **Relapsing MS**, patients experience symptoms and then remission, followed by a resurfacing or even worsening of the original symptoms, followed by remission. **Secondary MS** occurs in patients who have had relapsing MS, who then have gradual worsening symptoms between relapses, before merging into a general progression of the disease. **Primary MS** occurs with a gradual progression of the disease with no periods of remission.

- **Etiology**: Unknown, though it is suspected that genetics and environmental conditions set off an autoimmune response.

- **Symptoms**: Bladder and bowel dysfunction; unsteady gait and/or balance; dizziness/vertigo; difficulty with vision; fatigue, slurred speech, muscle spasms, tingling or a feeling of pins and needles; short-term memory loss; and/or depression.

- **Oral manifestations**: Swallowing problems, trigeminal neuralgia, ulcerations, xerostomia and gingival hyperplasia from medications.

- **Oral care**: Keep office visits brief and consider wheelchair transfer; provide oral hygiene adjuncts depending on the patient's dexterity.

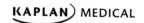

MUSCULAR DYSTROPHY

Muscular dystrophy (MD) is a genetic muscle disorder the causes the degeneration of skeletal muscles. It is a progressive and irreversible condition. In late stages, muscle fibers are replaced by fat and connective tissue. There are different types of MD; among the more common are Duchenne (pseudohypertrophic); facioscapulohumeral; myotonic; and limb-girdle.

Duchenne MD affects males (ages 3–5) who have a mutation of a gene that regulates dystrophin—a muscle-fiber protein that safeguards muscle-fiber integrity. The majority of those affected are unable to walk by the age of 12.

Facioscapulohumeral MD affects adolescents, characterized as a progressive weakness in facial, arm, and leg muscles.

Myotonic MD affects individuals of any age, and is characterized by myotonia or prolonged muscle spasm. It affects the fingers, facial muscles; and gait.

Limb-girdle MD affects the voluntary muscles of the hips, and the pelvic and shoulder girdles (limb girdles).

- **Etiology**: Genetics, with each type of MD involving different genetics. A mother may pass on an X-linked recessive gene. An autosomal recessive gene may be passed on by both parents. An autosomal dominant trait with only one faulty gene may have been passed along from parents.

- **Symptoms**: Weakness in the limbs, head, neck, and/or face; unsteady gait; lack of coordination; dizziness; frequent falling.

- **Oral manifestations**: Breathing through the mouth; thick lips with facioscapulo-humeral MD, periodontal disease, and possible resulting carious lesions

- **Oral care**: Provide oral hygiene instruction as per the patient's ability, providing the caregiver with instruction. For in-office visits, assist the patient with walking and with wheelchair transfer.

MYASTHENIA GRAVIS

Myasthenia gravis is an autoimmune disease affecting the neuromuscular system that causes weakness in the voluntary muscles of the body. Certain areas that may be affected include eyes, facial expression, chewing, or swallowing. Respiratory muscles can become affected causing serious breathing problems

The neuromuscular junction is where a nerve fiber ends just short of the muscle fiber to send acetylcholine to the muscle fiber for contraction. With myasthenia gravis, there are about 80% fewer receptor sites for acetylcholine to cross over to, causing the message to not get out to muscle fibers.

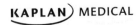

- **Etiology**: Autoimmune disease that produces antibodies against receptor sites. Patients with MG have abnormal antibodies in their blood. Stress or systemic illnesses can worsen this condition.

- **Symptoms**: Drooping eyelids, slurred speech with nasal tones, unsteady gait, difficulty in breathing, unable to sit up or hold head erect.

- **Oral manifestations**: Drooling, unable to speak well, unable to breath, difficulty with swallowing, food retention, difficulty chewing food.

- **Oral care**: Try to make short duration office appointments as stress free as possible. Maintain good oral hygiene with homecare instructions to prevent carious lesions and periodontal disease that require more frequent and possibly stressful visits. Keep airway open in an emergency situation with suction, and oxygen available.

PARKINSON'S DISEASE

Parkinson's disease is a chronic neurological disorder that affects the substantia nigra neurons of the brain. These dopamine-producing neurons die or else become impaired. Dopamine is a neurotransmitter that sends signals to the brain in places where muscle control and coordination are moderated. With the loss of dopamine, the striatum nerve cells fire out of control and cause loss of controlled movements.

> Parkinson's patients can have a back-and-forth rhythmic tremor of the thumb and forefinger, called "pilling."

- **Etiology**: Unknown but several theories suggest free radicals (oxidates), environmental toxins, genetics, or age

- **Symptoms**: Tremors of the hands, arms, legs, face and jaw with loss of coordination and imbalance, rigidity, and loss of spontaneous movement (bradykinesia).

- **Oral manifestations**: Speech changes, difficulty in swallowing, choking or drooling. Impaired oral hygiene care may result in periodontal disease and/or carious lesions. Xerostomia due to medications.

- **Oral care**: Loss of coordination may impair oral hygiene home care. Work with adjuncts and power-assisted toothbrushes, depending on the patient's ability.

RADIATION THERAPY

Radiation therapy, along with surgery and chemotherapy, is often used for cancer of the head and neck. Radiation helps to shrink the tumor prior to surgery. Therapy may be from an external beam, which can be less-penetrating orthovoltage for superficial lesions. Another external source is the linear accelerator which produces high-energy external radiation beams that penetrate the tissues and deliver the radiation dose deep in the area of the body where the cancer resides.

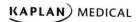

An internal delivery system of radiation with the use of implants is called brachytherapy, which delivers high radiation doses to specific cancer cells without damaging adjacent normal tissues.

- **Etiology**: Radiation treatment
- **Symptoms**: Dry skin, weight loss, dehydration, alopecia.
- **Oral manifestations**: Sore throat, loss of taste sensation, xerostomia, carious lesions, mucositis, trismus, and rarely, osteoradionecrosis.
- **Oral care**: Drink water, artificial saliva, fluoride treatments, carious lesion therapy, treat any fungal infections

RESPIRATORY PROBLEMS

Asthma

Asthma, also called reactive airway disease (RAD), is a chronic inflammatory respiratory disease. When the bronchi constrict, mucous plugs form, which then block-off the alveoli and trap air in the alveoli.

- **Etiology**: Precipitated by environmental factors, stress, foods, exercise, and drugs
- **Symptoms**: Difficulty in breathing, tight chest, wheezing, altered level of consciousness, cyanosis
- **Oral manifestations**: Oral candidiasis from inhaler use, mouth-breathing, carious lesions, xerostomia.
- **Oral care**: Remind patient to have inhaler on-hand for dental visits, schedule appointments in the late morning or late afternoon, and maintain a non-stress environment. With oral hygiene instruction, advise patient to rinse with water as soon as possible after inhalant usage.

Chronic Bronchitis

Chronic bronchitis is an inflammation of the bronchial tree where excessive mucous secretions are produced. Coughing and sputum production continues for months, with each successive episode lasting longer than the last, and with more frequent reappearance. The cough with sputum has occurred for 3 months per year for at least two consecutive years.

- **Etiology**: Smoking; air pollution and occupational exposure to inhaled substance. Rarely, genetics.
- **Symptoms**: Frequent episodes of mucus-producing cough; shortness of breath, and wheezing

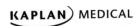

- **Oral manifestations**: None.
- **Oral care**: Review history along with medications; adapt appointment length to patient's ability; position chair for patient comfort.

Emphysema

Emphysema is the loss of elasticity in the alveoli of the lungs, making the alveoli more flaccid (like a deflated balloon with less surface area than an inflated balloon) to exchange carbon dioxide and oxygen.

- **Etiology**: Smoking
- **Symptoms**: Fatigue, shortness of breath (dyspnea), chronic mild cough, weight loss
- **Oral manifestations**: Periodontal disease and carious lesions.
- **Oral care**: Review history along with medications; adapt appointment-length to patient's ability; position chair for patient comfort.

SCLERODERMA

Scleroderma literally means "hardening of the skin and connective tissues." More common in women than in men, scleroderma causes the skin to lose its elasticity first and then to turn shiny as it stretches over bone and hardens. It can involve just the skin, which is not life threatening, but also can become systemic, in which case, organ failure can ensue.

- **Etiology**: Unknown
- **Symptoms**: Joint stiffness, pain or color change in fingers, toes, cheeks, nose and ears, poor food absorption in the digestive tract
- **Oral manifestations**: Microstomia, difficulty in brushing causing periodontal disease and carious lesions, speech impairment, mumbling, slurring, esophageal dysfunction, thin pale mucosa, radiographically widened periodontal ligaments.
- **Oral care**: Microstomia limits the patient's mouth opening for good home care and dental procedures. Denture or partials become more problematic to wear with disease progression. Focus on good home care.

SEIZURE

There are over 30 types of seizures, with two major divisions: partial and generalized seizures. Each division has subdivisions.

Partial seizures affect a single part of the brain and are categorized by where in the brain they originate. A **focal motor seizure** is a simple partial seizure that produces a spasm or clonus of a muscle or muscle group.

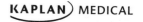

During a **simple partial seizure**, the patient **remains conscious**, but she may have an altered level of consciousness. Some people are aware of what is going on around them but cannot speak. There may be mood swings or some uncontrolled movement (blinking, twitching, rapid eye movement); these movements are called **automatisms**.

Complex partial seizures affect a larger portion of the brain than simple partial seizures. Here, there is a **partial or total loss of consciousness**. The patient may be in a dream-like state or may have amnesia regarding the episode. These seizures often occur in the temporal lobe and can also produce automatisms. The duration of the seizures may be just a few seconds.

Generalized seizures affect both cerebral hemispheres and are a result of abnormal neural activity. The subdivisions include absence (petite mal), generalized tonic clonic (grand mal), atonic, and myoclonic.

Absence seizures—once called **petite mal seizures**—are the result of a sudden pause of conscious thought or activity, with the patient seeming to stare into space. These seizures, which can last a few seconds to minutes, can be accompanied by clonic movements or automatisms.

General tonic clonic seizures—once called **grand mal seizures**—are characterized by a loss of consciousness accompanied by tonic convulsions (muscle stiffness), followed by clonic convulsions (bilateral jerking movements). A postictal phase usually follows these seizures, where the patient has a headache, is temporarily confused, or is extremely fatigued.

Atonic seizures cause a sudden loss of muscle tone, causing the person to "drop" from loss of muscle strength. Injury may occur as a result of this sudden fall.

With **myoclonic seizures**, the patient experiences sudden, brief jerks of a muscle or muscle group.

- **Etiology**: Focal or generalized disturbance of cortical function; drug or alcohol withdrawal; developmental defects; birth injuries; tumors; genetics; trauma; brain infection; or a metabolic disease. Febrile seizures occur from a high fever.

- **Symptoms**: An "aura" feeling, such as a smell or taste (depending on where in the brain the seizure occurs) prior to seizure, loss of consciousness or staring into space, tonic clonic movement, eye twitching, incontinence, or altered level of consciousness.

- **Oral manifestations**: Gingival hyperplasia from seizure medications, trauma to tissues during seizure activity, or erythema multiforme from taking carbamazepine, phenytoin, or ethosuximide.

- **Oral care**: Provide oral hygiene instruction to manage gingival hyperplasia.

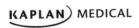

SPINA BIFIDA

Spina bifida is a neural tube defect caused by the failure of the spine to develop and close properly during the first month of pregnancy, causing incomplete development of the brain and spinal cord. Some infants are born with the spinal cord and meninges protruding through the backbone (**myelomeningocele**); they can be surgically repaired. Permanent nerve damage, however, causes different degrees of permanent paralysis. **Meningocele** is the protrusion of the meninges and cerebrospinal fluid only in a sac from an open bony defect of the spinal column. **Spinal bifida occulta** is a hidden spinal bifida that is a much smaller defect and does not involve the spinal chord itself.

Anencephaly is the failed closure of the neural tube at the brain level, causing a fatal congenital absence of most of the brain. Infant mortality rate is high with anencephaly.

- **Etiology**: Genetics, folic acid deficiency, anti-seizure medication, maternal illnesses
- **Symptoms**: Malformation of the brain and skull, hydrocephalus, learning disabilities, bowel and bladder problems, latex allergy
- **Oral manifestations**: None
- **Oral care**: **Latex allergy** occurs frequently from repeated exposure to latex in urinary catheterization and surgical procedures. Premedication with an antibiotic is necessary for ventriculoatrial shunt for dental procedures, though *not* necessary for ventriculoperitoneal shunts. Advise wheelchair transfer or assistance for patients on crutches.

THYROID PROBLEMS

The thyroid gland is a part of the endocrine system. Its function is to produce the thyroid hormones, thyroxine (T4) and triiodothyronine (T3), using iodine as a raw material. These hormones are released into the bloodstream and are transported to cells, where they control metabolism.

All cells of the body rely on thyroid hormones to regulate metabolism. The thyroid gland is stimulated by thyroid stimulating hormone (TSH) from the pituitary gland to produce thyroxine (T4) and triiodothyronine (T3).

Hypothyroidism

In hypothyroidism, the thyroid produces an insufficient amount of hormone. As a result, the pituitary gland produces more TSH in order to stimulate the thyroid. The barrage of TSH enlarges the thyroid gland, which then forms a goiter.

A child with hypothyroidism will develop **cretinism**, which can result in serious retardation of physical and mental development if left untreated.

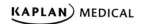

Myxedma is the result of hypothyroidism in adults. It is characterized by lethargy and slow body functions.

- **Etiology**: Autoimmune thyroiditis or medical treatments such as radioactive iodine to remove goiters or surgery to remove thyroid cancer. **Cretinism** is usually the result of a congenital defect but can develop later from a lack of iodine in the diet or if the thyroid is diseased. **Myxedema** can be the result of thyroid atrophy of unknown origin, surgical removal, or radiation treatments.

- **Symptoms**: Fatigue, cold intolerance, weight gain, dry rough skin, muscle cramps, constipation, irritable, depression. **With cretinism**: retardation, stunted growth, small stature of a dwarf, thick skin, flattened nose, protruded abdomen, bradycardia, and slow movement and speech. **With myxedma**: dry skin, slow speech and mental awareness, obesity, cold intolerance, fatigue, lethargy, and bradycardia

- **Oral manifestations**: Enlarged tongue (macroglossia), delayed tooth eruption, small jaw development, malocclusion.

- **Oral care**: Provide dental treatment after medical consultation and disease is under control,, and oral hygiene instruction for caregiver if patient is severely retarded.

Hyperthyroidism

In hyperthyroidism, the thyroid produces too much hormone, which in turn causes an increase in the body's metabolism. Patients often feel hot and slowly lose weight though their food consumption increases. Symptoms are so gradual that patients often don't recognize the symptoms until they become more severe.

Graves' disease is as an autoimmune disease caused by antibodies that attach to specific sites of thyroid gland. It causes the thyroid to produce too much hormone. The result is inflammation around the eyes, causing swelling (exophthalmos) and thick skin over the lower legs.

A thyroid storm (thyrotoxic crisis) may occur if hyperthyroidism is left untreated and is exacerbated by infection, trauma, or stress. In this state, patients tend to be sensitive to epinephrine and amines.

- **Etiology**: Graves disease, nodules within the thyroid gland, or thyroiditis.

- **Symptoms**: **Exophthalmos**, heat intolerance, fatigue, insomnia, dyspnea, chest pain and tachycardia, weight loss, trembling hands and muscle weakness

- **Oral manifestations**: Early loss of deciduous teeth and early tooth eruption of permanent teeth, large mandibles, osteoporosis of alveolar bone causing more progressive periodontal disease,

- **Oral care**: Avoid dental treatment until hyperthyroidism is under control.

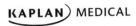

TOURETTE SYNDROME

Tourette syndrome is an inherited, neurological disorder characterized by involuntary body movements (tics) and uncontrollable vocal tics. These involuntary outbursts are not intentional, and can include blinking, arm-thrusting, kicking, shoulder shrugging, twirling, sniffing, grunting, or jumping.

- **Etiology**: Genetics. Research has found a possible problem with the neurotransmitter dopamine.

- **Symptoms**: Involuntary, rapid, sudden movements or vocalizations

- **Oral manifestations**: None

- **Oral care**: Provide oral home-care instruction. In the office, make the patient feel comfortable.

VISUAL IMPAIRMENT

Visual impairment can have many etiologies. For patients who lose their sight, retaining their independence is very important. "Legally blind" is defined as vision acuity of not more than 20/200 with correction.

Glaucoma is caused by damage to the optic nerve. It was once thought to occur from high intraocular pressure, but it is now believed other factors contribute to glaucoma. **Primary open angle glaucoma** occurs when the eye's drainage canals become clogged over time, causing intraocular pressure to rise because the correct amount of fluid can't drain out of the eye. **Angle closure glaucoma** also known as acute glaucoma or narrow angle glaucoma is much more rare. ACG is particularly distinctive from open angle glaucoma because the eye pressure usually goes up rapidly. **Secondary glaucoma** is the end product of an eye injury, drugs, inflammation, tumor, advanced cataracts or diabetes. **Normal tension glaucoma** occurs from damage by intraocular pressure although it is not very high.

Diabetic retinopathy occurs when small blood vessels that nourish the retina weaken and break down, or become blocked.

A **cataract** is an opacity within the lens of the eye that blocks the normal passage of light needed for vision.

Macular degeneration is a degenerative eye disease that causes atrophy or deterioration of the macula portion of the retina. The macula is responsible for central vision acuity for tasks such as reading, driving, or watching television. Side or peripheral vision is not affected so total blindness does not occur.

Strabismus, a double vision that occurs in infants and young children, is the inability of one eye to maintain binocular vision with the other eye. The eyes are misaligned.

Many glaucoma medications such as Timoptic or Occupress have hidden beta blockers that are absorbed into the bloodstream.

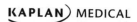

- **Symptoms**: Blindness; cloudy or fuzzy images

- **Oral manifestations**: None

- **Oral care**: Provide home care instruction since patient cannot monitor his tissues for gingivitis or periodontal disease. For in-office appointments, have the chair lowered to the appropriate height prior to the patient's entrance into the operatory. Blind people are used to being led into a certain side by one side, so allow them to take your arm. Some patients have guide dogs that can sit off to the side during the appointment.

WHEELCHAIR TRANSFER/SPINAL CORD INJURY

Spinal cord injuries and paralysis can result from many things, including trauma, infection by microorganisms, neoplasms, spine degeneration, and congenital defects. The location of the injury determines the extent of paralysis. Paralysis occurs in the areas of the cervical and thoracic vertebrae.

- **Symptoms**: Limited movement depending on area of injury the cord

- **Oral manifestations**: With limited arm usage possible, carious lesions and periodontal disease

- **Oral care**: If the patient has limited arm activity, provide oral hygiene instruction with adaptations as needed. Wheelchair transfer also depends on the extent of the injury.

Injury Site	Movement	Functional Goals
C-2, C-3	Limited head and neck movement.	Depends on ventilator, may be able to operate electrical wheelchair with a mouth or chin stick.
C-4	Arm & leg paralysis with initial respiratory problems	Weans from ventilator, specialized electric wheelchair.
C-5	Head and neck control, can shrug shoulder and has shoulder control. Can bend his/her elbows and turn palm.	Perform daily tasks of eating, bathing, grooming, etc. Ability to push a manual wheelchair for short distances on smooth surfaces. Power wheelchair with hand controls for daily activities.
C-6	Head, neck, shoulders, arms and wrists. Can shrug shoulders, bend elbows, turn palms up and down and extend wrists.	Much more independence of daily tasks of feeding, bathing, grooming, etc. Independently do transfers but often require a sliding board. Can use a manual wheelchair for daily activities.
C-7	Same as C-6 with added ability to straighten his/her elbows.	May need a few adaptive aids for independent living with manual wheelchair.
C-8	Finger and hand movement more precise.	Independent living without adaptive devices and manual wheelchair.
T-1–T-10	Normal motor function of head, neck, shoulders, arms, hands and fingers with increased use of rib, abdominal, and trunk control.	Total independence with limited walk with braces to prevent injuries and stress on muscles.

Stand & Pivot Transfer

- Patient can support own weight
- Wheelchair same direction/height as dental chair
- Patient places arms around assistant's neck
- Assistant reaches around patient, grasps safety-waist belt
- Patient lifted to standing position
- Patient pivots slowly into dental chair

Paraplegia refers to a spinal injury that causes paralysis in the lower portion of the body. **Quadraplegia** causes paralysis to all four limbs and the torso.

Immobile Patient 1 Assistant

- Patient cannot support his own weight
- Patient wears transfer safety belt
- Wheelchair same direction/height as dental chair
- Patient crosses arms, assistant reaches underneath them and grasps transfer belt
- Assistant lifts patient to standing position
- Patient pivoted toward dental chair to allow lowering into chair

Immobile Patient 2 Assistant

- Patient cannot support her own weight
- 2 assistants available
- Wheelchair same direction/height as dental chair
- Patient crosses arms while assistant #1 reaches underneath them and grasps the patient below the elbow
- Assistant #2 in front of patient and lifts legs into chair
- Patient pivoted toward dental chair to allow lowering into chair

Sliding Board Transfer

- Wheelchair same direction/height as dental chair
- Side arm of wheelchair removed
- Sliding board placed under patient's hips in wheel chair with other end of board on dental chair
- Patient slid across board connecting chairs
- Patient pivoted into seat

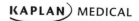

REVIEW QUESTIONS

1. A patient with severe hand arthritis and deformation of knuckles has poor oral hygiene. What would you suggest to help her with oral hygiene?

    A. Flossing instruction

    B. Electric toothbrush

    C. Interproximal toothbrush

    D. Use of chlorhexadine

    E. Fluoride rinse

2. Medical conditions requiring special diets include all of the following except one. Which one is this EXCEPTION?

    A. Diabetes

    B. Congestive heart failure

    C. Bradycardia

    D. Alcoholism

    E. Bulimia

3. Oral manifestations of sickle cell anemia include all the following except one. Which one is this EXCEPTION?

    A. Pallor of tissues

    B. Mucosal redness

    C. Hypoplastic enamel

    D. Delayed tooth eruption

4. Low blood pressure, extreme weakness, skin pigmentation, susceptibility to infections, and destruction of adrenocortical tissue are symptoms of

    A. DeQuervain's disease

    B. Crohn's disease

    C. Cushing's disease

    D. Addison's disease

    E. Peutz-Jegher syndrome

5. The immunological indication that signifies a patient's has AIDS is

    A. Suppression of humoral immunity

    B. Suppression of cellular immunity

    C. Loss of neutrophil production

    D. Loss of monocytes

6. All the following are characteristic traits of Sjogren's syndrome except one. Which one is this EXCEPTION?

    A. Coexists with Paget's disease

    B. Dry eyes and mouth

    C. Joint pain

    D. Fatigue and lethargy

    E. Body attacks its moisture-laden glands

7. The AIDS virus attaches to which of the following cells?

    A. B lymphocytes

    B. Suppressor T lymphocytes

    C. Helper T lymphocytes

    D. Neutrophils

    E. Platelets

8. Radiation therapy such as brachytherapy or linear accelerator therapy can have serious side effects, the MOST serious of which is

    A. Xerostomia

    B. Carious lesions

    C. Trismus

    D. Dysgeusia

    E. Osteoradionecrosis

9. A characteristic trait of von Recklinghausen's disease is

   A. Café-au-lait macules

   B. Dwarfism

   C. Buffalo hump and moon face

   D. Hemorrhage

10. Polycythemia is a stem-cell disorder that over-produces red blood cells. All of the following are symptoms of polycythemia except one. Which one is this EXCEPTION?

    A. Bleeding gingiva

    B. Epistaxis

    C. Active blood flow

    D. Thromboses

    E. GI bleeds

11. Your patient constantly wrings his hands in your operatory. He also reports that he brushes his teeth at least 10 times a day and flosses at least 4 times a day. This patient suffers from

    A. Obsessive-compulsive disorder

    B. Panic attacks

    C. Psychotic disorder

    D. Anxiety disorder

12. Which of the following disorders is characterized by periods of active symptoms, then remission when toxins that damage nerve fibers and replace the myelin sheath with sclerotic tissue?

    A. Muscular dystrophy

    B. Multiple sclerosis

    C. Myasthenia gravis

    D. Parkinson's disease

13. Which of the following special needs patients do not need to be premedicated with an antibiotic prior to dental treatment?

    A. Uncontrolled diabetes

    B. Spinal bifida

    C. End-stage renal failure

    D. Inflammatory rheumatoid arthritis

    E. Mitral valve prolapse with no regurgitation

14. A patient with pernicious anemia will suffer from which of the following symptoms?

    A. Glossitis

    B. Cheilosis

    C. Severe gingivitis

    D. Burning mucosa

15. Asperger syndrome occurs in individuals who seem of normal intelligence and communicate well with others, but suffer from

    A. ADHD

    B. Alzheimer disease

    C. Autism

    D. Bipolar disorder

    E. Cerebral palsy

16. A patient with mild Alzheimer's disease presents with high plaque levels and calculus. He lives in a nursing home, but is visited often by his family. What is the most important aspect of good home care for this patient?

    A. Chlorhexidine rinses

    B. Help with flossing instruction

    C. Use of an electric toothbrush

    D. Fluoride rinses

    E. Gearing the home-care instruction to the family members

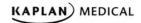

17. What is the appropriate order in which to transfer a patient from a wheelchair into the dental chair?

    A. Place transfer board under patient and onto dental chair, align wheelchair and dental chair to same height, remove arm from wheelchair, slide patient into dental chair, pivot patient into seat.

    B. Remove arm from wheelchair, place transfer board under patient and onto dental chair, align wheelchair and dental chair to same height, slide patient into dental chair, pivot patient into seat.

    C. Align wheel chair and dental chair to same height, remove arm from wheelchair, place transfer board under patient and onto dental chair, slide patient into dental chair, pivot patient into seat.

    D. Align wheelchair and dental chair to same height, remove arm from wheelchair, place transfer board under patient and onto dental chair, pivot patient, slide patient into dental chair.

18. Patients with visual impairments are often on topical medications, that contain a pharmaceutical that can be absorbed into the bloodstream. That pharmaceutical is

    A. Calcium channel blockers
    B. Beta blockers
    C. Depolarizing agents
    D. Adrenergic blockers
    E. Both adrenergic and beta blocking agents

19. If an individual has tight lips and skin, and cannot open wide enough, he likely has

    A. Bell's palsy
    B. Scleroderma
    C. Trigeminal neuralgia
    D. Cystic fibrosis

20. The congressional act that protects patients with disabilities and that allows them public access is

    A. Standard Rules on Equalization of Opportunities for Persons with Disabilities
    B. Special Rapporteur on Human Rights and Disability
    C. Americans with Disabilities Act
    D. Disabled People's Protection Policy

21. Which of the following indicates a protein in blood that mediates platelet cohesiveness when endothelium is injured?

    A. Stuart factor
    B. Thalassemia
    C. Von Willebrand factor
    D. Prothrombin deficiency
    E. Agranulocytosis

22. Which of the following disorders is characterized by blinking, arm thrusting, kicking, shoulder-shrugging, twirling, sniffing, grunting, and/or jumping?

    A. Anxiety disorder
    B. Brief psychotic disorder
    C. Post-traumatic stress disorder
    D. Tourette syndrome

23. Which of the following disorders features a "butterfly" on the bridge of the nose that can be raised, bright red, and edematous, though with time, the center becomes depressed as the color fades?

    A. Epidermis bullosa
    B. Pemphigoid
    C. Lupus erythematosus
    D. Pemphigus
    E. Behçets syndrome

24. All of the following are symptoms of myasthenia gravis except one. Which one is this EXCEPTION?

    A. Slurred speech with nasal tones
    B. Difficulty in breathing
    C. Difficulty chewing food
    D. Drooling
    E. Steady gait

25. For the patient in Question #24, your plan of treatment would include all the following except one. Which one is this EXCEPTION?

    A. Make office appointments as stress-free as possible.
    B. Keep airway open in an emergency situation with suction.
    C. Maintain patient airway.
    D. Schedule long appointments to decrease the number of visits.

ANSWER EXPLANATIONS

1. B

A patient with severe arthritis of the hands would benefit from the use of an electric toothbrush.

A. Flossing instruction would not help with severe deformation unless the patient could hold a floss holder.

C. An interproximal toothbrush could have a handle too small to hold with deformed hands.

D. Chlorhexidine will not penetrate plaque, which the patient is unable to remove.

2. C

Bradycardia does not require a special diet. It is a heart rhythm that is too slow, and requires medication to speed up the rate.

3. B

Sickle cell anemia would not manifest as mucosal redness, but rather, as pale gingiva.

4. D

Low blood pressure, extreme weakness, skin pigmentation, susceptibility to infection, and destruction of adrenocortical tissue indicate Addison's disease, the hyposecretion of cortisol from the adrenal glands.

A. DeQuervain's symptoms are severe pain on the radial or thumb side of the wrist.

C. Cushing's disease causes weight gain, fatty tissue deposits creating a "moon" face, buffalo hump, and large abdomen.

E. Peutz-Jegher syndrome causes gastrointestinal polyps and skin-freckling.

5. B

An individual who has AIDS will have a suppression of cellular immunity. The invading HIV attacks the T lymphocytes needed for cellular immunity.

A. Suppression of humoral immunity involves B lymphocytes, which create antibodies against invading pathogens. HIV happens to like T lymphocytes.

C. Neutrophils are involved in acute infectious responses with neutrophil-loss, and are not an indication of AIDS.

D. Monocytes become macrophages during chronic infection.

6. A

Sjogren's disease does not typically coexist with Paget's disease, a bone disease.

7. C.

HIV likes to multiply in the helper T lymphocytes or CD4 cells.

8. E

The most serious side effect of radiation therapy is osteoradionecrosis, the progressive devitalization of bone due to radiation exposure. This results in necrotic exposed bone, along with necrotic mucosa, pain, and parasthesia.

9. A

A trait of von Recklinghausen's disease (a neurofibromatosis) is café-au-lait macules.

B. Dwarfism occurs with cretinism of hypothyroidism.

C. Buffalo hump and moon face occur from Cushing's syndrome with hypercortisolism.

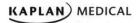

10. C

Polycythemia does not manifest as active blood flow, since blood sludges instead.

11. A

A patient who constantly brushes and flosses likely has obsessive-compulsive disorder.

D. Anxiety disorder occurs when the patient worries excessively about everything all the time.

12. B

When the myelin sheath of nerves is destroyed and replaced by sclerotic tissue, that is multiple sclerosis.

A. Muscular dystrophy is a muscle disease.

C. Myasthenia gravis is an that causes weakness in the voluntary muscles of the body, such as facial expression, chewing, and swallowing.

D. Parkinson's disease is a chronic neurological disorder that affects the substantia nigra neurons of the brain.

13. E

Patients with mitral valve prolapse with no regurgitation do not need premedication.

14. A

Someone with pernicious anemia will suffer from glossitis, since the stomach is unable to absorb vitamin B^{12}.

B. Cheilosis is from lack of vitamins B2, B3 and B6.

C. Severe gingivitis is from a lack of vitamin C.

D. Burning mucosa is from a lack of vitamin B1.

15. C

Asperger syndrome is a form of high-functioning autism.

16. E

Gearing the home care instruction to the family members is the most important task.

C. Use of an electric toothbrush may be helpful but only if the patient remembers to use it.

17. C

Align wheelchair and dental chair to same height, remove arm from wheelchair, place transfer board under patient and onto dental chair, slide patient into dental chair, pivot patient into seat.

18. B.

Ophthalmic medications that can be absorbed into the bloodstream are beta blockers that can cause tachycardia, vasodilation, and bronchodilation.

A. Calcium channel blockers can cause gingival hyperplasia.

C. Depolarizing agents can produce cardiac arrhythmias.

D. Adrenergic blockers decrease blood pressure.

E. Both adrenergic and beta blocking agents lower blood pressure.

19. B

Tight lips and skin that cause microstomia (inability to open wide) is scleroderma.

A. Bell's palsy will cause a drooping of the lip and facial muscles.

C. Trigeminal neuralgia is severe pain triggered by something.

20. C

The Americans with Disabilities Act allows patients with disabilities public access.

A. Standard Rules on Equalization of Opportunities for Persons with Disabilities is a United Nations proclamation to recognize disabled people.

D. Disabled People's Protection Policy is a policy in the United Kingdom.

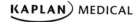

21. **C**

A blood protein that mediates platelet cohesiveness when the endothelium is injured is Von Willebrand factor.

A. Stuart factor is a lack of Factor X in the blood.

B. Thalassemia is a genetic disorder that impairs the creation of the alpha or beta hemoglobin chain, producing reduced or erroneous hemoglobin.

D. Prothrombin deficiency is an acquired or a rarely inherited autosomal recessive disorder that lacks Factor II.

E. Agranulocytosis is an insufficient number of white blood cells called neutrophils.

22. **D**

Tourette syndrome manifests with sudden, rapid jerking movements.

23. **C**

Lupus erythematosus manifests as a "butterfly" on the bridge of the nose that can be raised, bright red, and edematous, but it can also fade.

A. Epidermis bullosa manifests as blisters of the skin and oral mucosa that break open easily, especially mucous membrane blisters, leaving flat, painless reddish ulcer bed with no inflammatory halo.

B. Pemphigoid manifests as bullae that recur in the same area but most commonly the eyes and mucosa with a vast majority of oral involvement resulting in desquamative or erosive gingivitis.

E. Behçets syndrome is an autoimmune disease that yields painful oral ulcers, eye lesions, fever, and pallor.

24. **E**

A patient with myasthenia gravis will not have a steady gait since he has uncoordinated movements.

25. **D**

Patients with myasthenia gravis need short, not long, appointments, to eliminate stress which can cause breathing difficulties.

Chapter Twenty:
Medical Emergencies in the Dental Office

A medical emergency can occur in the dental office at any time. It can come in the form of anaphylaxis in a premedication patient who has never had a problem with an antibiotic, or of a reaction to local anesthesia. It may even be a sudden problem with a loved one waiting in the reception area. No matter what, knowing proper emergency procedures may save a life.

In this chapter, you will find "activate EMS" for many emergency treatment plans. It is always better to call 911 if anything serious is suspected. Waiting too long to get a heart-attack victim to the hospital can cause serious damage. Naturally, that can cause the patient to have a more difficult recovery.

The dental hygienist is responsible for providing a **standard of care** up to her level of training in emergency medical management and cardiopulmonary resuscitation (CPR) training. Updating a patient's medical history is vital in revealing conditions that may predispose a medical crisis.

PATIENT ASSESSMENT

Being able to recognize the signs of an unforeseen medical complication is an important responsibility of the dental hygienist. Patient assessment will help you to recognize those signs. The **primary assessment** is your basic evaluation of what the specific emergency is. The **secondary assessment** focuses on treating the given complication. A **symptom** is what the **patient says**. A **sign** is what **you observe**.

Primary Assessment

First you need to recognize that a medical emergency is taking place. Was the patient speaking normally a moment ago and he is now acting strangely? Did he lose consciousness? Is he having trouble breathing? Is he experiencing chest pain?

Then you must evaluate the patient's **level of consciousness**. Is he totally conscious and responding clearly to questions about his emergency? Is he explaining the source of the pain or is he not responding at all?

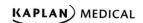

1. **Position the patient** correctly. Lying someone down who has left-sided heart failure, for example, and is having a hard time breathing will actually make it harder for her to breathe. Doing CPR on a padded dental chair also would not allow for good depth compressions. (Lie her down on a hard surface.) Maintaining her **airway** will prevent her from having another medical emergency that could lead to respiratory arrest, which leads to cardiac arrest.

2. **Assess her breathing** rate. Is it the proper rate? Are ventilations adequate? Is she getting enough oxygen?

3. **Assess her circulation**. Does she have a pulse? Is it too fast or too slow?

AVPU is new to the dental profession. It evaluates more in-depth the patient's level of consciousness.

- A stands for the patient being totally **alert**. She is talking and can answer questions appropriately.

- V stands for the patient being responsive to **verbal stimuli**. She may seem somewhat unconscious and responds only when you speak directly to her, or she may look conscious but cannot respond correctly. She is not sure about where she is or the correct day of the week.

- P stands for the patient being responsive to **painful stimuli** such as pinching. She becomes somewhat conscious only in response to painful stimuli and may go in and out of consciousness.

- U stands for **unresponsive**. No matter what you do, the patient does not respond.

Secondary Assessment

Details about a patient's medical status will help you in the **Secondary Assessment**, when you are assessing the medical crisis in-depth.

1. First, the patient may need **oxygen**. All medical offices should keep a bottle of oxygen in a visible place.

2. Then, monitor his **vital signs**. Monitor them often, since vital signs can change either way depending on which way the symptoms change.

3. Review the patient's **medical history** to see if there is a history with a current medical compromise. Review his list of medications, and have a photocopy of that list available for the EMT should one be summoned. With all the information in hand, the dentist will make a **differential diagnosis** on how to proceed.

4. **Reassess the patient**. Since vital signs can change, so can the patient's condition.

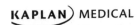

Primary and Secondary Assessment

Primary	AVPU	Secondary
Recognize the emergency	A = Alert Patient aware	Give oxygen
Assess consciousness	V = Verbal Patient responds to voice Patient not aware of surroundings	Monitor vitals
Position patient	P = Pain Patient responds to painful stimuli	Review medical history
Maintain airway	U = Unresponsive Patient totally unresponsive	Differential diagnosis
Assess breathing		Reassess
Assess circulation		
AVPU		

All medical offices must have a proper emergency kit, with drugs that are regularly monitored so that they are not out-of-date. Some companies supply emergency kits that are automatically monitored; when the drugs expire, the company sends new ones.

Following is a list of drugs that should be kept in a **Basic Life Support (BLS) kit.**

- Oxygen
- Epinepherine
- Benadryl
- Albuterol
- Glucose
- Nitroglycerine

VITAL SIGNS

Vital signs track a patient's blood pressure, pulse rate, and respiratory rate. During a medical emergency, vital signs can fluctuate depending on what complication is occurring. Getting a normal baseline set of vitals when the patient first enters the office will help in evaluation should an emergency occur. See Chapter 14 for more information on the taking of vital signs. A **sphygmomanometer** measures blood pressure in millimeters (mm) of mercury (Hg). The standard normal for blood pressure had been 120/80 but has been changed to 115/75.

CPR

Many states require cardiopulmonary resuscitation (CPR) for the maintenance of a dental hygiene license. Basic life-support CPR certification is offered to the public by the American Red Cross and the AHA. For someone who is not breathing, CPR sends oxygen and circulation to the brain, heart, and vital organs. This is usually sufficient until EMS support arrives. Some dentists may have advanced cardiac life support (ACLS) certification, in which case fluids and drugs can be administered intravenously along with defibrillation.

The **ABCs** of **CPR** should be initiated after you have established unresponsiveness and that there is no breathing or pulse, and after EMS has been called.

- A is for **airway** that needs to be opened. With the head tilted, lift the chin, unless there is a spinal injury. In that case, use the modified jaw thrust method.

- **B is for breathing.** After opening the airway, look, listen, and feel for breathing for 3–5 seconds. If there is no rise and fall of the chest, deliver two rescue breaths slowly over 1.5–2 seconds to prevent gastric distention. If air does not go in, re-tip the head and try giving two more rescue breaths. If air still does not go in, there is an obstructed airway, which will be discussed further on. Assume that the two breaths did go in, so the next step will be circulation.

- **C is for circulation.** For 5–10 seconds, check for a pulse at the carotid artery (if the patient is an infant under age 1, check for a pulse at the brachial artery). If there is no pulse, chest compressions need to be performed.

For **adult CPR**, the newest AHA guidelines are the same for one rescuer and two rescuers. After giving the patient the 2 initial breaths and confirming no pulse at carotid artery, the rate of 30 compressions is given followed by 2 breaths. The compression depth is 1.5-2 inches with both hands on the sternum.

The rate of 30 compressions to 2 breaths continues until an AED arrive or ALS arrives. If the AED arrives, the AED checks for a shockable rhythm and shocks when necessary. Rhythm is checked and if no pulse confirmed continue with **five** cycles of 30 compressions.

Chest compression rate is **100 per minute** for an adult, child, or infant. For **child CPR** (1–8 years old), the rate is **30 compressions** to **2 breaths**, with one person or two, and **one hand** over the sternum at a depth of $\frac{1}{3}$ to $\frac{1}{2}$ **the depth of the chest.** After 1 minute, check for a pulse. If not, continue CPR.

For **baby CPR** (under 1 year old) the rate is **30 chest compressions** to **2 breaths,** whether one person or two, and **two fingers** between the nipples at a depth of $\frac{1}{3}$ to $\frac{1}{2}$ **the depth of the chest.** After 1 minute, check for a pulse. If not, continue CPR.

Defibrillation

Semiautomatic defibrillation training is available to health care providers. While a team or individual is performing CPR, the semiautomatic defibrillator can be set up. The two leads are attached over the sternum and apex. Everyone should back away from the patient to allow the AED to **analyze** the rhythm, since the AED will detect movement by rescuers as cardiac rhythm. If the AED detects a shockable rhythm, it will tell everyone to stand clear.

When the AED is fully charged, it will announce that the patient can be shocked. When the **shock** button is pressed, the AED will determine whether the defibrillation was successful. Up to three shocks may be delivered by the AED. Check for a pulse after the third shock. If there is none, restart CPR for 1 minute and repeat sequence with the AED.

Obstructed Airway

Airway obstructions may be **partial or completely blocked**. If the patient is **talking** to you or **coughing**, then his airway is partially obstructed. In that case, **leave him alone** and allow him to cough.

If the airway is **completely blocked** on a **conscious patient**, you must initiate the **Heimlich maneuver**: Standing behind the patient, make a fist together with both hands. With thumbs up, place the fists up into the abdomen between the navel and xiphoid process. Use a swift **inward and upward thrust** until the object comes out. If the patient becomes unconscious, lower her to the floor and proceed as follows for an unconscious patient.

If the patient is **unconscious**, open airway, check for **breathing for 3–5 seconds**. If no breathing occurs, give **2 rescue breaths** over 1.5–2 seconds. If air does not go in, **re-tip the head and try 2 more rescue breaths**.

If air still does not go in, there is an obstructed airway. **Straddling** the patient, place one hand over the other with the heel of one hand on his abdomen between the navel and xiphoid process. **Administer 5 upward abdominal thrusts**. Check the patient's mouth by doing a **finger sweep** to see if the object was dislodged. If not, reopen the airway and **attempt ventilation**. If air does not go in, repeat the sequence.

For an **unconscious baby**, tilt the head slightly into the **sniffing position** and give **2 puffs of air**. If air does not go in, **retip the head** and **ventilate with 2 more puffs**. If those do not go in, there is an airway obstruction. Give **5 back blows** between the shoulder blades and **five chest thrusts** with 2 fingers between the nipples.

Check for an object. A finger sweep is performed on a **baby ONLY if you can see an object**. If no object present, **attempt ventilations**. If air still does not go in, repeat sequence. If the infant starts to breath again on her own, place her in the recovery position on her side. Remember that the tongue is the biggest airway obstructor.

OXYGEN ADMINISTRATION

Oxygen is necessary for cell life. During a medical emergency, the body may require more oxygen than normal. Everyone in the office should be aware of the oxygen tank location in case of an emergency.

Portable **oxygen tanks** are in **green cylinders** (size E is recommended) and have an adjustable flow meter. The **bag valve mask** is the correct equipment for **rescue breathing or CPR**: It is attached to the flow meter, which is turned up to 12 liters, and the reservoir is filled. The mask is placed securely over the patient's face for a tight fit. The bag should be compressed with positive pressure every 3–5 seconds, while chest rise is observed. If the patient is **conscious**, a **nasal cannula** may be used to administer oxygen at a rate of 2–4 liters or a **clear oxygen mask** may be used at a flow rate of about 10 liters.

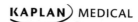

SYNCOPE

Syncope is a sudden transient loss of consciousness due to inadequate blood flow to the brain. A phobia about dental procedures or stress may prompt an episode.

- **Signs and symptoms:** Nausea, weakness, lightheadedness, ashen color, and diaphoretic (cold, clammy skin), rapid pulse initially, shallow breathing

- **Plan of treatment:** Activate EMS, supine position (Trendelenburg), maintain airway, provide rescue breathing every 3–5 seconds if needed, administer oxygen, administer ammonia capsule under patient's nose, monitor vital signs until patient regains consciousness

HYPOTENSION AND SHOCK

- **Orthostatic hypotension** is not a specific disease but a manifestation of an abnormal blood pressure. It occurs when a patient sits up too fast, causing a pooling of blood in the legs. The baroreceptors in the aortic arch and carotid artery do not have a chance to recover so there's a sudden drop of the blood pressure. It can be caused hypovolemia, side effects from drugs, prolonged bed rest, atherosclerosis, or neurological disorders.

  - **Sign and symptoms:** Dizziness, fainting, lightheadedness upon standing

  - **Plan of treatment:** Place patient back in supine position, monitor vitals signs, administer oxygen if necessary, and raise the patient slowly while monitoring vital signs. Release patient if all previous signs and symptoms are absent and vitals signs are normal.

- **Shock** is inadequate tissue profusion due a failure of the circulatory system. The **heart** may have failed, resulting in **cardiogenic shock**. Dehydration or blood loss—and a resulting **decrease in circulating blood** volume—may have occurred, resulting in **hypovolemic shock**. A **large infection** may have invaded the body, leading to the production of toxin that in turn caused organ failure (**septic shock**). The **autonomic nervous system** (that controls vasoconstriction) may have been disrupted, causing vasodilation and the pooling of blood in the peripheral system (**neurogenic shock**). **Psychogenic shock** is simple **fainting** and is the most easily correctable shock. Anaphylactic shock will be discussed further on.

  - **Signs and symptoms:** Altered mentation or level of consciousness, thirst, tachycardia, increased respiratory rate, diaphoresis (cool, clammy skin), cyanosis (blue), and hypotension or decrease in blood pressure

  - **Treatment plan:** Activate EMS, place patient in Trendelenburg position, maintain **airway** and administer **oxygen**, and monitor **vital signs**.

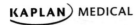

ALLERGIC REACTION AND ANAPHYLAXIS

- There are many things a patient may suddenly become allergic to: foods, medication, chemicals, insect bites, and environmental sources. A patient who has never before had a problem with anesthesia may develop an allergy in the dentist's chair. A premedicated patient (heart murmur, mitral valve prolapse or joint replacement, etc.) may develop an allergy to his medication out of the blue. Allergic reactions can range from **mild** (delayed) to **life-threatening**, as in **anaphylactic shock**.

  - **Signs and symptoms of delayed allergic reaction**: Skin rash, localized swelling, or urticaria (hives), along with respiratory difficulty (dyspnea) or wheezing

  - **Treatment plan**: For delayed reaction involving a skin rash, an oral antihistamine is indicated. Monitor patient for further symptoms. If airway is affected, oxygen is indicated. If the airway is blocked, administer epinephrine subcutaneously, followed by an intramuscular injection of diphenhydramine.

- **Anaphylaxis** is an immediate life-threatening reaction to an antigen that occurs within one hour of exposure to that antigen. The immune system is activated to encounter the invading antigen when the lymphocytes release B lymphocyte cells (B cells) and T lymphocyte cells (T cells). See chapter 6, Microbiology.

  - **Signs and symptoms of anaphylaxis**: Flushed skin or urticaria (hives), apprehension, anxiety, nausea, vomiting, difficulty breathing (dyspnea), obstructed airway from angioedema of the larynx

  - **Treatment plan**: Terminate the dental procedure, activate EMS, move patient into a supine position, maintain airway, administer oxygen, administer epinephrine and subcutaneous, intramuscular diphenhydramine, monitor vital signs, and perform basic life support procedures if necessary.

DRUG-RELATED EMERGENCIES

A drug-related emergency can also be an idiosyncratic response to a drug, overdose, or bad drug interaction in someone with a chemical dependency. In this last case, someone dependent on cocaine, for instance, could have a bad reaction to the epinephrine contained in local anesthetics.

- **Signs and symptoms**: Altered level of consciousness, change in mental activity, bradycardia, flaccid muscles, hypotension, and diaphoresis

- **Treatment plan:** Terminate dental procedure, activate EMS, administer oxygen, maintain airway, administer epinephrine subcutaneously followed by intramuscular diphenhydramine for anaphylaxis, if ALS-certified, administer naloxone (Narcan) for suspected overdose, and monitor vital signs.

> Naloxone (Narcan) is the medication of choice for a suspected drug overdose.

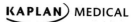
KAPLAN MEDICAL

CARDIOVASCULAR EMERGENCIES

A cardiovascular emergency in the dental office necessitates definitive treatment: **Coronary artery disease** increases a patient's risk for heart problems and stroke. **Atherosclerosis** is the narrowing or occlusion of blood vessels. **Arteriosclerosis** is the actual hardening of the arteries. Risk factors include obesity, smoking, hypertension, sedentary lifestyle, high cholesterol, and diabetes.

Congestive Heart Failure

Congestive heart failure occurs when the heart muscle is incapable of keeping up with the needs of supplying the body with blood. It may be caused by heart valve damage, hypertension, coronary artery disease, myocardial damage, or inflammatory disease.

■ **Right-sided heart failure** occurs when the right side of the heart (which receives blood back from the body) isn't functioning at full capacity to pump blood to the lungs. As a result, blood backs up in the body, and peripheral edema results.

- **Signs and symptoms**: Peripheral edema; weakness; fatigue; jugular vein distention; or cool extremities

- **Treatment plan**: Terminate the dental procedure, activate EMS, administer oxygen, monitor vital signs.

> Many CHF patients are on loop diuretics whose function is the removal excess water from the body. This takes place in the glomerulus of the kidney.

■ **Left-sided heart failure** occurs when the left side of heart (which receives blood back from the lungs) isn't functioning at full capacity. It isn't able to pump blood out the body. As a result, it causes fluid to build up in the lungs. Left-sided heart failure can lead to right-sided failure.

- **Signs and symptoms**: Weakness; fatigue; pulmonary edema; cyanosis; difficult breathing—especially lying supine

- **Treatment plan**: Terminate the dental procedure, activate EMS, sit patient upright, administer oxygen, monitor vital signs.

> Nitroglycerine lowers blood pressure, so the patient's blood pressure needs to be monitored carefully.

Angina Pectoris

Angina pectoris is transient chest pain or pressure caused by an insufficient supply of oxygen to the heart muscle. This happens when the coronary arteries have narrowed. The supply of blood is not keeping up with the demand that is brought on by stress or rigorous physical activity.

- **Signs and symptoms**: Substernal chest pain or pressure that can radiate out to the arms, neck, or mandible; difficulty in breathing

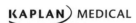

- **Treatment plan**: Terminate dental procedure, summon EMS, administer oxygen, assist with nitroglycerine sublingual, monitor vital signs especially blood pressure. Up to 3 nitroglycerine pills may be administered.

The symptoms of angina pectoris and myocardial infarction are very similar. If the pain is not relieved by the nitroglycerine, resting, or with oxygen, the patient is having a myocardial infarction.

Prinzmetal angina causes chest pain but it is not caused by an occluded artery. It is caused by a coronary artery spasm that causes a sudden constriction of that vessel.

Myocardial Infarction

When the heart muscle doesn't receive enough coronary arterial blood oxygenation, it becomes ischemic and **myocardial infarction** results. This means death (necrosis) to the heart muscle or myocardium. Naturally, this impairs the cardiac output, yet patients often say they simply experience indigestion.

- **Signs and symptoms**: Anxiety; substernal chest pain or pressure not relieved by nitroglycerine, rest, or oxygen; pain radiated into the arms, up the neck, into the mandible; diaphoresis (cool, clammy skin); difficulty in breathing
- **Treatment plan**: Discontinue dental procedure, activate EMS, maintain airway, administer oxygen, administer up to 3 doses of nitroglycerine, monitor vital signs carefully. Nitroglycerine will lower the blood pressure.

Sudden Death

Sudden cardiac death is the abrupt cessation of the heart, resulting in death. It can occur within minutes of the onset of symptoms. In 90 percent of individuals, it occurs from occluded arteries, though it may also occur in younger adults with heart abnormalities. Other causes are anaphylaxis, arrhythmias, drugs, or shock.

- **Signs and symptoms**: Cyanosis; loss of consciousness; no pulse; apnic (no breathing)
- **Treatment plan**: Activate EMS, open airway, give basic life support: CPR and oxygen.

> When opening a bottle of nitroglycerine, a fetid odor or powder indicates the nitroglycerin is not good.

> If the patient has been given 3 doses of nitroglycerin and the chest pain is not relieved, he is having a myocardial infarction.

Cerebrovascular Accident

A cerebrovascular accident or stroke occurs from an interruption of oxygen to the brain, causing death to some brain cells and damage to others. There are two types of strokes: ischemic and hemorrhagic.

Ischemia to the brain occurs from an artery occlusion that doesn't allow blood flow to that part of the brain. The occlusion may be the result of coronary artery disease or atrial fibrillation. This type of stroke occurs more often than the hemorrhagic stroke. **Hemorrhagic stroke** occurs from sudden bleeding from a blood vessel within the brain. Risk factors include age, race, family history, gender, hypertension, coronary artery disease.

- **Signs and symptoms**: Altered level of consciousness, uncoordinated muscle movement (**ataxia**), weakness on one side (hemiplegia), headache, numbness, dizziness, paralysis, slurring of speech
- **Treatment plan**: Discontinue dental procedure, activate EMS, maintain airway, administer oxygen, monitor vital signs, perform basic life support CPR if needed.

Transient Ischemic Attack

A **transient ischemic attack** is often called a ministroke. Unlike a stroke, however, it lasts for a much shorter duration. Usually, it lasts less than 24 hours and most often, less than 10 minutes. A transient ischemic attack places the patient at a higher risk for a cerebrovascular accident.

- **Signs and symptoms**: Weakness to one side of the body, confusion, speech disturbances, difficulty in walking, dizziness, loss of coordination
- **Treatment plan**: If symptoms subside, ask patient to seek medical advice. If symptoms persist, follow same procedure for stroke.

Aneurysms

Marfan's syndrome is an inherited connective disease disorder. People are usually taller in stature than most, are prone to the dislocation of an eye lens, may have a heart murmur, and are prone to dissecting aortic aneurysms.

An aneurysm is the dilation or ballooning out of a weakened arterial wall which has burst. It may occur in the aorta in the thoracic cavity, abdomen, or in the brain. Inherited factors like **Marfan syndrome** place a patient at risk for aneurysm.

- **Signs and symptoms**: Stabbing back pain for aortic aneurysm, sudden headache for cerebral aneurysm, diaphoresis, extreme drop in blood pressure, pulsation in the abdomen, difficulty swallowing
- **Treatment plan**: Terminate procedure, immediate activation of EMS, maintain airway, administer oxygen, monitor vitals, keep patient warm.

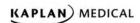

RESPIRATORY EMERGENCIES

Respiratory emergencies such as hyperventilation can occur in the dentist's office, particularly in patients with high anxiety. **Anoxia** is the lack of oxygen. **Hypoxia** is a deficiency of oxygen. **Apnea** is no breathing movement, while **dyspnea** is difficulty in breathing. **Hypoventilation** is not breathing fast enough. **Hyperventilation** is breathing too fast.

Hyperventilation

Hyperventilation, or rapid breathing, can occur in a patient experiencing great pain or anxiety. The rapid rate of breathing produces lower levels of carbon dioxide in the blood. That, in turn, results in respiratory alkalosis, which means a rise of body–fluid pH-balance.

- **Signs and symptoms**: Rapid breathing; light-headedness; altered level of consciousness; heart palpitations; tingling of extremities
- **Treatment plan**: Terminate dental procedure, coach the patient to relax and breath slower, have patient breathe into her cupped hands over her face.

Asthma

Asthma, also called reactive airway disease, is a recurrent inflammatory disorder when the bronchi constrict and mucous plugs block off the alveoli, trapping air in the alveoli. It can be precipitated by environmental factors, stress, foods, exercise, or drugs.

Status asthmaticus is a severe prolonged attack of asthma that is not eliminated by the use of each successive bronchodilator and is a true emergency. Patients with this condition are in imminent danger of total respiratory failure.

- **Signs and symptoms**: Wheezing; coughing; chest tightness; shortness of breath; cyanosis; anxiety
- **Treatment plan**: Terminate dental procedure, allow patient to use his bronchodilator. If symptoms worsen, activate EMS, maintain airway, administer oxygen and then albuterol by nebulizer mask.

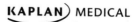

Chronic Obstructive Pulmonary Disease (COPD)

- **Chronic bronchitis** is an inflammation of the bronchial tree, where excessive mucous secretions are produced. Coughing and sputum production continues for months, with each successive episode longer and more frequent than the last.

  - **Signs and symptoms**: Mucus-producing cough; shortness of breath; frequent wheezing
  - **Treatment plan**: Terminate dental procedure, maintain airway, administer oxygen if needed, monitor vitals. If symptoms persist or worsen, activate EMS.

- **Emphysema** is the loss of elasticity in the alveoli of the lungs, making the alveoli more flaccid. Think of a deflated balloon that has less surface area than an inflated balloon to exchange carbon dioxide and oxygen.

  - **Signs and symptoms**: Fatigue, shortness of breath (dyspnea), chronic mild cough, weight loss
  - **Treatment plan**: Terminate dental procedure, maintain airway, administer oxygen if needed, monitor vitals. If symptoms persist or worsen, activate EMS.

DIABETES

If in doubt about whether a patient is hypoglycemic or hyperglycemic, give SUGAR. In hypoglycemia, glucose is used up extremely fast and the patient will die without immediate sugar.

Hyperglycemia is much slower; too much sugar is not good here due to the slow onset, but the situation can be managed more easily.

Diabetes occurs from **too much glucose** in the blood. The pancreas is not able to produce enough **insulin**—the hormone that unlocks the cell so that the glucose can enter. It is the β (beta) cells of the pancreas that produce insulin.

It is important to schedule diabetic patients when their blood glucose levels are optimal. In the morning, blood glucose is at its highest level. At this time, the insulin levels are low and will not use up the glucose too quickly. In the afternoon, it is just the opposite: The blood glucose level is low and the insulin level higher, predisposing the patient to a possible hypoglycemic attack. The patient should be told to notify the clinician if she feels any symptoms during the dental procedure.

Type 1 IDDM

Type 1 diabetes used to be called *juvenile diabetes* since it is diagnosed mostly in children. Type 1 diabetes is an autoimmune destruction of the β (beta) cells that produce insulin. Because the β cells are destroyed, the body does not produce insulin. Insulin is necessary for cell life, in that it allows glucose to enter into cells. Type I diabetes may be caused by hereditary factors from both parents or a virus. More cases seem to develop during the winter.

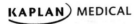

Type 2 NIDDM

- In **Type 2 diabetes**, insulin production occurs but is inadequate. The patient may be controlling her condition with proper diet or the ingestion of an oral hypoglycemic. Predisposing factors include genetics and obesity.

  - **Signs and symptoms for hypoglycemia**: Occurs very **rapidly**. Altered level of consciousness (combative, appears drunk, slurred speech), hunger, diaphoresis (cool, clammy skin), palpitations, weakness, headache

  - **Treatment plan for hypoglycemia**: Oral hyperglycemic such as a tube of icing, soda (not diet soda), orange juice with sugar added, maintain airway, oxygen if needed, monitor vitals. If symptoms worsen, activate EMS.

- **Hyperglycemia** occurs when there is too much glucose in the blood. This usually occurs when there is not enough insulin being produced, or when the patient has overeaten.

  - **Signs and symptoms of hyperglycemia**: Occurs **slowly**. Fruity (ketone) breath odor, increased urination, increased thirst, loss of appetite, weakness, dry flush skin, weak rapid pulse

  - **Treatment plan of hyperglycemia**: Terminate dental procedure, activate EMS, hospitalization to regulate sugar required.

- **Hypoglycemia** can occur with a diabetic or with a nondiabetic. With a **diabetic patient**, it is far more serious: Diabetics are prone to low blood sugar after taking their insulin or oral hypoglycemic, and need to eat right away.

With a **nondiabetic patient**, there are two types of hypoglycemia: **reactive** (or **postprandial**, occurring after a meal) and **fasting (postabsorptive)**. The signs and symptoms are very similar to a diabetic with hypoglycemia.

Reactive hypoglycemia occurs as something completely **unrelated to diabetes** with causes still open for debate. It may occur after excessive exercise has used up all the glucose. Patients who are stressed in the dental office and have not eaten can also use up their glucose quickly. It can also occur if too much insulin is produced. **Fasting hypoglycemia** is generally more involved with **disease**, such as hormonal deficiencies or non-beta tumors of the pancreas. Alternatively, it may be a side effect of drugs, alcohol, or illness.

  - **Signs and symptoms**: Headache, weakness, slurred speech, altered mentation, anxiety, hunger, shakiness, diaphoresis (cool, clammy skin), palpitations

  - **Treatment plan**: Terminate dental procedure. For conscious patient, administer oral hyperglycemic such as a tube of icing, soda (not diet soda), orange juice with sugar added. Monitor patient for 1 hour. For unconscious patient, activate EMS, maintain airway, oxygen, monitor vitals.

> If a patient suffers from polydypsia (thirst), polyphagia (hunger), and polyuria (frequent urination), he is likely diabetic.

> hyper = too much
> hypo = too low
> gly = glucose or sugar
> emia = in the blood

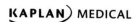

SEIZURES

Partial Seizures

Simple partial seizures occur when the patient is conscious, though he experiences an altered level of consciousness. There may be some uncontrolled movement such as blinking, twitching, or rapid eye movement.

Complex partial seizures affect a larger part of the brain, though they may last for just a few seconds. The patient may be in a dream-like state or completely unconscious. These seizures may also produce automatisms of blinking, twitching, and eye or mouth movements.

Generalized Seizures

- **Generalized seizures** affect both cerebral hemispheres and are a result of abnormal neural activity. **Absence seizures**—once called **petit mal seizures**—are an abrupt suspension of conscious thought or activity where the patient stares into space. These seizures are accompanied by clonic movements or automatisms of jerking, twitching, or eye movements, and may last a few seconds or minutes.

  - **Signs and symptoms absence seizure**: Unaware of surroundings, staring into space, rapid blinking

  - **Treatment plan**: Protect patient from injury, protect airway, administer oxygen if needed, monitor vital signs.

- **General tonic clonic seizures**—once called **grand mal seizures**—cause loss of consciousness and tonic convulsions (stiffening of muscles), followed by clonic convulsions (bilateral jerking movements). After that comes a postictal phase, where the patient may have a headache, be temporarily confused, or may be extremely tired.

  Status epilepticus is a continuous seizure that lasts more than 30 minutes. The longer the symptoms persist, the exponentially higher the mortality rate becomes. Also, the longer the duration of the seizure, the greater the neuron injury. This is a true medical emergency.

  - **Signs and symptoms**: Tonic convulsions (stiffening of muscles), clonic convulsions (bilateral jerking movements), post convulsive confusion, headache, fatigue.

  - **Treatment plan**: Protect patient from injury, protect airway, call EMS if prolonged, administer oxygen, monitor vital signs, allow patient to sleep in postictal state.

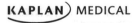

ADRENAL CRISIS (ADDISON'S DISEASE)

An adrenal crisis can occur when the adrenal glands produce insufficient gluco-cortoid, which maintains blood glucose levels. A patient who is tense in the dental chair may not be producing enough of this cortisol. If that is the case, he would need an immediate intravenous or IM injection of hydrocortisone.

- **Signs and symptoms**: Altered level of consciousness (confused, anxious, tense), dizziness, nausea/vomiting, abdominal pain, sweating, lethargy, tachycardia, rapid respiratory rate (tachypnea), eventually loss of consciousness, coma

- **Treatment plan conscious patient**: Terminate dental procedure, activate EMS and office response team, place patient in Trendelenburg position, administer oxygen, monitor vital signs.

- **Treatment plan unconscious patient**: Activate EMS, place patient in recovery position (as learned in CPR), maintain airway, monitor breathing, administer oxygen, monitor vitals.

HEMORRHAGE

Prolonged bleeding can result from many dental procedures. If blood is spurting, then an artery has been injured. If blood is oozing, a vein has been affected.

- **Treatment plans:**

  For extremity bleeding: Compress gauze over bleeding area, elevate the extremity, apply pressure to the pressure point of blood vessels in the area of the bleeding.

  For epistaxis (nose bleed): Apply cold pak to nose, apply pressure to nostril on affected side, instruct patient to avoid blowing nose afterward.

  For tooth-socket bleeding: Place folded gauze over socket and have patient apply a gentle biting pressure for 10 minutes. Instruct patient not to rinse or forcefully spit. If bleeding persists have patient bite on a moist tea bag.

EYE INJURIES

Eye injuries can occur in the dental operatory from flying debris and aerosols.

For foreign body in eye: Rinse with eye cup, gently pull lower lid down and inspect for foreign body, eliminate foreign body with damp cotton applicator. Or pull upper lid down over lower lid, then draw gently back upward.

For chemical burn to eye: Flush eyes at eyewash station for at least 10 minutes. Have eye examined by a physician.

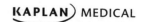

DISLOCATED MANDIBLE

A patient with temporomandibular joint dysfunction may suddenly lock open during a dental procedure. This condition is very painful.

- **Signs and symptoms**: Locked, open mouth that cannot close
- **Treatment plan**: Standing in front of patient, place protected thumbs on occlusal surfaces of mandibular molars with remaining fingers under the angle of the mandible. Press down and backward with thumbs while fingers draw upward and forward. Allow joint to slide back into place. Anesthesia may be required to manipulate the dislocation back into place. You may need to bandage the mandible in order to stabilize it and prevent wide-opening.

REVIEW QUESTIONS

1. To check a baby's pulse during CPR, you would check the _____ artery.

   A. Carotid

   B. Femoral

   C. Brachial

   D. Temporal

2. If a person is hyperventilating in the operatory, the first thing you should do is

   A. Give her oxygen by nasal canula

   B. Give her a paper bag to breath in

   C. Have her breathe into her cupped hands

   D. Perform BLS CPR

3. If a patient is suffering from bradycardia, his heart rate will be

   A. 90–100 beats per minute

   B. 100 + beats per minute

   C. Less than 60 beats per minute

   D. 60–80 beats per minute

4. A syncopal episode can best be described as

   A. The patient became dizzy as he sat up in the chair.

   B. A transient lack of blood to the brain.

   C. A postictal state.

   D. Difficulty in breathing.

5. According to the American Heart Association, once you have established that a person (an adult) is unconscious, the next step should be to

   A. Establish an airway

   B. Check for breathing

   C. Point to some one to call 911 to activate EMS

   D. Cover the patient up to keep her warm

6. A diabetic patient who initially appeared normal suddenly becomes confused and diaphoretic. He then lapses into unconsciousness. This patient is ailing from

   A. Ketoacidosis

   B. Diabetic coma

   C. Hyperglycemia

   D. Insulin shock

7. A patient suddenly has difficulty breathing and has audible inspirations that sound like wheezes. She is suffering from

   A. Chronic bronchitis

   B. Emphysema

   C. Asthma

   D. Left-sided heart failure

8. A patient is in your chair, and during the polishing, suddenly states that the polishing paste tastes different. This patient may be

   A. Hypoglycemic

   B. Experiencing an aura prior to a seizure

   C. Experiencing a transient ischemic attack

   D. None of the above

9. A patient begins to have sudden chest pain that radiates up into his mandible and neck. This may be a symptom of

   A. Right-sided heart failure

   B. A mandibular tooth abscess

   C. Myocardial infarction

   D. A cerebrovascular accident

KAPLAN) MEDICAL

10. Which of the following is not a type of shock?

    A. Hypovolemia

    B. Septicemia

    C. Chiasma

    D. Psychogenic

11. You are not sure if a patient is having a hypo-glycemic or hyperglycemic attack. You should

    A. Give her sugar anyway.

    B. Wait until the paramedics arrive to test the patient's blood sugar.

    C. Administer 50% dextrose.

    D. Wait until she becomes unconscious to know that it is hypoglycemia and then give her sugar.

12. The drug of choice for someone suffering from an acute asthma attack would be:

    A. Retrovir

    B. Albuterol

    C. Diphenhydramine

    D. Dramamine

13. Hyperventilation can cause

    A. Metabolic acidosis

    B. Metabolic alkalosis

    C. Respiratory acidosis

    D. Respiratory alkalosis

14. A patient who is not producing enough glucocor-toid becomes confused, diaphoretic, tachycardic, and hypotensive during a difficult extraction. 911 has been called, but now the patient becomes unconscious. This patient is suffering from

    A. Hypoglycemia

    B. Cerebrovascular accident

    C. Adrenal crisis

    D. Drug overdose

15. A patient who has pitting peripheral edema suffers from:

    A. Right-sided heart failure

    B. Left-sided heart failure

    C. Obesity

    D. None of the above

16. A patient who has been in the dental chair for over 2 hours stands up suddenly and becomes dizzy. This patient has experienced

    A. A syncopal episode

    B. Orthostatic hypotension

    C. Supine hypotensive syndrome

    D. Shock

17. Your perfectly cooperative patient suddenly has slurred speech with unequal pupils. He attempts to get up from the chair but cannot seem to use one leg. Your patient has experienced

    A. Allergic reaction

    B. Drug overdose

    C. Cerebrovascular accident

    D. Thyroid storm

18. All the following could cause hypertension except

    A. Not taking one's blood pressure medication regularly
    B. Hurrying in after being caught in traffic
    C. Regular exercise
    D. Having a child with Down syndrome and a parent who is an invalid.

19. If a patient suddenly suffers from a seizure in your chair, you would do all the following EXCEPT

    A. Put her in the recovery position
    B. Make sure she cannot injure herself
    C. Put in a tongue depressor
    D. Loosen her clothing

20. Your patient has had no symptoms of being ill. Suddenly, he loses consciousness and becomes pulseless, cyanotic, and apnic. Your patient is suffering from

    A. Hyperventilation
    B. Myocardial infarction
    C. Adrenal crisis
    D. Sudden death

21. When taking a medical history on a patient, which of the following questions is not necessary?

    A. Do you take any medications?
    B. Do you have any allergies?
    C. Do you exercise?
    D. Do you have a history of bleeding?

22. A patient has taken too much codeine for pain and is suffering from shallow breathing of 10 breaths per minute, a pulse rate of 56, has a blood pressure of 96/50, and is diaphoretic. Which of the following drugs would you administer?

    A. Atropine sulfate
    B. Naloxone
    C. Albuterol
    D. Epinepherine

23. If your patient has a blood pressure of 146/98, what would be your plan for dental treatment?

    A. Recheck annually.
    B. Recheck next 3 subsequent visits and refer for medical consultation if unchanged.
    C. Recheck in 5 minutes and if unchanged refer for medical consultation.
    D. No dental treatment, refer for medical consultation.

24. Your patient has a pulse rate of 102, a respiratory rate of 24, and a blood pressure of 122/76. Which of the following statements is true?

    A. All readings are within normal limits.
    B. Pulse rate is high, respiratory rate is normal, blood pressure is high.
    C. Pulse rate is normal, respiratory rate is high, blood pressure is normal.
    D. Pulse rate is high, respiratory rate is high, blood pressure is normal.

25. Which of the following hormones is released in the body during times of stress?

    A. Prolactin
    B. Thyroxin
    C. Cortisol
    D. Calcitonin

ANSWER EXPLANATIONS

1. C

During CPR, a baby's pulse should be checked at the brachial artery.

A. The carotid artery would be checked if the situation involved an adult or child.

2. C

If a patient is hyperventilating, try to calm her down and have her breathe into her cupped hands.

A. Giving her oxygen by nasal canula is contraindicated.

B. Giving her a paper bag to breathe into would have been the remedy of choice years ago.

D. Performing BLS CPR is not necessary for someone who is breathing.

3. C

If a patient is suffering form bradycardia, his heart rate will be less than 60 beats per minute

A. 90–100 beats per minute is high normal.

B. 100 + beats per minute is tachycardia.

D. 60–80 beats per minute is normal.

4. B

A syncopal episode can best be described as a transient lack of blood to the brain.

A. If a patient becomes dizzy while sitting up in a chair, that is orthostatic hypotension.

C. A postictal state occurs after a seizure.

D. Difficulty in breathing can indicate a variety of things.

5. C

If you have established that you have an unconscious adult patient, the next step should be to call 911.

A. Establish an airway would be the next step after calling 911.

B. Check for breathing comes after that.

D. Covering the patient is not a part of the AHA protocol

6. D

A patient who initially seems normal and then suddenly becomes confused and diaphoretic, and lapses into unconsciousness is suffering from insulin shock.

A. Ketoacidosis goes with hyperglycemia which is too much blood sugar, which occurs more slowly.

B. Diabetic coma occurs slowly from too much blood sugar.

C. Hyperglycemia is too much blood sugar that occurs more slowly.

7. C

Asthma is a sudden onset of difficulty in breathing along with audible inspirations that sound like wheezing.

A. Chronic bronchitis is a chronic obstructive pulmonary disease where the patient produces too much mucus in her lungs.

B. Emphysema is also a chronic obstructive pulmonary disease when the alveoli lose elasticity.

D. Left-sided heart failure does not occur suddenly since it is a chronic illness.

8. B

A change in taste of the polishing agent is an aura that may precede a seizure. The aura may be not only a change in taste but also halos around lights or an odor in the patient's nose depending on where in the brain the electrical activity is interrupted.

A. Hypoglycemia is a sudden onset of blood sugar that is too low.

C. Staring off into space is a symptom of someone experiencing a transient ischemic attack .

9. C

If a patient has sudden chest pain that radiates up into his mandible and neck, it may be a symptom of a myocardial infarction.

A. Right-sided heart failure is characterized by pitting edema in the extremities where fluid is building up.

B. A mandibular tooth abscess does not involve chest pain.

D. A cerebrovascular accident is a stroke which is characterized by slurred speech, altered level of consciousness, and loss of motor function on one side of the body.

10. C

Chiasma is an anatomical term. This answer choice was included as a distractor. It is a decussation or X-shaped crossing in tissues such as nerves.

11. A

Giving sugar to a hypoglycemic is very important since he will lose sugar extremely fast. For hyperglycemia, the onset is slow.

B. Waiting until the paramedics arrive will be too long if the patient is hypoglycemic.

C. 50% dextrose is an advanced life support (ALS) drug which can be used if anyone on the office staff is ALS certified.

D. Waiting until she becomes unconscious to give sugar may cause her to aspirate the sugar.

12. B

The drug of choice in this list for someone suffering from an acute asthma attack would be albuterol. Epinepherine is not on this list but can also be used in an acute attack.

A. Retrovir is an antiviral medication.

C. Diphenhydramine can follow the albuterol if needed. Getting the bronchioles open right away is important.

D. Dramamine is a drug for motion sickness..

13. D

Hyperventilation can cause respiratory alkalosis from loss of too much CO_2.

A. Metabolic acidosis occurs when too much acid spills into the extra-cellular fluid. This can occur from lactic acidosis or diabetic ketoacidosis.

B. Metabolic alkalosis can occur when a patient ingests larges of amount of antacids, takes too much diuretic, or has been vomiting a lot.

C. Respiratory acidosis retains too much CO_2 from respiratory depression such as respiratory arrest.

14. C

An adrenal crisis occurs when the adrenal glands do not produce enough glucocortoid. The patient becomes confused, diaphoretic, tachycardic, and hypotensive.

A. Hypoglycemia is low blood sugar that happens suddenly.

B. Cerebrovascular accident is a stroke that is characterized by sudden slurred speech with unequal pupils and paralysis on one side of the body.

D. In a drug overdose, the patient's pupils will react equally whether constricted or dilated; it will also result in bradycardia, flaccid muscles, hypotension, and diaphoresis.

15. A

A patient who has pitting peripheral edema suffers from right-sided heart failure due to fluid accumulating in the extremities.

B. Left-sided heart failure results in difficulty in breathing due to a build-up of fluid in the lungs.

C. Obesity is a weight problem.

16. B

Standing up and suddenly becoming dizzy is a symptom of orthostatic hypotension.

A. A syncopal episode results in fainting.

C. Supine hypotensive syndrome occurs in pregnant females who have been laying back too long, causing the baby to put pressure on the vena cava, lessening blood flow back to the heart.

D. Shock has many more signs and symptoms than just dizziness.

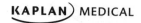

17.   C

Cerebrovascular accident is characterized by sudden slurred speech with unequal pupils and paralysis on one side of the body.

A. Allergic reaction symptoms include difficulty in breathing, rash, hives, and tachycardia.

B. Drug overdose will make both pupils equal whether dilated or constricted.

D. Thyroid storm symptoms include restlessness, chest pain, palpitations, shortness of breath, tremor, nervousness, and hypertension.

18.   C

The patient who exercises regularly will have low blood pressure. Patients who are under stress can suffer from high blood pressure.

19.   C

You would not insert a tongue depressor in the mouth of someone having a seizure. You might get bitten, or else the depressor might be bitten off, causing an airway obstruction.

A. Putting the patient in the recovery position is correct so that the tongue does not become an airway obstruction.

20.   D

Suddenly losing consciousness and becoming pulseless, cyanotic (blue), and apnic (not breathing) is a sign of sudden death

A. Hyperventilation is rapid breathing

B. Myocardial infarction results in difficulty in breathing and chest pain, which are not mentioned in this question.

C. During an adrenal crisis, the patient becomes confused, diaphoretic, tachycardic, and hypotensive.

21.   C

It is not necessary to ask about one's exercise in a health history.

22.   B

Naloxone is the drug of choice for an overdose.

A. Atropine sulfate can be used in a nebulizer mask for difficulty in breathing, but can also be used intravenously for a heart rate that is too slow.

C. Albuterol is used for difficulty in breathing.

D. Epineperine can be used for an allergic reaction or asthma attack, and can used intravenously for heart-related problems.

23.   B

Recheck next 3 subsequent visits and refer for medical consultation if unchanged.

A. Recheck annually would be correct if the pressure is < 140 systolic and < 90 diastolic.

C. Recheck in 5 minutes would be correct if pressure is 160-200 systolic and 100-115 diastolic.

D. No dental treatment would be correct if pressure is >200 systolic and >115 diastolic.

24.   D

The pulse rate of 102 is high, the respiratory rate of 24 is high, and the blood pressure of 122/76 is normal.

C. Normal blood pressure for adults varies depending on weight, illnesses, and exercising which lowers blood pressure. For adults, 120/80 has been the standard, with the new standard being normal at 115/75.

25.   C

Cortisol is released by the adrenal glands to control stress.

A. Prolactin is released by the pituitary gland to stimulate mammary glands to produce milk.

B. Thyroxin is released by the thyroid to control metabolic rate.

D. Calcitonin is released by the thyroid to stimulate calcium to be deposited into bone.

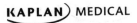

Chapter Twenty-One:
Legal and Ethical Issues

Dental hygiene is a profession dedicated to disease prevention and the promotion of good dental health. A code of ethics governs how duties are performed. Dental practice acts established by individual states grant the authority for dental personnel to perform these duties.

DENTAL ETHICS

Ethics is a principle of moral beliefs and values mandating what is good and what is bad. Though based on theory, ethics guide our conduct and the decisions we choose to make.

Morals describe the beliefs of what is right and what is wrong by expressing a view of correct behavior. Actions taken are measured against what is accepted.

Values place an importance or worth on what is right and what is wrong. Things we desire are among the things we value and are motivated by.

LEGAL TERMINOLOGY

Dental practice acts or statutes are established by state legislatures. These legislatures then empower their state board of dental examiners to adopt rules and regulations for dental professionals.

The State Board of Dental Examiners establishes licensure requirements by instituting a minimal level of competency for an individual to become licensed in his profession. The Board also has the ability to regulate, grant, and revoke licenses, as well as institute continuing-education standards for each profession.

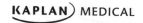

Laws are binding rules of conduct that express community expectancies and needs. A controlling authority enforces these rules and regulations.

Civil law is created by a legislature with rules and regulations that protect private people. It allows individuals to use the court system in private matters to settle a dispute.

Criminal law is also created by a legislature with rules and regulations but is an offense against society. Criminal law is punishable by fines and/or imprisonment. **Misdemeanors** are typically punishable by fines of less than $1,000 and/or less than 1 year of imprisonment. **Felonies** are typically punishable by fines of more than $1,000 and/or more than 1 year of imprisonment.

State and federal courts clarify legal disagreements by **judicial law**. These rulings may be based upon past similar legal cases in the same legal jurisdiction.

The **judicial process** utilizes a jury or judge to hear evidence in a court case to determine settlement, guilt, or innocence.

Due process is a formal procedure that protects individuals from random exploitation by a state or jurisdiction. Due process ensures that individuals are treated equally and fairly.

Tort law is concerned with civil wrong actions committed against an individual or his property. **Unintentional torts** are concerned with negligence and malpractice. **Negligence** is the absence of prudent care that an individual should receive in the dental setting. **Malpractice** is the failure to perform professional standards of care resulting in injury, loss, or damage.

Intentional torts are deliberate acts that result in harm or injury. **Assault** is the threat of causing bodily harm. **Battery** is the actual infliction of harm, placing the person in danger.

Defamation, also an intentional tort, includes libel and slander. Both of these convey false assertions regarding an individual. **Libel is written** defamation while **slander is verbal**.

Invasion of privacy is the offensive interference of an individual's private space or circumstances. This will be discussed further below in HIPAA.

Contracts are legal and binding agreements comprised of a promise or set of promises made by one party to another. They can be between two or more individuals. An **express contract** is one in which the terms are expressed verbally or in writing. An **implied contract** is one in which some of the terms are not expressed in words. **Breach of contract** occurs when the binding agreement is not honored by one of the parties to the contract.

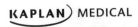

Patient confidentiality is the protection by state and federal laws of an individual's private information. Unauthorized disclosure of a person's information may be construed as breach or invasion of her privacy. The patient may consent in writing to the disclosure of information to a named person or entity.

Informed consent is an intelligent decision based on full disclosure of choices that the patient has regarding dental treatment. It includes the diagnosis, treatment plan, alternative choices, risks, and prognosis if treatment is received or refused. A written signature on the consent form signifies that the patient fully understands the treatment plan.

Informed refusal occurs when the patient refuses the treatment proposed. The patient must also be given details on the diagnosis, treatment plan, alternative choices, risks, and prognosis if treatment is refused. Careful documentation of the refusal and the reasons for it are a necessary part of the patient's record.

Fraud or **misrepresentation** is the deliberate misdirection of the truth to deceive another person. The imposter may represent himself wrongly, causing harm or loss to someone else.

Preceptorships have been proposed by a number of dental boards to train dental personnel in the performance of dental hygiene duties. Currently, the state of Alabama has the only preceptorship program. Kansas presently allows trained dental assistants to perform supra-gingival scalings.

Feasance is the performing of an act.

Malfeasance is a wrong doing, misconduct, or doing something legally unjust causing intentional damage.

Misfeasance is performing an act inadequately or poorly.

Nonfeasance is not performing, omitting, or neglecting to do an act.

Proximate cause is an event that results in injury due to negligence or an intentional wrongful act

Factual cause is an event that causes loss or damage to person

Legal cause is a considerable factor that allows harm

Breach of duty is a failure bring about ethical, moral or legal obligations in which a person has a right to demand satisfaction.

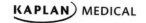

STANDARD OF CARE

As professionals, dental hygienists provide a **standard level of care**. All patients are granted the same level of attentiveness they would be afforded in any other dental setting. Dental hygienists are obligated to carry out the **lawful** standard of care as described in their individual state laws, and as instructed by the dentist whose supervision they are under.

With a goal of optimal health through prevention, dental hygienists provide care on three levels:

1. The **primary level of prevention** is to hinder the beginning of disease. This would include such things as fluoridated water, rinse-and-spit programs at schools, education of the public, and sealants.

2. The **secondary level of prevention** is to correct what the disease process has begun to destroy in the oral cavity. This would include fillings, inlays, onlays, crowns, periodontal treatment, and health care screenings.

3. The **tertiary level of prevention** restores the patient back to normalcy by replacing lost structures. This could include bridges, partials, dentures, and implants.

HIPAA

The Health Insurance Portability and Accountability Act (HIPAA) established in 1996 has a two-fold purpose. The first is to protect health insurance coverage for workers and their families should they change or lose their jobs. The second is to protect the privacy of the patient's personal and health information, given the submission of electronic insurance claims between health care organizations. This Act also states that group health plans cannot deny your application for coverage based solely on your health status.

The privacy portion of HIPAA guarantees patient access to one's own medical records, allowing for more authority on how one's protected health information is used. If the patient's privacy is compromised, there is an explicit path for legal recourse.

Dental health care providers who transmit dental health care information electronically are included in the Privacy Rule.

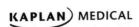

REVIEW QUESTIONS

1. All of the following are true about HIPAA except one. Which one is this EXCEPTION?

   A. Patients are guaranteed access to their own medical records.

   B. Health insurance coverage for workers and their families is protected.

   C. The privacy of patients' personal and health information is protected.

   D. Group health plans cannot deny an application for coverage based solely on one's health status.

   E. A patient can be denied coverage because of mental illness, genetic information, disability, or the claims that have been filed in the past.

2. If a new dental hygienist has just passed her National and State Board Exams and is asked to start working prior to receiving her license, she may be guilty of

   A. Violating civil law

   B. Violating state and federal law

   C. Breach of contract

   D. Negligence

3. The correction of the disease process that has begun to destroy structures in the oral cavity is called

   A. Primary level of prevention

   B. Secondary level of prevention

   C. Tertiary level of prevention

   D. None of the above

4. When a patient is granted the same level of attentiveness that would be afforded to her in any other dental setting, it is called

   A. Dental practice acts

   B. Express contract

   C. Implied contract

   D. Appropriation

   E. Standard of care

5. A patient was unhappy when the dentist told her she needed a root canal on Tooth #5 because she could not afford it. Before she had a chance to explain, the dentist proceeded to administer anesthesia and start the treatment. The legal claim that this patient could have against the dentist is

   A. Assault

   B. Battery

   C. Breach of contract

   D. Invasion of privacy

   E. Malpractice

6. When a dentist provides a patient with all the information necessary to make a decision about his own oral health, it is called

   A. Beneficence

   B. Veracity

   C. Informed consent

   D. Non-malfeasance

7. You are practicing dental hygiene in a rural area where all of the patients know one another. Your patient, Ms. Jones, arrives for her regular 6-month recall. During the medical history update, Ms. Jones reveals that she has recently been diagnosed with breast cancer. After the appointment, you join your coworkers at the local coffee shop and tell them about Ms. Jones's breast cancer. One of Ms. Jones's neighbors overhears the conversation. You have just committed

   A. Breach of confidentiality
   B. Slander
   C. Libel
   D. Negligence

8. If the dental board cites a dental hygienist for a violation of a dental law in that particular state, then the dental hygienist would be entitled to which of the following?

   A. Judicial process
   B. Lawful standard of care
   C. Judicial law
   D. Default judgment

9. Your 9:45 patient is an 8-year old girl. Because of traffic, she and her mother arrive at 10:00. As they rush in, the patient's mother excuses herself to go park the car. As you seat the child, you notice that she is in need of bitewing radiographs. Your next patient is scheduled for 10:15 and you are short on time, so instead of waiting for the mother to return, you go ahead and take the films. Your feeling is that she would indeed approve of this procedure. When the mother returns, however, she becomes upset that the radiographs were taken without her knowledge. What has occurred?

   A. Breach of confidentiality
   B. Assault
   C. Informed consent
   D. Implied consent
   E. Battery

10. As a newly licensed graduate, you have started practicing in a dental office as a full-time dental hygienist. There is another dental hygienist there as well, who has worked there for 20 years. All patients are on a 30-minute schedule, regardless of their treatment needs. After a few weeks, you notice that several of the patients have Class II periodontal disease with moderate amounts of deposit and bleeding. You also notice that several have not had a full periodontal charting in more than 5 years, and a few have not ever had periodontal charting. No documentation is present that would suggest that the patients have been advised about additional root debridement procedures or oral hygiene. When you ask the other hygienist about the lack of periodontal charting, she tells you not to worry, that the patients will never change their oral hygiene habits, and that she has been practicing long enough to know. What has occurred in this situation?

    A. Breach of standard of care
    B. Beneficence
    C. Veracity
    D. Non-maleficence
    E. All of the above

11. Of the following types of values, which one represents attitudes or beliefs that are not necessary for life?

    A. Extrinsic
    B. Intrinsic
    C. Terminal
    D. Instrumental

12. Which of the following statements best describes ethics?

    A. Ethics represents the customs of a group or sect.

    B. Ethics represents standards of thought and conduct.

    C. Ethics represents a study of regulations that oversee a profession.

    D. Ethics represents beliefs and values.

13. Against the dentist's advice, a patient has decided not to have a certain procedure performed. This patient's option to deny treatment is called

    A. Informed consent

    B. Informed refusal

    C. Fraud or misrepresentation

    D. Implied contract

    E. Negligence

14. The governmental agency that protects employees is

    A. HIPAA

    B. OSHA

    C. FDA

    D. ADHA

    E. ADA

15. A criminal investigation has shown that a dentist has practiced as an oral surgeon but has not in fact had any training in oral surgery. Which of the following terms does this concern?

    A. Violation of ethics

    B. Defamation

    C. Malpractice

    D. Misrepresentation

    E. All of the above

16. A patient seems to be experiencing a medical emergency but she is refusing to be treated. You have closed the door and will not allow her to leave. This could be called

    A. Illegal detainment

    B. Assault

    C. Battery

    D. Intrusion upon seclusion

17. If you physically held the patient in Question #16 down in the chair, what would have been done to the patient?

    A. Illegal detainment

    B. Assault

    C. Battery

    D. Intrusion upon seclusion

18. Which of the following describes on-the-job training of a dental hygienist without a formal education?

    A. Censorship

    B. Internship

    C. Apprenticeship

    D. Indentured assistantship

    E. Preceptorship

19. If a patient becomes unconscious while in the dental chair and you begin emergency procedures to correct the problem, this is called

    A. Informed consent

    B. Implied consent

    C. Express contract

    D. Implied contract

20. If a patient is unhappy with his treatment and posts this fact on a public billboard, he has committed

    A. Negligence
    B. Slander
    C. Libel
    D. Misrepresentation

21. A crime that is punishable by imprisonment for more than 1 year is called

    A. Tort law
    B. Felony
    C. Misdemeanor
    D. Due process
    E. Statutory law

22. Morals refer to

    A. Standards that govern the conduct of a profession, based on theory.
    B. Standards of conduct and thought, based on religious and ethical fundamentals.
    C. Beliefs and manners that prompt good actions.
    D. Cultural basics of a group.
    E. None of the above

23. According to HIPAA laws, a dental office is permitted to release confidential information to

    A. The insurance carrier
    B. A husband or wife
    C. The employer
    D. All of the above

24. State dental boards have the ability to perform all of the following functions except one. Which one is this EXCEPTION?

    A. Revoke licenses.
    B. Grant licenses.
    C. Determine continuing education standards.
    D. Grant authority to the dental board.
    E. Regulate license applications.

25. Laws made up by the legislative branch of government are called

    A. Administrative law
    B. Statutory law
    C. Constitutional law
    D. Judicial law
    E. None of the above

ANSWER EXPLANATIONS

1. E

One *cannot* be denied health coverage because of mental illness, genetic information, disability, or the claims that have been filed in the past.

2. B

Without receipt of a license, she may have violated state and federal law.

3. B

Secondary level of prevention

4. E

Standard of care

5. B

Battery is the actual physical touching of the person

6. C

Informed consent takes place when a practitioner provides the patient with all the needed information to make a decision about his oral health.

D. Non-malfeasance is the obligation of the health care provider to do no harm.

7. A

You have just committed breach in confidentiality, since you have revealed confidential medical information to individuals who do not directly treat the patient.

B. Slander is verbal defamation of an individual.

C. Libel is written defamation of an individual.

8. A

Judicial process is the evidential hearing that determines the guilt or innocence of a violation of law.

B. Lawful standard of care is a patient concern, not a hygiene-violation concern.

C. Judicial law is how a state or federal court clarifies discrepancies in laws.

D. Default judgment is the failure to act on something that is required by law.

9. E

Battery has occurred because treatment was rendered on a minor without parental consent.

A. Breach of confidentiality has not occurred since there was no discussion of the patient in an inappropriate manner.

C. Informed consent has not occurred since neither the mother nor the child gave consent for the radiographs to be taken.

D. Implied consent has not occurred since the mother never consented—verbally or in writing—to the taking of radiographs in her absence.

10. A

Breach in the standard of care has taken place here. The standard of care requires that all patients would have a full oral assessment, including periodontal charting at each dental exam.

11. A

Extrinsic value represents attitudes or beliefs that are not necessary for life.

B. Intrinsic values are necessary to sustain life.

C. Terminal values represent attitudes or beliefs associated with an outcome or result.

D. Instrumental values represent attitudes or beliefs associated with a course of action.

12. D

Ethics represents beliefs and values that mandate what is good versus bad.

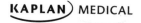

13. B

If a patient refuses to heed dental advice, it is called informed refusal.

A. Informed consent is concerned with intelligent information given to the patient regarding necessary treatment.

D. Implied contract is one in which some of the terms are not expressed in writing.

14. B

OSHA (Occupational Safety and Health Administration) is the government agency that protects employees.

A. HIPAA protects the privacy of the patient.

15. D

A dentist who misrepresents himself in a specialty practice where there has been no focused training is guilty of misrepresentation.

A. Violation of ethics is a breach of the rules governing the conduct of a profession. In this case, the dentist did violate rules but he misrepresented his abilities.

C. Malpractice is the failure to perform professional standards of care resulting in injury, loss, or damage.

16. B

If you threaten to hold a patient against her will, that is called assault.

A. Illegal detainment is an act done by law enforcement.

17. C

If you hold the patient down in the chair, that is considered battery.

18. E

A trained person who has not had a formal education yet who performs a dental prophylaxis on the job is called a preceptor.

B. An intern performs work under the supervision of an advanced, educated professional.

C. An apprentice is an indentured person who is learning a trade or craft.

19. B

If a patient becomes unconscious in the chair, implied consent would allow you to perform emergency procedures. When the patient is clearly not able to give her consent, it is implied that she would allow for help.

20. C

A patient who displays his negative feelings on a billboard is guilty of libel, since it is in written form.

B. Slander is verbal defamation.

21. B

This type of crime is a felony.

22. B

Morals are the standards of conduct and thought based on religious and ethical fundamentals.

A. Ethics are standards that govern the conduct of a profession based on theory.

C. Values are beliefs and manners that prompt good actions.

23. A

According to HIPAA laws, a dental office may release confidential information to the insurance carrier.

B. Release of information to a husband or wife is not allowed.

C. Release to an employer is not allowed even though it is the party who pays for the insurance.

24. D

State dental boards may not grant authority to the dental board, since that is the function of the state legislators.

25. B

Statutory law is legislation made up by the legislative branch of government.

Full-Length Practice Test

This examination is comprised of 2 components:

- **Component A, 200 test items in random order**
- **Component B, 150 test items based on 12 to 15 case studies**

You will be given 4 hours to complete this exam. You are not allowed to use reference sources.

For each test item, decide which choice is best and circle it. Record only one answer per test item. All test items are scored on an equal basis.

You may begin with Component A. When you have finished Component A, you may proceed directly to Component B.

Following the exam, you will find the answer explanations for every test item.

Full-Length Practice Test:
Component A: Multiple-Choice Questions

DIRECTIONS

Following are 200 multiple-choice questions, on varying topics of dental hygiene. Circle the answer you think is best.

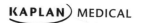

1. The dentist had prescribed Percodan for a patient after a difficult extraction. The patient arrives back with a family member somewhat confused and short of breath. He also has low blood pressure, slowed heart rate, nausea, and pinpoint pupils. The patient mostly likely

   A. Developed flu-like symptoms secondary to the extraction.
   B. Is suffering from tachycardia.
   C. Has overdosed on the Percodan.
   D. Is suffering from myasthenia gravis.

2. The antagonist pharmacological agent that should be used to treat the patient in Question #1 is

   A. Nubain
   B. Naldecon
   C. Naloxone
   D. Nizoral
   E. Nabilone

3. A diabetic patient on Humulin might experience all of the following side effects except one. Which one is this EXCEPTION?

   A. Too much (insulin) may cause him to have too low blood sugar.
   B. Too little (insulin) can cause symptoms of high blood sugar.
   C. He might become allergic.
   D. Too little (insulin) can cause rapid breathing and a fruity breath smell.

4. Intensifying screens in panoramic cassettes do all of the following things except one. Which one is the EXCEPTION?

   A. They contain phosphor to emit light when x rays strike it.
   B. They can contain rare-earth screens that are faster than calcium tungstate screens.
   C. They need more radiation for exposure.
   D. They emit blue light.
   E. They emit green light.

5. What type of radiation effect produces an ion when the atom is missing an electron and takes on a net-positive charge of an ion?

   A. Compton effect
   B. Classical scattering
   C. Thompson effect
   D. Indirect effect
   E. Photoelectric effect

6. A child presents as an emergency patient to the office with fever, lymphadenopathy, malaise, and ulcers in the mouth. The oral lesions began as small, yellow vesicles, but are now beginning to coalesce into gray centers with red borders. The doctor diagnoses this patient with

   A. Acute herpetic gingivostomatitis
   B. Juvenile periodontitis
   C. Rapid progressive periodontitis
   D. Necrotizing ulcerative periodontitis

7. With respect to the overall well-being of the child in Question #6, what would be the most serious concern about which to warn the parent?

   A. Malnutrition
   B. Dehydration
   C. Gingivitis
   D. Vesicular lesions

8. Upon performing an EDE/IOE oral cancer screening, you find a lesion on a patient's tongue that you suspect is a neoplasm. You refer the patient to an oral surgeon. If the lesion is malignant and is composed of muscle tissue of the tongue, it would be called

    A. Leiomyosarcoma

    B. Schwannoma

    C. Rhabdomyosarcoma

    D. Neurosarcoma

    E. Chondrosarcoma

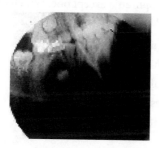

9. The smooth uniocular radiolucency in the illustration above originates from the reduced enamel epithelium and is associated with a tooth. This type of cyst is likely to be a

    A. Residual cyst

    B. Dentigerous cyst

    C. Primordial cyst

    D. Globulomaxillary cyst

    E. Median mandibular cyst

10. Which of the following rigid impression materials is a beta hemi-hydrate with regular particles that require little water when mixing?

    A. Gypsum

    B. Sodium borate

    C. Stone

    D. Plaster

11. Bulimics eat but purge their food. All of the following are characteristics of bulimia except one. Which one is this EXCEPTION?

    A. Esophageal inflammation

    B. Perimylolysis

    C. Parotid gland enlargement

    D. Burning tongue

    E. Lanugo

12. Which of the following is radiographically seen as a heart-shaped cyst that develops within the incisive papillae of the anterior palatal gingiva or in bone and soft tissue?

    A. Globulomaxillary cyst

    B. Median palatine cyst

    C. Nasopalatine cyst

    D. Residual cysts

13. Tuberculosis has become resistant to drugs because many patients do not complete their full regimen of antibiotics. Which of the following drugs is NOT used for the treatment of tuberculosis?

    A. Rifampin

    B. Ethambutol

    C. Isoniazid

    D. Pyribenzamine

    E. Pyrazinamide

14. Items that may corrode in an autoclave can be dry-heat sterilized. What time and temperature would be appropriate for dry heat sterilization?

    A. 15–20 minutes at 225° F

    B. 20–30 minutes at 250° F

    C. 20–30 minutes at 275° F

    D. 30–60 minutes at 300° F

    E. 60–120 minutes at 320° F

15. Every tooth is unique in its own way. Which of the following permanent teeth has an oblique ridge?

   A. Maxillary first molar

   B. Maxillary second premolar

   C. Mandibular second premolar

   D. Mandibular first molar

16. While dining out, you decide to have a piece of cake that is 180 g and is 33% carbohydrates. How many kilocalories are derived from the carbohydrates?

   A. 120 kilocalories

   B. 210 kilocalories

   C. 240 kilocalories

   D. 270 kilocalories

   E. 300 kilocalories

17. The human body has the ability to manufacture things in many ways. What organ synthesizes triglycerides?

   A. Pancreas

   B. Liver

   C. Gallbladder

   D. Spleen

18. After a new dental hygienist enters a school system in a small town, she notices generalized fluorosis. The water supply is fluoridated at 0.8 PPM. The majority of the students see the same pediatrician. What would be the most likely reason for the generalized fluorosis?

   A. Excess fluoride in the water supply

   B. Swallowing of toothpaste

   C. Excess topical fluoride

   D. Fluoride supplements

19. Which of the following conditions has an onset in adolescence or early adulthood and is characterized by disordered thinking, loss of contact with reality, and false beliefs?

   A. Post-traumatic stress disorder

   B. Bipolar disorder

   C. Schizophrenia

   D. Anxiety disorder

   E. Psychotic disorders

20. All of the following drugs are used in the treatment of schizophrenia except one. Which one is this EXCEPTION?

   A. Amitriptyline

   B. Chlorpromazine

   C. Haloperidol

   D. Resperidone

   E. Triflupromazine

21. Malnutrition can occur in a HIV-infected patient as a result of

   A. Intestinal malabsorption

   B. Cachexia

   C. Alterations in metabolism

   D. Alteration in adrenal and thyroid hormones

   E. All of the above

22. Carcinoma in-situ may best described as

   A. Atypical layers of slightly raised or flat, thickened areas in the middle or upper epithelium

   B. Immature basaloid cells of abnormal differentiation located toward the prickle and keratinizing layers in the lower two-thirds of epithelium

   C. Encapsulated high-grade epithelium that is hypercellular with no cell maturation at the surface and an intact basement membrane

   D. Fibrillar connective tissue that is irregularly shaped with coarse fibers

23. A patient has presented to your office with a brown lesion on her upper lip at the vermillion border that looks like a mole. This lesion is most likely

    A. Keratoacanthoma
    B. Melasma
    C. Melanoma
    D. Papilloma

24. On a periapical x-ray of #2 and #3, you find a radiopaque well-defined bony looking mass at the apices of both teeth. This mass is most likely a(n)

    A. Concrescence
    B. Osteoma
    C. Stafne's bone cyst
    D. Fibroma
    E. Torus palatinus

25. A dental material ideal for use on someone under-going radiation therapy and prone to Class V carious lesions is

    A. Glass ionomers
    B. Composites
    C. Hybrid ionomers
    D. Compomers

26. Diabetic patients tend to heal slowly from injury or disease. One reason they cannot fight off disease so easily is because they have fewer

    A. Basophils
    B. Erythrocytes
    C. Eosinophils
    D. Monocytes
    E. Polymorphonuclear leukocytes

27. A patient discusses some general health complaints that cause you to suspect he has diabetes. Oral manifestation of an undiagnosed diabetic would include all the following except one. Which one is this EXCEPTION?

    A. Magenta enlarged papillae
    B. Burning mouth
    C. Xerostomia
    D. Fast healing with periodontal treatment

28. Acetaminophen is an analgesic, antipyretic, and anti-inflammatory. Excessive acetaminophen can have adverse effects on the liver and kidney.

    A. Both statements are true.
    B. The first statement is true. The second statement is false because acetaminophen does not damage the kidneys or liver.
    C. The first statement is false because acetaminophen is not an anti-inflammatory. The second statement is true.
    D. Both statements are false.

29. All of the following microbiota EXCEPT ONE produce sulfur and are associated with halitosis. Which one is the EXCEPTION?

    A. *Atopobium parvulum*
    B. *Eubacterium sulci*
    C. *Fusobacterium nucleatum*
    D. *Actinomyces* group

30. The immune system defense that actually breaks down the connective tissue in periodontal disease is

    A. Interferon
    B. Interleukin
    C. Lymphokine
    D. Chemokine
    E. Cytokines

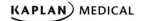

31. A patient with a history of heart disease has sudden chest pain in the office. He takes out his nitroglycerine pills which come out of the bottle as a powder with a strong fetid smell. The office emergency kit has nitroglycerine spray, which is sprayed under the tongue. After 3 doses of metered nitroglycerine spray, the patient is still experiencing chest pain. The patient is mostly likely suffering from

    A. First-degree heart block
    B. Angina pectoris
    C. Myocardial infarction
    D. Congestive heart failure

32. An agar-agar impression was taken on a patient who is having two crowns made for #20 and #19. To prevent distortion, the impression must be removed in what way?

    A. Slowly eased out
    B. Quickly
    C. With a quick snapping motion
    D. Pried out with gloved fingers

33. The maximum safe dosage of lidocaine for a 30 kg child is

    A. 60 mg
    B. 13.2 mg
    C. 0.15 mg
    D. 132 mg
    E. 150 mg

34. For the child in Question #33, how many cartridges is this?

    A. 1
    B. 2
    C. 2.5
    D. 3
    E. 3.6

35. How does secondary hypertension differ from primary hypertension?

    A. 5–10% of hypertension cases are thought to result from secondary causes, such as renal disease, Cushing's syndrome, or endocrine disorders.
    B. 80% of primary hypertension is of unknown origin.
    C. Secondary hypertension is more common than primary hypertension.
    D. Secondary hypertension must be treated first before finding its cause.

36. Which of the following types of amelogenesis imperfecta (a genetic disorder) features enamel with a normal thickness and occlusal thirds of the teeth white in color?

    A. Type 1
    B. Type 2
    C. Type 3
    D. Type 4

37. As teeth develop, the different tissues become specialized. The enamel organ, dental papillae, and dental sac are derived from which of the following tissues?

    A. Ectoderm
    B. Mesoderm
    C. Endoderm
    D. Ectomesenchyme

38. As the dental follicle undergoes change into specialized tissues to produce a crown of a tooth, which tissues lie between the inner and outer enamel epitheliums and provide support for the developing tooth?

    A. Tomes' process and stellate reticulum
    B. Dental lamina and stratum intermedium
    C. Tomes' process and dental lamina
    D. Stellate reticulum and stratum intermedium
    E. Dental lamina and stellate reticulum

39. Deficiencies in vitamins can cause oral manifestations such as cheilosis. Cheilosis might indicate a deficiency in all of the following EXCEPT

   A. Folic acid
   B. Riboflavin
   C. Niacin
   D. Pyridoxine
   E. Biotin

40. A patient with a lower partial denture has an irritation of the vestibule adjacent to where #30 and #31 used to be. It is exophytic, red in color, firm to palpation, and elongated. This lesion is most likely

   A. Giant cell granuloma
   B. Epulis fissuratum
   C. Myxoma
   D. Irritative fibromatosis
   E. Herpangina

41. Certain drugs can induce gingival hyperplasia. Which of the following statements is true about gingival hyperplasia?

   A. Hyperplasia changes the DNA of a cell.
   B. Hyperplasia is an increase in the number of cells.
   C. Hyperplasia is an increase in individual cell size.
   D. Hyperplastic tissues can metastasize.

42. If a patient has a hyper-erupted tooth that is being traumatized, what can occur with the periodontal ligament?

   A. It can atrophy.
   B. It will widen.
   C. The PDL fibers will regenerate.
   D. There will be no change.

43. As plaque forms in the mouth, it undergoes changes in microbiota. As plaque spreads coronally, by what time frame does a more mixed flora of rods, filamentous forms, and fusobacteria thicken?

   A. Day 1–2
   B. Day 2–4
   C. Day 4–7
   D. Day 7–14
   E. Day 14–21

44. Black hairy tongue can occur in smokers and alcoholics as papillae elongate. This condition affects which of the following papillae on the tongue?

   A. Circumvallate
   B. Filiform
   C. Foliate
   D. Fungiform

45. The cranium has many foramina for nerves and blood vessels to pass through. Which cranial bone contains the foramen rotundum and foramen ovale?

   A. Ethmoid
   B. Occipital
   D. Lacrimal
   D. Palatine
   E. Sphenoid

46. A new office employee is offered a hepatitis B vaccination, something mandated by OSHA. What type of immunization is HBIG?

   A. Natural active
   B. Natural passive
   C. Artificial active
   D. Artificial passive

47. New CDC guidelines emphasize maintaining mechanical barriers in the prevention of infection. Which of the following is not a preventative measure?

   A. Keeping intact skin on hands.
   B. Preventing mucous membrane contamination.
   C. Limiting droplet contamination with a saliva ejector.
   D. Washing hands before and after glove removal.
   E. Wearing personnel protective equipment.

48. A patient presents with an acute periodontal infection. Which of the following blood cells is the first line of defense for acute infections?

   A. Eosinophils
   B. Basophils
   C. Erythrocytes
   D. Neutrophils
   E. Monocytes

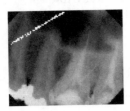

49. What technical error has occurred in the above radiograph?

   A. Bent film
   B. Scratch
   C. Herringbone
   D. Elongation

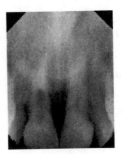

50. In the radiograph above, the radiopaque elongated area between #8 and #9 is called the

   A. Median palatine suture
   B. Maxillary sinus
   C. Inverted Y
   D. Nasal septum
   E. Maxillary tuberosity

51. A patient who smokes a pack of cigarettes a day presents today with heavy stain. This type of stain is

   A. Exogenous extrinsic
   B. Exogenous intrinsic
   C. Endogenous intrinsic
   D. None of the above

52. Which of the following permanent mandibular teeth can develop with a bifurcated root?

   A. Canine
   B. Lateral
   C. Central
   D. First bicuspid

53. A child with a history of epidermis bullosa has presented to the office with a toothache. Epidermis bullosa manifests as ulcers and blisters. In treating the patient's toothache, you could apply all of the following treatments EXCEPT

    A. Topical anti-inflammatory and immuno-suppresant therapy
    B. Topical anesthesia
    C. Injections of collagen
    D. Pad the dental chair to protect elbows, kness and buttocks

54. The pH of fluorides varies, with the strongest being acidulated phosphate fluoride. With acidulated fluoride, the pH is

    A. 3.0–3.5
    B. 4.5–5.0
    C. 5.5–6.5
    D. 8.5–9.0
    E. 9.5–10.0

55. When treating a patient with chronic periodontal disease, the best way to remove endotoxins is through

    A. Polishing
    B. Curet use
    C. Scaling
    D. Ultrasonic scaling
    E. Irrigation

56. Dental hygienists play an important role in educating parents on the value of sealant placement. What would allow for the best retention of a sealant?

    A. Tooth isolated with a rubber dam
    B. Use of a 37% phosphoric acid
    C. Properly etched surface
    D. Tooth rinsed for the proper amount of time

57. Humans have different types of connective tissue throughout their body. Which type of connective tissue is the most abundant?

    A. Reticular fibers
    B. Collagen fibers
    C. Elastic fibers
    D. Ground substance

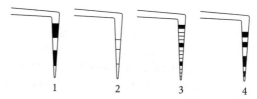

58. In the above diagram, image 3 represents which of the following types of periodontal probes?

    A. Michigan
    B. PSR
    C. Williams colored
    D. PCPUNC
    E. Marquis

59. The electrical activity that initiates a heartbeat begins where in the heart?

    A. AV node
    B. Purkinje fibers
    C. Bundle of His
    D. SA node

60. Of the following microbiota, which organism is the latent virus form of chicken pox that can manifest as shingles?

    A. Epstein Barr
    B. Varicella zoster
    C. B. burgdorferi
    D. S. dysenteriae
    E. C. tetani

61. Autoclaves, statims, and dry heat accomplish sterilization in most dental offices. Which of the following reasons MOST often accounts for incomplete sterilization?

    A. Types of packaging
    B. Misreading the indicators on the packages
    C. Overpacked loads
    D. Incomplete ultrasonic time

62. Your patient has arrived for her recare appointment with a herpes lesion on his lower lip that is in the healing stages. Which of the following lymph nodes is the main drainage for the lower lip?

    A. Submandibular nodes
    B. Submental nodes
    C. Facial nodes
    D. Retroauricular
    E. Occipital

63. Antibiotics can cause various side effects, such as photosensitivity. Which of the following pharmaceuticals can cause photosensitivity?

    A. Doxycycline and minocycline
    B. Azithromycin and clarithromycin
    C. Cefuroxime and cephalexin
    D. Acyclovir and zidovudine
    E. Rifampin and isoniazid

64. Which of the following teeth usually erupts first in the mouth?

    A. Mandibular first molars
    B. Mandibular central incisors
    C. Maxillary first molars
    D. Maxillary central incisors

65. A patient who requested a gold tooth on #8 has arrived for the insertion appointment. After the tooth has arrived from the lab, you polish it with _____ before taking it to the operatory.

    A. Tin oxide
    B. Pumice
    C. Rouge
    D. Sand disk
    E. Diatomaceous earth

66. Which of the following disinfectants should not be used for a reversible hydrocolloid impression?

    A. Glutaraldehyde
    B. Phenolic glutaraldehyde
    C. Iodophors
    D. Chlorine bleach 1:10

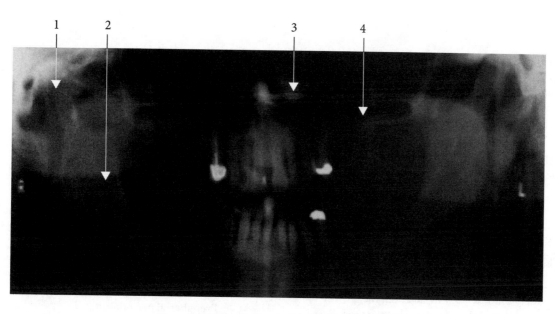

Panographic radiograph for Questions 67–70

67. In the panographic radiograph above, arrow #1 is pointing to which anatomical landmark?

   A. Coronoid process
   B. Meniscus
   C. Condyle
   D. Zygomatic arch
   E. Submandibular fossa

68. In the panographic radiograph above, arrow #2 is pointing to the anatomical landmark of the

   A. Internal oblique ridge
   B. External oblique
   C. Mental foramen
   D. Mandibular canal
   E. Lingual foramen

69. In the panographic radiograph above, arrow #3 is pointing to the anatomical landmark of the

   A. Maxillary torus
   B. Anterior nasal spine
   C. Median palatine suture
   D. Hamular process
   E. Maxilla

70. In the panographic radiographabove, arrow #4 is pointing to the anatomical landmark of the

   A. Nasal fossa
   B. Maxillary sinus
   C. Inverted Y
   D. Maxillary tuberosity

71. Your patient is being evaluated for an orthodontic referral. You find that the buccal groove of the mandibular first molar is distal to the mesiobuccal cusp of the maxillary first molar by at least the width of a premolar. The mandible is retruded with one or more of the maxillary incisors being retruded. What classification should be written on the referral slip?

    A. Class I
    B. Class II Division I
    C. Class II Division II
    D. Class III

72. A patient's mother is worried about the growth pattern of her child's profile. Which of the following occlusions does this child have if the distal of the mandibular canine is mesial to the mesial surface of the maxillary canine by at least half the width of a premolar?

    A. Class I
    B. Class II
    C. Class III
    D. None of the above

73. All of the following patients EXCEPT one could require an antibiotic premedication. Which of the following is the EXCEPTION?

    A. Someone with spina bifida
    B. An uncontrolled diabetic
    C. Someone with any autoimmune disease
    D. Someone with inflammatory rheumatoid arthritis
    E. Someone with systemic lupus erythematosis

74. What fluorosis classification as described by Dean would include opaque white areas that cover less than 50% of the tooth surface?

    A. Very mild
    B. Mild
    C. Moderate
    D. Severe

75. According to the American Academy of Periodontology, which of the following is not considered to be an aggressive periodontitis?

    A. Necrotizing periodontitis
    B. Juvenile periodontitis
    C. Prepubertal periodontitis
    D. Rapid progressive periodontitis
    E. Abscesses of the periodontium

76. A custom-fabricated implant that fits over the bone and under the periosteum is a(n)

    A. Endosseous implant
    B. Ceramic implant
    C. Subperiosteal implant
    D. Transosteal implant

77. According to Heifetz and Horowitz, the Certainly Lethal Dose (CLD) of fluoride can become toxic for ALL children at what dose?

    A. 320 mg
    B. 422 mg
    C. 538 mg
    D. 655 mg
    E. 500 mg

78. When taking radiographs, if you are changing from an mA of 16 at 5 impulses to an mA of 8, how many impulses would you need for the new mA?

    A. 2 impulses
    B. 10 impulses
    C. 18 impulses
    D. 26 impulses

79. When modifying a BID from 6" at 3 seconds to a 1" BID, what is the new exposure time?

    A. 0.09 seconds
    B. 0.08 seconds
    C. 0.02 seconds
    D. 0.1 seconds
    E. 0.2 seconds

80. Hemophilia is a genetic disorder passed on to males by females who are carriers of the gene. Hemophilia B patients lack which protein factor necessary for blood clotting?

    A. Factor VIII
    B. Factor IX
    C. Factor XI
    D. Stuart factor

81. Radiographic film magnification is affected by

    A. Umbra
    B. Penumbra
    C. Object-to-film distance
    D. Source-to-film distance

82. Which of the following medications is a loop diuretic that a patient with hypertension might be prescribed?

    A. Propranolol
    B. Furosemide
    C. Lidocaine
    D. Diltiazem
    E. Provastatin

83. The medication in Question #82 is a diuretic that affects which part of the kidney?

    A. Arterioles
    B. Loop of Henle
    C. Glomerulus
    D. Nephrons
    E. Cortex

84. Von Willebrands disease is a genetic disorder that affects

    A. Factor XI
    B. Platelet cohesiveness
    C. Lipids released by the lining of blood cells
    D. Men only

85. Antipyretic agents affect the

    A. Thyroid
    B. Parathyroid
    C. Hypothalamus
    D. Gallbladder
    E. Pituitary gland

86. Your patient suddenly becomes unconscious, with her eyes rolling back in her head. There had been no prior symptoms. What would you do first?

    A. Use ammonia aromatics
    B. Place her in a recovery position
    C. Start CPR
    D. Give 100% oxygen by bag valve mask

87. Which of the following is NOT a symptom of Parkinson's disease?

    A. Loss of coordination and imbalance
    B. Difficulty in swallowing with possible choking
    C. Fixed facial stare with decreased facial mobility
    D. Limp muscles
    E. Head-nodding

KAPLAN) MEDICAL

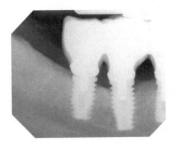

88. Which of the following types of implants is pictured here?

    A. Endosseous
    B. Subperitoneal
    C. Transosteal
    D. Ceramic

89. Etching materials can be applied in different ways. When applying a gel, what is the best method for obtaining a properly etched surface?

    A. Gently dab the surface
    B. Apply and leave alone
    C. Etch for 10 seconds
    D. Dab vigorously for 20 seconds

90. Which of the following cardiac pharmaceuticals can cause gingival hyperplasia?

    A. Amyl nitrate
    B. Procainimide
    C. Nifedipine
    D. Bretylium
    E. Atorvastatin

91. Many arteries and veins carry blood to and from the head and neck region. The external carotid artery supplies blood to all the following except one. Which of the following is the EXCEPTION?

    A. Muscles of the face
    B. Floor of the mouth
    C. Lower and upper lips
    D. Soft palate and palatine muscles
    E. Brain

92. All of the following things are associated with Vitamin K except one. Which of the following is the EXCEPTION?

    A. Blood clotting
    B. Normal liver function
    C. Dark green leafy vegetables
    D. Prevent night blindness

93. What type of immunity occurs when the B cells release antibodies that interact with microbes?

    A. Humoral
    B. Acquired immunity
    C. Cell mediated immunity
    D. GALT

94. All of the following stains except one are removed by a routine polishing during a pediatric prophylaxis. Which of the following is the EXCEPTION?

    A. Green stain
    B. Orange stain
    C. Brown stain
    D. Yellow stain

95. Under the Health Insurance Portability and Accountability Act (HIPAA) of 1996, all of the following statements are true except one. Which of the following is the EXCEPTION?

    A. A patient's medical history may be shared with another health professional for treatment purposes.
    B. Denial of an individual's medical insurance is based upon health status.
    C. A patient's information is kept confidential.
    D. A patient's treatment information may be submitted electronically for payment of services.

96. An enzyme-linked immunosorbent assay screens human blood serum. If a patient is suspected of being HIV-positive, what test would he be given?

    A. Mantoux
    B. ELISA
    C. PTT
    D. PPD
    E. Western blot

97. The tooth-desensitizing agent that works best and is recommended for all patients is

    A. Potassium nitrate
    B. Stannous fluoride
    C. Sodium fluoride
    D. Calcium hydroxide
    E. None of the above

98. Which of the following foods is not a source of vitamin E?

    A. Wheat germ
    B. Dark leafy vegetables
    C. Carrots
    D. Vegetable oil

99. What is a contraindication of using the push stroke for calculus removal?

    A. Lateral pressure with a push stroke removes heavy calculus deposits only.
    B. Adaptation to concave root surfaces may be difficult.
    C. Calculus deposits may become burnished.
    D. Calculus deposits may become embedded in soft tissue.

100. Zinc oxide and eugenol could be used for all the following except one. Which one is this EXCEPTION?

    A. Temporary filling
    B. Periodontal pack
    C. Oil based cement
    D. Class II restoration
    E. Impression

101. Your patient states that she feels "funny" and suddenly becomes unconscious. Upon checking the pupils, you see that one is dilated and the other constricted. This patient has most likely experienced

    A. Seizure
    B. Cerebrovascular accident
    C. Drug overdose
    D. Diabetic coma
    E. Insulin shock

102. The periodontal dressing placed after a periodontal surgery does all the following things except one. Which one is this EXCEPTION?

    A. Supports clot formation
    B. Prevents irritation to the surgical site
    C. Supports mobile teeth
    D. Retains sutures in place
    E. Stains teeth

103. Of the following foramina of the cranial bones, from which does the mandibular branch of the trigeminal nerve exit?

    A. Foramen ovale
    B. Foramen rotundum
    C. Foramen magnum
    D. Foramen spinosum

104. The main component of a reversible hydrocolloid impression is

    A. Polymer
    B. Agar
    C. Zinc
    D. Gypsum
    E. Sodium alginate

105. Which of the following is true of the acquired pellicle?

    A. It does not provide a barrier to protect against acids.
    B. It is a nidus for bacteria.
    C. Calculus is unable to attach there.
    D. It is always stained.

106. Which of the following gingival conditions is typically associated with a temporary hormonal imbalance, and can occur in both males and females?

    A. Kaposi sarcoma
    B. Fistula
    C. Pyogenic granuloma
    D. Wickham's striae

107. The safest time to take radiographs on a pregnant female is

    A. First trimester
    B. Second trimetster
    C. Third trimester
    D. None of the above

108. In autoclaves, heat sterilization takes place at 250° F for 20-30 minutes. Which of the following biological indicators is used with autoclaves to verify heat sterilization?

    A. *Aeromonas hydrophila*
    B. *Bacillus stearothermophilus*
    C. *Neisseria lactamica*
    D. *Bacillus subtilis*
    E. *Bacillus lentus*

109. A single tooth that is experiencing premature contact when occluding with the opposite arch is most likely in

    A. Mesioversion
    B. Infraversion
    C. Buccoversion
    D. Supraversion
    E. Distoversion

110. If a patient experiences a pulmonary embolism, the first local effect to the tissue of the lung would be

    A. Ischemia
    B. Necrosis
    C. Dysplasia
    D. Hypertrophy
    E. Hemorrhage

111. A patient has arrived with a facial lesion that has fluid inside and is movable. This lesion is a(n)

    A. Ulcer
    B. Papule
    C. Macule
    D. Bulla
    E. Caruncle

112. The least effective method for detecting calculus on the lingual aspect of the maxillary 1st molars and maxillary 2nd premolars is

    A. Explorer
    B. Bitewing radiograph
    C. Appearance of adjacent gingival tissue
    D. Air

113. A mucocele is a blocked minor salivary gland. The most common common site for a mucocele is the

    A. Palate
    B. Upper lip
    C. Buccal mucosa
    D. Lower lip
    E. Tongue

114. Which of the following is the chief reason that sealants are placed as soon as possible on a tooth after it erupts into the mouth?

    A. They cover the pits and fissures.
    B. They act as a hinderance or barrier.
    C. They prevent bacteria from entering the pits and fissures.
    D. They help to prevent cavities.

115. Where does collimation actually start in the dental x-ray unit?

    A. The tungsten
    B. The target
    C. The focusing cup
    D. Diaphragm
    E. Collimator

116. Which of the following is NOT typically an oral characteristic of a Down syndrome patient?

    A. Fissured tongue
    B. Class II malocclusion
    C. Delayed eruption
    D. Enamel dysplasia
    E. Short crown to root ratio

117. A patient returns for her 6-week evaluation after a root debridement. The tissue around #30 and #31 seems not to have responded very well. When evaluating this area, what is the MOST important criterion to consider with respect to its prognosis?

    A. Edematous tissue
    B. Tissue contour
    C. Bleeding upon probing
    D. Loss of attachment
    E. Presence of purulence

118. An otherwise healthy college student home for spring break presents with bleeding gingiva, catered punched out-papillae, and a gray pseudo-membrane. Radiographically, the bone levels are normal. This patient most likely suffers from

    A. Periodontal abscess
    B. Necrotizing periodontitis
    C. Juvenile periodontitis
    D. Necrotizing ulcerative gingivitis

119. Palliative measures for the patient in Question #118 would include all the following except one. Which one is this EXCEPTION?

    A. Mechanical debridement
    B. Topical anesthesia
    C. Reappoint in 1 week for second debridement.
    D. Oral hygiene instructions
    E. Repair any defective margins on any restorations

120. Cell immunity takes place in many parts of the body. What part of the body matures the T lymphocytes for immunity?

    A. Hypothalamus
    B. Bone marrow
    C. Thymus
    D. Spleen
    E. Liver

Scenario for Questions 121–125

A 43-year-old woman has generalized, chronic, moderate to severe periodontitis, and subgingival calculus with moderate to heavy bleeding upon probing throughout the mouth. During the first appointment with the dental hygienist, she states that she is brushing 3 times daily and flosses when she remembers. She has a history of a heart murmur, and hypertension, and was recently diagnosed with diabetes. The patient is also 75 pounds overweight. The patient is currently taking Toprol XL 50 mg, once daily, HCTZ 100 mg, once daily and glucophage 100mg BID. The patient verified that she took her prophylactic premedication prior to today's visit.

121. What should be the first step in treating this patient?

    A. Root debridement
    B. Prophylaxis
    C. Tell the patient that flossing daily is essential
    D. Patient counseling and education

122. The least effective way to instruct on flossing is to

    A. Demonstrate flossing first on a manikin
    B. Demonstrate flossing in the patient's mouth
    C. Have the patient demonstrate flossing in her own mouth
    D. Dispense a pamphlet

123. Which of the following conditions most often requires premedication prior to dental treatment?

    A. Heart murmur
    B. Hypertension
    C. Diabetes
    D. All of the above

124. During the patient education and counseling portion of the appointment, the dental hygienist uses disclosing solution. The lingual surfaces of the mandibular molars and buccal surfaces of the maxillary molars show a considerable amount of plaque. Which of the following would be the most likely reason?

    A. The patient is not being honest about her oral hygiene regime.
    B. The patient is inadvertently missing this area.
    C. The patient is not flossing.
    D. The patient is using a toothbrush that is soft.

125. The patient is taking glucophage for

    A. Hypertension
    B. Heart murmur
    C. Diabetes
    D. Obesity

126. A dry mouth can be caused by all the following pharmaceutical compounds except one. Which one is this EXCEPTION?

    A. Levadopa
    B. Molindone
    C. Atropine
    D. Pilocarpine
    E. Haloperidol

127. A patient is sent to the oral surgeon for the difficult extraction of #1 with general anesthesia. What is the drug of choice to relax the larynx and laryngeal muscles so that the patient can be intubated during surgery?

    A. Succinylcholine
    B. Pentothal
    C. Versed
    D. Halothane
    E. Nitrous oxide

128. A topical anesthetic is rapidly absorbing into the bloodstream and should be applied to a very large area. An example of a topical anesthetic is Benzocaine, which is an ester.

    A. Both statements are true.
    B. The first statement is true. The second statement is false because Benzocaine is an amide.
    C. The first statement is false because topical anesthetics should be applied to a small area. The second statement is true.
    D. Both statements are false.

129. Bone has varying degrees of density. Which of the following structures is not seen radiographically?

    A. Trabecular bone
    B. Alveolar bone
    C. Cancellous bone
    D. Lamina propria
    E. Lamina dura

130. During fetal development, what tooth structure is NOT developed within the dental sac?

    A. Dentin
    B. Periodontal ligament
    C. Alveolar bone
    D. Cementum

131. If the medial nasal process fails to fuse with the maxillary process as a baby develops, when would this occur?

    A. Weeks 4–7 of the embryonic period
    B. Weeks 4–7 of the fetal period
    C. Weeks 8–12 of the embryonic period
    D. Weeks 8–12 of the fetal period
    E. Weeks 12–16 of the fetal period

132. Which of the following best describes the difference between ultrasonic and sonic instruments?

    A. Ultrasonics use vibrations.
    B. Sonic scalers are more efficient than ultrasonics.
    C. Ultrasonics use a higher frequency than sonic scalers.
    D. Ultrasonics use a lower frequency than sonic scalers.

133. The distal aspect of the maxillary canine has a 4 mm pocket. What type of shank would be found on the dental instrument best suited removal of subgingival deposits?

    A. Long and straight
    B. Long and angulated
    C. Short and straight
    D. Short and angulated

134. Ultrasonic instrumentation would be MOST beneficial for which of the following conditions?

    A. Stain
    B. Overhanging margins of amalgam restorations
    C. Supragingival and subgingival calculus deposits
    D. Supragingival calculus only

135. Sharp instruments help dental hygienists on a daily basis. What best explains why having a sharp instrument is so important?

    A. It is easier to remove deposits.
    B. It is easier to perform debridement.
    C. Patient comfort.
    D. It lessens clinician tedium.
    E. It retains the integrity of the instrument.

136. Which of the following terms features a bent root?

    A. Fusion
    B. Attrition
    C. Dilaceration
    D. Enamel pearl
    E. Gemination

137. Fluorides come in different forms and strengths. Acidulated phosphate fluoride solutions should be stored only in containers that are

    A. Etched glass
    B. Clear glass
    C. Polyethylene
    D. All of the above

138. Trisomy means having one or a few diploid chromosomes become triploid chromosomes. Trisomy 13, trisomy 18, and trisomy 22 have all of the following things in common except one. Which one is this EXCEPTION?

    A. Cleft lip or palate
    B. Mental retardation
    C. Congenital heart defects
    D. Anencephaly
    E. Rocker bottom feet

139. Some dental hygiene students are putting together a caries control program for a local orphanage. All of the following are essential in creating a caries control program except one. Which one is this EXCEPTION?

    A. Routine oral prophylaxis
    B. Routine personal hygiene
    C. Routine dental exam and treatment
    D. A balanced diet that is low in fermentable carbohydrates
    E. Fluoridation of drinking water or topical applications of fluoride

140. A patient presents to your office with a 7 mm pocket on the mesial aspect of #14. The instrument most appropriate for subgingival deposit removal is

    A. Columbia 13/14
    B. Gracey 7/8
    C. Gracey 11/12
    D. Gracey 13/14
    E. Gracey 17/18

141. A reduction in the number of infectious agents on a dental unit is known as

    A. Asepsis
    B. Attenuation
    C. Sterilization
    D. Disinfection

142. To keep a curet tip from breaking, what would help the MOST?

    A. Design of the blade
    B. Flexibility of the shank
    C. Sterilization process used
    D. Sharpening technique used

143. Universal curets can be used both supragingivally and subgingivally for debridement. What is the total number of cutting edges on a universal curet?

    A. 2
    B. 3
    C. 4
    D. 6

144. Egg contains albumin. The biologic value of eggs is high because the proteins

    A. Are rich in biotin.
    B. Are destroyed when cooked.
    C. Are low in cholesterol.
    D. Contain all essential amino acids.
    E. Contain the proper amount of calcium.

145. Six weeks post-root debridement treatment, your periodontal patient returns for evaluation. What sign would best indicate that the patient still has active periodontal disease?

    A. A change in tissue color
    B. A loss of stippling
    C. Tooth sensitivity
    D. Bleeding upon probing
    E. Pocket depth greater than 3 mm

146. When sharpening an instrument, what is the best way to determine that you have achieved sharpness?

    A. The blade has a wire edge.
    B. The edge of the blade reflects light.
    C. The edge of the blade does not reflect light.
    D. None of the above

147. Ultrasonic scalers make life easier for a dental hygienist. All of the following conditions except one would be contraindicated for the use of the ultrasonic scaler. Which one is this EXCEPTION?

    A. Susceptibility to infections
    B. Veneers
    C. Tuberculosis
    D. Difficulty swallowing
    E. Shielded pacemaker

148. Patients can have different degrees of sensitivity while receiving dental treatment. Which of the following would produce excessive heat during polishing?

    A. Use of an air-water syringe
    B. Using a low speed with a fine powder
    C. Using a high speed with a dry agent
    D. Using light intermittent pressure
    E. Using high speed suction

149. Which of the following instruments would best remove moderate supragingival deposits from #25 and #26 lingual?

    A. Gracey curet
    B. Jaquette 33
    C. Columbia 12/13
    D. 204SD

150. When instructing your dental patient on oral hygiene, your goal is to

    A. Make him aware of his needs
    B. Help him to overcome dental fears
    C. Help him to accept his dental treatment plan
    D. Help prevent disease

151. A nurse at a local detention center for juveniles has recently contacted the county public health hygienist to present an oral health care program. The detention center has 35 juveniles aged 8-12, a director, a nurse, and a doctor who visits weekly. After contacting the appropriate personnel, what should be the first step in establishing the program?

    A. Determine the needs of the target population
    B. Develop a program goal
    C. Design the program
    D. Collect baseline information

152. After completing the project in Question #153, the administrator decides to report the results in a statewide governmental report on the oral health status of juvenile delinquent residents. She mails the results, including the dental records of each juvenile in the facility. By doing so, she is violating which of the following legal or ethical responsibilities?

    A. Previous approval by the dental hygienist
    B. Confidentiality of the juvenile delinquent residents
    C. Consent by state officials
    D. None of the above

153. The pharyngeal tonsils drain primarily through the

    A. Superior deep cervical lymph nodes
    B. Inferior deep cervical lymph nodes
    C. Retropharyngeal lymph nodes
    D. Retroauricular lymph nodes

154. Stenson's duct of the encapsulated parotid gland passes through which of the following facial muscles?

    A. Masseter
    B. Buccinator
    C. Depressor anguli
    D. Lateral pterygoid
    E. Zygomaticus major

155. Pilocarpine is used to stimulate saliva flow. What type of central nervous system stimulation occurs with this pharmaceutical?

    A. Sympathomimetic
    B. Sympatholytic
    C. Parasympathomimetic
    D. Parasympatholytic

156. Tetracycline is an oral medication that should be avoided by all of the following individuals except one. Which one is this EXCEPTION?

    A. Children under 12 years of age
    B. Nursing mothers
    C. Pregnant females
    D. A 14-year old with aggressive juvenile periodontitis

157. Tetracycline has a longer half-life in gingival crevicular fluid. Which of the following micro-biota of periodontal disease is particularly susceptible to tetracycline?

    A. *Porphyromonas gingivalis*
    B. *Prevotella intermedia*
    C. *Streptococcus mitis*
    D. *Actinobacillus actinomycetemcomitans*
    E. *Bacteroides forsythus*

158. Transient bacteremias may occur from all of the following dental procedures except one. Which one is this EXCEPTION?

    A. Root debridement
    B. Dental extractions
    C. Orthodontic wire placement
    D. Tooth crown preparation
    E. Subgingival antibiotic placement

159. When exposing radiographs, which of the following kVp's is ideal for the detection of bone loss with periodontal disease?

    A. 60 kVp
    B. 70 kVp
    C. 80 kVp
    D. 90 kVp

160. Kilovoltage is controlled by which part of a dental x-ray unit?

    A. Anode
    B. Cathode
    C. Target
    D. Collimator
    E. Focusing cup

161. If a nasopalatine duct cyst is not excised, all of the following can occur except one. Which one is this EXCEPTION?

    A. Tooth displacement
    B. Sub-labial swelling
    C. Produce an ameloblastoma
    D. Palatal swelling

162. A patient who seems to have a moon-shaped face, buffalo hump, and large abdomen probably suffers from

    A. Hyperthyroidism
    B. Hypothyroidism
    C. Hypercortisolism
    D. Hypocortisolism

163. Gingival indices are irreversible indices. Gingival indices measure gingival inflammation.

    A. Both statements are true.
    B. The first statement it true. The second statement is false because it measures gingival recession.
    C. The first statement is false because it is a reversible index. The second statement is true.
    D. Both statements are false.

164. Parkinson's disease is a disorder of the central nervous system. Patients with this disease lack which of the following neurotransmitters?

    A. Acetylcholine
    B. Epinephrine
    C. Norepinephrine
    D. Dopamine
    E. Serotonin

165. Insulin produced in the pancreas is intended to

    A. Break down the glycogen in the liver when the blood sugar gets too low.
    B. Unlock the cells to allow glucose into the cells.
    C. Produce glycogen.
    D. Produce glucagon.

166. Which of the following microbiota is transmitted by airborne droplets, and produces a mononucleosis-like illness in adults and severe illness in children?

    A. Rhinovirus
    B. Cytomegalovirus
    C. Connavirus
    D. Bordetella pertussis
    E. Adenovirus

KAPLAN MEDICAL

167. In the healing process of a wound, what blood cell is the most numerous with chronic infections?

    A. Eosinophils
    B. Monocytes
    C. Neutrophils
    D. Basophils
    E. Platelets

168. Which of the following microorganisms causes an illness that can result in mulberry molars?

    A. Varicella zoster
    B. *Treponema pallidum*
    C. Rubella virus
    D. Rubeola virus
    E. *Bordetella pertussis*

169. A secondary intention healing could occur from which of the following periodontal procedures?

    A. A surgical incision
    B. Periodontal flap surgery
    C. Palatal donor site
    D. None of the above

170. Transmissible spongiform encephalopathies or prions are new microbiota that the CDC is unsure of as far as the disease transmission route. Prions are associated with which of the following conditions?

    A. Creutzfeldt-Jakob disease
    B. Peutz-Jegher syndrome
    C. Papillon-Lefèvre syndrome
    D. Pierre Robin syndrome

171. Cretinism is a hormonal problem caused by

    A. Hyperthyroidism
    B. Hypothyroidism
    C. Hypercortisolism
    D. Hypocortisolism

172. A papule or vesicular lesion that has changed to a bulla begins to look like a bull's-eye target. This lesion occurs with which of the following conditions?

    A. Pemphigoid
    B. Pemphigus
    C. Erythema multiforme
    D. Epidermis bullosa

173. Which of the following positioning errors causes elongation of a radiograph?

    A. Not enough vertical angle
    B. Too much vertical angle
    C. Incorrect horizontal angle
    D. Incorrect patient positioning
    E. None of the above

174. A patient on a loop diuretic may need which of the following supplemental medications as well?

    A. Sodium bicarbonate
    B. Adenosine
    C. Digitalis
    D. K-Dur

175. A patient arrives in a wheelchair. He cannot move his lower extremities and needs help into the dental chair. This patient is

    A. Hemiplegic
    B. Paraplegic
    C. Quadraplegic
    D. None of the above

176. When gathering information to produce a dental index, all of the following are criteria for a good dental index EXCEPT one. Which of the following is the EXCEPTION?

    A. Reliability
    B. Validity
    C. Ease of calibration
    D. Flexibility

177. After teaching a 3rd grade class, a dental hygienist gives a quiz to determine the effectiveness of instruction. The mean score is 8 and a standard deviation is 1. Which of the following interpretations can be made?

    A. The lowest score is 8
    B. The highest score is 9
    C. The lowest score is 7
    D. The highest score is 10
    E. Most of the scores are between 7 and 9

178. Which of the following correlation coefficients indicates a strong relationship in a statistical measure?

    A. −0.30
    B. +0.50
    C. −0.95
    D. −0.05
    E. +0.05

Questions 179–182 refer to the following scenario:

A nurse at a local orphanage has asked the county public health hygienist to present an oral health care program. The orphange has 50 children, aged 2–10, a nurse, and a doctor who visits biweekly.

The dental hygienist consults with the administration and interviews the healthcare staff, and finds that they feel ill equipped to convey oral hygiene instruction to the children. Dental care visits to the residents are infrequent, available oral hygiene aids are nominal, and mobile equipment for preventive care is non-existent here. The entire staff meets monthly to address issues that face the facility.

179. After determining the needs of the target population, what should be the next step to establishing the oral health care program?

    A. Survey the needs
    B. Goal identification
    C. Design the program
    D. Finance the program
    E. Prioritize the list

180. To determine the caries incidence in this population, which of the following indices would be used?

    A. deft
    B. Deft
    C. DMFT
    D. dmft
    E. DEFT

181. All of the following items except one are considered in program evaluation. Which one is this EXCEPTION?

    A. Inter-rater reliability deals
    B. Intra-rater reliability deals
    C. Validity of measuring instrument
    D. Randomization of the population

182. Which of the following would NOT be appropriate for assessing the outcome of the oral hygiene program?

    A. Comparisons of pre and post indices
    B. Inventory of oral hygiene aids and mobile dental equipment
    C. Survey with the administration, and staff.
    D. Comparisons of this program with other programs the dental hygienist has administered.

KAPLAN) MEDICAL

183. The most cost-efficient way to determine the needs of dental patients is to

    A. Distribute a questionnaire.
    B. Conduct personal interviews.
    C. Observe oral hygiene practices.
    D. Use an oral hygiene index.

184. Which scenario makes most efficient use of a public dental hygienist's time?

    A. Providing oral hygiene instruction to elementary and middle school classrooms.
    B. Instructing faculty at elementary and middle schools on the proper administration of fluoride for the school's fluoride-rinse program.
    C. Conducting oral health screenings.
    D. Providing preventive services to elementary and middle school children.
    E. Educating parents.

185. Which of the following is a long-term study?

    A. Randomized study
    B. Longitudinal study
    C. Double blind study
    D. Systemic random study

186. Food poisoning occurred at one of the local restaurants where 80 dental hygienists were holding their ADHA meeting. After the health department completes its investigation, what type of study will it use to determine the cause of the illness?

    A. Retrospective
    B. Experimental
    C. Prospective
    D. Longitudinal

187. When examiners collected data of an oral health screening of 1,000 patients, they found the following results. From this data, what was the average DMF for this group?

    | Carious lesions | 3,380 |
    | Extracted teeth | 385 |
    | Filled teeth | 2,135 |

    A. 2.5
    B. 2.9
    C. 5.5
    D. 5.9
    E. 7.7

188. An index that measures a stable variable consistently at different intervals is called

    A. Valid
    B. Acceptable
    C. Objective
    D. Reliable

189. A group of dental hygiene students was asked to write a study on the decay rate of a certain tribe of native Americans in a western state. Where would the students go to research the latest statistics on dental disease?

    A. Library of Congress
    B. National Institute of Health
    C. Dental abstracts from JADA
    D. American Dental Association
    E. Medline

190. A patient's radiograph reveals a carious lesion on the mesial of #29. What classification of restoration would this be?

    A. Class I
    B. Class II
    C. Class III
    D. Class IV
    E. Class V

191. A public health dental hygienist is working with a school system to offer healthier snacks in vending machines. Cold vending machines now distribute vegetables and fruits. The public health hygienist examines the students over a period of time to track the rate of carious lesions. During the study, what type of group is this school system considered?

  A. Stratified sampling
  B. Experimental group
  C. Control group
  D. Probability sample

192. Of the following values, which is the mode?

    3, 2, 5, 3, 7, 6, 3, 2, 7, 6, 2

  A. 7
  B. 6
  C. 3
  D. 2
  E. Both 2 and 3

Community Dental Health Case Study

You live in a rural community with a population under 40,000. The median income is $55,000 per year for a family of 4. Since this is a rural community, 80% of the population is using well water. The community's water supply is not fluoridated due to the cost. The primary crop grown in this community is tobacco. A large percentage of the population is transient due to it being a farming community that has many migrant workers that live in the area during the spring through autumn as farm workers. Most of the workers speak primarily Spanish. Untreated dental disease is prominent here because access to dental care is difficult. 75% of the men in this community use some form of tobacco, and many started to use chew in their teens. Last year cancer and heart disease were the number one cause of death in this community.

The dental public health department is launching a dental department that will help to address the needs of this community. As the public health hygienist, your role is to design and implement a preventive program that would benefit this population. Answer the following questions based upon the above scenario.

193. What would be the first step to determining the needs of this population?

  A. Implementation
  B. Evaluation
  C. Assessment
  D. Treatment

194. Which of the following indices would be used to determine the periodontal needs of this community?

  A. OHI-S
  B. GI
  C. DMFT
  D. Deft
  E. The Community Periodontal Index of Treatment Needs

195. All of the following are access to care issues for this population EXCEPT one. Which of the following is the EXCEPTION?

  A. Finance
  B. Language
  C. Fluoridation of the water supply
  D. Transportation

196. What would be the best way for the health department to initially address the tobacco use issue?

    A. Provide free oral cancer screenings at a local public health fair.

    B. Place posters in public locations that show what a cancerous lesion in the oral cavity would look like.

    C. Send out pamphlets to all homes in the community about the dangers of tobacco use.

    D. Enlist the help of other health care workers in the community to participate in a health fair for the community with a focus on cancer.

197. In order to determine the unmet caries rate of the adult populations, which index would you, the public health hygienist, use?

    A. Deft

    B. deft

    C. Dmft

    D. DMFT

    E. DEMT

198. Since most of the population does not receive the benefit of fluoridated water, what would be the most cost effective way to supply preventive treatment to the community?

    A. Start a sealant program in the elementary schools

    B. Start a monthly fluoride mouth rinse program

    C. Have all students receive an examination, prophylaxis, and professional fluoride treatment once a year.

    D. Fluoridation of the school's water supply

199. When educating the public about the dangers of oral cancer and teaching individuals to perform self-screenings on a monthly basis, what level on the learning ladder is reached?

    A. Unawareness

    B. Self interest

    C. Physiologic

    D. Involvement

    E. Social

200. Upon further study of the community, the public health hygienist discovers that the mean starting age for tobacco is age 16, with a standard deviation of 2 years. What range would support the average starting age for tobacco?

    A. 15–17

    B. 14–17

    C. 14–18

    D. 15–19

Answer Explanations: Component A

1. **C**

The patient has probably overdosed on the Percodan. These symptoms include confusion, shortness of breath, low blood pressure, slowed heart rate, nausea, and pinpoint pupils.

A. Flu-like symptoms would not include pinpoint pupils.

B. Tachycardia is a heart rate that is too fast and does not cause pinpoint pupils.

D. Myasthenia gravis is a chronic autoimmune neuromuscular disease characterized by a weakness of the skeletal muscles.

2. **C**

Naloxone should be used to unlock the Percodan (agonist) from the cells.

A. Nubain would be used for pain.

B. Naldecon is an antihistamine.

D. Nizoral is an antifungal.

E. Nabilone is an antiemetic.

3. **D**

Rapid breathing and a fruity (ketonees) breath smell are not side effects of too little insulin. Too *much* insulin can cause these things in diabetics.

4. **C**

Intensifying screens do not need more radiation for exposure; they need less. There are 2 intensifying screens in each cassette. Less radiation—not more—is needed since the screens contain phosphor. The phosphor emits light onto the film when the radiation ions collide with it, exposing the film.

5. **E**

Radiation that produces an ion when the atom is missing an electron and takes on a net-positive charge is called photoelectric effect.

A. Compton effect occurs when a photon with sufficient energy collides with an outer electron, ejecting it from its orbit without transferring all of its energy to the recoil electron. The photon then goes off in a different direction with less energy.

B. Classical scattering occurs when a low energy photon that is unable to eject an electron excites it instead by transferring its low energy. The photon ceases to exist while the vibrating electron becomes an x-ray photon that exits that atom.

C. Thompson effect is the same thing as classical scattering.

D. Indirect effect is the effect of x-ray photons on free radicals in the body to cause radiolysis.

6. **A**

This child likely has acute herpetic gingivostomatitis.

B. Juvenile periodontitis is an early onset aggressive periodontitis characterized by extreme bone loss in usually localized areas. These patients have neither high plaque levels nor systemic symptoms.

C. Rapid progressive periodontitis might be seen in a young adult aged 20–30 with rapid bone and connective tissue loss. Systemic symptoms do not occur.

D. Necrotizing ulcerative periodontitis presents with gray pseudomembrane, and punched-out papillae with fever and malaise.

7. B

The most serious concern for this child would be dehydration, since he will have a hard time swallowing.

A. Malnutrition is a secondary concern since dehydration occurs first.

C. Gingivitis is an oral concern but is not as serious as dehydration.

D. Vesicular lesions that extend onto the face are not life-threatening.

8. C

Cancer of the tongue is called rhabdomyosarcoma, a striated muscle cancer that affects skeletal muscle and the tongue.

A. Leiomyosarcoma is smooth muscle cancer of the digestive tract, blood vessels, or respiratory system.

B. A Schwannoma is a tumor of the myelin sheath covering nerve cells.

D. Neurosarcoma is cancer of nerve cells.

E. Chondrosarcoma is cancer that affects cartilage.

9. B

This is a dentigerous cyst, the kind of cyst that arises from the reduced enamel epithelium.

A. Residual cyst occurs after a tooth is extracted if the radicular cyst at the root apex was not also removed.

C. Primordial cyst arises from the odontogenic epithelium and is often located in the mandibular 3rd molar region.

D. Globulomaxillary cyst arises from odontogenic epithelium and is located between the maxillary lateral and canine.

E. Median mandibular cysts originate from mesenchyme, and develop at the midline of the merger of the two mandibular prominences.

10. C

Stone is a rigid material that is a beta hemi-hydrate. The particles are more regularly shaped so they require little water, making the material stronger.

A. Gypsum is what plaster and stone are derived from.

B. Sodium borate is a retardant that can be added to rigid impression materials.

D. Plaster is an alpha hemi-hydrate of irregular particles; it requires a lot of water, thus decreasing its strength.

11. E

Patients with bulimia do not usually have lanugo, the downy hairy growth seen in many anorexia nervosa patients.

12. C

A nasopalatine cyst is heart-shaped, though it is truly an ovoid cyst. It appears heart-shaped because of the radiopacity of the nasal septum.

A. Globulomaxillary cyst is pear-shaped; it develops in the area of the maxillary lateral and canine.

B. Median palatine cyst occurs in the posterior nasopalatine canal.

D. Residual cyst occurs in the site of an extracted tooth.

13. D

Pyribenzamine is an antihistamine and so is not used to treat tuberculosis.

14. E

Dry heat sterilization requires 60–120 minutes at 320° F.

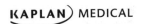

15. **A**

The maxillary first molar has an oblique ridge that is formed by the merger of the triangular distal and triangular lingual ridges.

B. Maxillary second premolar is hexagonal shaped and has a transverse ridge.

C. Mandibular second premolar can have 3 different occlusal presentations with a square shaped occlusal surface.

D. Mandibular first molar has 5 cusps making it pentagonal in shape and has a concavity on the facial surface.

16. **C**

240 kilocalories are derived from the carbohydrates. 33% of 180 g is 60 g of carbohydrates. Four kilocalories is 1 g of carbohydrate, so 60 g × 4 kilocalories/g equals 240 kilocalories.

17. **B**

The liver synthesizes triglycerides from left-over carbohydrates and proteins, which then become fat.

A. The pancreas produces digestive enzymes, insulin, and glucagon.

C. The gall bladder stores and concentrates bile from the liver.

D. The spleen filters red blood cells.

18. **D**

Fluoride supplements distributed by the same pediatrician are the most likely reason, since the fluorosis is generalized.

A. Excess fluoride in the water supply would not be the answer since the water is monitored for optimal fluoridation at 0.8 PPM.

B. Swallowing of toothpaste may cause some fluorosis but here, it is generalized in the school population.

C. Topical fluoride does not cause fluorosis.

19. **C**

Schizophrenia is characterized by disordered thinking, loss of contact with reality, and false beliefs. It has an early onset in adolescents.

B. Bipolar disorder or manic depression is a mood disorder characterized by varying cycles of extreme highs to extreme lows.

E. Psychotic disorders are characterized by delusions and hallucinations.

20. **A**

Amitriptyline is an antidepressant, and is not used to treat schizophrenia. Chlorpromazine (Thorazine), haloperidol (Haldol), resperidone (Risperdal), and triflupromazine (Vesprin) are all used to treat schizophrenia.

21. **E**

In an HIV-infected person, malnutrition can be caused by all of the listed conditions. Intestinal malabsorption, cachexia (physical wasting away), altered metabolism, and altered hormones all occur from HIV invading the body.

22. **C**

Carcinoma in-situ is encapsulated high-grade epithelium. It is hypercellular with no cell maturation at the surface, and it has an intact basement membrane.

A. Atypical layers of slightly raised or flat, thickened areas in the middle or upper epithelium would be mild dysplasia.

B. Immature basaloid cells of abnormal differentiation located toward the prickle and keratinizing layers in the lower two-thirds of epithelium would be moderate dysplasia.

D. Irregularly shaped fibrillar connective tissue with coarse fibers would be polyostotic fibrous dysplasia.

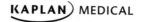

23. B

The lesion is most likely melasma, a brown hyperpigmentation of the cheeks, forehead, and upper lip due to sun exposure.

A. Keratoacanthoma is a cutaneous tumor that presents predominantly in sun-exposed skin of elderly patients.

C. Melanoma is a skin cancer.

D. Papilloma is an intraoral lesion.

24. E

A radiopaque mass at the roots of #2 and #3 would be torus palatinus.

A. Concrescence is the fusion of two teeth at the cementum.

B. Osteoma is a radiopaque mass rarely found in the maxilla or mandible.

C. Stafne's bone cyst is radiolucent.

D. Fibroma is a soft-tissue lesion.

25. A

Glass ionomers contain fluoride within the material, and so are recommended for those with high-risk caries—especially root caries.

C. Hybrid ionomers could be used but they would not be the ideal choice.

D. Compomers are recommended for moderate-risk caries.

26. E

Diabetics have fewer polymorphonuclear leukocytes that are involved with the first line of defense in acute infections.

A. Basophils produce heparin in an allergic reaction.

B. Erythrocytes are red blood cells that transport oxygen and carbon dioxide.

C. Eosinophils are involved in fighting parasitic infections and in allergic responses.

D. Monocytes are involved in chronic inflammation and produce macrophages.

27. D

Fast healing with periodontal treatment would not be an indication of diabetes. A diabetic patient would heal slowly.

28. C

The first statement is false because acetaminophen is not an anti-inflammatory. The second statement is true.

29. D

Actinomyces group does not produce the sulfur smell of bad breath.

30. E

Cytokines overproduce an enzyme called collagenase, which breaks down proteins, including the proteins of connective tissue.

A. Interferon is a group of cytokines that activates protection against viruses.

B. Interleukin is a type of cytokine that stimulates lymphocytes.

C. Lymphokine is a soluble molecule that allows communication between lymphocytes.

D. Chemokines are soluble molecules that chemically attract lymphocytes and other cells.

31. C

If the chest pain is not relieved after 3 doses of nitroglycerine, the patient probably has a myocardial infarction.

A. First-degree heart block would have no signs or symptoms.

B. Angina pectoris would be relieved with nitroglycerine.

D. Congestive heart failure is the inability of the heart to work proficiently. Someone with CHF can lead a relatively normal life.

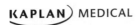

32. C

To prevent distortion, the agar-agar impression should be removed with a quick snapping motion.

33. D

Not more than 132 mg of lidocaine should be given to a 30 kg child. Lidocaine is 2% or 0.02 g per cc (or ml), which equals 20 mg per cc (or mL). Each cartridge holds 1.8 cc (or mL). So 1.8 cc × 20 mg/cc is 36 mg per cartridge.

The maximum safe dose of lidocaine for a child is 4.4 mg/kg. So 4.4 mg/kg × 30 kg equals 132 mg for this child.

34. E

This is 3.6 cartridges. 132 mg is divided by 36 mg/cartridge, resulting in 3.6 cartridges.

35. A

5–10% of hypertension cases are thought to result from secondary causes such as renal disease, Cushing's syndrome, or endocrine disorders.

B. This figure is incorrect; in fact, 90% of primary hypertension is of unknown origin.

C. Secondary hypertension is not more common than primary hypertension—it is less common.

D. This statement is incorrect. Secondary hypertension does not have to be treated before its cause is found.

36. C

Type 3 amelogenesis imperfecta features enamel with normal thickness and white occlusal thirds.

A. Type 1 features enamel hypoplasia, a defect in the enamel matrix. Enamel is thin or absent.

B. Type 2 features enamel hypocalcification, a defect in enamel mineralization.

D. Type 4 features enamel hypomaturation and is associated with taurondontism.

37. D

The enamel organ originates from ectoderm, while the dental papillae (which produces dentin and pulp) forms from mesenchyme. The dental sac produces the cementum, periodontal ligament, and alveolar bone, also from mesenchyme. Ectomesenchyme fits all of these categories, so it is the answer.

38. D

The star-shaped stellate reticulum and stratum intermedium of compressed cuboidal cells lie between the inner and outer enamel epitheliums. These tissues support tooth development.

A. Tomes' process is a 6-sided pyramid that makes up the prism shaped rods of enamel and stellate reticulum.

E. Dental lamina connects the ectomesenchyme with the oral epithelium and stratum intermedium.

39. A

Cheilosis would not be caused by a deficiency of folic acid.

40. B

Epulis fissuratum is exophytic, red, firm, elongated, and found under a partial denture. It is caused by flange irritation.

A. Giant cell granuloma is caused by a local irritant and occurs anterior to the molars.

C. Myxoma is a deep lesion that is a radiolucency in the bone.

D. Irritative fibromatosis occurs from mouth breathing or orthodontic appliances

E. Herpangina is a viral infection caused by the Coxsackie virus, seen in the palate, uvula, tongue and tonsils.

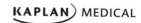

41. B

Hyperplasia is an increase in the number of cells.

A. Hyperplasia does not change the DNA of a cell.

C. Hypertrophy is an increase in individual cell size.

D. Hyperplastic tissues cannot metastasize.

42. B

Trauma to a tooth will cause widening of the PDL.

A. The PDL can atrophy if not in occlusion.

C. The PDL fibers will not regenerate.

D. There will indeed be a change in the PDL with trauma.

43. C

By days 4–7, there will be an increase in rods, filamentous forms, and fusobacteria.

A. Days 1–2: gram-positive cocci with *S. sanguis* and *S. mutans* are prevalent.

B. Days 2–4: cocci are prominent with a proliferation of filamentous forms and rods.

D. Days 7–14: vibrios and spirochetes emerge along with white blood cells to fight infection, as gram-negative anaerobes surface.

E. Day 14–21: vibrios and spirochetes predominate along with cocci and filamentous forms that become more dense.

44. B

Black hairy tongue occurs from the elongation of the filiform papillae, which fill in the spaces of the other papillae.

45. E

The sphenoid bone in the skull contains the foramen ovale, foramen rotundum, and the supraorbital fissure.

46. D

The hepatitis B vaccination (HBIG) is an artificial passive imunization, something short-lived and requiring a booster shot.

A. Natural active vaccine occurs after an exposure to the disease. In that case, the body builds it own antibodies against the disease.

B. Natural passive vaccine occurs when a mother passes her antibodies to her infant.

C. Artificial active vaccine is one of inactive treated organisms. This type of vaccine gives permanent immunity.

47. C

Droplet contamination will be limited if done with a high-speed suction tip—not a saliva ejector.

48. D

Neutrophils are involved with the first line of defense, especially in acute infections.

A. Eosinophils are involved in parasitic infections.

B. Basophils are involved in allergic reactions.

C. Erythrocytes are red blood cells that transport oxygen.

E. Monocytes are involved in chronic inflammation and produce macrophages.

49. B

A scratch has occurred, as seen in the white line. The emulsion was scratched off the film before it was developed.

A. Bent film is a black streak

C. Herringbone appears on one end of the film from placing the film backwards.

D. Elongation is not in this radiograph but occurs when there is not enough vertical angle.

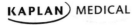

50. D

The radiopaque area is the nasal septum, located between the central incisors, that divides the nasal cavity into two parts.

A. Median palatine suture is radiolucent between #8 and #9.

B. Maxillary sinus is radiolucent and not pictured in this radiograph.

C. Inverted Y is a radiopacity at the juncture of the anterior sinus with the floor of the nasal fossa.

E. Maxillary tuberosity is a radiopaque area at the most posterior end of the maxilla.

51. A

Smoking causes exogenous extrinsic stain, originating from an outside source. Extrinsic staining stains the outer surface.

52. A

The permanent mandibular canine has the greatest chance of developing with a bifurcated root.

B. Lateral teeth rarely have two roots.

C. Central teeth rarely have two roots.

D. First bicuspid is not known to develop with a bifurcated root.

53. C

A collagen injection is not a dental procedure, so it would not be used.

54. A

The pH of acidulated fluoride is very acidic, at 3.0–3.5.

55. D

Ultrasonic scaling would be the best way to remove the endotoxins. An ultrasonic scaler not only removes deposits, it also flushes the pockets at the same time.

A. Polishing passses over the supragingival area and does not remove endotoxins.

B. Curets have value but the ultrasonic is better to flush endotoxins out of the pocket.

C. Scaling is a supragingival procedure that does not go into pockets.

E. Irrigation with an oral irrigator has limited value.

56. C

The most important factor in sealant retention is a properly etched surface.

A. When the tooth is isolated with a rubber dam, the field keeps from getting contaminated, though the sealant retention is not affected.

B. Use of a 37% phosphoric acid provides the retentive surface, but does not play a direct role in retention.

D. Rinsing the tooth properly would not affect retention.

57. B

Collagen fibers are the most abundant type of connective tissue.

A. Reticular fibers consist of collagen and fill in the spaces between cells and fibers.

C. Elastic fibers are in tissues such as ligaments that are subject to stretching, but are also found with collagen in tendons, arteries, and skin.

D. Ground substance acts as a lubricant and protective barrier as it fills the space between connective tissue cells and fibers.

58. D

The periodontal probe in image #3 is the PCPUNC probe.

A. Image #2 is the Michigan probe.

C. Image #4 is the Williams colored probe.

E. Image #1 is the Marquis probe.

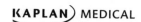

59. D

Electrical impulses from the medulla oblongota of the brain initiate the heartbeat at the SA node, which is at the very top of the heart. The SA node is the natural pacemaker of the heart.

A. AV node is at juncture of the atrium and ventricle and would be the second place that the heart would conduct electricity if the SA node stops functioning.

B. Purkinje fibers are at the outermost reaches of the ventricles and will try to keep the heart beating as a last resort if all other conduction routes stop functioning.

C. Bundle of His is after the AV node and splits the heart's electrical conduction into the left and right bundles to supply electrical conduction to the right and left ventricles.

60. B

The microorganism that is the latent form of chicken pox that produces shingle is the Varicella zoster virus.

A. Epstein-Barr produces mononucleosis.

C. *B. burgdorferi* produces Lyme disease.

D. *S. dysenteriae* produces shigellosis dysentery.

E. *C. tetani* produces tetanus.

61. C

Incomplete sterilzation usually occurs from overpacked loads that do not allow the steam to properly circulate.

A. Types of packaging is not the best choice.

B. The indicators on the packages represent that the temperature was achieved but do not indicate sterility.

D. Incomplete ultrasonic time does not affect sterilization.

62. B

The submental nodes drain the mandibular incisors, lower lip, apex of the tongue, soft palate, tonsillar area, and soft palate.

A. Submandibular nodes drain the maxillary teeth, maxillary sinus, mandibular canine and posterior teeth (except third molars), floor of the mouth, sublingual and submandibular glands, tongue, and hard palate.

C. Facial nodes drain the facial area and then drain into the submandibular nodes.

D. Retroauricular nodes drain the ear.

E. Occipital drains the scalp.

63. A

The tetracycline relatives of doxycycline (Vibramycin) and minocycline (Minocin) can cause photosensitivity.

B. Azithromycin (Zithromax) and clarithromycin (Biaxin) are members of the macrolide group of antibiotics.

C. Cefuroxime (Cephtin) and cephalexin (Keflex) are antibiotics of the cephalosporin group.

D. Acyclovir (Zovirax) and zidovudine (AZT, Retrovir) are antiviral medications.

E. Rifampin (Rifadin) and isoniazid (INH) are antituberculins.

64. B.

The *primary* mandibular central incisors erupt at 6–10 months.

A. Mandibular first molars erupt at 14-18 months.

C. Maxillary first molars erupt at 13-19 months.

D. Maxillary central incisors erupt at 8-12 months.

65. C

In the dental laboratory, rouge would be used to polish the crown before placement.

A. Tin oxide is for polishing amalgams.

B. Pumice is not the answer since it can scratch.

D. Sand disk will scratch the surface.

E. Diatomaceous earth comes from minute aquatic plants and is too abrasive.

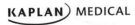

66. A

Glutaraldehyde should not be used for a reversible hydrocolloid impression, since it is not recommended by the manufacturer.

67. C

Arrow #1 is pointing to the condyle.

68. D

Arrow #2 is pointing to the mandibular canal.

69. E

Arrow #3 is pointing to the maxilla.

70. B

Arrow #4 is pointing to the maxillary sinus.

71. C

Class II Division II occurs when the mesiobuccal cusp of the maxillary first molar is retruded by at least the width of a premolar and the mandible, with one or more of the maxillary incisors being retruded.

A. Class I is neutrocclusion, with the mesiobuccal cusp of the maxillary first molar occluding with the buccal groove of the mandibular first molar.

B. Class II Division I occurs when the buccal groove of the mandibular first molar is distal to the mesiobuccal cusp of the maxillary first molar by at least the width of a premolar, and the maxillary anterior teeth protrude more facially away from the mandibular anterior teeth.

D. Class III occurs when the buccal groove of the mandibular first molar is mesial to the mesiobuccal cusp of the maxillary first molar by at least the width of a premolar.

72. C

Class III occurs when the distal of the mandibular canine is mesial to the mesial surface of the maxillary canine by at least half the width of a premolar.

A. Class I occurs with the maxillary canine occludes with the distal half of the mandibular canine and also the mesial half of the mandibular first premolar.

B. Class II occurs when the distal surface of the mandibular canine is distal to the mesial surface of the maxillary canine by at least the width of a premolar.

73. C

Someone with any autoimmune disease is the exception, since not all autoimmune diseases carry systemic effects.

74. B

Mild fluorosis occurs when less than 50% of the tooth has opaque areas.

A. Very mild fluorosis consists of small opaque, paper-white areas covering less than 25% of the tooth surface.

C. Moderate fluorosis consists of all tooth surfaces affected; marked wear on biting surfaces; brown stain may be present.

D. Severe fluorosis means all tooth surfaces are affected; discrete or confluent pitting; brown stain is present.

75. A

According to the AAP, necrotizing periodontitis demonstrates less loss of clinical attachment and destruction of alveolar bone than necrotizing ulcerative periodontitis (NUP).

B. Juvenile periodontitis (JP) results in rapid loss of attachment and bone destruction, often localized in first permanent molars and permanent incisors.

C. Prepubertal periodontitis is characterized by severe gingival inflammation, rapid bone loss, mobility, and early loss of deciduous teeth.

D. Rapid progressive periodontitis occurs in young adults age 20–30 and results in severe inflammation, rapid bone and connective-tissue loss, and tooth loss.

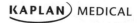

76. C

A subperiosteal implant is a custom-fabricated metal framework created by an impression of the exposed (by surgical flap) underlying bone or designed by computer tomography of the patient.

A. Endosseous implant is a screw-shaped, cylindrical, or blade implant that serves as an anchor for a crown or bridge.

B. Ceramic implant, which had greater success than earlier polymer implants, was used prior to titanium implants.

D. Transosteal implant is not as widely used because of the success of the osseointegrated implant.

77. E

500 mg exceeds the CLD for all children, according to Heifetz and Horowitz.

A. 320 mg would be toxic for a 2-year-old.

B. 422 mg would be fatal for a 4-year-old.

C. 538 mg would be toxic for a 6-year-old.

D. 655 mg would be toxic for an 8-year-old.

78. B

The new mA of 8 would require 10 impulses. Take the original 16 mA × 5 impulses and divide that by 8 (new) mA to get 10 impulses.

79. B

The new exposure time is 0.08 seconds. Changing from a 6" BID to a 1" BID decreases the distance by $\frac{1}{6}$. The inverse square law states that $(\frac{1}{6})^2 = \frac{1}{36} \times 3$ seconds = 0.08 seconds.

80. B

Patients with hemophelia B lack Factor IX, necessary for clotting.

A. Factor VIII is related to hemophilia A.

C. Factor XI is related to hemophilia C.

D. Stuart factor is involved with intrinsic and extrinsic blood coagulation.

81. C

Radiographic magnification is affected by the object-to-film distance. An object that is farther away from the film will have more distortion, while an object that is closer will reduce distortion.

A. Umbra is the full shadow on the radiographs.

B. Penumbra is the partial shadow on the radiographs.

D. Source-to-film distance affects image sharpness.

82. B

A loop diuretic such as furosemide eliminates sodium in the loop of Henle of the glomerulus of the kidney.

A. Propranolol is ß blocker.

C. Lidocaine is a sodium channel blocker.

D. Diltiazem is a calcium channel bocker.

E. Provastatin (Pravachol) is an antihyperlipidemic.

83. B

The loop of Henle is part of the glomerulus where the electrolyte of sodium is variably removed from filtrate. When most sodium is removed from filtrate, water then follows the sodium out of the system, reducing excess fluid.

A. Arterioles supply blood to the kidney.

C. Glomerulus filters electrolytes and waste in the loop of Henle.

D. Nephrons contain the glomeruli.

E. Cortex contains the nephrons.

84. B

Von Willebrand's disease is a genetic disorder that affects platelet cohesiveness, when the endothelium is injured

A. Factor XI is related to hemophilia C.

C. Von Willebrand's does not affect lipids; it affects proteins.

D. Von Willebrand's affects both men and women.

85. C

The hypothalamus regulates body temperature. This is where antipyretic drugs take effect to reduce body temperature or fever.

A. The thyroid regulates metabolism and calcium levels.

B. The parathyroid regulates calcium and phosphorus.

D. The gallbladder stores bile released from the liver.

E. The pituitary gland regulates growth and many other functions.

86. B

Place her in a recovery position since the tongue is the biggest airway obstruction.

C. CPR would be premature if the pulse has not been checked.

D. Oxygen would be acceptable if she is not breathing on her own, though that wasn't established here.

87. D

With the tremors of Parkinson's disease, muscles become rigid, not limp.

88. A

The implant pictured is an endosseous implant.

B. Subperitoneal goes over the bone and under the periosteum.

C. Transosteal goes through the mandible.

D. Ceramic is a coating that may cover an implant.

89. B

Apply the gel and leave it alone. This helps prevent the break-up of the micropores created by the etch.

C. Etching for 10 seconds is not long enough. It should be etched for 15–60 seconds, depending on product type and manufacturer's recommendation.

D. Dabbing vigorously for 20 seconds will break up the newly etched surface.

90. C

Calcium channel blockers such as nifedipine can cause gingival hyperplasia.

A. Amyl nitrate is an antianginal medication.

B. Procainimide is an antiarrhythmic medication.

D. Bretylium is a potassium channel blocker medication.

E. Atorvastatin (Lipitor) is an antihyperlipidemic medication.

91. E

The external carotid artery doees not supply blood to the brain. The *internal* carotid artery is responsible for that task.

92. D

Vitamin K does not prevent night blindness; Vitamin A prevents it.

93. A

Lymphocyte B cells release antibodies during humoral immunity for specific antigens or microbes.

B. Acquired immunity involves antibodies against any invasive antigens either by active or passive means.

C. Cell mediated immunity occurs when the T lymphocytes are stimulated.

D. GALT is an old immunity term for **g**ut-**a**ssociated **l**ymphoid **t**issue that lines and protects the digestive tract from invading pathogens.

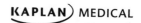

KAPLAN MEDICAL

94. A

Chromogenic bacteria produce green stain, which embeds in areas of decalcification, so care is needed in its removal. Hydrogen peroxide may be utilized for its removal.

B. Orange stain is based upon poor oral hygiene habits.

C. Brown stain is based upon poor oral hygiene habits.

D. Yellow stain is based upon poor oral hygiene habits.

95. B

According to HIPAA, a patient may not be denied medical insurance based upon current or past medical status.

A. When conferring with another professional regarding treatment, the patient's health status may be revealed.

C. Patient information is kept confidential.

D. Information about the patient may be submitted electronically to a third-party payer in order to acquire payment for services rendered.

96. B

An enzyme-linked immunosorbent assay or ELISA tests for enzymes of HIV or AIDS.

A. Mantoux test is used for detecting TB.

C. PTT is the prothrombin time test for blood clotting.

D. PPD is another skin test for TB.

E. Western blot follows up the ELISA test to validate the ELISA test.

97. E

None of the above. There is no *one* agent that will desensitize everyone.

98. C

Carrots are not a source of vitamin E, but rather, vitamin A.

99. D

A push stroke can cause calculus deposits to become embedded in soft tissue, an undesired effect.

A. A lateral stroke and pressure should be used to remove large deposits.

B. Adaptation is difficult on convex surfaces, not concave.

C. Calculus deposits are crushed when a pull stroke is used, therefore the chances of burnishing the deposit is minimal to non-existent.

100. D

Zinc oxide and eugenol would not be used for Class II restorations. ZOE should be limited to non-stress bearing areas, and Class II restorations bear stress.

101. B

Unequal pupils occur when a cerebrovascular accident affects one side of the brain.

A. With a seizure, pupils would be equal.

C. Drug overdose would affect both pupils in the same way.

D. Diabetic coma is slow onset with equal pupils.

E. Insulin shock is sudden onset but the pupils would be equal.

102. E

Periodontal dressings do not cause teeth to stain.

103. A

The mandibular branch of the trigeminal nerve exits the brain by way of the foramen ovale of the sphenoid bone.

B. The maxillary branch of the trigeminal nerve exits the brain by way of the foramen rotundum.

C. The spinal chord exits the cranium by way of the foramen magnum.

D. The middle meningeal artery enters the cranial cavity by way of the foramen spinosum.

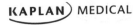

104. B

Agar is the main component of a reversible hydrocolloid impression. It is derived from seaweed.

A. Polymer is contained in polysulfide impression materials.

C. Zinc is contained in zinc oxide–eugenol impressions.

D. Gypsum is contained in impression plaster.

E. Sodium alginate is contained in alginate impressions.

105. B

The acquired pellicle is a nidus or breeding area for bacteria to multiply.

A. The acquired pellicle does provide a barrier to protect against acids.

C. Calculus is, in fact, able to attach there.

D. It can be stained or unstained.

106. C

Pyogenic granuloma is most commonly associated with hormonal changes that take place during pregnancy and is due to a local irritant. It can also occur in males.

A. Kaposi sarcoma is associated with HIV-positive patients.

B. Fistula is associated with an abscess.

D. Wickham's striae is associated with lichen planus.

107. C

The third trimester is the safest time to take radiographs on a pregnant female. All of the organs of the fetus have formed by then, and are just growing in size

A. The first trimester is the most dangerous time, since all the organs are differentiating.

108. B

The biological indicator used to verify heat sterilization in autoclaves is *Bacillus stearothermophilus*

A. *Aeromonas hydrophila* is a species of bacterium present in all fresh-water environments.

C. *Neisseria lactamica* is part of the normal flora of the human upper respiratory tract.

D. *Bacillus subtilis* checks dry heat sterilization.

E. *Bacillus lentus* is an organism that produces an alkaline protease.

109. D

Premature contact can cause a tooth to move into supraversion as the tooth extends further away from the alveolus and the plane of occlusion.

A. Mesioversion refers to a tooth that has moved to a position that is mesial to its normal position.

B. Infraversion refers to a tooth that has not fully erupted and is not in occlusion

C. Buccoversion indicates a tooth that has moved buccal to its normal position.

E. Distoversion indicates a tooth that has moved distally to its normal position.

110. A

In a pulmonary embolism, ischemia occurs first. The tissue lacks oxygen due to the thrombosis, which eventually leads to necrosis.

B. Necrosis is dead tissue.

D. Hypertrophy occurs when the tissue cells become larger in size.

E. Hemorrhage would not occur in an occluded artery.

111. D

A bulla is an elevated lesion containing serous fluid.

B. A papule is a small solid, superficial elevation of skin that is circumscribed.

C. A macule is a flattened skin patch that is altered in color.

E. A caruncle or caruncula is a small, fleshy eminence that can be normal or abnormal.

112. B

Bitewing radiographs would not be effective. They detect interproximal decay, bone loss, and calculus deposits, not lingual or buccal deposits. Explorers, air, and the color and consistency of adjacent tissues are all acceptable means for calculus detection on the lingual aspects of teeth.

113. D

Mucoceles are commonly found on the lower lip.

114. B

Sealants are placed right away because they act as a hindrance (barrier) to cover the tooth surface. They prevent bacteria from entering the pits and fissures, which could then cause carious lesions.

115. D

Collimation begins in the diaphragm, which shapes and directs the beam toward the collimator.

A. The tungsten of the cathode is where radiation starts.

B. The target receives radiation from the cathode.

C. The focusing cup of the cathode directs it to the anode.

E. Collimator uses lead diaphragms to restrict beam size through a round or rectangular aperture.

116. B

Down syndrome patients typically have a Class III malocclusion with a prognathic mandible.

117. D

A refactory or unresponsive area may best be evaluated by the loss of tissue attachment. which would show the progression or apical migration of tissue.

A. Edematous tissue indicates swollen gingiva which can create a pseudopocket without the apical migration of tissue.

B. Tissue contour is scalloped in healthy individuals but can be blunted, flattened, or cratered in nonhealthy mouths.

C. Bleeding upon probing can be seen in early disease without loss of attachment.

E. Presence of purulence indicates active disease in a site but it does not signify periodontal tissue loss.

118. D

The patient likely suffers from necrotizing ulcerative gingivitis, since he is otherwise healthy. He may just be under stress.

A. Periodontal abscess is not generalized throughout the mouth.

B. Necrotizing periodontitis occurs over a longer period, destroying bone.

C. Juvenile periodontitis occurs with extreme bone loss, typically around the first molars and anterior teeth.

119. C

The patient should be reappointed 1–2 days after the first debridement, not a full week after.

120. C

The thymus matures the T cells for cell-mediated immune reactions.

A. The hypothalamus produces oxytocin and regulates body temperature.

B. Bone marrow matures B lymphocytes to act against specific antigens.

D. The spleen filters out old red blood cells.

E. The liver has many functions but maturing T-cells is not one of them.

121. D

Patient counseling and education are the first steps in treating this patient. This may motivate her.

A. Root debridement and use of the ultrasonic are indicated during the treatment phase for this patient, but they are not the first steps.

B. Prophylaxis is not indicated because of the patient's periodontal condition.

122. D

The least effective way to instruct on flossing is to dispense an impersonal written pamphlet.

123. A

A heart murmur is a risk for endocarditis and an indication for premedication.

C. Diabetes would not require premedication unless the patient has out-of-control diabetes.

124. B

The patient is inadvertently missing this area. Her toothbrushing technique is not adequately removing the plaque and so must be modified.

C. Flossing will not remove plaque from the buccal and lingual surfaces.

125. C

Glucophage is commonly prescribed for patients with non-insulin dependent diabetes melitus (NIDDM).

A. Toprol XL and HCTZ are prescribed for hypertension.

B. An antibiotic premedication would be taken for the heart murmur.

126. D

Pilocarpine helps in the production of saliva.

A. Levadopa treats Parkinson's disease.

B. Molindone is an antidepressant.

C. Atropine is prescribed for the patients with copious amounts of saliva to dry them up for dental procedures.

127. A

Succinylcholine helps the larynx to relax for the purposes of intubation.

B. Pentothal is an ultra-short acting barbiturate.

C. Versed is an IV anesthetic for conscious sedation.

D. Halothane is an inhalation anesthetic.

E. Nitrous oxide is an inhalation anesthetic.

128. C

The first statement is false because topical anesthetics should be applied to a small area, not a large one. The second statement is true.

129. D

Lamina propria is a highly vascular layer located between the basement membrane and epithelial lining of connective tissue and is not seen radiographically.

130. A

Dentin is produced by the dental papillae, not by the dental sac.

131. A

If the the medial nasal process fails to fuse with the maxillary process, it would happen in weeks 4–7 of the embryonic period. In that case, a cleft lip occurs.

C. During weeks 8–12 of the embryonic period, a cleft palate can occur.

132. C

Ultrasonic scalers use a higher frequency than sonic scalers.

A. Ultrasonic and sonic scalers use vibrations but in different ranges.

B. Sonic scalers are less—not more—efficient than ultrasonics.

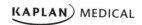

133. C

To debride the distal aspect of a maxillary canine, a curet with a short and straight shank should be used. Long shanks may be used in deeper pockets. Angulated shanks are found in posterior intruments.

134. C

Ultrasonic instrumentation is best used for supragingival and subgingival calculus deposits.

A. Stain that is not easily removed by hand instrumentation can be removed with ultrasonics, though the ultrasonic works best on calculus deposits.

D. Ultrasonics can be utlilized with subgingival calculus as well as supragingival calculus.

135. E

Retaining the integrity or shape of the instrument is the best—and broadest—reason why sharp instrumentation is important. All of the other answer choices are subsets of this answer: A sharp instrument will help to maintain patient comfort and in deposit removal and debridement, and it will lessen clinician tedium or fatigue.

136. C

Dilaceration is a sharp bend or angulation of the root.

A. Fusion is the union of two teeth from separate tooth germs, usually due to external pressure.

B. Attrition is tooth-to-tooth wear.

D. Enamel pearl usually occurs at the CEJ, when the ameloblasts produced excess enamel.

E. Gemination is the development of two teeth from one tooth germ.

137. C

Acidulated phosphate fluoride solutions should be stored in polyethylene or plastic containers so that they can remain stable compounds.

138. D

Trisomy 13, trisomy 18, and trisomy 22 patients do not commonly have anencephaly, the incomplete formation of the brain and skull.

139. A

Routine oral prophylaxis does not aid in caries prevention. A caries control program helps the orphans with the daily routine of personal hygiene and a balanced diet to prevent caries. Routine examinations and treatment helps to control caries as well as systemic and topical applications of fluoride.

140. C

A 7 mm pocket on the mesial aspect of #14 should be debrided with a Gracey 11/12.

A. Columbia 13/14 is a posterior distal aspect instrument.

B. Gracey 7/8 is an anterior instrument.

D. Gracey 13/14 is a posterior distal aspect instrument.

E. Gracey 17/18 is a posterior distal aspect instrument.

141. D

To prevent cross-contamination on dental units, disinfection should be performed between patients.

A. Asepsis is the prevention of contact with microorganisms.

B. Attenuation is the reduction of the virulence of pathogenic organisms.

C. Sterilization kills all life forms and is not used on dental units.

142. D

The sharpening technique used keeps the curet tip in its best condition and decreases its chances of breakage.

A. The design of the blade is important to where the specific instrument is used.

B. The flexibility of the shank aids in a tactile sense.

C. Heat sterilization can eventually cause stress on metal.

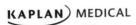

143. C

In a universal curet, there are 4 cutting edges— 2 cutting edges per end.

144. D

Eggs contain all essential amino acids.

A. Eggs have some biotin but are not rich in it.

B. Egg proteins are not destroyed when cooked.

C. Eggs are high, not low, in cholesterol.

E. Eggs contain some but not all of the calcium required.

145. D

If the patient bleeds upon probing, the disease is likely still active.

A. A change in tissue color indicates some response of the tissue to disease but bleeding upon probing is a better indicator.

B. Loss of stippling indicates collagen fibers are being broken down but it is not the best choice.

C. Tooth sensitivity is not a soft tissue disease indicator.

E. Pocket depth greater than 3 mm would not be a sign since some patients can maintain healthy pockets.

146. C

When the edge of an instrument does not reflect light, it is safe to say it is sharp.

A. An instrument blade that has a wire edge is undesired.

B. If the edge of an instrument blade reflects light, the instrument is dull.

147. E

An ultrasonic instrument can be used with a patient who has a shielded pacemaker.

148. C

Use of a high speed with a dry agent would cause dental hypersensitivity.

149. B

To remove supragingival calculus from #25 and #26, a Jaquette 33 scaler should be used.

A. A Gracey curet is a site-specific subgingival instrument.

C. Columbia 12/13 should be a Columbia 13/14.

D. 204SD is a posterior instrument.

150. A

By making your patient aware of his needs, he will be able to overcome any fears he may have, to accept his dental treatment plan, and to prevent disease. All of the other answer choices are subsets.

151. A

The first step in establishing an oral health program is to determine the needs of the juvenile population.

152. B

By sharing the dental records of each juvenile, breach of confidentiality was committed.

153. A

The superior deep cervical nodes drain the pharygeal tonsils.

B. Inferior deep cervical nodes are the secondary drainage of the tonsils.

C. Retropharyngeal nodes drain the paranasal sinuses and the hard and soft palates.

D. Retroauricular drains the scalp and external ear.

154. B

Stenson's duct passes through the buccinator muscle.

A. The masseter, a muscle of mastication, is not penetrated by Stenson's duct.

C. Depressor anguli is in the chin.

D. Lateral pterygoid, a muscle of mastication, is not penetrated by Stenson's duct.

E. Zygomaticus major is not penetrated by Stenson's duct.

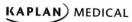

155. C

Pilocarpine stimulates the CNS to mimic the para-sympathetic system as a parasympathomimetic, thus stimulating salivation.

D. Parasympatholytic inhibits salivation.

156. D

A 14-year old with aggressive juvenile periodontitis can be treated with tetracycline since all of his permanent teeth—except the thrid molars—are formed.

157. D

Actinobacillus actinomycetemcomitans are particularly susceptible to the action of tetracycline. Tetracycline blocks protein synthesis of the microbes.

158. C

Transient bacteremias are not typically created by the placement of orthodontic wires, so premedication with an antibiotic is not needed.

159. D

To detect bone loss with periodontal disease radiation should be set at 90 kVp for better bone contrast.

B. 70 kVp is ideal in the detection of caries.

160. A

Kilovoltage is controlled by the anode of a dental radiograph unit.

B. The cathode controls milliamperage.

C. The target accepts electrons from the cathode.

D. The collimator shapes and directs the beam.

E. The focusing cup directs the electrons toward the target.

161. C

A nasopalatine duct cyst does not produce an ameloblastoma which can occur with a dentigerous cyst.

162. C

A moon-shaped face, buffalo hump, and large abdomen occurs with hypercortisolism which is excessive cortisol produced from the adrenal glands.

A. Hyperthyroidism is excessive thyroid hormone that causes Graves disease.

B. Hypothyroidism causes myxedema in adults and cretinism in children.

D. Hypocortisolism is a lack of cortisol production by the adrenal glands and results in dark skin pigmentations.

163. C

The first statement is false because it is a reversible index. The second statement is true.

164. D

Parkinson's disease results from a lack of dopamine produced by the brain as a neurotransmitter. It acts on peripheral receptors such as blood vessels.

165. B

Insulin is produced by the beta cells of the pancreas to unlock the cells and allow glucose into the cells.

A. Glucagon produced by the alpha cells of the pancreas go after the glycogen stored in the liver when the blood sugar gets too low.

C. Glycogen storage is a function of the liver.

D. Glucagon is produced by the alpha cells in the pancreas.

166. B

Cytomegalovirus causes a mononucleosis-like illness in adults that can become severe in children.

C. Connavirus causes the common cold and also the SARS-CoV.

D. *Bordetella pertussis* causes whooping cough.

E. Adenovirus causes the common cold.

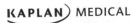

167. B

Chronic infections have an influx of monocytes into the area.

A. Eosinophils are involved in allergic responses.

C. Neutrophils are involved with acute infection.

D. Basophils are involved with allergic responses.

E. Platelets take part in blood clotting.

168. B

Mulberry molars occur from acquired syphilis due to the *Treponema pallidum* microbe.

A. Varicella zoster causes chicken pox.

D. Rubeola virus causes measles.

E. *Bordetella pertussis* causes whooping cough.

169. C

It could occur from palatal donor site, since the edges of the wounds are not within close proximation, and the wound has to fill in from the base outward.

170. A

Prions infect patients who have Creutzfeldt-Jakob disease.

B. Peutz-Jegher syndrome is a rare, autosomal-dominant, inherited condition that results in gastrointestinal polyps along the length of the bowel and mucocutaneous pigmentation of the lips, skin, and mouth.

C. Papillon-Lefèvre syndrome is a rare, autosomal recessive disorder characterized by palmoplantar keratoderma and rapid progressive periodontitis.

D. Pierre Robin syndrome is a birth defect that results in a smaller lower jaw, cleft palate, and tongue that "balls up" in the back of the mouth.

171. B

Hypothyroidism produces myxedema in adults and cretinism in children.

A. Hyperthyroidism is excessive thyroid hormone that causes Graves disease.

C. Hypercortisolism is excessive cortisol production in the adrenal glands.

D. Hypocortisolism is a lack of cortisol production by the adrenal glands, resulting in dark skin pigmentation.

172. C

A lesion that looks like a bull's-eye target is due to erythema multiforme.

A. Pemphigoid is an autoimmune disease that manifests as bullous lesions intraorally, rupturing and leaving scars.

B. Pemphigus is an autoimmune disease that manifests first as a mucosal lesion that also affects the skin with vesciles or bulla that collapse. Nikolsky's sign shows that desmosomes lose contact.

D. Epidermis bullosa is an autoimmune disease that manifests as blisters within the basement membrane predisposing the patient to both squamous and basal cell carcinoma.

173. A

Elongation occurs on radiographs due to not enough vertical angle.

B. Too much vertical angle causes foreshortening.

C. Incorrect horizontal angle causes overlap.

174. D

A patient on a loop diuretic might need a potassium supplement such as K-Dur.

A. Sodium bicarbonate causes sodium retention.

B. Adenosine is a medication that slows the heart rate.

C. Digitalis increases cardiac contractile force.

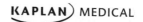
KAPLAN MEDICAL

175. B

A patient who cannot move his lower extremities and needs help into the dental chair is a paraplegic.

A. Hemiplegic is paralysis of half the body on either the right or the left side, which is usually the result of a stroke.

C. Quadraplegic is paralysis of all the extremities.

176. D

Flexibility is the exception since it allows for undesired changes.

177. E

Most of the scores are between 7 and 9, since the standard deviation is 1. The mean is 8, with +1 or −1 on either side of 8 as the deviation.

178. C

−0.95: a strong correlation will fall between +1.0 and −1.0 so the closer to 1, the stronger the correlation

179. E

Prioritizing the list comes after establishing the needs.

A. Surveying the needs is the same as determining the needs.

B. Goal identification occurs after prioritizing the list.

C. Designing the program is the last step.

D. Financing the plan comes after designing the program.

180. A

Caries incidence is determined by the deft, which is for children.

B. Deft does not exist

C. DMFT is adults

D. dmft does not exist

E. DEFT does not exist

181. D.

Randomization of the population is the exception since the population is limited to the facility.

A. Inter-rater reliability deals with consistency between examainers.

B. Intra-rater reliability deals with the same person doing the scoring.

C. Validity of measuring instrument means the numbers can be reproduced.

182. D

Comparisons of this program with other programs the dental hygienist has administered is not appropriate since there is a specific group in the facitliy being evaluated.

183. A

A questionnaire is the most cost-efficient way to determine the needs of dental patients.

184. B

The most efficient use of a public dental hygienist's time would be instruction of faculty at elementary and middle schools on the proper administration of fluoride. The faculty is with the students almost daily.

185. B

A longitunidal study is conducted over a long period of time.

A. A randomized study occurs with an unbiased cross-section of the population and is the desired study.

C. A double-blind study removes the examiners' bias since it is not known which is the control group being studied.

D. A systemic random study occurs when the participants are numbered.

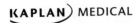

186. A

The health department will use a retrospective study since it will be conducted after the fact of the incident.

B. An experimental study occurs with an experiment that is controlled.

C. A prospective study is one in the planning stages.

D. A longitudinal study examines an extended period from the present into the future.

187. D

The average DMF is 5.9.

Carious lesions	3,380
Extracted teeth	385
Filled teeth	2135
	5,900

5,900 divided by 1,000 is 5.9.

188. A

A valid index measures a stable variable consistently at different intervals. It measures what it is intended to measure.

B. An acceptable index is safe for the subjects involved in the study.

D. A reliable index measures consistently at different times.

189. A

The latest statistics on current studies in dental disease can be found at the Library of Congress.

190. B

A carious lesion on the mesial of # 29 would call for a Class II restoration which is for the proximal surfaces of posterior teeth.

A. Class I is for pits and fissures.

C. Class III is for proximal surfaces of anterior teeth.

D. Class IV is for proximal and incisal surfaces of anterior teeth.

E. Class V is for cervical lesions.

191. B.

These students are in the experimental group since they are all involved in the study.

A. Stratified sampling is random selection and this is an intact group.

C. The control group usually receives the placebo, but there is no group here receiving a placebo.

D. Probability sampling occurs when there is a wide range of willing population who get involved. This is an intact group.

192. E

Both 2 and 3 since they occur three times each.

193. C

Assessment is the first step in program planning. The needs of the community will be determined during this phase.

A. Implementation is getting the program started.

B. Evaluation appraises the program after it has been implemented.

D. Treatment is just that, treating the problems.

194. E

The Community Periodontal Index of Treatment Needs would be used to screen for the periodontal treatment needs of this community.

A. OHI-S is used to determine the amount of oral debris found on specific teeth.

B. GI is used to determine the severity and location of gingivitis based upon color, consistency, and bleeding upon probing.

C. DMFT determines the number of decayed, missing, and filled teeth in the adult populations respectively.

D. deft determines the number of decayed, missing, and filled teeth in the juvenile populations respectively.

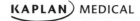

195. C

Fluoridation of the water supply is not an access to care issue. Communication would be an issue since a percentage of the population speaks only Spanish.

A. Finance is an issue that directly affects access to care.

B. Language is an issue that directly affects access to care.

D. Transportation is an issue that directly affects access to care.

196. B

Place posters in public locations that show how a cancerous lesion in the oral cavity looks. Media are the most effective initial way to reach the community.

A. Providing free oral cancer screenings is secondary. Education is first.

C. Sending out pamphlets would reach patients, but if the pamphlets are not written in Spanish as well as English, then the population will not be adequately reached.

D. Setting up a health fair is essential but only after the population has been reached with the information.

197. D

The DMFT is used for all individuals over age 14.

A. Deft does not exist.

B. deft is used for individuals under age 14.

C. Dmft does not exist.

E. DEMT does not exist.

198. D

Fluoridation of the school's water supply is the most cost effective way to deliver fluoride to the community.

A. A sealant program in the elementary schools would provide occlusal surface protection but would not supply fluoride to developing teeth.

B. A monthly program would help existing teeth but it would not supply fluoride to developing teeth.

C. Giving all students an exam, prophylaxis, and professional fluoride treatment once a year would not supply fluoride to developing teeth.

199. D

Involvement is when the individual actively takes part in the self exam.

B. Self realization occurs when the individual is determined to be at the top.

C. Physiologic achieves survival needs.

E. Social occurs when the person has met the physiologic and security needs and wants to be loved and accepted.

200. C

If the median age is 16 with a standard deviation of 2 years for starting tobacco use, then 14–18 would be the range.

Full-Length Practice Test:
Component B: Case-Based Questions

DIRECTIONS

1. The following test items are presented in 14 cases. Each case includes the following components:

    A. Patient History

    B. Periodontal Chart

    C. Radiographs and Clinical Photographs when necessary

These materials should be reviewed before answering the test questions.

> For the Radiographs and Clinical Photographs for each case, please turn to the color insert at the back of this book. Make sure you turn to the correct case.

2. The periodontal charts represent each patient's clinical findings. Restorations have not been charted; some carious lesions that might be visible on radiographs have been charted.

3. The sequencing of items within cases parallels actual practice. So, as the treatment proceeds, new information might be given in subsequent items to guide you in making future treatment decisions. When this new information is provided, it should not influence your answers to prior items.

CASE 1

PATIENT STATISTICS

Age **40**

Sex **F**

Height **5'6"**

Weight **125**

PATIENT VITALS

Blood Pressure **124/76**

Pulse Rate **62**

Respiration Rate **14**

MEDICAL HISTORY

Past Medical History **Heart murmur, back pain**

Hospitalized last 5 Years? **X** Yes ___ No

Why? **Gall bladder removed last year**

Current medications **Synthroid, Prozac, Advil**

Allergies **Penicillin**

Women ___ Pregnant ___ Lactating

Smoker **One pack a day for 21 years**

Smokeless tobacco **No**

Other habits **None**

DENTAL HISTORY

Regular Check-Ups **6-month recare**

TMJ **WNL**

Oral tissue exam

Pink, firm, maintaining pockets 2–5 mm, excellent OH

Oral cancer screening

Patient presented today with round lesion on lower lip, left of midline, raised border, dried white center. Photo taken today.

Plaque Index **0**　　Calculus Index **1**

CHIEF COMPLAINT

Patient in for routine check-up states she has had a "bump" on her lip for the past 2 months, though it does not hurt. No other complaints.

SOCIAL/CAREER BACKGROUND

Married mother of 2 teenage children. Works as computer programmer. Likes horseback riding and playing golf. Has a beach house. Drinks socially.

Clinical Examination

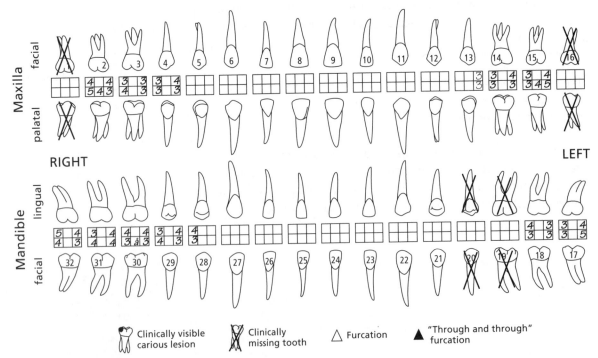

CASE 1: Questions 1–11

1. If this patient's heart murmur is organic, what would be the premedication of choice?

   A. Cephalexin 2 g
   B. Amoxicillin 2 g
   C. Erythromycin 1 g
   D. Azithromycin 1 g
   E. Tetracycline 1 g

2. Which of the following habits may have contributed to this patient's lesion?

   A. Tanning
   B. Alcohol consumption
   C. Smoking
   D. None of the above

3. Your patient is on Synthroid for

   A. Hyperthyroidism
   B. Hypothyroidism
   C. Hyperparathyroidism
   D. Hypoparathyroidism

4. This patient's lesion could possibly be diagnosed as

   A. Chancre
   B. Squamous cell carcinoma
   C. Solar cheilosis
   D. Keratotic plaque
   E. Leukoplakia

5. If this lesion has metastasized, the main lymph node for drainage of the lower lip is

   A. Submandibular nodes
   B. Superior cervical nodes
   C. Submental nodes
   D. Parotid nodes
   E. Postauricular nodes

6. Squamous cell carcinoma on the lip may also be mistaken for

   A. Herpes labialis
   B. Syphilitic chancre
   C. Verruca vulgaris
   D. All of the above

7. Of the medications that this patient is taking, which is a serotonin-specific reuptake inhibitor?

   A. Advil
   B. Prozac
   C. Synthroid
   D. None of the above

8. The patient's pulse rate would be considered

   A. Below normal
   B. On the low side of normal
   C. In the normal range
   D. On the high side of normal
   E. Higher than normal

9. Your patient is concerned by an article she read on disease transmission in the dental office. You tell her that this office applies the rules of "standard precautions." Which of the following statements would you present to her as a definition of "standard precautions"?

   A. Extra precaution is taken for every patient that you know has a specific contagion.

   B. Extra precautions are taken with HIV patients.

   C. All patients are considered to be potentially infectious for bloodborne pathogens.

   D. The CDC has established new standard precautions for dentistry.

   E. Patients who enter the office that seem ill are sent home.

10. Your patient notices a white spot on her radiographs. The round radiopaque area near the distal of #29 is

    A. Cervical abrasion

    B. Temporary restorations

    C. Resin fillings

    D. Cervical burnout

    E. Excess amalgam

11. When performing an EDE/IOE cancer screening, you notice two spongy, white circular lesions on the gingiva in the mucobuccal fold near the apex of #11. They do not resemble the lesion on the lip. These lesions might be

    A. Lichen planus

    B. Linear alba

    C. Papule

    D. Furuncle

    E. Nevus

CASE 2

PATIENT STATISTICS

Age **41**
Sex **M**
Height **5'11"**
Weight **178**

PATIENT VITALS

Blood Pressure **126/88**
Pulse Rate **90**
Respiration Rate **24**

MEDICAL HISTORY

Past Medical History **Chronic bronchitis**

Hospitalized last 5 Years? **X** Yes ___ No

Why? **Difficulty breathing 4 years ago**

Current medications **Azmacort, Albuterol, ASA**

Allergies **None**

Women ___ Pregnant ___ Lactating

Smoker **Two packs a day but quit 4 years ago**
Smokeless tobacco **Holds chewing tobacco in teeth**
Other habits **None**

DENTAL HISTORY

Regular Check-Ups **6-month recare**

TMJ **Slight deviation to right upon opening**

Oral tissue exam
Good OH, flosses 3 times daily, brushes multiple times daily, pink, stippled, firm

Oral cancer screening
Gray, corrugated area buccal mucosa fold noted in past visits is more pronounced today.

Plaque Index **1** Calculus Index **1**

CHIEF COMPLAINT

Patient in for routine check-up.

SOCIAL/CAREER BACKGROUND

Married male, one of 5 children. Tobacco farmer for past 23 years. Diagnosed with emphysema 4 years ago, so quit smoking but took up chewing tobacco.

Clinical Examination

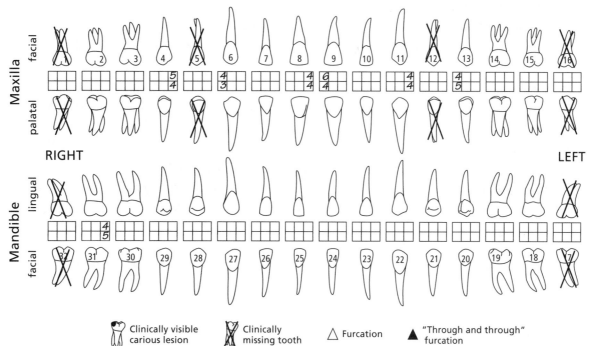

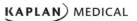

CASE 2: Questions 12–23

12. This patient's use of bronchodilator can cause

    A. Dry mouth
    B. Bad taste
    C. Urinary retention
    D. Tachycardia
    E. All of the above

13. When looking at the periapical radiograph of #8 and #9, you observe a radiolucent area. This radiolucency is a(n)

    A. Nasal septum
    B. Inverted Y
    C. Fracture
    D. Median palatine suture

14. You notice a flaky red lesion on patient's cheek that he states appeared 4 months ago. This lesion may be due to

    A. Sun exposure
    B. Medications he takes for emphysema
    C. His chewing tobacco habit
    D. A skin irritation from new soap detergent

15. The lesion in the vestibule may be diagnosed as

    A. Bulla
    B. Desquamative gingivitis
    C. Nicotine stomatitis
    D. Leukoplakia
    E. Verruca vulgaris

16. What is the most appropriate amount of time for a recall of this patient?

    A. 3 months
    B. 6 months
    C. 9 months
    D. 12 months

17. Upon examination, you find that the patient has 6 new cavities. Last recall, he had 4 cavities. This may be due to

    A. Chewing tobacco
    B. Inhaler use
    C. The ASA
    D. Both A & B
    E. None of the above

18. Which of the following oral hygiene aids would help this patient the most?

    A. Flossing instructions
    B. Chlorhexidine
    C. Home fluoride
    D. Chlorine dioxide

19. Being on a steroid inhaler such as Azmacort can cause all of the following side effects EXCEPT

    A. Cough
    B. Dysphagia
    C. Oral candidiasis
    D. Excessive saliva production
    E. Tachycardia

20. If you were to do periodontal scalings on this patient, what might you advise him with respect to his medication?

    A. That dry mouth can increase caries incidence.

    B. That erosion can occur.

    C. There can be increased bleeding with the deep scalings.

    D. None of the above.

21. Loss of gingival attachment can occur from

    A. Albuterol usage

    B. Patient's occupation

    C. Bruxing

    D. Tobacco habit

22. On the periapical radiograph of #3 which has had root canal therapy, there is a radiolucency that may be described as a(n)

    A. Radicular cyst

    B. Periapical abscess

    C. Residual cyst

    D. Maxillary sinus

23. Your patient has parents with periodontal disease and is aware that the inhalants that he is taking can cause problems with xerostomia and carious lesions. He brushes and flosses multiple times a day. This patient's desire to be meticulous with his oral hygiene is considered to be

    A. Bipolar disorder or manic depression

    B. A psychotic disorder

    C. An anxiety disorder

    D. A brief psychotic disorder

    E. Obsessive compulsive disorder

CASE 3

PATIENT STATISTICS

Age **39**

Sex **F**

Height **5'3"**

Weight **162**

PATIENT VITALS

Blood Pressure **140/92**

Pulse Rate **56**

Respiration Rate **16**

MEDICAL HISTORY

Past Medical History **Psychiatric treatment**

Hospitalized last 5 Years? **X** Yes ___ No

Why? **Complete hysterectomy 4 years ago**

Current medications **Lithium, Ativan, Premarin**

Allergies **None**

Women ___ Pregnant ___ Lactating

Smoker **No**

Smokeless tobacco **No**

Other habits **Chews on pencils while reading. Sucks on Life-Saver candies.**

DENTAL HISTORY

Regular Check-Ups **First visit in 5 years**

TMJ **WNL**

Oral tissue exam

Patient wears upper denture and lower partial; both are over 15 years old. Tissues beneath denture and partial are red with white area on mandibular ridge. All other tissues WNL.

Oral cancer screening **WNL**

Plaque Index **1**   Calculus Index **2**

CHIEF COMPLAINT

Patient states she has had a sore under lower partial for last 2 months. It hurts when she eats. Lower left tooth hurts.

SOCIAL/CAREER BACKGROUND

Single mother of 2 teenage children. On disability for depression. Likes to read mystery novels. Does not get out much.

Clinical Examination

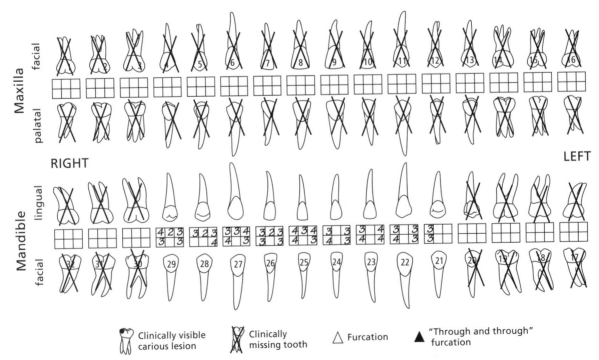

Clinically visible carious lesion

Clinically missing tooth

△ Furcation

▲ "Through and through" furcation

CASE 3: Questions 24–34

24. Your patient tells you that she removes her dentures only once a day for scrubbing. Additionally, she wears them at night while sleeping. On the topic of daily home care, you suggest that she

   A. Use a denture brush.
   B. Brush on a nightly fluoride before going to sleep.
   C. Remove her dentures at night.
   D. Get more frequent recalls.
   E. Not be embarrassed about having her denture out for cleaning.

25. The red areas under the denture and partial can be described as

   A. Caruncle
   B. Cellulitis
   C. Hemangioma
   D. Erythematous
   E. Nodule

26. This patient's Life Saver habit may be due to

   A. Anxiety
   B. Dry mouth due to drug side effects
   C. Trauma to tissue
   D. Inadequate hygiene

27. With regard to the patient's blood pressure, what would be your plan for treatment?

   A. Medical consultation with physician before treatment.
   B. Recheck blood pressure in 5 minutes.
   C. Question patient why her blood pressure is high.
   D. Postpone treatment until blood pressure under control.

28. This patient is at risk for caries because of

   A. Infrequent removal of denture/partial
   B. Life Saver habit
   C. Gingival recession
   D. All of the above

29. The lower partial may be irritating the patient because of

   A. Bone loss due to osteoporosis
   B. Age of the partial/denture
   C. Pencil biting habit
   D. Increased saliva flow due to Life Saver habit

30. The lesion under the partial might be diagnosed as

   A. Chemical burn
   B. Pleomorphic adenoma
   C. Fibroma
   D. Hyperkeratosis
   E. Carbuncle

31. The most critical information needed to provide appropriate nutritional counseling for this patient is

    A. Counseling the person responsible for meal preparation
    B. Discussing the effects of frequent carbohydrate intake
    C. Discussing her cultural food preferences
    D. All of the above

32. Which of the following instruments would you use to remove deposits of subgingival calculus for Tooth #28?

    A. Gracey curet 1/2
    B. Gracey curet 7/8
    C. Gracey curet 11/12
    D. Sickle scaler
    E. Hoe

33. On the patient's radiographs, the bone loss on the distal of #29 could be characterized as

    A. Slight horizontal
    B. Slight vertical
    C. Moderate horizontal
    D. Moderate vertical

34. On the radiograph of the central incisors, what is the radiopaque area at the bottom?

    A. Mental ridge
    B. Inferior border of the mandible
    C. Mandibular torus
    D. Internal oblique ridge
    E. Genial tubercles

CASE 4

PATIENT STATISTICS

Age   *28*
Sex   *F*
Height   *5'2"*
Weight   *130*

PATIENT VITALS

Blood Pressure   *110/70*
Pulse Rate   *80*
Respiration Rate   *15*

MEDICAL HISTORY

Past Medical History   *OB/GYN, expecting*

Hospitalized last 5 Years?   *X* Yes   No

Why?   *Son born 4 years ago*

Current medications   *Prenatal vitamins*

Allergies   *Erythromycin*

Women   *X* Pregnant   Lactating

Smoker   *No*
Smokeless tobacco   *No*
Other habits   *None*

DENTAL HISTORY

Regular Check-Ups   *Yes*

TMJ   *Slight unremarkable deviation to the right*

Oral tissue exam
   *Marginal inflammation, 4–7mm posterior readings.
   Patient does not like to floss.*

Oral cancer screening   *WNL*

Plaque Index   *1*   Calculus Index   *1*

CHIEF COMPLAINT

*Patient bit her cheek 1 month ago, and though she still
bites it, this "thing" on her cheek keeps getting bigger.*

SOCIAL/CAREER BACKGROUND

*A stay-at-home mother of a 4-year-old boy. Is 5 months
pregnant. Former Miss North Carolina. Likes to sing and
scuba dive.*

Clinical Examination

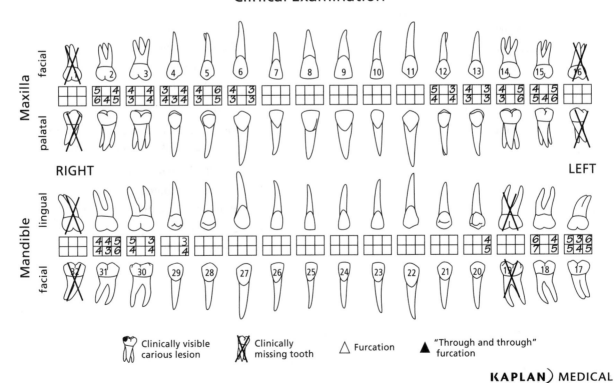

Maxilla — facial / palatal

RIGHT   LEFT

Mandible — lingual / facial

♥ Clinically visible carious lesion   ✕ Clinically missing tooth   △ Furcation   ▲ "Through and through" furcation

KAPLAN) MEDICAL

CASE 4: Questions 35–46

35. While discussing your patient's pregnancy and home life, you discover that she has just moved into a home with well water. For her 4-year-old son, you should suggest

    A. Fluoride drops 0.25 mg
    B. Fluoride vitamins 0.5 mg
    C. Fluoride vitamins 1.0 mg
    D. None of the above

36. The patient's gingival inflammation may be due to inadequate hygiene and/or hormonal changes. To help her improve her hygiene, you would counsel/instruct her to

    A. Floss at a different time of day
    B. Use an irrigating device
    C. Use a Perio-Aid
    D. Use a floss holder

37. Should you need to prescribe antibiotics for this patient, which drug would not be safe to use during pregnancy?

    A. Amoxicillin
    B. Azithromycin
    C. Clindamycin
    D. Cephalexin
    E. Tetracycline

38. Which drug(s) should be avoided during pregnancy?

    A. NSAID
    B. Aspirin
    C. Metronidazole
    D. Acyclovir
    E. All of the above

39. A differential diagnosis of this lesion may be called

    A. Mucocele
    B. Giant cell granuloma
    C. Papilloma
    D. Pyogenic granuloma
    E. Nevus

40. What might be some general causes for this lesion?

    A. Calculus
    B. Poor restorations
    C. Response to injury
    D. Hormones
    E. All of the above

41. In general, clinical characteristics of this lesion would include all of the following EXCEPT

    A. Pedunculated or sessile
    B. Deep red in color
    C. Hard upon palpation
    D. Lobulated
    E. Freely movable

42. Treatment for this patient's lesion would include

   A. Excision
   B. Removal of the irritant
   C. Leave it alone
   D. Both A & B
   E. All of the above

43. If this pregnant patient were to lay back in the chair too long and get dizzy upon arising, it would be due to

   A. Orthostatic hypotension
   B. Supine hypotensive syndrome
   C. Adrenal crisis
   D. Syncope

44. In which trimester is it safest to take radiographs if needed?

   A. First
   B. Second
   C. Third
   D. None of the above

45. The radiopaque curvature near the root tips of #3 and #14 is best described as

   A. External oblique ridge
   B. Maxillary tuberosity
   C. Maxillary sinus
   D. Hamular process
   E. Zygomatic arch

46. In the radiograph of #20, what has caused the abnormal shape of the crown?

   A. Congenital defect
   B. Calculus
   C. A filling designed to close the contact
   D. An overhang

CASE 5

PATIENT STATISTICS

Age **56**
Sex **M**
Height **6'1"**
Weight **260**

PATIENT VITALS

Blood Pressure **150/94**
Pulse Rate **74**
Respiration Rate **12**

MEDICAL HISTORY

Past Medical History   **HTN, Angina**

Hospitalized last 5 Years?   **X** Yes _____ No

Why?   **Kidney stones 3 years ago, angina 2 years ago**

Current medications   **Procardia, Aspirin daily**

Allergies   **Latex**

Women _____ Pregnant _____ Lactating

Smoker   **One pack a day for 38 years but quit 8 days ago**

Smokeless tobacco   **No**

Other habits   **None**

DENTAL HISTORY

Regular Check-Ups   **New patient, last visit 3 years ago**

TMJ   **Bilateral popping sounds upon opening**

Oral tissue exam
   Generalized inflammation, generalized pocketing, gingival hyperplasia

Oral cancer screening
   Red-white lesion #31 distal

Plaque Index   **1**   Calculus Index   **0**

CHIEF COMPLAINT

Patient states he has had a sore spot distal to #31 for the past 3 weeks. Also, he is concerned about the stain on his teeth. Additionally, his gums bleed.

SOCIAL/CAREER BACKGROUND

Divorced male, air traffic controller, fisherman. Likes to hang out with his buddies on weekends and drink beer.

Clinical Examination

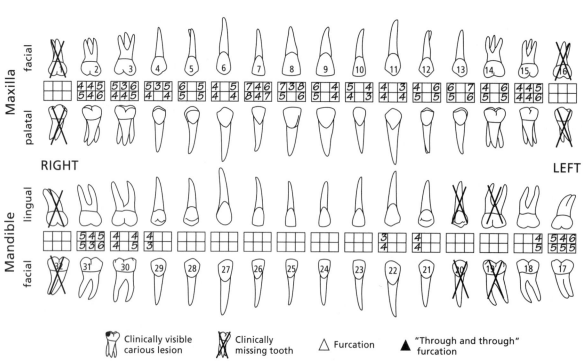

RIGHT   LEFT

🦷 Clinically visible carious lesion   ✗ Clinically missing tooth   △ Furcation   ▲ "Through and through" furcation

CASE 5: Questions 47–60

47. According to the classifications of the American Academy of Periodontology, the periodontal status of this patient is

    A. Type I
    B. Type II
    C. Type III
    D. Type IV
    E. Type V

48. This patient's gingival hyperplasia is most likely due to

    A. His smoking habit
    B. Hormonal changes
    C. A side effect of aspirin
    D. A side effect of Procardia
    E. None of the above

49. This patient is at risk for cancer because of his

    A. Alcohol consumption
    B. Being overweight
    C. Smoking habit
    D. Both A & B
    E. Both A & C

50. Based upon this patient's periodontal charting and radiographs, what kind of bone loss do you observe?

    A. No bone loss
    B. Generalized horizontal and vertical bone loss
    C. Localized horizontal and vertical bone loss
    D. Generalized vertical bone loss
    E. Localized vertical bone loss

51. Based upon the medications this patient is taking, which of the following conditions may occur?

    A. Xerostomia
    B. Candidiasis
    C. Increased bleeding
    D. Hyperpigmentation

52. In formulating a treatment plan for this patient, all of the following are necessary EXCEPT

    A. Radiographs
    B. Intra/extraoral examination
    C. Periodontal evaluation
    D. Diet history
    E. Current medical status & medications

53. The soft tissue lesion distal to Tooth #31 may be diagnosed as

    A. Candidiasis
    B. Epulis fissuratum
    C. Squamous cell carcinoma
    D. Angular stomatitis
    E. Aphthous ulcer

54. How would you categorize the patient's blood pressure?

    A. High normal
    B. Stage 1
    C. Stage 2
    D. Stage 3

KAPLAN MEDICAL

55. On the anterior periapicals radiograph of Tooth #8, what is the radiopacity on the mesial aspect?

    A. Overlap
    B. Resin filling
    C. Carious lesion
    D. Amalgam filling

56. Your patient states that #18, #19, and #21 have become cold-sensitive in the past few months. Nothing is found radiographically or clinically. Your next step is to use a desensitizing agent. You would do all the following EXCEPT

    A. Clean the teeth prior to apply agent
    B. Dry the teeth with an air-water syringe
    C. Isolate the area with cotton rolls and dry angles
    D. Use iontophoresis to apply desensitizing agent
    E. Remove excess agent to prevent ingestion

57. The radiopacity seen on the periapical radiograph of the apices of #28 and #29 is

    A. Mental foramen
    B. Submandibular fossa
    C. Pterygoid fovea
    D. Lingula
    E. Mandibular torus

58. If you were to perform root debridement, what might you caution this patient?

    A. That he will need to perform proper home care to obtain a good result.
    B. If he quits smoking, there will be a decrease in his bleeding.
    C. That there may be excessive bleeding due to the daily aspirin.
    D. That the root debridement will improve the gingival hyperplasia.

59. This patient has bilateral joint sounds upon opening. Which of the following is NOT a symptom of temporomandibular disorders (TMD)?

    A. Migraine headache
    B. Tooth sensitivity with no dental problem
    C. Pain when yawning
    D. Fibromyalgia symptoms
    E. An earache and infection

60. For treatment of TMD disorders, the Academy of General Dentistry recommends all of the following EXCEPT

    A. Equilibration
    B. Stress management
    C. Massage
    D. Eating hard foods to exercise the jaw
    E. Night guard

CASE 6

PATIENT STATISTICS

Age | **12**
Sex | **M**
Height | **4'11"**
Weight | **140**

PATIENT VITALS

Blood Pressure | **114/78**
Pulse Rate | **62**
Respiration Rate | **14**

MEDICAL HISTORY

Past Medical History | *Down syndrome, atrial septal defect (ASD), seizures, leukemia*

Hospitalized last 5 Years? ___ Yes **X** No

Why?

Current medications | *Dilantin*

Allergies | *None*

Women ___ Pregnant ___ Lactating

Smoker | *No*
Smokeless tobacco | *No*
Other habits | *Bilateral cheek-chewing for past 2 months as per staff at group home*

DENTAL HISTORY

Regular Check-Ups | *Yearly recare*

TMJ | *Deviation to the left upon closure*

Oral tissue exam
Gingival hyperplasia, poor oral hygiene due to patient's lack of cooperation

Oral cancer screening | *WNL*

Plaque Index **3** | Calculus Index **0**

CHIEF COMPLAINT

Group home staff noticed patient has been drooling lately and has been sucking in cheeks bilaterally, chewing on cheeks

SOCIAL/CAREER BACKGROUND

Moderately retarded patient who lives in group home. Likes to watch baseball. Cooperative with group home staff, except for oral hygiene care.

Clinical Examination

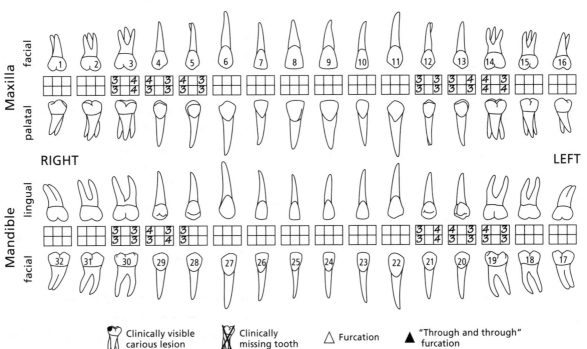

| | Clinically visible carious lesion | | Clinically missing tooth | △ Furcation | ▲ "Through and through" furcation |

CASE 6: Questions 61–70

61. Premedication for ASD would be

    A. Clindamycin 2 g , 1 hour prior to appointment

    B. Azithromycin 1 g, 1 hour prior to appointment

    C. Clarithromycin 2 g, 1 hour prior to appointment

    D. Amoxicillin 2 g, 1 hour prior to appointment

    E. Cephalexin 2 g 1 hour prior to appointment

62. The patient is being premedicated for

    A. Leukemia

    B. Seizures

    C. Atrial septal defect

    D. Down syndrome

63. Another name for Down syndrome is

    A. Trisomy 13

    B. Trisomy 18

    C. Trisomy 21

    D. Trisomy 22

    E. Trisomy 27

64. What are some of the oral concerns for this patient?

    A. Swallowing problems

    B. Dry tissues due to mouth breathing

    C. Tongue thrusting

    D. All of the above

65. Down syndrome patients are at increased risk for

    A. Hemophilia

    B. Cushing's syndrome

    C. Cleidocranial dystosis

    D. Hepatitis

    E. Leukemia

66. What can you discuss with the health care providers to help this patient with home care?

    A. Patient is stuck in a "groove" for not doing home care, needs motivation

    B. Macrodontia makes home care difficult

    C. Patient at low risk for caries

    D. Periodontal disease uncommon in DS patients

    E. Frequent repetition does not work well with DS patients

67. Preventive measures for this patient should include all the following EXCEPT

    A. Sealants

    B. Fluoride treatments

    C. Fluoride supplements

    D. Oral hygiene instructions

68. This patient has a bilateral bulbous blue areas distal to #3 and #14, which are soft and spongy upon palpation. These areas are most likely

    A. Eruption hematomas

    B. Bulla

    C. Furuncle

    D. Macule

    E. Pyogenic granuloma

69. The microorganism most prevalent in this patient's mouth could be

    A. *Prevotella intermedia*

    B. *Streptococcus sanguis*

    C. *Lactobacilli*

    D. *Streptococcus salivarius*

70. Down syndrome patients are at increased risk of all the following oral manifestations EXCEPT

    A. Enamel dysplasia

    B. Adenoid and tonsil hyperplasia

    C. Delayed tooth eruption

    D. Large nasomaxillary complex with closed mouth

    E. Fissured tongue

CASE 7

PATIENT STATISTICS

Age **65**
Sex **F**
Height **5'6"**
Weight **135**

PATIENT VITALS

Blood Pressure **120/80**
Pulse Rate **88**
Respiration Rate **20**

MEDICAL HISTORY

Past Medical History **Cancer, GERD, radiation therapy**

Hospitalized last 5 Years? **_X_** Yes ___ No

Why? **Mastectomy 2 years ago**

Current medications **Prilosec, Tamoxifen**

Allergies **Erythromycin**

Women ___ Pregnant ___ Lactating

Smoker **One pack a day, is trying to quit**
Smokeless tobacco **No**
Other habits **None**

DENTAL HISTORY

Regular Check-Ups **Regular 6-month check-up**

TMJ **WNL**

Oral tissue exam
 Recession, excellent OH

Oral cancer screening
 Pharyngeal redness

Plaque Index **0**   Calculus Index **1**

CHIEF COMPLAINT

Patient complains of dry mouth. Also, a red spot that appeared on her lower lip 4 months ago is getting slightly larger.

SOCIAL/CAREER BACKGROUND

Recently retired female EMS dispatcher who is married with 3 children and 5 grandchildren. Belongs to quilting club. Likes to bowl.

Clinical Examination

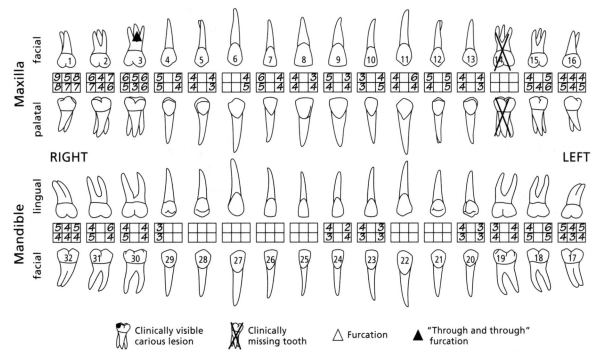

Clinically visible carious lesion   Clinically missing tooth   △ Furcation   ▲ "Through and through" furcation

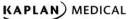

CASE 7: Questions 71–81

71. According to ASA, this patient's medical history would categorize her as

    A. ASA I
    B. ASA II
    C. ASA III
    D. ASA IV
    E. ASA V

72. This patient is at a higher risk for caries due to

    A. Recession
    B. Effects of gastric acid on teeth
    C. Dry mouth
    D. All of the above

73. Based upon this patient's medical history, which condition may be noted?

    A. Increased saliva production
    B. Decreased varices
    C. Decreased risk for esophageal problems
    D. Pharyngeal inflammation
    E. Back pain

74. Side effects from tamoxifen include all the following EXCEPT

    A. Xerostomia
    B. Nausea & vomiting
    C. Mucosal ulcerations
    D. Staining
    E. Inhibition of oogenesis

75. If GERD is left untreated, it can lead to all the following EXCEPT

    A. Problems with asthma
    B. Esophageal ulcers
    C. Esophageal strictures
    D. COPD
    E. Pneumonia

76. This patient's pigmented lesion is most likely

    A. Hemangioma
    B. Erythroplakia
    C. Herpangina
    D. Dysplasia
    E. Melanotic macule

77. After performing a routine prophylaxis on this patient, you would recommend which office fluoride?

    A. Sodium fluoride
    B. Acidulated fluoride
    C. Stannous fluoride
    D. Sodium monophosphate

78. The patient has generalized stain with moderate stain on her mandibular incisors. The best technique for removal would be

    A. Porte polisher
    B. Air polisher
    C. Ultrasonic scaler
    D. Curet
    E. File

79. Your patient has complained of a dry mouth and has asked you to recommend something to alleviate the xerostomia. Which of the following would you NOT suggest?

   A. Home fluoride therapy

   B. Saliva producing rinses

   C. Glycerin aerosol spray

   D. Chlorine dioxide

80. The patient's original lesion began to change after 1 year and she went to the oral surgeon for a biopsy. This lesion might have become

   A. Hyperplastic candidiasis

   B. Chronic hyperplasia from smoking

   C. Erythroplakia

   D. Wheal

   E. Lymphoma

81. A radiopacity appears on the periapical radiographs of #6–#11. Which of the following conditions might this be?

   A. Nasal septum

   B. Hamular process

   C. Maxillary tuberosity

   D. Median palatine suture

   E. Palatal tori

CASE 8

PATIENT STATISTICS

Age	24
Sex	F
Height	5'9"
Weight	140

PATIENT VITALS

Blood Pressure	90/60
Pulse Rate	60
Respiration Rate	12

MEDICAL HISTORY

Past Medical History *Perioral dermatitis*

Hospitalized last 5 Years? ___ Yes _X_ No

Why?

Current medications *Orthotricycline, Tetracycline, Corticosteroid cream*

Allergies *None*

Women ___ Pregnant ___ Lactating

Smoker	No
Smokeless tobacco	No
Other habits	None

DENTAL HISTORY

Regular Check-Ups

New patient appointment. Patient presented with full mouth x-rays

TMJ *WNL*

Oral tissue exam

Excellent OH, pockets 1–4mm, pink, strippled

Oral cancer screening *WNL*

Plaque Index *0*   Calculus Index *1*

CHIEF COMPLAINT

Patient complains of cold sensitivity, Patient is in for a new patient visit.

SOCIAL/CAREER BACKGROUND

Newlywed female, just moved to the area with her new husband. Works as a paralegal, has 3 dogs and 1 cat. She just joined a gym and likes to ski. Has had past orthodontic treatment and surgery for the orthodontics.

Clinical Examination

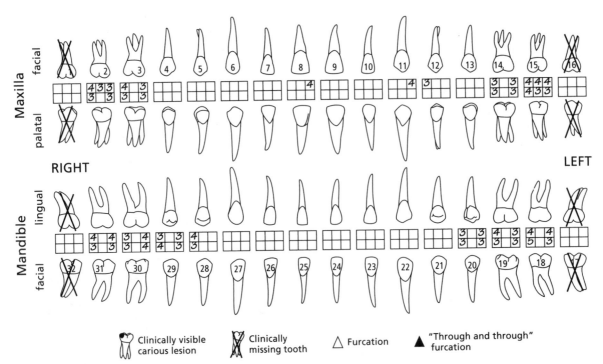

Clinically visible carious lesion

Clinically missing tooth

△ Furcation

▲ "Through and through" furcation

CASE 8: Questions 82–91

82. For the patient's blood pressure, you would

   A. Recheck the pressure in 5 minutes and get a medical consult if pressure is not elevating.

   B. Have her get a medical consultation regarding her pressure.

   C. Release her without treatment that day.

   D. Check with the dentist about the patient's blood pressure.

   E. Check with the patient to see how often she exercises at the gym.

83. The patient is being treated by a dermatologist for perioral dermatitis. What should you caution her about?

   A. Check to see if she is allergic to the antibiotic.

   B. Check to see if her prescription plan covers brand names over generic.

   C. Tell her that the orthotricycline may not be as effective as another type of birth control.

   D. None of the above

84. What else may you want to caution the patient with respect to the tetracycline she is taking?

   A. Tetracycline might constipate her.

   B. Tetracycline should be taken with food.

   C. If she should become pregnant, tetracycline shouldn't be used the last half of the pregnancy since it stains teeth in unborn children.

   D. Tetracycline does not have photosensitivity as do some of the antibiotics in the macrolide group.

   E. Superinfection with this drug is uncommon.

85. The white circular radiopacity inferior to the mandibular incisors is most likely due to a(n)

   A. Past orthognathic surgery for orthodontics

   B. Possible past fracture of the mandible

   C. Artifact

   D. None of the above

86. There is a radiolucency on the bitewing of #12 mesial. This radiolucency will most likely be mistaken for

   A. Carious lesion

   B. Cervical burnout

   C. Radiolucent restoration

   D. Temporary restoration

   E. Open margin

87. The radiolucency on the periapical of #11 is a(n)

   A. Artifact

   B. Nasopalatine cyst

   C. External root resorption

   D. Internal tooth resorption

88. Perioral dermatitis may be mistaken for

   A. Alopecia

   B. Hypertrichosis

   C. Psoriasis

   D. Seborrheic dermatitis

   E. Rosacea

89. When cautioning the patient about use of a corticosteroid cream, you would include all of the following EXCEPT

   A. Long-term use of corticosteroids suppresses the immune system.

   B. Corticosteroids do not cure the disease but rather alleviate symptoms.

   C. Since she has low blood pressure, she should have it monitored; one side effect of steroids is a drop in blood pressure.

   D. Use of steroids can contribute to periodontal disease since they interfere with the body's response to pathogens.

   E. She might gain weight.

90. How would you categorize the patient's pulse rate and respiratory rate in relation to normal heart and respiratory rates?

   A. They are both below normal.

   B. They are both on the low side of normal.

   C. They are both in the normal range.

   D. They are both on the high side of normal.

   E. The pulse rate is low, the respiratory rate is normal.

91. Which of the following dentifrice ingredients would you temporarily not recommend for this patient?

   A. Pyrophosate

   B. Sodium fluoride

   C. Potassium nitrate

   D. Citroxain

CASE 9

PATIENT STATISTICS

Age **72**
Sex **F**
Height **5'7"**
Weight **145**

PATIENT VITALS

Blood Pressure **160/108**
Pulse Rate **74**
Respiration Rate **14**

MEDICAL HISTORY

Past Medical History **Cancer, hypertension, recent ear infection, osteopenia**

Hospitalized last 5 Years? **X** Yes ___ No

Why? **Thyroid cancer surgery, radiation treatment**

Current medications **Lasix, Catapress, Septra**

Allergies **None**

Women ___ Pregnant ___ Lactating

Smoker **No**
Smokeless tobacco **No**
Other habits **None**

DENTAL HISTORY

Regular Check-Ups
Because of side effects from radiation therapy, patient has not returned for 2 years.

TMJ **Crepitus right side**

Oral tissue exam
Good OH

Oral cancer screening
WNL

Plaque Index **0**   Calculus Index **1**

CHIEF COMPLAINT

Patient complains of a white area in the muccobuccal fold of her upper lip.

SOCIAL/CAREER BACKGROUND

Single female who never married. Has a loving family of 3 siblings, 3 nieces, and 4 nephews. Former restaurant owner. Likes to go dancing at the seniors center.

Clinical Examination

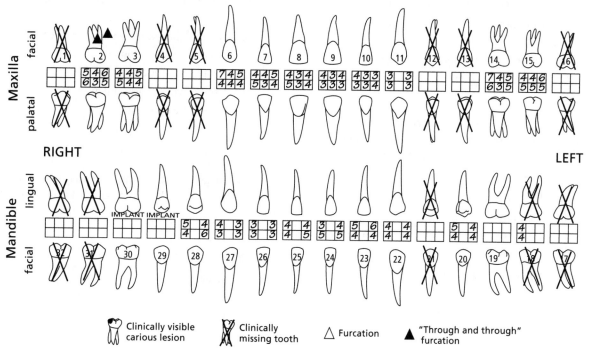

Maxilla — facial / palatal

| | 5 4 6 / 6 3 5 | 4 4 5 / 5 4 4 | | | 7 4 5 / 4 4 4 | 4 4 5 / 5 3 4 | 4 3 4 / 3 3 3 | 4 3 4 / 3 3 4 | 4 3 3 / 3 3 4 | 3 / 3 / 3 / 3 | | | 7 4 5 / 6 3 5 | 4 4 6 / 5 5 5 | |

RIGHT   **LEFT**

Mandible — lingual / facial

IMPLANT IMPLANT

| | | | | 5 4 4 / 4 6 | 4 3 / 3 3 | 3 3 / 3 3 | 3 4 / 4 5 | 3 4 / 4 4 | 5 6 / 4 4 | 4 4 / 4 4 | | 5 4 / 4 4 | | | 4 4 / 4 4 | |

Clinically visible carious lesion
Clinically missing tooth
△ Furcation
▲ "Through and through" furcation

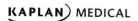

CASE 9: Questions 92–105

92. Upon examining the patient's creamy white lesion, you notice that it can be removed, though it leaves a raw red area. This lesion is

    A. Angular cheilitis
    B. Desquamative gingivitis
    C. Erythematous candidiasis
    D. Pseudomembranous candidiasis
    E. Lichen planus

93. This lesion has appeared in the last 2 months and was caused by all of the following EXCEPT

    A. Immune-compromised state of the patient
    B. Xerostomia due to medications
    C. Antibiotic for ear infection
    D. Melanin pigmentation

94. Upon performing a periodontal pocket probing, you notice that Tooth #2 is mobile. Which of the following best describes this type of bone loss?

    A. Vertical loss with furcation involvement
    B. Horizontal bone loss with furcation involvement
    C. Vertical and horizontal bone loss
    D. Normal bone loss

95. This patient has not been in recently due to radiation therapy side effects. You would suggest the following adjuncts to help this patient EXCEPT

    A. Rinse with Listerine
    B. Sodium fluoride
    C. Interproximal brush with plastic-coated wire
    D. Perio-Aid
    E. Sip water frequently

96. Radiation therapy has all of the side effects EXCEPT

    A. Difficulty in swallowing
    B. Dysgeusia
    C. Burning sensation with spicy foods
    D. Exostosis
    E. Mucositis

97. Which of the following fluorides might you suggest for this patient?

    A. Brush-on gel
    B. Stannous fluoride
    C. Neutral sodium
    D. Acidulated phosphate

98. While reviewing your patient's diet, you discover that she drinks soda to relieve her xerostomia. You would recommend instead that she do all of the following EXCEPT

    A. Brush with a soft toothbrush to remove deposits
    B. Drink a glass of red wine daily since it contains antioxidant
    C. Avoid spicy foods
    D. Use sugarless candy and gum
    E. Use a salivary substitute

99. You are going to curet the mesial aspect of the distal root of #2. Which curet would you choose?

    A. Gracey 1/2
    B. Gracey 7/8
    C. Gracey 11/12
    D. Gracey 13/14
    E. Gracey 17/18

100. What would be your next step with respect to this patient's blood pressure?

    A. Recheck in 5 minutes
    B. Recheck the next three subsequent visits and if not improved get medical consultation
    C. Medical consultation
    D. No treatment or medical consultation

101. Which of the following microorangisms is this patient especially prone to orally?

    A. Candida
    B. Proteus
    C. Borrelia
    D. Escherichia

102. In which ASA category would you place this patient?

    A. Type I
    B. Type II
    C. Type III
    D. Type IV
    E. ASA V

103. Crepitus of the temporomandibular joint is likely due to

    A. Whiplash
    B. Stress
    C. Psychosocial factors
    D. Internal derangement of the joint
    E. Degenerative joint disease

104. In the periapical radiograph, you notice a radiolucency on the roots of #8. This radiolucency is a(n)

    A. Internal resorption
    B. External resorption
    C. Fracture
    D. Root caries
    E. Radicular cyst

105. Which of the following types of implants does this patient have?

    A. Transosteal
    B. Subperiosteal
    C. Endosseous
    D. Ceramic
    E. Titanium

CASE 10

PATIENT STATISTICS

Age **69**
Sex **F**
Height **5'5"**
Weight **168**

PATIENT VITALS

Blood Pressure **170/100**
Pulse Rate **92**
Respiration Rate **18**

MEDICAL HISTORY

Past Medical History **Type I diabetes, CVA, hypertension**

Hospitalized last 5 Years? **_X_** Yes ____ No

Why? **Stroke, uncontrolled diabetes**

Current medications **Humulin, Coumadin, Accupril, Synthroid**

Allergies **Tetracycline**

Women ____ Pregnant ____ Lactating

Smoker **No**
Smokeless tobacco **No**
Other habits **None**

DENTAL HISTORY

Regular Check-Ups
Patient on irregular recare due to nursing home limitations

TMJ **WNL**

Oral tissue exam
Poor OH, patient had successful periodontal surgery 4 years ago

Oral cancer screening **WNL**

Plaque Index **2**   Calculus Index **2**

CHIEF COMPLAINT

Patient wants her teeth cleaned and complains of a sore under her tongue.

SOCIAL/CAREER BACKGROUND

Retired female nurse, has 6 children and 15 grandchildren. Lives in a nursing home since her stroke 18 months ago. She was an avid golfer and active in her church until her stroke.

Clinical Examination

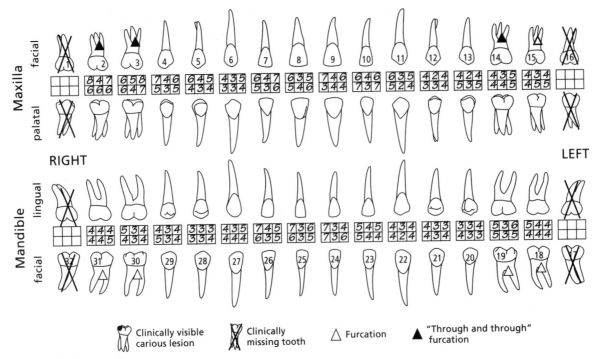

Maxilla — facial / palatal
Mandible — lingual / facial

RIGHT   LEFT

| | | | | | | | | | | | | | | |
847 | 658 | 746 | 645 | 647 | 635 | 746 | 646 | 635 | 424 | 424 | 435 | 434
666 | 647 | 535 | 434 | 536 | 546 | 344 | 737 | 524 | 334 | 535 | 445 | 455

444 | 534 | 434 | 333 | 435 | 745 | 734 | 545 | 434 | 433 | 334 | 536 | 544
445 | 434 | 534 | 334 | 444 | 635 | 736 | 544 | 424 | 434 | 433 | 535 | 444

Legend:

🦷 Clinically visible carious lesion   ✕ Clinically missing tooth   △ Furcation   ▲ "Through and through" furcation

CASE 10: Questions 106–117

106. Your patient has not been in the office since her stroke. She had been through successful periodontal surgery but has not been able to keep up with her home care due to partial paralysis. Which of the following adjuncts would most help with her home care?

   A.   A thicker floss such as ribbon

   B.   A floss holder

   C.   Power-assisted toothbrush

   D.   A Velcro strap on a toothbrush

   E.   An electric toothbrush

107. What is the difference between diabetes mellitus and diabetes insipidus?

   A.   Both types of diabetes are both characterized with polyuria and polyphagia, but not polydipsia.

   B.   Both types of diabetes occur due to an autoimmune response but only one requires medication.

   C.   Both types of diabetes are characterized by polyuria and polydipsia, but diabetes insipidus is induced by an antidiuretic hormone deficiency.

   D.   In both types of diabetes, the beta cells are destroyed but with diabetes mellitus, the alpha cells take over.

108. Diabetics tend to have fewer _____ blood cells.

   A.   Polymorphonuclear leukocytes

   B.   Platelet

   C.   Lymphocyte

   D.   Monocyte

   E.   Basophil

109. What is the best time of day to schedule a diabetic patient?

   A.   First thing in the morning before she has eaten breakfast

   B.   First thing in the morning after she has eaten breakfast

   C.   Just before lunch

   D.   Mid-afternoon

   E.   At the end of the day

110. Your patient is complaining about a tenderness on the ventral surface of her tongue. Upon inspection, you find a white lesion surrounded by a red halo. This lesion is most likely

   A.   Fistula

   B.   Apthous ulcer

   C.   Macule

   D.   Verruca vulgaris

   E.   Petechiae

111. This patient's blood pressure can be categorized as

   A.   High normal

   B.   Stage 1

   C.   Stage 2

   D.   Stage 3

112. A typical diabetic's blood pressure is usually normal or slightly elevated, but the pulse rate is usually

    A. Below normal and regular
    B. Below normal and irregular
    C. Normal
    D. Above normal and irregular
    E. Above normal and regular

113. There is significant bone loss on the bitewing radiograph of #14. How would this be categorized according to classifications of furcation involvement?

    A. Class I
    B. Class II
    C. Class III
    D. Class IV

114. What type of bone loss do you see on the radiographs?

    A. Generalized horizontal
    B. Localized horizontal
    C. Localized vertical and horizontal
    D. Generalized vertical and horizontal

115. This patient would be placed in which periodontal category?

    A. Type I
    B. Type II
    C. Type III
    D. Type IV

116. What are the bilateral radiopacities on the mandibular anterior periapical radiograph?

    A. Odontogenic cyst
    B. Nasopalatine duct cyst
    C. Myxoma
    D. Mandibular tori
    E. Odontogenic keratocyst

117. Typically, which classifications of mobility can you expect to find on all the anterior teeth?

    A. Class I
    B. Class II
    C. Class III
    D. Class IV

CASE 11

PATIENT STATISTICS

Age	**48**
Sex	**M**
Height	**6'2"**
Weight	**172**

PATIENT VITALS

Blood Pressure	**161/104**
Pulse Rate	**78**
Respiration Rate	**16**

MEDICAL HISTORY

Past Medical History **HTN, kidney dialysis for end-stage renal disease**

Hospitalized last 5 Years? __X__ Yes ___ No

Why? **Kidney failure, patient on transplant list**

Current medications **Diovan, Allopurinol**

Allergies **Aspirin**

Women ___ Pregnant ___ Lactating

Smoker	**No**
Smokeless tobacco	**No**
Other habits	**None**

DENTAL HISTORY

Regular Check-Ups **Recare appointment overdue**

TMJ **WNL**

Oral tissue exam
  Marginal redness

Oral cancer screening
  WNL

Plaque Index **2**   Calculus Index **2**

CHIEF COMPLAINT

None. Patient is here for his recare appointment and refuses any radiographs today. Full mouth radiographs were taken one year ago.

SOCIAL/CAREER BACKGROUND

Father of 2 small chidren who is currently on disability for end stage renal disease and is awaiting a transplant. On dialysis twice a week. Used to drive a cement truck.

Clinical Examination

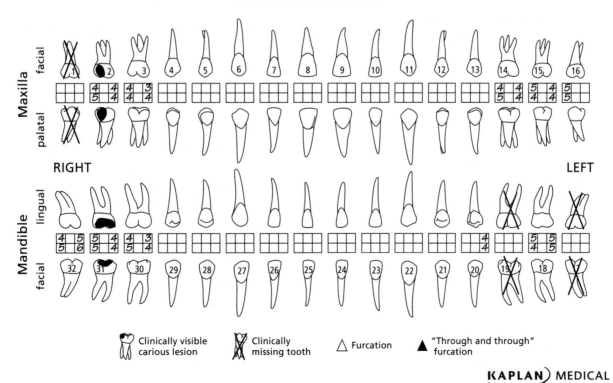

RIGHT   LEFT

Clinically visible carious lesion	Clinically missing tooth	△ Furcation	▲ "Through and through" furcation

KAPLAN MEDICAL

CASE 11: Questions 118–125

118. This patient has not been into the office for some time because of ill health. Upon updating his medical history, you tell the patient that a medical consultation with his physician is necessary before any treatment and you can only update his radiographs today. When you attempt to administer them, he becomes upset and wants to refuse them. You would

   A. Have the patient sign a release form for not having radiographs today.
   B. Have the dentist talk the patient into radiographs.
   C. Dismiss the patient.
   D. Inquire about the patient's concerns over radiographs.

119. Your patient is on Diovan for hypertension. Which of the following is the most serious side effect of antihypertension medications?

   A. Cough
   B. Abdominal pain
   C. Severe drop in blood pressure
   D. Runny nose
   E. Diarrhea

120. Antihypertensives can cause all of the following common symptoms EXCEPT

   A. Dizziness
   B. Insomnia
   C. Muscle cramping
   D. Fatigue
   E. Decreased urine output

121. With respect to the patient's blood pressure level, what would be the next step for treatment?

   A. Retake the blood pressure in 5 minutes.
   B. Recheck the next three subsequent visits.
   C. Do a medical consultation and provide dental treatment today.
   D. Do a medical consultation and provide no dental treatment today.

122. How would you classify this patient's hypertension?

   A. High normal/high
   B. Stage 1
   C. Stage 2
   D. Stage 3

123. The most important step for the patient's next recare visit is to

   A. Prescribe an antibiotic premedication.
   B. Check his blood pressure prior to treatment.
   C. Review his medical history.
   D. Review his oral hygiene care and give any adjuncts that would aid in better home care.
   E. Create a treatment plan for root debridement.

124. The drug Allopurinol is classified as an

   A. Antianxiety drug
   B. Antihypertensive drug
   C. Antineoplastic drug
   D. Antihyperuricemia drug
   E. Antihyperlipidemic

125. Should your patient need pain relief, the dentist would NOT want to prescribe

   A. Percoset
   B. Percodan
   C. Naloxone
   D. Tylenol #3
   E. Meperidine

CASE 12

PATIENT STATISTICS

Age **16**
Sex **F**
Height **5'0"**
Weight **109**

PATIENT VITALS

Blood Pressure **118/72**
Pulse Rate **65**
Respiration Rate **14**

MEDICAL HISTORY

Past Medical History **Sports-induced asthma**

Hospitalized last 5 Years? **_X_** Yes ___ No

Why? **Orthoscopic knee surgery**

Current medications **None**

Allergies **Penicillin**

Women ___ Pregnant ___ Lactating

Smoker **No**
Smokeless tobacco **No**
Other habits **None**

DENTAL HISTORY

Regular Check-Ups **Check-Ups 6 month recare**

TMJ **WNL**

Oral tissue exam
Slight marginal redness

Oral cancer screening
WNL

Plaque Index **1**   Calculus Index **0**

CHIEF COMPLAINT

Patient's gums bleed so she is afraid to floss.

SOCIAL/CAREER BACKGROUND

A female high school junior. Lives at home with an older brother and younger sister. Is on the varsity cheerleading squad and also works part-time at a veterinary hospital.

Clinical Examination

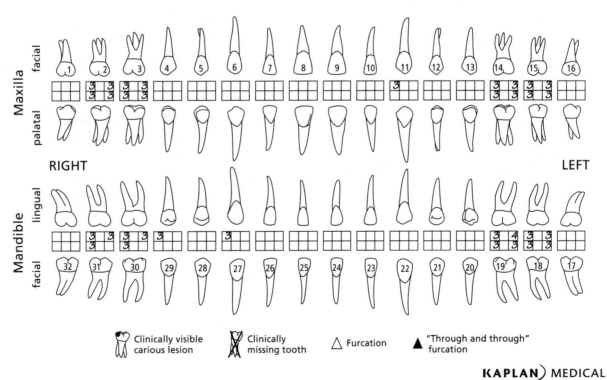

Maxilla — facial / palatal

RIGHT   LEFT

Mandible — lingual / facial

🦷 Clinically visible carious lesion   🦷 Clinically missing tooth   △ Furcation   ▲ "Through and through" furcation

KAPLAN MEDICAL

CASE 12: Questions 126–132

126. Your patient got her tongue pierced 5 months ago and does not want her parents to find out. The mother, however, suspects something, and asks you to reveal why her daughter is secretive about her oral hygiene when she is in the bathroom. You would

    A. Tell the mother about the tongue piercing since the patient is a minor.

    B. Not tell the mother, since the patient asked you not to.

    C. Not tell the mother, since, when a state law permits patient confidentiality, it prohibits telling a parent.

    D. None of the above

127. You need to take a panorex radiograph on this patient to evaluate her wisdom teeth. The patient states she has never taken out the piercing and would not even know how. You would

    A. Leave it in place and take the panorex.

    B. Tell her she needs to take it out no matter what.

    C. Instruct her on how to unscrew the end with her fingers.

    D. Take two pieces of gauze and guide her on how to unscrew the piercing.

    E. Ask the dentist for help.

128. Tongue piercing can cause many types of complications, but which type would be the most serious?

    A. Cracked teeth

    B. Cyst formation

    C. Scarring

    D. Speech impediments

    E. Toxic shock syndrome

129. Who would be at greatest risk for infection with a tongue piercing?

    A. Someone who had once had endocarditis

    B. A diabetic

    C. Someone with asthma

    D. Someone with COPD

    E. Someone with an allergic reaction to titanium

130. Apart from endocarditis, what is the most serious oral problem a tongue piercing could cause?

    A. A cyst

    B. Nerve damage

    C. Ludwig's angina

    D. Speech impediment

    E. Inflammation and oozing

131. If an infection of the tongue occurs, the main lymph node drainage for the body of the tongue would be

    A. Submental node

    B. Submandibular node

    C. Superior deep cervical node

    D. Retropharyngeal node

132. Your patient is afraid of flossing since it causes her gums to bleed. What can you do to assure her it's to her benefit to floss?

    A. Demonstrate flossing technique

    B. Demonstrate brushing technique

    C. Explain that she is not cutting her gums when flossing

    D. Show patient how to use a Perio-Aid

    E. Explain that gingivitis causes ulcers that bleed

CASE 13

PATIENT STATISTICS

Age **53**
Sex **F**
Height **5'9"**
Weight **155**

PATIENT VITALS

Blood Pressure **148/95**
Pulse Rate **67**
Respiration Rate **19**

MEDICAL HISTORY

Past Medical History **Von Willebrand's disease, rosacea**

Hospitalized last 5 Years? ___ Yes **X** No

Why?

Current medications **Minocycline**

Allergies **Eggs**

Women ___ Pregnant ___ Lactating

Smoker **No**
Smokeless tobacco **No**
Other habits **None**

DENTAL HISTORY

Regular Check-Ups **6 month recare, jaw pain**

TMJ **WNL**

Oral tissue exam
Mucosa

Oral cancer screening
Purpuric spots on left buccal mucosa

Plaque Index **1**   Calculus Index **0**

CHIEF COMPLAINT

Patient has had jaw pain for the past 2 days.

SOCIAL/CAREER BACKGROUND

Single female CPA with several nephews and nieces. Enjoys hiking, gardening, watching football, and her parakeet.

Clinical Examination

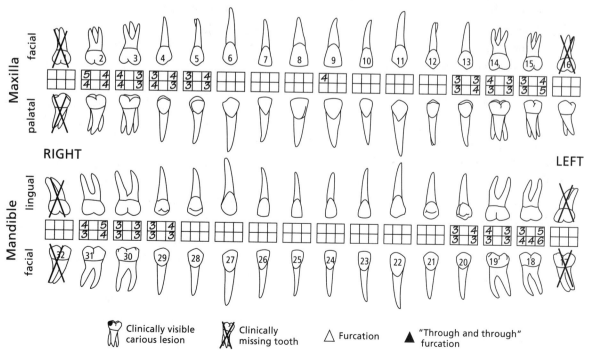

Maxilla — facial / palatal

RIGHT   LEFT

Mandible — lingual / facial

🦷 Clinically visible carious lesion   ✕ Clinically missing tooth   △ Furcation   ▲ "Through and through" furcation

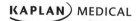
KAPLAN MEDICAL

CASE 13: Questions 133–141

133. Since the patient has an egg allergy, she would NOT want to

    A. Eat eggplant
    B. Get a flu vaccine
    C. Eat peanut butter
    D. Get a tetanus shot

134. A side effect of minocycline is

    A. Tooth discoloration
    B. Hemolytic anemia
    C. Red pigmentation of the alveolar bone and hard palate
    D. Photosensitivity
    E. Angioneurotic edema

135. Your patient has many bruises on her arms as a result of the Von Willebrand's disease. This disease affects what blood factor?

    A. Factor V
    B. Factor VIII
    C. Factor IX
    D. Factor XI
    E. Stuart factor

136. Oral implications from Von Willebrand's disease include all the following EXCEPT

    A. Purpuric spots
    B. Prolonged bleeding after dental procedures
    C. Hematomas
    D. Neurofibromatomas
    E. Petechiae

137. Von Willebrand's disease occurs more often in

    A. Women
    B. Men
    C. Both men and women
    D. None of the above

138. The picture of this patient's buccal mucosa can be described as

    A. Hematoma
    B. Petechia
    C. Purpuric spots
    D. Hemangioma
    E. Cellulitis

Scenario for Questions 139–141

Your patient complains of having had lower jaw pain for 2 days. Radiographs taken of the area were negative for oral pathology. After the radiographs are exposed, she lies back in the chair and becomes dizzy, but then she improves. The oral exam is negative for pathology in the complaint area. The patient also states that when she got out of bed this morning, she was dizzy, but then was well. As she gets out of the chair, she again becomes dizzy.

139. Your patient is likely suffering from

    A.   Orthostatic hypotension

    B.   Supine hypotensive syndrome

    C.   Low blood sugar

    D.   Myocardial infarction

140. Which of the following procedures would you perform first to help this patient?

    A.   Open the airway

    B.   Place the patient in Trendelenburg position

    C.   Administer oxygen

    D.   Take vital signs

    E.   Call 911

141. The patient wants to get up and drive home since she is feeling better. What is the best medical advice you could give her?

    A.   If when driving home you still feel dizzy, pull the car over and call 911 on your cell phone.

    B.   Call a neighbor or friend to drive you home.

    C.   That you are calling the paramedics to check her.

    D.   That you will have to hold her down in the chair if she tries to leave.

CASE 14

PATIENT STATISTICS

Age	64
Sex	M
Height	5'10"
Weight	222

PATIENT VITALS

Blood Pressure	182/112
Pulse Rate	92
Respiration Rate	22

MEDICAL HISTORY

Past Medical History   *Arthritis, spinal degeneration, UTI, glaucoma*

Hospitalized last 5 Years?   _X_ Yes   ___ No

Why?   *Spinal surgery and disc removal*

Current medications   *Bactrim, Dolobid, Timoptic*

Allergies   *Codeine*

Women ___ Pregnant ___ Lactating

Smoker	*Quit smoking 15 years ago*
Smokeless tobacco	*No*
Other habits	*None*

DENTAL HISTORY

Regular Check-Ups   *6 month recare*

TMJ   *Right deviation upon opening that is asymptomatic*

Oral tissue exam
Lesion on lower right lip that has been there for 2 years; another lesion under the tongue that the patient says goes up and down

Oral cancer screening
WNL

Plaque Index   **2**   Calculus Index   **1**

CHIEF COMPLAINT

Patient is concerned about a new lesion under his tongue that swells up and down, though doesn't hurt.

SOCIAL/CAREER BACKGROUND

Retired male newspaper editor who lives in a retirement community with his wife and 3 cats. Enjoys sailing and playing the stock market.

Clinical Examination

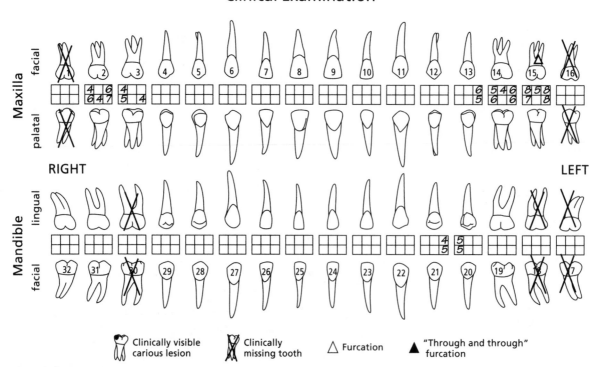

Clinically visible carious lesion   Clinically missing tooth   △ Furcation   ▲ "Through and through" furcation

CASE 14: Questions 142–150

142. This patient is on Bactrim for

    A. Disc removal

    B. Arthritis

    C. Glaucoma

    D. UTI

143. With respect to this patient's blood pressure, what should be the next step for dental treatment?

    A. Recheck the blood pressure the next 3 subsequent visits.

    B. Recheck the blood pressure in 5 minutes.

    C. Recheck the blood pressure in 5 minutes and if not better, have patient get a medical consultation.

    D. No dental treatment; patient should get a medical consultation.

144. This patient is on Timoptic for glaucoma. What substance in glaucoma medication can affect the heart?

    A. Calcium channel blockers

    B. Beta blockers

    C. Antiadrenergic agents

    D. ACE inhibitors

145. The lesion on the patient's lower lip may be diagnosed as

    A. Furuncle

    B. Pyogenic granuloma

    C. Macule

    D. Epulis fissuratum

    E. Irritative fibroma

146. The lesion under the patient's tongue, to the right of the lingual frenum, may be diagnosed as

    A. Sialolith

    B. Ranula

    C. Nodule

    D. Papule

    E. Nevus

147. The radiopacity distal to #31 is

    A. Staphne bone cyst

    B. Tooth #32

    C. Genial tubercles

    D. Condylar head

    E. Odontoma

148. Which of the following pain medications could be prescribed for this patient?

    A. Tylenol #3

    B. Percoset

    C. Percodan

    D. Oxycodone

    E. Acetylsalicylic acid

149. The artery that supplies blood to Tooth #31 is the

    A. Buccal artery

    B. Greater palatine artery

    C. Sphenopalatine artery

    D. Inferior alveolar artery

150. The nerve that supplies sensation to Tooth #2 is the

    A. Posterior superior alveolar nerve

    B. Lesser palatine nerve

    C. Greater palatine nerve

    D. Mental nerve

    E. Accessory nerve

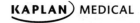

Answer Explanations: Component B

CASE 1

1. A

Cephalexin 2 g would be best, since the patient is allergic to penicillin.

B. Amoxicillin is not correct due to the patient's penicillin allergy.

C. Erythromycin used to be the old drug of choice for a penicillin allergy, but many people got upset stomachs from erythromycin.

D. Azithromycin is a choice for penicillin allergy, but the dosage was incorrect and should be 500 mg.

2. C

Smoking is the obvious answer.

A. Tanning may be a contributing factor but her history does not discuss tanning.

B. While alcohol can be a risk factor, the patient's history says she drinks socially.

3. B

Synthroid treats hypothyroidism, when the thyroid does not produce enough thyroxine.

A. Hyperthyroidism occurs when the thyroid produces too much thyroxine. There would be no need to add more of the hormone with medication, which is what Synthroid does. It results in Grave's disease and exophthalmos. It can lead to a thyroid storm.

C. Hyperparathyroidism occurs when the parathyroid produces too much parathyroid hormone (PTH), and there is an increase in calcium levels in the blood serum. Treatment of choice is removal of the parathyroid glands which cures 95% of cases.

D. Hypoparathyroidism occurs when the parathyroid does not produce enough PTH, and there is a decrease in calcium levels in blood serum. Treatment of choice is calcium and vitamin D supplements.

4. B

The lesion could be squamous cell carcinoma, which arises from the epidermis and resembles the squamous cells that make up the outermost layers of skin. If not treated, it can penetrate underlying tissues.

A. A chancre occurs from syphilis.

C. Solar or actinic cheilosis is the result of sun damage to the lip. It can be hard to differentiate from squamous cell carcinoma. Solar cheilosis loses the vermilion border of the lip initially and then becomes pale with a bluish background but may go on to develop dry scaly areas.

D. WHO defines keratotic plaque as a white lesion, which cannot be scraped off and is not caused by smoking. It can lead to leukoplakia. It is generally found intra-orally or on pharyngeal mucosa.

E. Leukoplakia is a tobacco-related white patch or plaque that cannot be rubbed off. Initially the lesion is nonpalpable, faintly translucent, and has white discoloration, but it can become a diffuse, slightly elevated, opaque white plaque that develops irregular outlines.

5. C

The main lymph nodes for drainage are the submental nodes, which also drain the mandibular incisors and associated tissues.

A. Submandibular nodes drain the maxillary 1st and 2nd molars and premolars, and associated tissues.

B. Superior cervical nodes drain the tongue base, palatine tonsils, and lingual tonsils.

D. Parotid nodes drain the middle ear and the parotid gland.

E. Postauricular nodes drain the ear.

6. D

Squamous cell carcinoma on the lip could be mistaken for all of the answer choices.

7. B

Prozac is a serotonin-specific reuptake inhibitor.

A. Advil is an analgesic.

8. B

The patient's pulse rate is a bit low.

9. C

"Standard precautions" means that all patients are considered to be potentially infectious for bloodborne pathogens.

10. E

The area near the distal of #29 is excess amalgam filling in the tissue.

A. Cervical abrasion would be radiolucent.

B. Temporary restorations may have some radiopacity.

C. Resin fillings are variably radiopaque, not bright white.

D. Cervical burnout is radiolucent.

11. E

The lesions might be nevi. A nevus is a diffuse, white, and spongy lesion that is also smooth and flat.

A. Lichen planus has white, lacy lines.

B. Linear alba occurs on the buccal mucosa.

C. Papule is a small solid, superficial elevation of skin that is circumscribed.

D. Furuncle is a boil or painful skin nodule that has a circumscribed area of inflammation.

CASE 2

12. E

A bronchodilator (albuterol) can cause all of the listed side effects: dry mouth, bad taste, urinary retention, and tachycardia.

13. D

The radiolucency between #8 and #9 is the median palatine suture.

A. The nasal septum is between #8 and #9 but it is radiopaque.

B. The inverted Y is a radiolucency that is the juncture of the nasal floor and the maxillary anterior sinus.

C. A fracture may be mistaken for the median palatine suture.

14. A

The lesion was probably caused by sun exposure, since the patient is a farmer and works outside.

C. Chewing tobacco will change tissues intraorally.

15. D

The lesion is likely leukoplakia, which is caused by tobacco chewing. Chewing tobacco can lead to oral cancer if the tissue changes and invades the lower layers of the dermis.

A. A bulla is a blister.

B. Desquamative gingivitis is a white lesion that can be rubbed off with a 2 × 2.

C. Nicotine stomatitis is caused by the heat of smoking and occurs in the hard and soft palates. The minor salivary glands become inflamed, initially red in color but then become a diffuse gray–white area with a red center.

E. Verruca vulgaris is a wart caused by the papilloma virus. It is found on the lips, tongue, or mucosa.

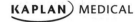

16. A

This patient should be recalled in 3 months, since he has tissue changes that should be monitored.

17. D

Answer choices A and B would have caused a sharp increase in cavities. Chewing tobacco has a high sugar content, and albuterol causes xerostomia that can lead to a higher decay rate.

18. C

Home fluoride would help this patient greatly, because of the high decay rate.

A. Flossing instruction would help, though the patient already has good oral hygiene.

B. Chlorhexidine is prescribed for gingival disease, but the tissues are in good health.

D. Chlorine dioxide has no therapeutic value, but it is effective for halitosis.

19. D

Azmacort can cause rapid heart rate, cough, dysphagia, and/or oral candidiasis. It does not, however, cause excessive saliva.

20. C

You would advise him that there might be increased bleeding with the deep scalings. This is because of the daily aspirin (ASA) he is taking.

A. Dry mouth can increase caries incidence but that would not affect deep scaling in pockets.

21. D

Loss of gingival attachment can result from chewing tobacco.

22. D

The radiolucency is the maxillary sinus.

A. A radicular (or periapical) cyst is a slow-growing odontogenic cyst caused by caries, trauma, or pulpitis. It is a fluid-filled sac of epithelium that undergoes necrosis due to a lack of blood supply, causing the granuloma to become a cyst.

B. Periapical abscess or periapical granuloma is an acute or chronic inflammation of tissues at the apex of a tooth, resulting in a collection of pus after a pulpal infection. It is the result of a carious lesion or injury causing pulp necrosis, resulting in the formation of a periapical granuloma.

C. Residual cysts appear in the area of an extracted tooth.

23. E

Extreme meticulousness with oral hygiene would be the result of an obsessive compulsive disorder.

C. An anxiety disorder occurs when the patient worries excessively about everything all the time.

CASE 3

24. C

You recommend that she remove her dentures at night. Since the patient has reddened areas under both the partial and the denture, this will allow the tissue to heal. These red areas are a form of candidiasis.

A. Using a denture brush would be a good adjunct, though it is of secondary importance.

B. Brushing on a nightly fluoride gel would help, but it is of secondary importance to the tissues.

25. D

The reddened areas are erythematous.

A. A caruncle is a small, red, fleshy eminence.

B. A cellulitis is a very diffuse area that is not well-defined, and the reddened areas in this case perfectly outline the denture and partial.

26. B

It is likely that the patient uses Life Savers as a way to relieve dry mouth. Antidepressants such as lithium can cause dry mouth, and hard candy would keep the saliva flowing.

27. B

Treatment should be to recheck the blood pressure in 5 minutes, since the patient has anxiety to begin with. The pressure is within the guidelines for rechecking.

A. Medical consultation with the physician before treatment is not an absolute in this case, since it is within the guidelines for rechecking.

D. Treatment does not need to be postponed with the given blood pressure.

28. D

There are several things that put this patient at high risk for caries: infrequent removal of denture/partial; Life Saver habit; gingival recession; and non-removal of the partial at night.

29. B

The irritation may be due to the age of the partial/denture. The fit might have changed and is thus interfering with the lesion.

A. Bone loss from osteoporosis was not mentioned in the patient's medical history.

C. The pencil biting habit could be a contributing factor, but the age of the denture is the more likely cause.

30. D

The lesion is hyperkeratosis, since it is white in color.

A. An oral chemical burn would be caused by holding an aspirin against a painful tooth, for instance. It is usually a white lesion surrounded by an inflammatory halo.

B. Pleomorphic adenoma is a benign salivary gland tumor and would not be found on the mandibular ridge.

C. A fibroma is a pink projection usually found on the buccal mucosa, gingiva, floor of the mouth, tongue lips, or palate.

E. A carbuncle is necrotizing skin infection made up of a cluster of boils or furuncles.

31. B

Discussing the frequency of the Life Saver habit would be the most important item. The patient should use sugarless candy or drink water for the xerostomia.

A. Nutritional counseling could be important, but nothing was mentioned in the history to indicate abnormal eating habits.

C. Cultural food preferences may be significant if they involve a high carbohydrate intake; however, that was not mentioned in the history.

32. A

To remove deposits of subgingival calculus, you would use a Gracey curet 1/2.

B. A Gracey curet 7/8 is for the facial and lingual surfaces of posterior teeth.

C. A Gracey curet 11/12 is for the mesial aspect of posterior teeth.

D. A sickle scaler is not a subgingival instrument.

E. A hoe cannot be adapted to a curved tooth surface and is used to primarily remove heavy supragingival calculus. The radiographs do not show heavy calculus.

33. B

The bone loss is a slight vertical bone loss.

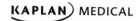

34. E

The radiopaque area indicates genial tubercles.

A. Mental ridge is a radiopaque line that travels along the anterior aspect of the mandible.

B. Inferior border of the mandible is not included in this radiograph.

C. Mandibular torus is usually not located in this area.

D. Internal oblique ridge is a posterior landmark.

CASE 4

35. B

With respect to the water for her child, you should suggest fluoride vitamins 0.5 mg, which is the recommended dosage for 3–6 year-olds.

A. Fluoride drops 0.25 mg would be appropriate for children 6 months–3 years old.

C. Fluoride vitamins 1.0 mg would be for children aged 6–16.

36. D

A floss holder would be beneficial.

A. Flossing at a different time of day would be good advice in the first trimester of pregnancy, when morning sickness is common.

B. Using an irrigating device would control gingival disease, where the gingiva is loosely attached.

C. Using a Perio-Aid would help the patient trace along the gingiva nicely but would not reach plaque interproximally under the gingiva.

37. E

Tetracycline would be the only unsafe antibiotic during pregnancy.

38. E

All of the answer choices should be avoided during pregnancy: NSAID, aspirin, metronidazole, and acyclovir.

39. D

The lesion could be described as a pyogenic granuloma, brought on by the irritation of the patient's constant biting.

A. A mucocele is a plugged minor salivary gland found typically on the lower lip.

B. A giant cell granuloma is normally found in the anterior segment of the mouth.

C. A papilloma is usually found on the soft palate. It is a wart-like, cauliflower structure.

E. A nevus is a circumscribed raised area of gray-white pigmentation (mole).

40. E

The lesion might have been caused by any of the answer choices: calculus, overhangs, hormonal response, or injury.

41. C

The lesion would not be hard upon palpation, but rather, soft.

42. D

Even though the patient is pregnant, the lesion should be removed, because her constant biting is making it larger.

43. B

Supine hypotension occurs when a pregnant patient lies back for too long. The baby presses on the vena cava, restricting blood flow back to the heart. That, in turn, lowers the patient's blood pressure.

A. Orthostatic hypotension occurs from laying back too long, but it is due a blood reflex problem.

C. Adrenal crisis will lower the blood pressure but other symptoms would be observed as well.

D. Syncope will also lower the blood pressure but it is a transient loss of consciousness.

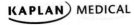

44. C

For taking radiographs on a pregnant female, the last trimester is safest. By that time, all the vital organs are formed and the baby is growing in size. Do not confuse this with the safest time to perform a dental procedure on a pregnant patient—the second trimester.

45. E

The radiopaque curvature is a zygomatic arch.

A. External oblique ridge is a mandibular landmark.

B. Maxillary tuberosity is posterior to the molars.

C. Maxillary sinus is radiolucent.

D. Hamular process is posterior to the molars near the medial pterygoid plate.

46. C

The reason the crown has an abnormal shape is that a filling was designed to close the contact of #29 and #31. That was because #31 had drifted and tilted mesially.

CASE 5

47. B

This patient has Type II status, chronic periodontitis.

A. Type I is gingivitis.

C. Type III is aggressive periodontitis.

D. Type IV is periodontitis due to systemic condition of either a hematologic or genetic disorder.

E. Type V is necrotizing periodontitis.

48. D

Gingival hyperplasia is a side effect of Procardia, which is a calcium channel blocker.

49. E

This patient's drinking and smoking habits put him at greater risk for cancer.

50. B

You would likely find generalized horizontal and vertical bone loss.

51. C

Since the patient takes aspirin daily, you would likely observe increased bleeding.

52. D

Diet history is not typically a part of treatment planning, though it should be addressed if appropriate. All of the other factors would be required for treatment planning: radiographs; examination; periodontal evaluation; and medical information.

53. C

The lesion distal to # 31 might be squamous cell carcinoma if biopsied. This is because of the patient's high risk factors.

A. Candidiasis is an opportunistic infection that is white, soft, creamy plaque that leaves a red ulcerated or eroded area at the base.

B. Epulis fissuratum is caused by an irritation from a phlange on a denture.

D. Angular stomatitis occurs at the angles of the mouth.

E. Aphthous ulcer is an oval/round lesion with an ulcer floor. Initially yellow in color, it takes on a gray hue surrounded by an erythematous halo.

54. B

The patient's blood pressure categorizes him a Stage 1, hypertension.

	Systolic		Diastolic
Optima	< 120 mmHg	and	< 80 mmHg
Normal	< 130 mmHg	and	< 85 mmHg
High normal/ High	130-139 mmHg	or	85-89 mmHg
Stage 1	140-159 mmHg	or	90-99 mmHg
Stage 2	160-179 mmHg	or	100-109 mmHg
Stage 3	> or = 180 mmHg	or	> or = 110 mmHg

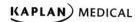

55. B

What you see on the mesial aspect is a resin filling that is radiopaque.

A. Overlap is on the distal of # 8 and # 7.

C. A carious lesion would be radiolucent.

D. An amalgam filling is much more radiopaque than resin.

56. B

You would not dry the teeth with an air-water syringe before applying the desensitizing agent. That would be very painful.

A. Cleaning the teeth before application helps the desensitizing agent to penetrate the tooth surface.

C. Isolating the area with cotton rolls and dry angles helps to apply the agent better.

D. Iontophoresis utilizes a low electrical current to impregnate the ion into the tooth.

57. E

The radiopacity here is mandibular torus.

A. Mental foramen is radiolucent.

B. Submandibular fossa is radiolucent.

C. Pterygoid fovea is a radiolucent depression anterior to the condyle.

D. Lingula is a radiopacity inferior to the ramus on the lingual surface.

58. C

You would caution the patient that there may be excessive bleeding. This is because of the daily aspirin intake.

B. If the patient were to quit smoking, there would be an increase in bleeding since smoking constricts vessels.

D. The root debridement will improve the gingival hyperplasia though that is not the most important concern.

59. E

An earache along with infection is not a symptom of TMD. Rather, it would be an earache without infection.

60. D

Eating hard foods is not recommended in cases of TMD. Rehabilitation exercises, instead, are recommended by the Academy.

CASE 6

61. D

Premedication for ASD is amoxicillin 2 g, 1 hour before the appointment.

A. Clindamycin 2 g is the wrong dosage; it should be 600 mg.

B. Azithromycin 1 g is the wrong dosage; it should be 500 mg.

C. Clarithromycin 2 g is the wrong dosage; it should be 500 mg.

E. Cephalexin 2 g would be for joint replacement.

62. C

The premedication is for atrial septal defect, a hole between the right and left atria.

B. You would not premedicate for seizures.

D. Down syndrome patients are susceptible to periodontal disease but that is not a reason to premedicate this patient.

63. C

Another name for Down syndrome is Trisomy 21.

64. D

All of the answer choices are of concern: swallowing problems (because they often have large tongues); dry tissue (because they are mouth breathers); and tongue thrusting.

65. E

Down syndrome patients are 10–15 times more likely to develop leukemia than normal children.

D. Down syndrome patients are at slightly increased risk for hepatitis due to lack of proper hygiene.

66. A

Down syndrome patients often get stuck in a "groove" of their own and need to be motivated.

B. Macrodontia is not a Down syndrome trait.

C. Down syndrome patients are at a high risk—not low—for caries.

D. Periodontal disease is common—not uncommon—in Down syndrome patients.

E. Frequent repetition does in fact work well with Down syndrome patients.

67. A

Sealant would normally be ideal but since this patient is a gagger and cannot tolerate intraoral films, he wouldn't tolerate sealant application well. And since he is a drooler, you would not be able to keep the field dry.

68. A

The bilateral bulbous blue areas distal to #3 and #14 are eruption hematomas. Look at the age and location of these areas as well.

B. Bulla is a serous-filled blister that may contain blood.

C. Furuncle is a boil.

D. Macule is a skin patch unaltered in color, flat, and not elevated.

E. A pyogenic granuloma can occur in males as well but it is bright red.

69. A

Prevotella intermedia is most prevalent. It is a periodontal microorganism, and Down syndrome patients are prone to periodontal disease. All of the other microorganisms listed here are associated with caries.

70. D

Down syndrome patients tend to have small nasomaxillary complexes with open mouths, not large nasomaxillary complexes with closed mouths.

CASE 7

71. C

The ASA would categorize this patient as ASA III since she has a history of cancer and GERD.

B. ASA II is a healthy patient with minor problems such as allergies.

72. D

Recession, gastric acid effects on teeth, and dry mouth all put this patient at high risk for caries.

73. D

Pharyngeal inflammation might be observed. It comes from the acid of GERD.

74. D

Tamoxifen does not cause staining. Xerostomia (dry mouth), nausea & vomiting, mucosal ulcerations, inhibition of oogenesis (egg production) are all side effects.

75. D

COPD would not result from untreated GERD. COPD is a long-range respiratory problem of emphysema or chronic bronchitis.

A. Asthma can develop from inhaling the acid.

76. E

The flat, localized, pigmented lesion is a melanotic macule.

B. Erythroplakia is a red, velvety macule.

C. Herpangina is caused by the Coxsackie virus and is found in the palate.

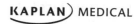

77. A

Sodium fluoride should be used; it would not bother the inflamed tissues from GERD.

B. Acidulated fluoride is too harsh on inflamed tissues.

C. Stannous fluoride is too harsh on inflamed tissues.

D. Sodium monophosphate is found in toothpaste.

78. C

Ultrasonic scaling would remove the deposits most quickly.

A. A porte polisher would take too long.

B. An air polisher with baking soda may irritate the inflamed tissues.

79. D

You would not recommend chlorine dioxide for xerostomia, since it contains alcohol and would dry the tissues even more.

80. B

The lesions might have been chronic hyperplasia as a result of her smoking.

A. Hyperplastic candidiasis occurs in the buccal mucosa from a fungal infection.

C. Erythroplakia is a red velvet macule.

D. Wheal is a sudden elevation of the skin.

E. Oral lymphomas are typically found on the palate, tongue, or gingiva.

81. E

The condition might be palatal tori.

B. Hamular process is found posteriorly from this location.

C. Maxillary tuberosity is posterior to the molars.

D. Median palatine suture is radiolucent.

CASE 8

82. E

You would ask the patient how often she exercises. Patients who work out will have low blood pressure, low pulse, and respiratory rates.

83. C

You would caution the patient that the orthotricycline she is taking might not be very effective, and that she should use another type of birth control.

A. Checking to see if she is allergic to the antibiotic should have been done before prescribing the antibiotic.

84. C

If the patient were to become pregnant, tetracycline should not be used in the last half of the pregnancy. One side effect of this drug is that it stains teeth in unborn children.

A. Tetracycline would not constipate her; rather, it can cause diarrhea.

B. Tetracycline should be taken without food, not with food.

D. Tetracycline can indeed cause photosensitivity.

E. Superinfection with this drug is extremely common.

85. A

The white circular radiopacity is a past orthognathic surgery for orthodontics.

86. B

This radiolucency could easily be mistaken for cervical burnout.

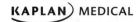

87. **D**

The radiolucency on the periapical of #11 is internal tooth resorption.

A. An artifact is something that appears to be there but is not.

B. A nasopalatine cyst is a heart-shaped radiolucency in the nasal area.

C. This is internal resorption, not external.

88. **E**

Perioral dermatitis may be mistaken for rosacea and acne.

C. Psoriasis is a chronic skin condition in which the body produces skin cells at an abnormally fast rate—and before old cells can exfoliate—causing a build-up.

D. Seborrheic dermatitis is a dermatitis involving fat glands.

89. **C**

You would not caution her that a side effect of steroids is a drop in blood pressure. In fact, it is an increase in blood pressure: hypertension, not hypotension.

B. Corticosteroid use can suppress the immune system; the disease is not cured but symptoms are alleviated.

90. **B**

Pulse and respiratory rate are both on the low side of normal.

91. **D**

You would advise against using citroxain, a tooth whitening agent that causes tooth sensitivity.

CASE 9

92. **D**

Since the lesion is removable, it is pseudomembranous candidiasis, found on the buccal and labial mucosa. The clue here is that it is creamy white in color.

A. Angular cheilitis occurs at the angles of the mouth.

B. Desquamative gingivitis wipes off with a 2 × 2 and leaves a raw, red area, but it is a sloughing-off of gingiva tissue.

C. Erythematous candidiasis is a small, flat, red lesion.

E. Lichen planus is a benign asymptomatic, autoimmune mucositis that is characterized by a white, lacy lesion.

93. **D**

Melanin pigmentation has nothing to do with this lesion.

94. **A**

The bone loss is vertical loss with furcation involvement.

95. **A**

You would not recommend rinsing with Listerine, which has a high alcohol content.

96. **D**

Radiation therapy has nothing to do with exostosis, which is extra-bony growth on the facial surfaces.

97. **A**

Brush-on gel would be the best for this patient.

B. Stannous fluoride is too acidic.

C. Neutral sodium is a good second choice for this patient.

D. Acidulated phosphate is too acidic

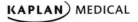

98. B

You would advise that she stop drinking alcohol, since it is not advisable with xerostomia.

99. C

Gracey 11/12 is the instrument of choice for any mesial aspect, even though it is the distal root.

A. Gracey1/2 is an anterior curet.

B. Gracey 7/8 is for the facial and lingual aspects of posterior teeth.

D. Gracey 13/14 is not appropriate; even though this is the distal root, we are deep scaling the mesial aspect.

E. Gracey 17/18 is not appropriate; even though this is the distal root, we are deep scaling the mesial aspect.

100. C

In response to this patient's blood pressure, medical consultation is needed.

101. A

The patient is particularly prone to *Candida*, because of her age and medical status.

B. *Proteus* usually results in UTI.

C. *Borrelia* are spread by vectors or bugs.

D. *Escherichia* usually results in UTI.

102. C

This patient would be considered Type III because of her history of cancer and hypertension.

103. E

Crepitus of the TMJ was almost surely caused by degenerative joint disease; it is the primary cause.

104. C

The radiolucency in the radiograph is a fracture.

A. Internal resorption is more diffuse internally and not a clear line.

B. External resorption is more diffuse externally and not a clear line.

D. Root caries do not occur so deep.

E. Radicular cyst occurs at the apex and not at the middle of the root.

105. C

The patient has an endosseous implant.

A. Transosteal implant is stapled into the inferior border of the mandible.

B. Subperiosteal is custom fabricated to the mandible.

D. Ceramic is a type of material for some implants and also for coating titanium.

E. Titanium is the material used to make implants.

CASE 10

106. D

A Velcro strap on a toothbrush that holds her hand tight to the toothbrush would be most helpful. Many stroke victims lack dexterity as a result of partial paralysis.

A. A thicker floss might still be a problem with hand paralysis.

B. A floss holder would be helpful if she could hold it.

C. A power-assisted toothbrush would be helpful.

E. An electric toothbrush is good only if she could hold the brush mechanism.

107. C

Both types of diabetes are characterized by polyuria and polydipsia, but diabetes insipidus is induced by an antidiuretic hormone deficiency.

108. A

Diabetics tend to have fewer polymorphonuclear leukocytes, which fight acute infection.

B. Platelets are necessary for clotting.

C. Lymphocytes are the second most common blood cell, used as cell mediators in immunity.

D. Monocytes are involved with chronic infection as macrophages.

E. Basophils produce heparin with acute immune responses.

109. B

The best time of day to see a diabetic patient would be first thing in the morning after he has eaten breakfast.

110. B

The lesion is likely an aphthous ulcer, a white lesion with red halo.

A. Fistula is from an abscess.

C. Macule is a flat lesion with altered color.

D. Verruca vulgaris is a wart-like lesion.

E. Petechiae are minute, round purplish red spots on the palate that are the inflamed orifices of mucous glands caused by intradermal or submucous hemorrhage.

111. C

This patient's blood pressure is considered Stage 2.

112. D

Though most diabetics usually have normal or slightly elevated blood pressure, their pulse rate tends to be above normal and irregular.

113. C

This bone loss would be considered Class III furcation involvement.

114. D

The bone loss seen on the radiographs is generalized vertical and horizontal.

115. B

The patient would be placed in a Type II category for chronic periodontitis.

116. D

The bilateral radiopacities are mandibular tori.

A. Odontogenic cysts are varied.

B. Nasopalatine duct cyst is a midline maxillary radiolucency.

C. A myxoma is a benign, infiltrative odontogenic lesion that is difficult to distinguish from an ameloblastoma.

E. Odontogenic keratocyst arises from the remnants of the dental lamina as a small uniocular radiolucency. It is more often detected radiographically as a large, multiocular radiolucency producing a soap bubble appearance.

117. C

The anterior teeth typically have Class III, since there is such a great amount of bone loss.

CASE 11

118. D

If the patient refuses radiographs, you should inquire about his concerns.

A. Having him sign a release form might be done only after his concerns were addressed.

B. Having the dentist speak talk him into having the radiographs would not help in alleviating the patient's concerns.

C. Dismissing him may have an adverse effect on his return to your office.

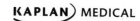

119. C

The most serious side effect of antihypertension medications is a severe drop in blood pressure.

120. E

Decreased urine output is not a common sympton of antihypertensives. Rather, they cause increased urine production.

121. A

You would retake the blood pressure after 5 minutes. This is recommended for blood pressure 160–180/100–110; if it is not better with a second reading, you should consider a medical consultation.

B. Rechecking the next three subsequent visits would be the next step for blood pressure 140–160/90–100.

C. Treatment should not be an option for a person with this blood pressure.

D. No treatment would be for blood pressure >180/ >110.

122. C

This patient has Stage 2 hypertension.

123. A

This patient should be premedicated with an antibiotic next time because of his end-stage renal disease.

124. D

Allopurinol is classified as an antihyperuricemia drug. It helps in the treatment of gout.

125. B

Percodan should not be prescribed, since it is oxycodone and aspirin. As per the patient's history, he is allergic to aspirin.

A. Percoset is oxycodone and acetaminophen.

C. Naloxone is an opioid antagonist.

D. Tylenol #3 is acetaminophen and codeine.

E. Meperidine is of little use in dentistry.

CASE 12

126. C

In this case, you would not reveal any information to the mother. As per most state laws, minors have the right to keep a confidence—even from a parent.

127. D

You would take two pieces of gauze and help her to unscrew the piercing.

A. Leaving it in place and taking the panorex is not an option.

B. Telling her that she must take it out won't work if she has no idea about removal.

C. Instructing her on how to unscrew the end with just fingers may not work since the piercing can slip.

E. Asking the dentist for help is not feasible.

128. E

The most serious infection that can result from a tongue piercing is toxic shock syndrome.

129. A

Someone who had had an endocarditis would be at greatest risk for infection with a tongue piercing.

B. Diabetics are prone to many things but a past endocarditis takes priority here.

C. Asthma can affect breathing problems but the past history of endocarditis is the greatest risk factor.

D. COPD is a chronic ailment.

E. Titanium allergies are rare.

130. C

A tongue piercing could cause Ludwig's angina, which occurs when the tongue swells and cuts off the airway.

B. Nerve damage, though serious, would not be as significant as an obstructed airway.

131. B

The main lymph node drainage for the body of the tongue is the submandibular node.

A. Submental node drains the tongue apex, floor of the mouth, lower lip, and chin.

C. Superior deep cervical node drains the base of the tongue, tonsils, and maxillary third molars.

D. Retropharyngeal node drains the pharynx, palate, nasal cavity, and nasal sinuses.

132. E

The most important thing you can advise her is that flossing helps to prevent gingivitis. With gingivitis, ulcers occur, causing bleeding gingiva. So flossing will help to heal the ulcers of gingivitis.

C. Explaining that she isn't in fact cutting her gums when flossing would help but won't necessarily motivate her to change.

D. Showing her how to use a Perio-Aid is of little benefit in the absence of flossing.

CASE 13

133. B

The patient would not want to get a flu shot. Eggs are used to incubate the flu vaccine.

D. Tetanus vaccine is prepared by Cohn cold-ethanol fractionation of human plasma of voluntary blood donors.

134. D

Minocycline causes photosensitivity.

C. A black pigmentation of the alveolar bone and hard palate—not a red one—can result from Minocycline use.

E. Angioneurotic edema is a side effect of Clindamycin.

135. B

Von Willebrand's disease affects Factor VIII and therefore, affects hemophilia A.

A. Factor V is a parahemophilia.

C. Factor IX occurs with hemophilia B patients.

D. Factor XI occurs with hemophilia C patients.

E. Stuart factor effects factor X, which is involved with intrinsic and extrinsic blood coagulation.

136. D

Neurofibromatomas result from Von Recklinghausen disease, not Von Willebrand's disease.

137. C

Von Willebrand's disease occurs in both men and women.

138. C

The buccal mucosa could be described as purpuric spots, ecchymoses, or small hemorrhages of the skin or mucous membranes.

B. Petechia are pinpoint, nonraised, purplish red spots caused by submucous hemorrhage.

D. Hemangioma is a proliferation of blood vessels.

E. Cellulitis is more diffuse.

139. D

This patient most likely is suffering from a myocardial infarction, which can manifest as jaw pain.

A. Orthostatic hypotension occurs when a patient rises suddenly but not when lying back.

B. Supine hypotensive syndrome occurs with pregnant females.

C. Low blood sugar can make a person dizzy, but does not manifest as jaw pain.

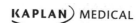

140. B

The first thing to do would be to place the patient in the Trendelenburg position.

A. The airway is already open.

C. Administering oxygen can be of benefit, but laying the patient down comes first.

E. Calling 911 should be assigned to a staff member while laying the patient down.

141. C

The best advice is to call the paramedics to check her. In most states, if paramedics are summoned and find nothing wrong, the patient can sign an emergency medical waiver that releases the dental office from potential legal action. If the paramedics do find something wrong, they can assist with treatment.

A. Driving is not an option since she might become dizzy while driving and have an accident.

B. Calling a friend to drive her home is not the best option.

D. Holding her down in the chair can be considered battery.

CASE 14

142. D

Bactrim treats urinary tract infections (UTIs).

143. D

The patient's blood pressure reading of 182/112 indicates that no dental treatment should be performed at this appointment. This blood pressure level is Stage 3 and could go higher during a stressful dental treatment, so the patient should get a medical consultation.

144. B

Glaucoma medications may affect the heart with hidden beta blockers that can get absorbed systemically.

145. E

Since the lesion on the lower lip has been there for 2 years, it may be an irritative fibroma.

A. Furuncle is a boil or painful skin nodule that has a circumscribed area of inflammation.

B. Pyogenic granuloma is much redder in color.

C. Macule is a skin patch that is flattened—not elevated—and is altered in color.

D. Epulis fissuratum is a denture flange irritation.

146. B

The lesion under the tongue might be ranula, which is the blockage of salivary gland by stone or sialolith. It typically occurs in Wharton's duct in the floor of mouth. It can block saliva drainage, causing swelling if the stone blocks the duct, but can also become less noticeable if the stone moves and allows the saliva to drain.

A. Sialolith is a salivary stone or calculus.

C. Nodule is a small knot or node that is a minute collection of tissue.

D. Papule is a small solid, superficial elevation of skin that is circumscribed.

E. Nevus is a circumscribed raised area of gray-white pigmentation (mole).

147. B

The radiopacity distal to #31 is tooth #32.

A. Staphne bone cyst is radiolucent.

C. Genial tubercles is anterior anatomy.

D. Condylar head is more superior to #31.

E. Odontoma is an irregular calcified radiopaque mass surrounded by radiolucent band.

148. E

You could prescribe acetylsalicylic acid. All of the other answer choices are opioid derivatives (as is codeine), which the patient is allergic to.

149. D

The inferior alveolar artery supplies blood to Tooth #31. It supplies the mandibular teeth, the floor of the mouth, and mental area.

A. Buccal artery supplies the buccinator muscle and buccal area.

B. Greater palatine artery supplies the hard and soft palate.

C. Sphenopalatine artery supplies the nasal cavity and anterior hard palate.

150. A

The posterior superior alveolar nerve supplies sensation to Tooth #2.

B. Lesser palatine nerve supplies the soft palate and palatine tonsils.

C. Greater palatine nerve supplies the maxillary posterior gingiva and posterior hard palate.

D. Mental nerve supplies the mandibular labial mucosa.

E. Accessory nerve supplies the trapezius and sternocleidomastoid muscles.

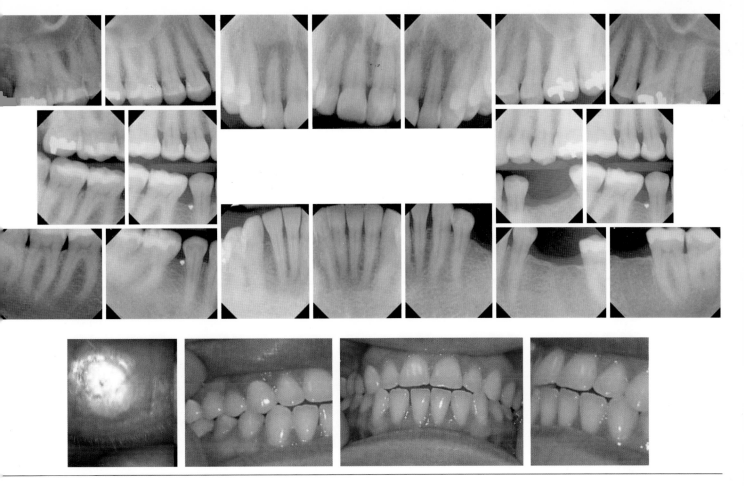

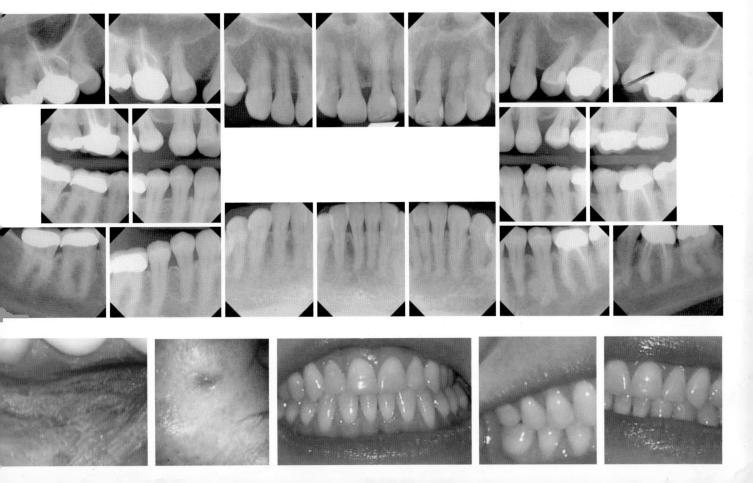

CASE STUDY 3

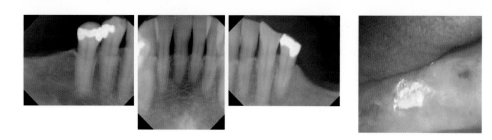

CASE STUDY 4

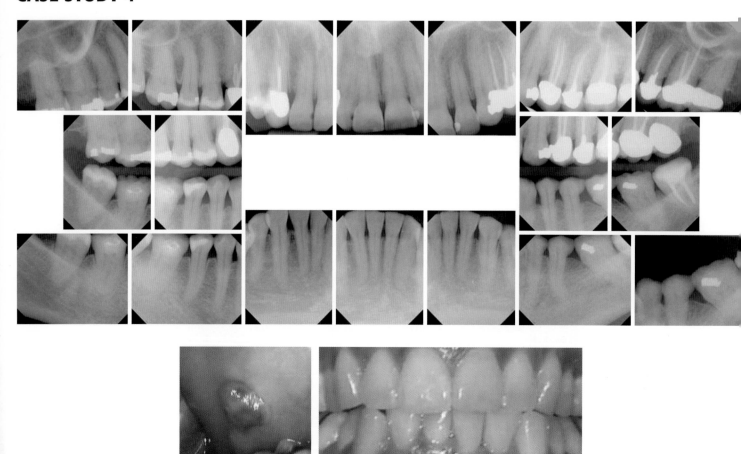

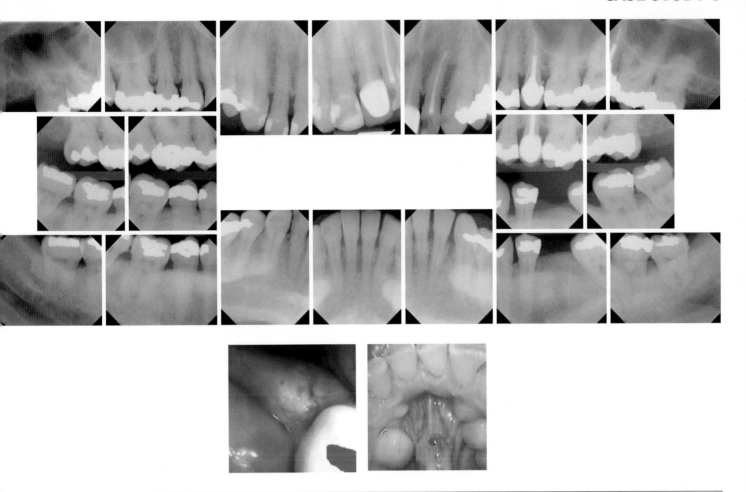

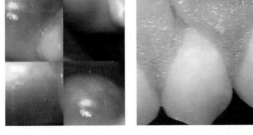

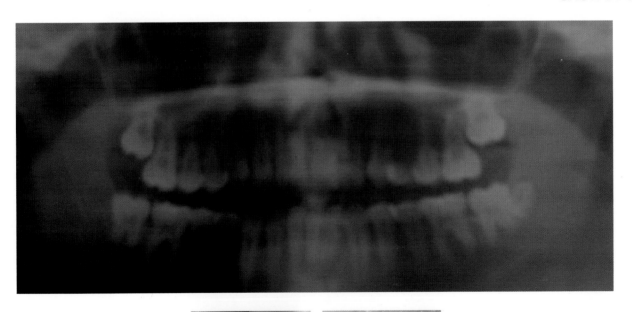

CASE STUDY 7

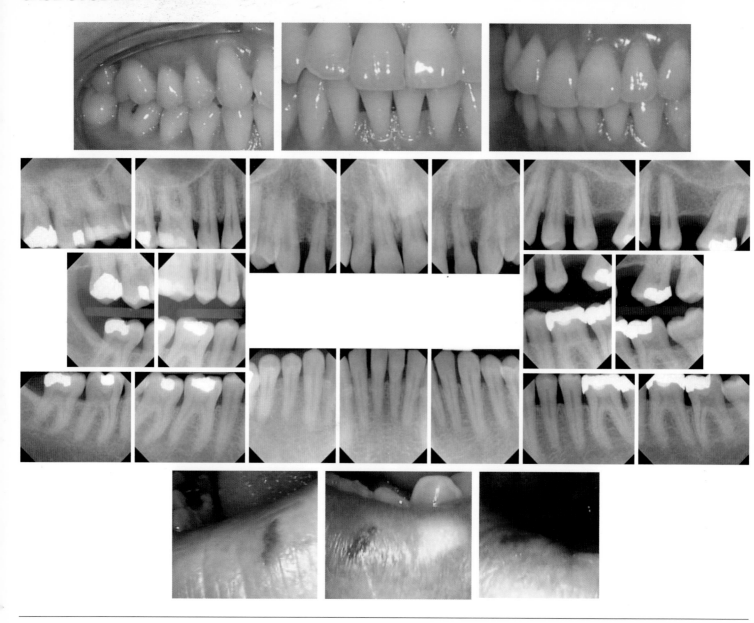

CASE STUDY 8

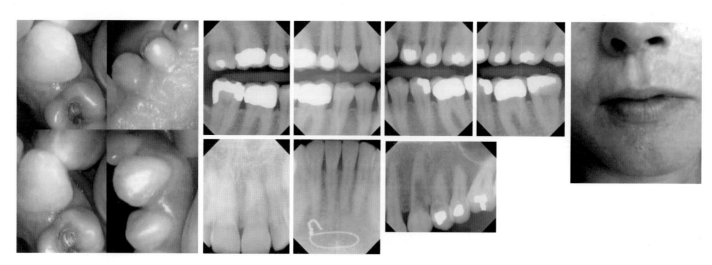

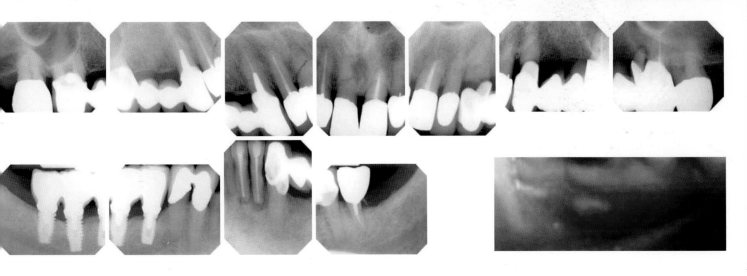

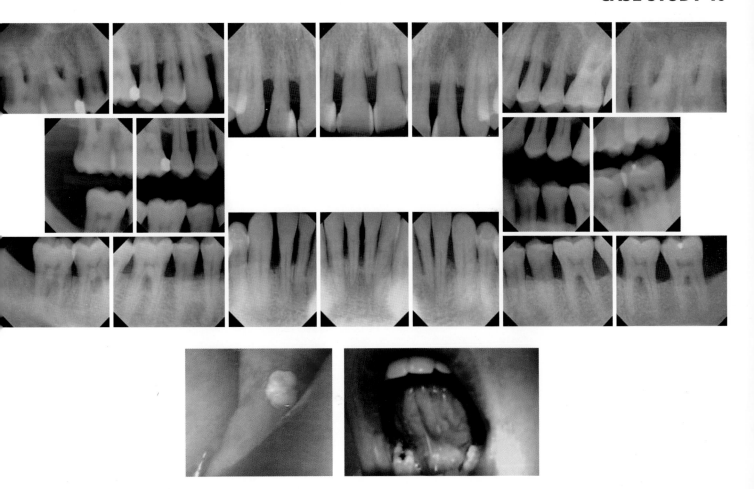

CASE STUDY 11

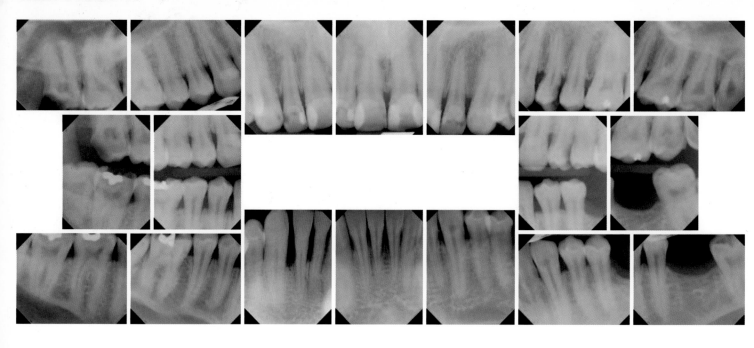

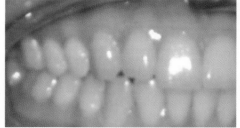

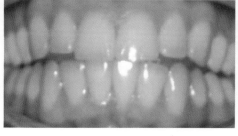

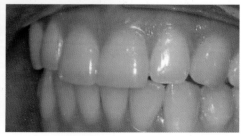

CASE STUDY 12

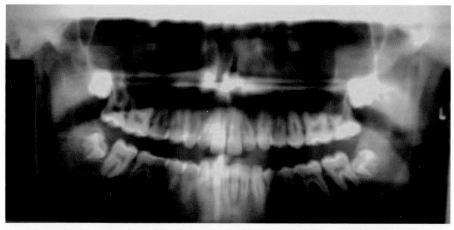